Asinou across Time

Dumbarton Oaks Studies XLIII

Asinou across Time

Studies in the Architecture and Murals of the Panagia Phorbiotissa, Cyprus

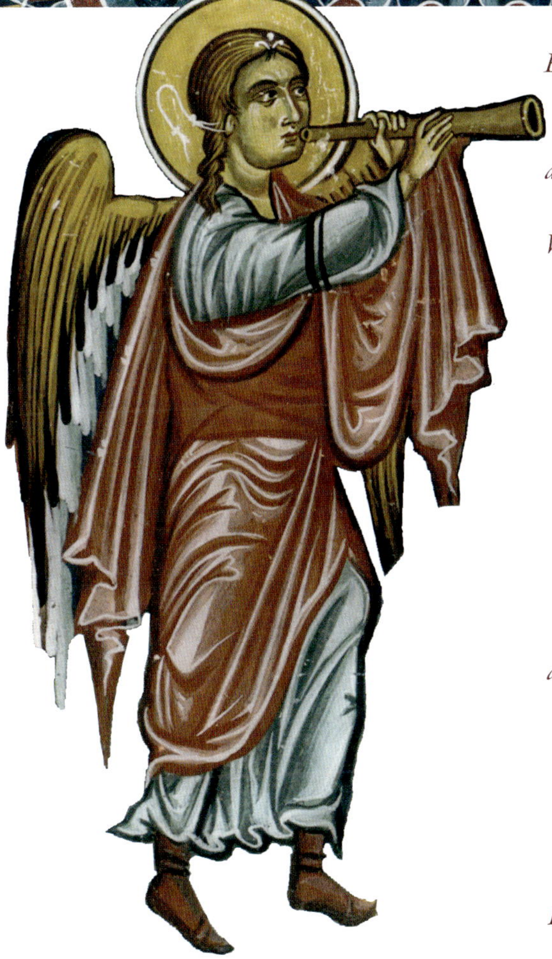

Edited by

Annemarie Weyl Carr

and Andréas Nicolaïdès

With contributions by

Annemarie Weyl Carr,

Gilles Grivaud,

Ioanna Kakoulli,

Sophia Kalopissi-Verti,

Andréas Nicolaïdès,

Athanasios Papageorgiou,

Nancy Patterson Ševčenko,

and David Winfield

Published by

DUMBARTON OAKS RESEARCH LIBRARY AND COLLECTION

Printed in China by Everbest Printing Company, Ltd.

19 18 17 16 15 14 13 12 1 2 3 4 5

Library of Congress Cataloging-in-Publication Data

Asinou across time : studies in the architecture and murals of the Panagia Phorbiotissa, Cyprus / edited by Annemarie Weyl Carr and Andréas Nicolaïdès ; with contributions by Annemarie Weyl Carr . . . [et al.].
p. cm. — (Dumbarton Oaks studies ; 43)
Includes bibliographical references and indexes.
ISBN 978-0-88402-349-4 (cloth : alk. paper)
1. Panayia Phorviotissa (Church : Asinou, Cyprus) 2. Architecture, Byzantine—Cyprus—Asinou. 3. Mural painting and decoration, Byzantine—Cyprus—Asinou. 4. Asinou (Cyprus)—Antiquities. I. Carr, Annemarie Weyl. II. Nicolaïdès, Andreas.
NA5593.A75 2012
726.5095693—dc23

2012021970

Managing Editor: Joel Kalvesmaki
Book and Jacket Design and Composition: Melissa Tandysh
Art Direction: Kathleen Sparkes

www.doaks.org/publications

Contents

Preface

This volume of studies on the history, architecture, and post-1105/6 paintings of the church of the Panagia Phorbiotissa in Asinou marks another step in the long process of publishing the major fieldwork and restoration projects carried out by Dumbarton Oaks on the island of Cyprus in the 1960s and 1970s. It contributes to the substantial progress made on that front in recent years, with the appearance of David and June Winfield's *The Church of the Panaghia tou Arakos at Lagoudhera, Cyprus: The Paintings and Their Painterly Significance* (2003); *Kourion: Excavations in the Episcopal Precinct* (2007), by A. H. S. Megaw and colleagues; and lengthy monographic articles by Andréas Nicolaïdès ("L'église de la Panagia Arakiotissa à Lagoudera, Chypre: Étude iconographique des fresques de 1192") and Tassos Papacostas ("The History and Architecture of the Monastery of Saint John Chrysostomos at Koutsovendis, Cyprus") in *Dumbarton Oaks Papers* 50 (1996) and 61 (2007). Much of the credit for the revival of efforts to publish Lagoudera and Kourion should go to my predecessor as Director of Byzantine Studies (1991–1996), Henry Maguire, who oversaw the preparation of *Lagoudhera* and laid the groundwork for the realization of *Kourion*.

For various reasons, publication plans for Asinou did not materialize until the late 1990s, when the project was revived, thanks to the initiative of Andréas Nicolaïdès. The Senior Fellows of Dumbarton Oaks entrusted a new scholarly team, led by Annemarie Weyl Carr and Dr. Nicolaïdès, with the preparation of a comprehensive study of the mural decoration that had been cleaned and conserved by David Winfield and Ernest Hawkins, to be accompanied by chapters on historical and architectural context, and a technical examination of the paintings. Although it has proved impossible to include the initial 1105/6 phase of the paintings in this volume, the decision was made to proceed with publication of the later phases of mural decoration, so as not to delay even longer the presentation of this World Heritage site to the scholarly public. It is anticipated that the early twelfth-century painting program will be published at a later date. I should like to express the gratitude of Dumbarton Oaks to all the scholars who have contributed to the volume, and to the funding institutions which have supported their research and made possible both the physical analyses used in the technical study of the paintings and the lavish color illustrations.

Alice-Mary Talbot
Director of Byzantine Studies
July 2008

Acknowledgments

In preparing this book, our team of eight contributors has drawn upon the generosity of a number of institutions and individuals, and we extend our thanks to each of them for enabling our work. First and most fundamentally, our sincere gratitude goes out to the late Konstantinos Leventis, whose enthusiastic interest lay at the genesis of this project. He provided the funds for Professor Ioanna Kakoulli's technical analyses of the frescoes, which underlie many conclusions in this volume. We are grateful to the A. G. Leventis Foundation in Nicosia, and to its director, Dr. Vassos Karageorgis, for making possible the ample use of full-color reproductions in the book, both by a grant to fund the printing and by giving us permission to reproduce transparencies of Asinou's murals made by the Foundation. The transparencies are now housed in the Archaeological Research Unit of the University of Cyprus, and we are grateful to its director, Professor Demetrios Michaelides, for his help in making them available. We extend our warm thanks, too, to the Samuel F. Kress Foundation in New York, for support that made possible two periods of study together as a team on-site in Cyprus. Through the generosity of Dr. Sophocles Hadjisavvas, Director of the Department of Antiquities of Cyprus, we were able to use scaffolding, lights, and a generator provided by the Department. Most particularly, we have drawn fully and heavily upon the photographs and notes that are archived at Dumbarton Oaks. We owe special thanks for access to the meticulous records of the inscriptions made in 1967 by Professor Ihor Ševčenko. Every member of the team has relied upon his work. We have received valuable technical support in scanning images from the Laboratoire d'Archéologie Mediévale et Moderne en Mediterranée—CNRS, Aix-Marseille Université, and precious financial support for Charles Dibble's skilled translation of Gilles Grivaud's text from the Université de Rouen. We express our sincere gratitude to the UCLA Materials Science and Engineering Department and the Cotsen Institute of Archaeology at the University of California, Los Angeles, and to the Getty Conservation Institute for assistance in the physical analyses of pigments and materials used in Dr. Kakoulli's chapter on the technical analysis of Asinou's frescoes. Both the University of Athens and Southern Methodist University have given valuable administrative and technical support to the project. The State Archive of the Republic of Cyprus permitted our reproduction of the vintage photograph of the church of Asinou from 1909 (Fig. 1.6). We owe thanks to all these institutions.

Many individuals, too, have been crucial to this effort. We extend heartfelt and respectful thanks to His Reverence Neophytos, the Bishop of Morphou, for his steady support and insightful interest in our project. We owe our particular thanks to the priest of the church of Asinou, Father Kyriakos Christophi. Father Kyriakos's generosity, perceptivity, and keen enthusiasm facilitated our work and gave it a very special warmth and resonance. Dr. Marina Solomidou-Ieronymidou of the Department of Antiquities has provided guidance and insight. Crucial assistance was offered by Professor emeritus Robin Cormack, who provided his archives of the restoration work done by David and June Winfield. We owe thanks to Professor Henry Maguire, with whom negotiations for the publication were begun. We thank Dr. Gerald Carr for his many photographs. Finally, and most fully, we owe our unqualified thanks to Dr. Alice-Mary Talbot, the Director of Byzantine Studies at Dumbarton Oaks until 2009, for holding the project on course through many vicissitudes.

Annemarie Weyl Carr
Newark, Delaware

Andréas Nicolaïdès
Aix-en-Provence

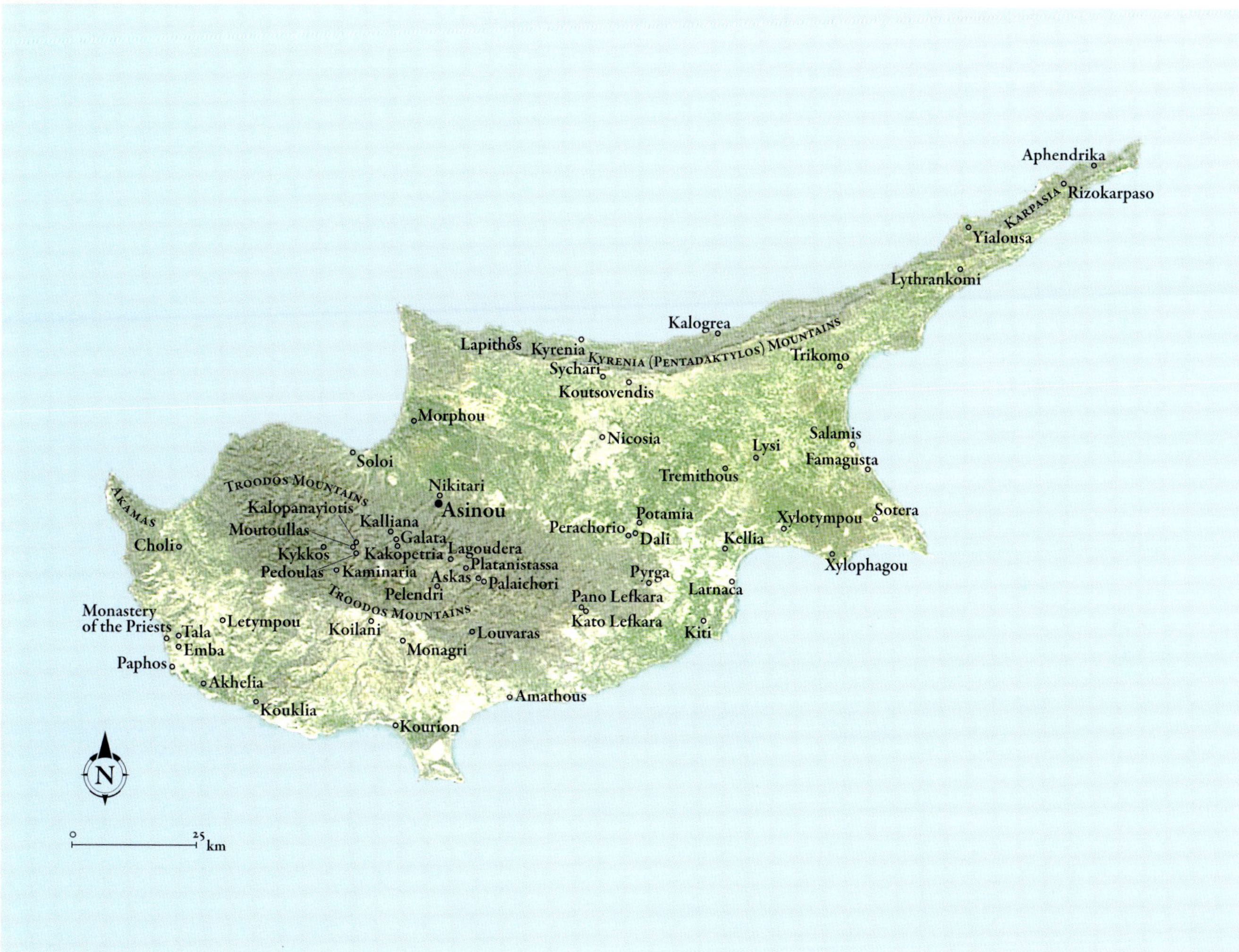
Aphendrika
Rizokarpaso
Karpasia
Yialousa
Lythrankomi
Kalogrea
Kyrenia (Pentadaktylos) Mountains
Lapithos
Kyrenia
Sychari
Koutsovendis
Trikomo
Morphou
Nicosia
Salamis
Lysi
Famagusta
Soloi
Tremithous
Troodos Mountains
Nikitari
Asinou
Kalopanayiotis
Akamas
Kalliana
Moutoullas
Galata
Potamia
Xylotympou
Sotera
Perachorio
Dali
Kellia
Choli
Lagoudera
Kykkos
Kakopetria
Platanistassa
Xylophagou
Pedoulas
Kaminaria
Askas
Palaichori
Pyrga
Pelendri
Larnaca
Troodos Mountains
Pano Lefkara
Monastery of the Priests
Tala
Letympou
Koilani
Louvaras
Kato Lefkara
Kiti
Emba
Monagri
Paphos
Akhelia
Amathous
Kouklia
Kourion
N
0
25
km

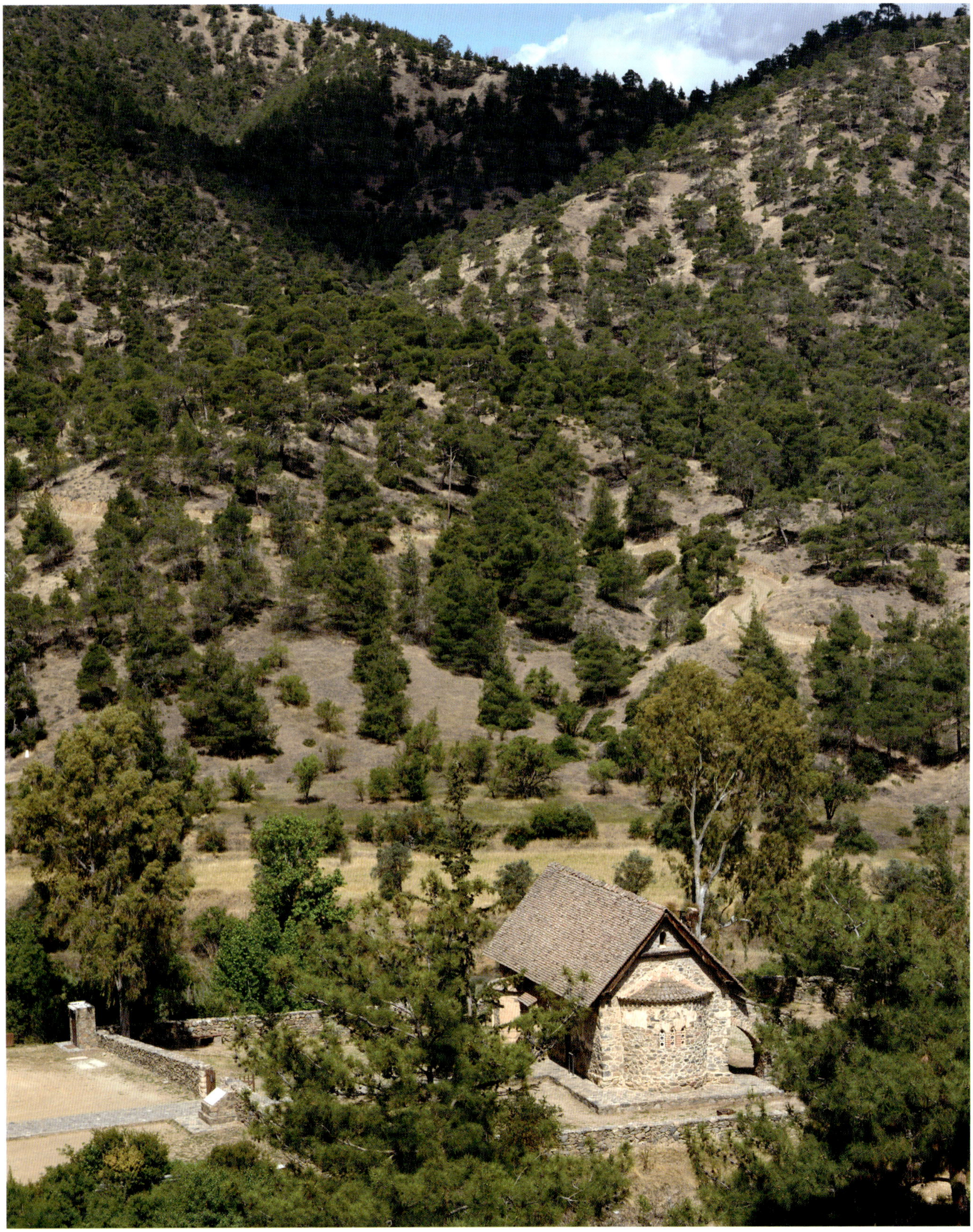

The church of Panagia Phorbiotissa from the hill of the Cross
(photo courtesy of G. L. Carr)

Introduction

Annemarie Weyl Carr

Lapped by the golden meadows of a mountain valley, the little church of the Mother of God Phorbiotissa seems suspended in time (Intro. Fig. 1). Isolated, it stands out alone against the layered green of the lower Troodos, the mountain massif that dominates Cyprus's inland center. The village of Asinou that gave the building its familiar nickname had vanished already in Ottoman times; the monastery it served had ceased to function by 1825; and today only the church remains, a lone, intensely picturesque survivor. It enfolds its visitors in tranquil isolation already well before they step into the enveloping color of its interior. It is the paintings indoors that they come to see (Intro. Fig. 2). Whether as pilgrims who venerate the ring of saints before the bema or as tourists who turn their backs on the bema to venerate the Asinou Master's art in the western bay, those who come are doubly seduced, first by its solitude and then by its color. Asinou is among the most cherished sites in Cyprus.

The building is in fact far from isolated. Since 1985 it has been a UNESCO World Heritage Site, one of ten churches comprising the Troodos Painted Churches group.[1] This designation ensures not only its protection but also its constant visitation. Located some forty-five kilometers from the periphery of Nicosia, Cyprus's capital, and readily accessible by well-graded roads, it is visited by some thirty thousand tourists a year and by many thousands of Cypriots who come to celebrate baptisms there. The appeal of the church rests partly upon its comparatively easy accessibility, low in the foothills of the Troodos, and partly upon its picturesque setting. But above all it rests upon the interior of the building, which is covered throughout with mural paintings. The paintings are the subject of this book.

The frescoes in Asinou are the product of different periods, patrons, and purposes (Intro. Fig. 3). Their chronological diversity has shaped this book. This is the first monograph on one of Cyprus's major diachronic churches, adorned not just

1. Report Maison de l'UNESCO, SC-85/CONF.008/9; http://whc.unesco.org/en/list/351; http://whc.unesco.org/cyprus2009/index-en.html; see also pp. 36, 66, below.

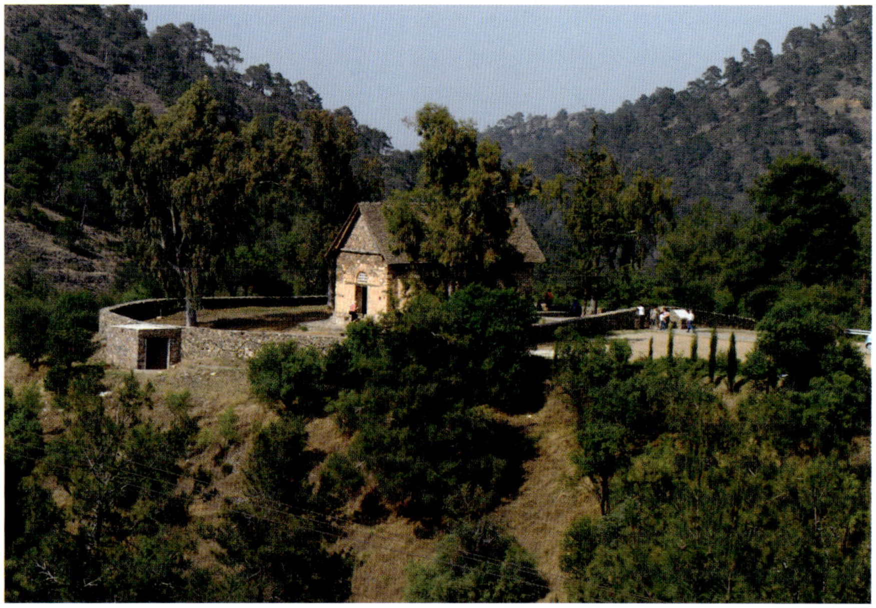

INTRO. FIG. 1
The church of Panagia Phorbiotissa, exterior from the southwest (photo courtesy of G. L. Carr)

with isolated images but with whole image programs dating from different periods.[2] Asinou's successive programs reshaped its interior to serve different eras and needs. No one phase sums up its functional life. Rather, each phase articulated anew both the space and the other images within it. The church as initially built around 1100 CE was modest in the extreme. Its first frescoes, by contrast, were by a painter so outstanding that history has not allowed him to remain anonymous. He is known as the "Asinou Master." His paintings, dated by an inscription to 1105/6, cloaked the whole interior of the church and at least two overdoors on its exterior. For most readers, the work of 1105/6 *is* Asinou. But in fact, it is not; that is just Asinou's first phase, the starting point of its long life.

This life as it emerges from the frescoes is the focal concern of this book. The chapters present successive phases in the articulation of Asinou's space, each with its images, its ideas, and its distinctive ways of addressing the era's needs. The frescoes of 1105/6 will be presented separately. The present volume addresses the imagery that encrusted and slowly remade the program of 1105/6. Thus it reframes the Asinou Master's cycle not as *the* church of Asinou, but as one of the phases whose aggregate makes Asinou's interior so concentrated, so dense in time. This is the study of a church not so much suspended as deeply layered in time.

The frescoes studied in this volume range from the late twelfth to the early seventeenth century.

2. Most monographs on Cypriot churches have examined structures with one dominant phase of painting. This is the case with Perachorio (Megaw and Hawkins, "Church of the Holy Apostles"); the Holy Trinity church in the monastery of St. John Chrysostom, Koutsovendis (Mango, "Monastery of St. Chrysostomos" and most recently Papacostas, "History and Architecture of the Monastery"); the Enkleistra of St. Neophytos (Mango and Hawkins, "Hermitage of St. Neophytos"); the Panagia tou Arakos in Lagoudera (Nicolaïdès, "Étude iconographique"; Winfield and Winfield, *Church of the Panaghia tou Arakos*); the Panagia Amasgou in Monagri (Boyd, "Church of the Panagia Amasgou"); the church of the Archangel Michael in Kato Lefkara (Papageorgiou, "Ἡ ἐκκλησία τοῦ Αρχαγγέλου"); St. Themonianos, Lysi (Carr and Morrocco, *Byzantine Masterpiece*); and the church of the Panagia in Moutoullas (Mouriki, "Wall Paintings of the Church of the Panagia"). The major exception is the church of the Panagia Kanakaria in Lythrankomi, which is famous for its early Christian apse but adorned fitfully with images of diverse periods: see Megaw and Hawkins, *Church of the Panagia Kanakaria*.

Throughout these centuries the church of Asinou served the monastery of the Mother of God ton Phorbion (τῶν Φορβίων). "Mother of God" is the standard epithet in the Orthodox Church for the Virgin Mary, designating her as the mother not only of the human Jesus but of the God-man Jesus Christ. Another widely-used epithet for Mary is "Panagia": that is, All-Holy. The church at Asinou is customarily referred to by this name. As in many Cypriot churches, Mary's name is linked with that of a plant, in this case spurges. Thus the church is known as the Panagia ton Phorbion: the All-Holy [Mother of God] of the Spurges.

The monastery attracted new sponsors throughout the medieval centuries, their sponsorship registered visibly in the steady accretion of mural paintings in the church. New paintings gathered above all in the narthex, which had been added to the original church in the course of the twelfth century and so did not participate in its initial fresco program. The images seem at first to have appeared in the narthex one by one. But eventually, in 1332/33, a comprehensive program draped the entire narthex in a coat of color as all-enveloping as that of the 1105/6 program in the naos. Fresh paintings were applied to the church's main apse conch and triumphal arch after the original conch collapsed at an undetermined date, most probably in the thirteenth century. Somewhat later, portions of the central bay of the naos were repainted in the wake of structural repairs to the walls and vault. The date at which these additions began, the pace of their accretion, and their relation both to one another and to the dated campaign of 1332/33, are points addressed in this book; chronology is a concern throughout. A second concern is to identify the sources, themes, subjects, and messages of the successive mural programs. And a third is to relate them to the social conditions of Cyprus during the building's active period as a village church or monastery chapel. Cyprus was a prosperous, strategically important bulkhead of Byzantine naval power when the earliest of the church's frescoes were produced. The island was seized in 1191 during the Third Crusade, becoming an independent kingdom ruled by the

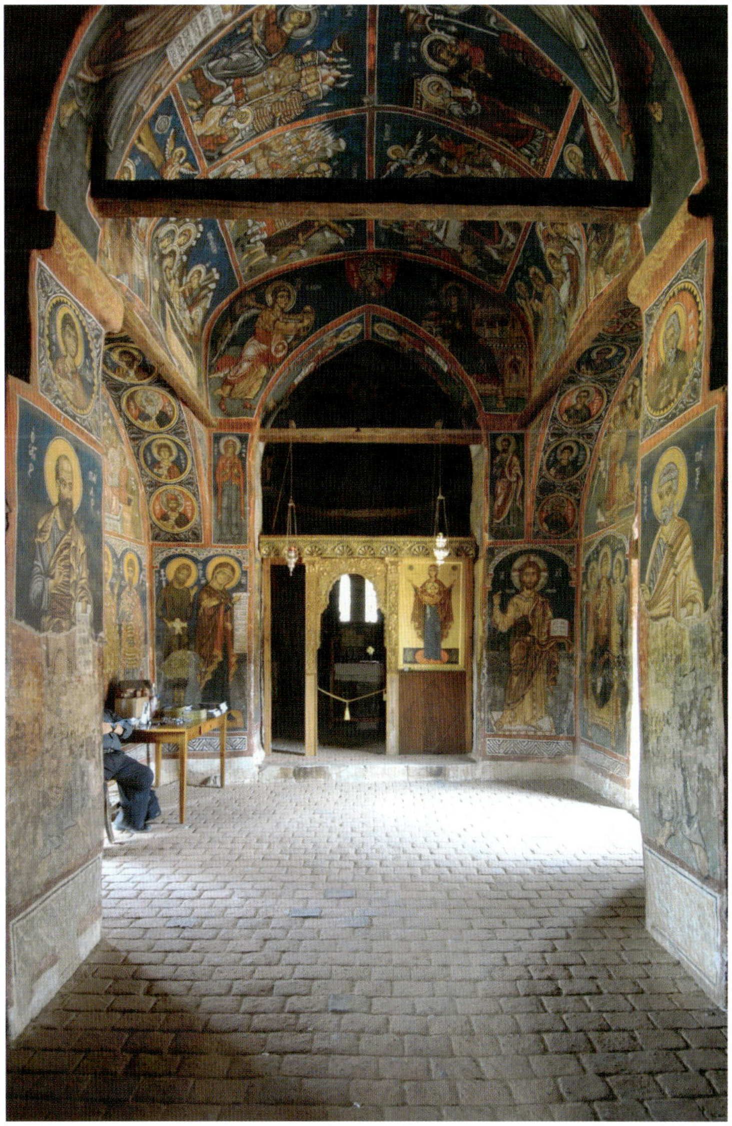

INTRO. FIG. 2 The church of Panagia Phorbiotissa, interior toward the east (photo courtesy G. L. Carr)

Roman Catholic Lusignan family of French crusaders until 1474. From that point the island was a colony of Venice until its conquest by the Ottomans, in 1570/71. The frescoes illuminate the life of an Orthodox monastic institution through this sequence of shifting regimes.

To treat the multiple dimensions of Asinou, the book draws upon scholars of varied discipline and method. The first three chapters set the stage for the frescoes. They open with a chapter by Gilles

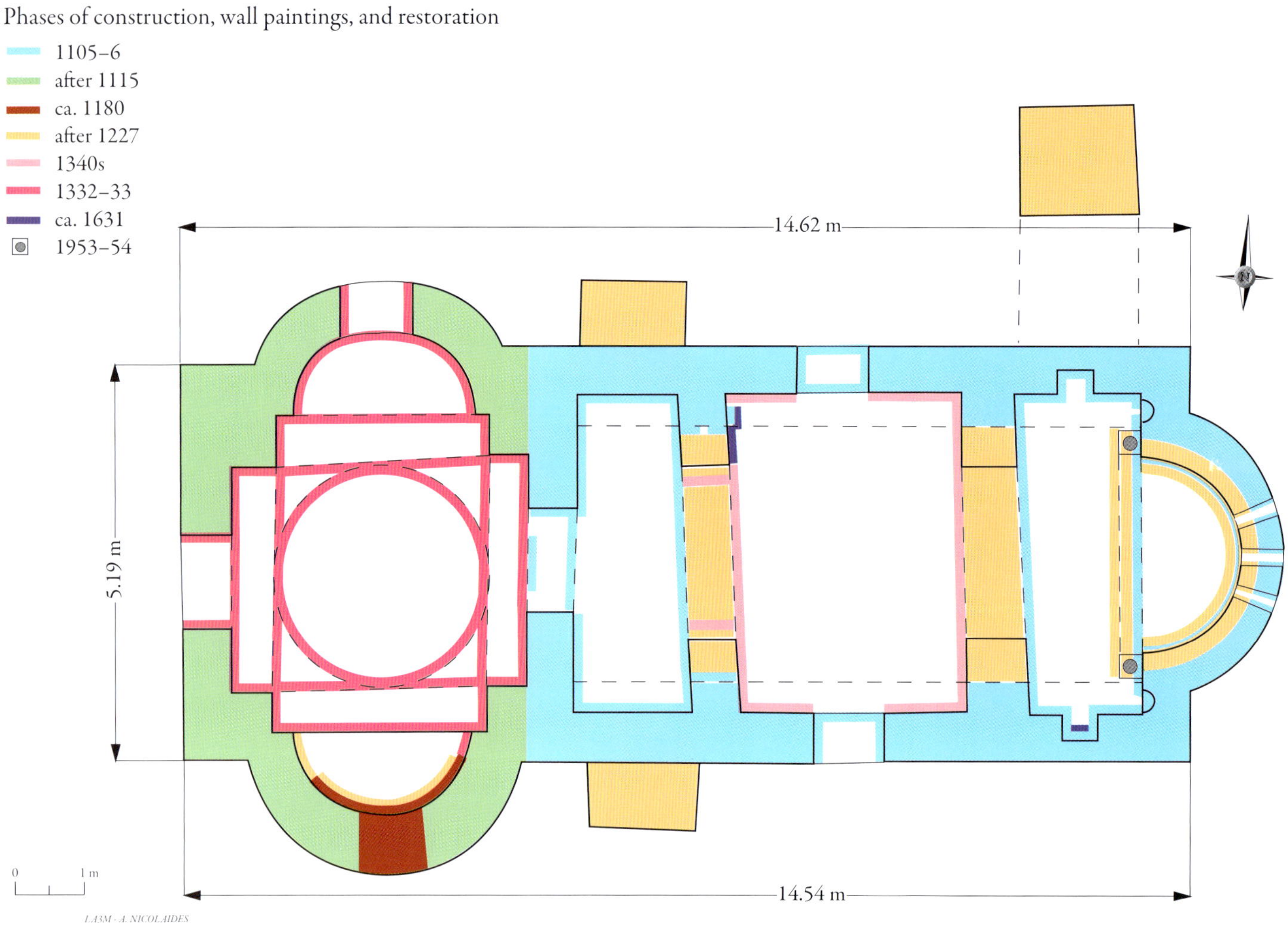

INTRO. FIG. 3 Ground plan of the church of Panagia Phorbiotissa with color indicating the successive phases of construction, mural painting, and restoration. Drawing by Andréas Nicolaïdès

Grivaud on the history of the church and monastery, the first attempt ever at a continuous history for the institution. This study offers a methodological paradigm for the historical analysis of a mountain monastery like Asinou that has, by and large, eluded written documentation, though attesting in its physical fabric to a sustained vitality and significance to its community. The second chapter, by Athanasios Papageorgiou, examines the architecture of the church. Simply constructed as a barrel-vaulted rectangle of three bays with an eastern apse, the building was modified both by the addition of a narthex, surely required for its monastic functions, and by substantial structural repairs in the apse and the central bay of the naos (Intro. Fig. 3). Neither modification is dated; both raise questions about the functional and economic history of the church; and each is important for the frescoes, for they presented fresh surfaces for new frescoes that significantly altered the building as a painted interior. The third chapter, by Nancy Patterson Ševčenko, analyzes the poetic inscriptions that accompany the paintings. Inscriptions in twelve-syllable verse appear in four of the phases of painting. They are fundamental to establishing dates and identifying donors. But they are also significant in coloring the messages of the images they accompany, and in illuminating the climate of culture and literacy in which the images were commissioned and conceived. These three chapters create a foundation for the ensuing three chapters, which are devoted to the phases of fresco painting that followed 1105/6.

The chapters on the fresco programs address the way in which the interior spaces were shaped or defined by the paintings. The most significant of these spaces, the narthex, is addressed in two chapters. Chapter four examines the surviving evidence for the earliest phase of ornament in the narthex. It focuses on the most outstanding of the paintings, the mural icon of St. George that fills the southern apse, presenting it both iconographically, in the analysis of Andréas Nicolaïdès, and technically, in that of its conservator, David Winfield. Along with the fresco icon of St. George, however, are fragments of both ornamental and figural painting that underlie the program of 1332/33. These are probed for information about the chronological relation of the narthex's construction to its initial adornment, about the character and content of this adornment, and about the relation of the surviving fragments to one another and to the St. George. The second chapter on the narthex, chapter five, is by Sophia Kalopissi-Verti. It treats the resumption of painting in the narthex during the Lusignan period. This phase of painting began fitfully in the late thirteenth century with the addition of new votives near the fresco of St. George. It culminated in 1332/33 in a new, comprehensive campaign strongly anchored in the central dome. This phase is by far the most significant addition to the painted interior of Asinou. Approximating a church interior in its own right and dotted with the portraits of its sponsors, this phase points to a new community of participants in the monastery's life and raises a range of questions about the identity, class, and religious confession of the people who are represented here; about the painter(s) whom they chose; about the sources of the styles and imagery that they selected; and about the functions that their imagery served. The last of the three chapters on the painting, by Annemarie Weyl Carr, looks at the renewal of the areas inside the church. The conch and the triumphal arch of the main apse and the central bay of the naos were repainted in the later thirteenth and fourteenth centuries. These paintings replaced, in some cases literally effaced, frescoes by the Asinou Master of 1105/6. But it is they that produce the seamless sweep of color that dominates visitors' impression of Asinou. Much of the appeal of Asinou's interior is due to the murals' warm color and to the message they signal as each visitor enters: that this is an interior dense with the layered aggregate of successive lives and times.

Chapter seven offers a comparative technical examination of the successive phases of painting. It presents physical and chemical analyses of the pigments, the binding media, and the plaster; it also examines the layering of the plaster in areas with images from diverse painting campaigns. Such analyses are crucial to an understanding of both the procedural methods of the medieval painters and the effective modes of modern conservation. They have proved equally fundamental to the chronological attributions adopted in this book.

The volume concludes with an illustrated inventory of the paleographic forms used in the successive phases of painting. Unparalleled as yet in other monographs, it offers a basis for future comparative analyses of the letter forms in Cypriot frescoes, whether in tracing conventions of epigraphy, or in tracing workshops and individual artists' hands.

This book fulfills an obligation assumed by Dumbarton Oaks in 1965–67, when it undertook the restoration and consolidation of Asinou's paintings with the expectation that this work would yield publishable material. The project brought to successful conclusion a half-century-long effort to preserve the church and its murals. The demise of the monastery in the early nineteenth century had left the building unprotected, its paintings exposed to wear and abrasion by shepherd squatters and to water damage from the structurally compromised wooden roof. The lower walls of the central bay suffered especially extensive abrasion from animals and equipment, still very perceptible in the church today, while the frescoes in the western vault were undermined by water seepage. Between 1907 and

1922, George Jeffery, the committee of the Cyprus Museum, and above all Hieronymos Peristianes initiated efforts to preserve the building, drawing repeated attention to its deteriorating condition (see below, pp. 65–66). In 1922, after more than a decade of petitions, the Bishop of Kyrenia agreed to finance the replacement of the church's severely decayed wooden roof (compare Fig. 1.6 with Fig. 1.5), thus ensuring the preservation of the murals. That same year, Peristianes' book on the history of the Asinou valley presented the first published description of the church and its paintings.[3] His book remains fundamental for its ethnographic information and its photographs of the church and the site before the old roof was removed.

A new chapter in Asinou's history opened in March 1931, when Harold Buxton, soon to be consecrated bishop of Gibraltar, walked the ten miles from Evrykhou to Asinou and entered the church, surveying its paintings with appreciative fascination. He later wrote:

> Entering by the west door into the narthex, I stood and held my breath. For in spite of some broken furniture and an accumulation of dust and rubbish, my eyes were caught and held by the warmth and harmony of the colouring on the walls. Looking this way and that, looking up into the dome, I saw the whole surface from dome to floor as a gallery of very remarkable paintings. Nothing comparable to this had I ever seen elsewhere, except (if my memory serves me aright) at Boyana, in the Balkans, twenty years earlier. First the colouring, then the vigour of the drawing, then the sense of mystical reflection which the interior with its unique painting inspires, seemed to rivet one to the spot.[4]

Buxton—who appreciated Cyprus's Byzantine antiquities and later left a fund for their preservation[5]—clearly responded at once to the special value of Asinou's painted interior. The building's life as an art-historical monument really begins with him. He arranged for the paintings to be photographed and sought out scholars to publish them, settling on William H. Buckler and his wife, the Byzantine scholar Georgina Buckler.[6] The Bucklers published the first art-historical study of the monument in the journal *Archaeologia* in 1933.[7] William Buckler described and laid out a chronology for all frescoes visible at that time; his text was accompanied by forty-eight black-and-white photographs commissioned by Buxton from the Mangoian brothers of Nicosia, ten section drawings of the church by Major Vivian Seymer showing the placement of the images and the area included in each of the photographs, and translations of the major inscriptions. Although Buckler's chronology of the later frescoes—especially those in the central bay of the naos—would eventually be discarded, his inventory of images and inscriptions gave scholars access to data about Asinou that was equaled by few Byzantine monuments. In an accompanying "Historical Note," Georgina Buckler proposed that the church's initial patron, Nikephoros Ischyrios, should be identified with Nikephoros, son of the Constantinopolitan governor of Cyprus, Constantine Euphorbenos Katakalon, because the family name [Eu]phorbenos could explain the monastery's name, "ton Phorbion." While her suggestion has since been abandoned, the questions she raised—of Nikephoros's identity, his relationship to the monastery, and the source of the name τῶν Φορβίων—remain vital issues today. The Bucklers' analysis of the church was adopted almost verbatim four years later by Rupert Gunnis in the entry on Asinou in his *Historic Cyprus*, thus lodging the

3. Peristianes, *Μονογραφία τῆς ἀρχαίας πόλεως καὶ ἐκκλησίας*.
4. Buxton et al., "Church of Asinou," 328.
5. See the reference to the Harold Buxton Trust for the preservation of Byzantine paintings in the *ARDAC* for 1950, 5.
6. For more on the engagement of Harold Buxton and the Bucklers with Asinou, see Roueché, "Prehistory," 155–66.
7. Buxton et al., "Church of Asinou," 327–50.

study firmly in the historiography of the building.[8] Gunnis spoke of the church as disused, saying that "[N]o human habitations are near, and it must be many years since a service was celebrated within its walls."[9] The characterization, though exaggerated, contrasts emphatically with the more recent activity recorded by Gilles Grivaud, who in this volume notes that, during Holy Week alone in 1989, some twenty thousand pilgrims visited Asinou for services (see below, p. 36).

The Bucklers' early interest in and engagement with Asinou played a role in this transformation. As one of the major forces behind the creation of a Cypriot department of antiquities, William Buckler used his illustrated lectures on Asinou and its frescoes to stimulate interest in Cyprus and support for the protection of its antiquities, presenting the monument to audiences not only in London and Oxford but also in the United States, at The Johns Hopkins University and at Harvard University's Fogg Art Museum.[10] He also circulated its photographs to a range of scholars, including not only Byzantinists Norman Baynes and Hippolyte Delehaye but also art historian Bernard Berenson. In view of the longstanding ambivalence about the date of the paintings in the central bay of the naos, it is a credit to Berenson's keen eye that he associated the contrapposto of the Virgin in the scene of the donor portrait at Asinou with the frescoes of the church of the Savior in Chora, very near the date currently accepted for it. Late in 1932, in Oxford, Buckler also showed the photographs of Asinou to Mrs. Royall Tyler and her son, William R. Tyler, the future director of Dumbarton Oaks from 1969 to 1977. Thus occurred, as Charlotte Roueché writes, "the first link in a chain which would lead to Dumbarton Oaks' engagement in Cyprus."[11]

The phase of restoration to which Dumbarton Oaks eventually contributed so substantially began in the 1950s with work undertaken by the Department of Antiquities. In 1953, under the department's director, A. H. S. Megaw, the side walls were reinforced, cavities in the rubble fill were grouted, and the twelfth-century portion of the building was ringed with a reinforced collar to withstand the thrust of the roof beams, which were also repaired. Significantly, this was the last time the exterior surface of the vault was actually visible (Fig. 2.15). At the same time, two reinforcing piers—which had masked the original paintings on either side of the apse since the thirteenth century—were removed and replaced with slender shafts that exposed the paintings.[12] Thus the original Annunciation and the figures of Mary of Egypt and Zosimas became known to the world (Figs. 2.32, 6.5, 6.11). The small image of Christ in a Eucharistic chalice with twenty seventeenth-century signatures, painted on one of these piers, was moved to its present position on the south wall of the bema (Fig. 1.7). In 1955, Megaw invited Ernest Hawkins, who was then in Cyprus, to make a trial cleaning of the frescoes in the western bay of the naos, after which Megaw reported enthusiastically that "the gain in visibility was quite spectacular."[13] Hawkins worked with the Byzantine Institute, a privately funded American foundation that had cleaned and restored major Byzantine buildings, frescoes, and mosaics in Istanbul since 1930.[14] Hawkins himself had restored the mosaics of Hagia Sophia. At the death of the institute's founder, Thomas Whittemore, in 1950, the work was taken over by Dumbarton Oaks; and so it was that, in 1959, Dumbarton Oaks, as the Byzantine Institute's heir, signed an agreement with the Department of Antiquities to clean and repair paintings in the Byzantine churches of Cyprus. Work at Asinou, delayed by unrest on Cyprus in 1963, finally got underway in April 1965 with an examination of the frescoes by Ernest Hawkins.

8. Gunnis, *Historic Cyprus*, 180–82.
9. Ibid., 180.
10. Roueché, "Prehistory," 158–60.
11. Ibid., 158.
12. *ARDAC* for 1953, 10.
13. *ARDAC* for 1955, 10.
14. A sketch of Dumbarton Oaks' relation to the Byzantine Institute is given in Constable, "Dumbarton Oaks and Byzantine Field Work."

Work was directed at intervals by Ernest Hawkins and by David Winfield with the assistance of June Winfield and two of the Byzantine Institute's specially trained workmen, Kostas Zaferiades and Yannis Makridis. The conservation was completed in 1967. In the same year Dumbarton Oaks scholar Ihor Ševčenko visited Asinou to review the work and to make the epigraphic transcriptions that have served the authors of this volume so well.

Summarizing the restoration campaign, Cyril Mango wrote in 1969:

> One trait in particular is deserving of close attention: These paintings—I am referring here to the ones made before the Latin conquest—have nothing provincial about them. The paintings of St. Chrysostomos, Asinou and Trikomo embody the early Comnenian style in all its purity. . . . [T]here can be no doubt that the decorations made known in the last ten years constitute a most important contribution to the study of Byzantine art.[15]

The aim of Dumbarton Oaks' field work, to clarify the culture that lay at Byzantium's center, emerges clearly in this appreciation of the twelfth-century frescoes at Asinou. The importance of those frescoes has only grown since this assessment was made. If it is among the most regularly visited archaeological sites in Cyprus, Asinou is also among the most regularly cited monuments of Middle Byzantine art. It has a vast bibliography,[16] stimulated by the reproduction of its images in numerous publications: the Bucklers' article; the *Dumbarton Oaks Papers*;[17] the twice-expanded "bible" of Cypriot wall painting, *The Painted Churches of Cyprus* by Andreas Stylianou and Judith A. Stylianou;[18] Marina Sacopoulo's iconographic study of the twelfth-century paintings published in 1966;[19] and the large-scale images published by Athanasios Papageorgiou and A. H. S. Megaw.[20]

The later murals at Asinou drew less attention from Mango. Nonetheless, he and Ihor Ševčenko had discovered dated graffiti of 1446 and 1450 in the plaster layer of the central bay of the naos. These established a mid-fifteenth-century *terminus ante quem* for the plaster, and seemed unlikely to have been scratched into surfaces freshly painted in the decades just before 1450. Thus they undermined the widely accepted fifteenth-century date for these frescoes, and opened the way to the earlier, fourteenth-century attribution that is accepted today. Of this discovery Mango wrote:

> If the last conclusion is correct, the evolution of painting in Cyprus under Lusignan rule will have to be reconsidered, the more so as the late frescoes of Asinou may be matched in other churches of the island.[21]

His prediction that the Lusignan period would demand closer attention has been fully borne out in this publication. Dumbarton Oaks in 1967 had focused on the Byzantine center, and Asinou served this interest with the outstanding art of the Asinou

15. Mango, "Summary of Work."
16. Both Robin S. Cormack and Annabel Jane Wharton have included cogent observations on Asinou in books on Byzantine art: see Wharton, *Art of Empire*, 76–79; Cormack, *Writing in Gold*, 170–74. Articles devoted specifically to Asinou include Drossoyianni, "Some Observations on the Asinou Frescoes"; Frigerio-Zeniou, "Μονὴ τῶν Φορβίων à Asinou"; and, most recently, Georgiou, "Περί του κτίτορος της Μονής," with exhaustive bibliography.

17. Winfield and Hawkins, "Church of Our Lady at Asinou"; Hawkins, "Summary of Work;" Mango, "Summary of Work."
18. First published in 1964 as a sparsely illustrated, 171-page pocket guide by A. Stylianou and J. A. Stylianou, *The Painted Churches of Cyprus* was published in an expanded form in 1985 as an amply illustrated, 517-page volume titled *The Painted Churches of Cyprus: Treasures of Byzantine Art*. That volume was reissued in 1997.
19. Sacopoulo, *Asinou en 1106*.
20. Papageorgiou, *Masterpieces of the Byzantine Art of Cyprus*; Megaw and Stylianou, *Cyprus: Byzantine Mosaics and Frescoes*.
21. Mango, "Summary of Work," 103.

Master. The present volume, by contrast, focuses on Byzantine culture at work in a society that had been politically severed from the empire and become its own center. The parity given in this volume to the later stages of Asinou's painting permits a fuller exploration than hitherto of the frescoes' place in the art of Lusignan Cyprus itself. More than on their relation to the capital, it throws light on the frescoes' relation to other mural programs in Cyprus. The decorative programs of the island's churches appear to have been in constant dialogue with one another, building up over the centuries a distinctive repertoire of themes and programmatic schemes. Asinou both contributed to and drew upon this dialogue, and as much as it belongs to the broad discourse of Byzantine imagery, it was also integral to an evolving and distinctively local Cypriot tradition.

The conclusions reached on the basis of Dumbarton Oaks' restoration work were published with skeletal clarity in David Winfield's slender but indispensable *Asinou: A Guide*, published in Nicosia in 1969.[22] Moving figure by figure over the frescoed surfaces of the building, he corrected iconographic identifications made by both the Bucklers and by Sacopoulo, and for the first time sorted out the disputed chronological sequence of the many fresco campaigns. The chronology that Winfield laid out has been the basis of this volume. Our attributions, based on technical, stylistic, and iconographic analyses, support Winfield's conclusions, differing only in the somewhat later attribution of the paintings in the central bay of the naos.[23]

If the chronology itself is little altered, the scope of the present volume is deliberately wide. Its purpose is to provide clear and accurate information on as full a range of the church's defining characteristics as possible. The broad disciplinary scope of these chapters should help to make information about Asinou useful to scholars working in varied disciplinary contexts. The chapters on the history, architecture, inscriptions, and technical analysis approach Asinou's paintings from a range of methodological perspectives, enriching our grasp of the institution, its painters, and its community of sponsors and users. As we have previously looked to the paintings of 1105/6 to illuminate the life and culture of Byzantium's provinces under full imperial control on the brink of the Crusades, so Asinou's staunch institutional continuity and renewed artistic vitality during the centuries of Lusignan rule offer a particularly revealing prism through which to study the implications of Latin rule for the island and its Orthodox community. In turn, the chapters devoted to art-historical analysis of the successive fresco programs both align the church's iconographic and stylistic particularities with developments elsewhere in the Byzantine cultural world, and examine with novel intensity the artistic developments specific to fourteenth-century Cyprus. No other study explores so fully the extraordinary variety of sources and styles that combined at Asinou to produce the distinctive art of fourteenth-century Cyprus. The varied iconographic sources seen in Asinou's programs bespeak a steady interchange not only with Byzantine but with broader Mediterranean traditions. Stylistically, in turn, the "maniera cypria"—so often treated as exemplifying the Lusignan centuries as a whole—falls back here into a defined period on either side of 1300. This style was displaced around the 1340s by a more exuberant manner that, while still strongly affected by the Mediterranean interchange of the Crusader era, was responsive to Palaiologan developments as well. These stylistic changes were widely disseminated on the island by painters too numerous to be just a workshop: they must instead reflect a period style.

In many cases the range of skills offered by the team of authors made it possible to resolve long-debated questions. This was especially true of deciphering inscriptions, determining the sequence and chronology of fresco layers, and understanding historical conditions. On the other hand, there were serious questions that we could not investigate.

22. Winfield, *Asinou: A Guide*.

23. It was adopted, too, in the 2002 volume by Hadjichristodoulou and Myriantheus, *Church of Our Lady of Asinou*, which was published in multiple languages and is available to visitors at the church itself.

Neither the Church of Cyprus nor the Department of Antiquities was prepared to undertake the radical surgery that would have allowed us to remove the fourteenth-century murals from the walls of the naos and the narthex. Thus, we could not ascertain the extent or character of the paintings beneath them. Valuable as it would be to uncover what (if anything) remains of the twelfth-century imagery on the naos vault, and to see whether the narthex was indeed largely unadorned before the late thirteenth century, these revelations will have to wait for another time and the availability of less-invasive technology.

It was equally impossible to remove enough of the wooden roof to confirm or reject A. H. S. Megaw's judgment that the present naos vault is original to the building and was not a replacement for one that had collapsed when the east end fell, taking its original frescoes with it. Similarly, we were unable to make geophysical soundings under the naos and the narthex to determine whether there were accommodations for burials under the church, or to dig a trench under the narthex floor to identify the cavity detected in an earlier magnetic survey. From the record of the death of the enigmatic Gephyra in the naos,[24] through the themes of death and judgment in the narthex, to the fourteenth-century portrait of Nikephoros Ischyrios in the naos, a funerary association hovers over the whole span of the church's medieval centuries, but we were not able to find a concrete confirmation in places of interment. By the same token, it was not possible to make a geophysical survey of the area around the church to establish the location and configuration of the monastic buildings, or to confirm arrangements for inhumations outside the church. The dendrochronological analysis that we advocated promises to be carried out in the future.[25]

The volume's research team has had sustained access to the painted surface of Asinou's walls. No problems were encountered with excessive inpainting or overpainting from the restoration campaign of 1965–67. On the contrary, the testimony of the mural surfaces has been eloquent. At a number of places in the lower walls close observation reveals that the images are stained by reddish marks of a recurrent, slender oval form. As it turns out, these marks were left by candle flames; they are the tangible traces of veneration. To have at one's fingertips the very acts these walls were designed to motivate evokes a sharp sense of immediacy. This volume is offered with the hope that the keen, close scrutiny of the team can be made immediate to those who can know these surfaces only through our eyes.

24. See below, pp. 22–23 and 53–54.

25. Professor Maria Parani of the University of Cyprus is overseeing an extensive dendrochronological project with Professor Peter Kuniholm of Cornell University.

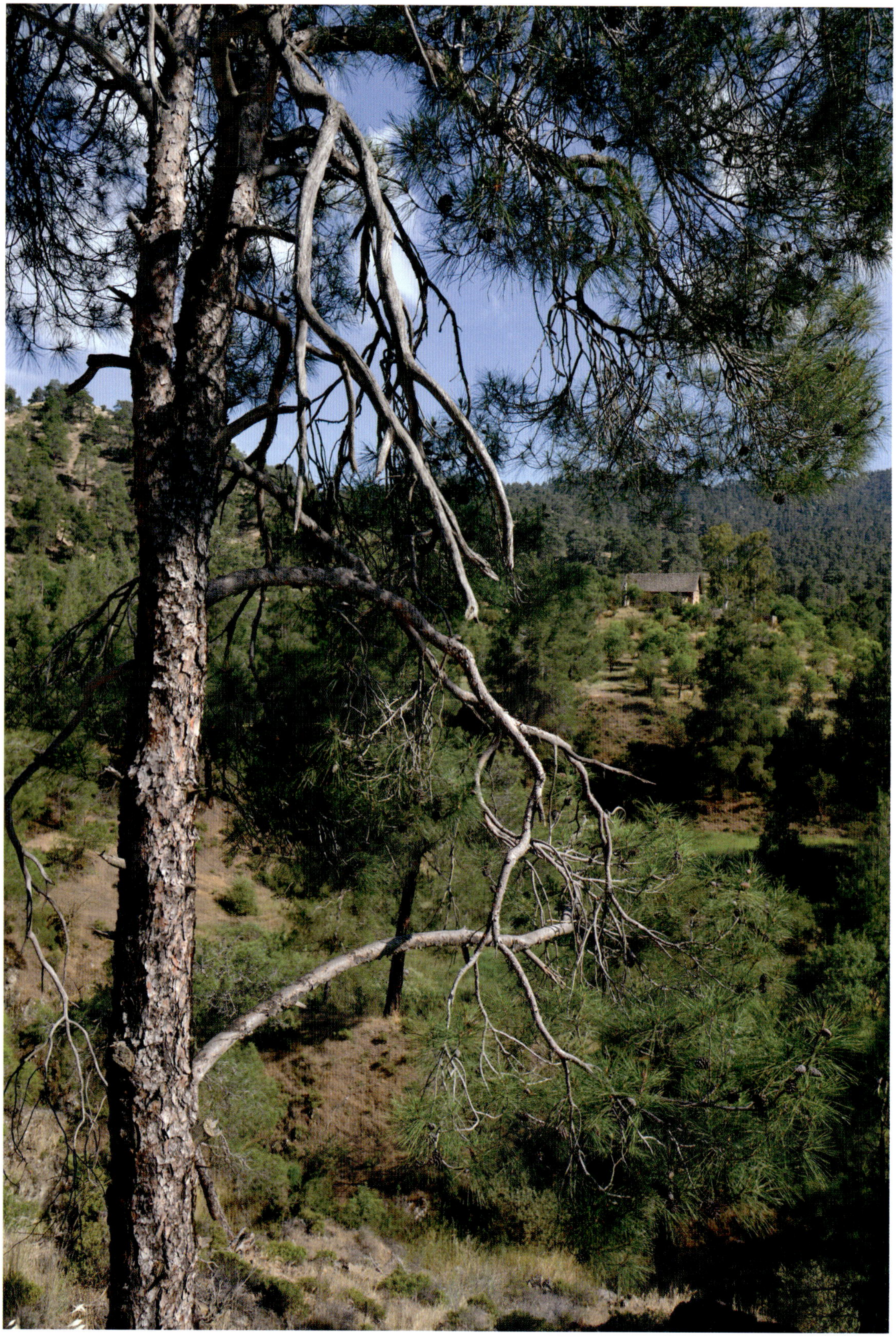

The church of Panagia Phorbiotissa seen across the Asinou River
(photo courtesy of G. L. Carr)

CHAPTER ONE

Fortunes and Misfortunes of a Small Byzantine Foundation

Gilles Grivaud
Translated by Charles Dibble

To this day, the path that leads to the church of the Panagia Phorbiotissa casts an indescribable charm on the traveler coming from Nicosia. After a slow crossing over the dry and monotonous plain of the Morphou Basin, one passes through the little village of Nikitari toward the foothills of the Troodos Mountains. The nearer slopes, which fall off abruptly, can be negotiated along a gorge carved out by the Asinou River (Asinou Potamos). There, the vegetation, shaded by pines, grows thicker and greener. After a short ascent, the path widens and the valley opens out at the foot of a small amphitheater capped by a series of low crests, obscured by the Adelphi forest. At the valley's entrance, on a natural rise, the Byzantine monument of Asinou nestles in the landscape.

The Site

The toponym "Asinou" describes the narrow alluvial valley that emerges at the juncture of the Rotson and the Chandakia (Figs. 1.1, 1.2). These two streams—the former approximately six kilometers long, the latter extending some four kilometers—are fed by small brooks; they form the drainage basin of the Asinou River, whose bed occupies the valley floor over an expanse of three kilometers. Downstream, the river has worn a passage between two hills; at its outlet, it flows unobstructed toward Nikitari, emptying into the Potamos tes Elias three kilometers to the north, after the village of Pano Koutraphas.

Because of its relative seclusion, the valley of Asinou is a world unto itself, its economy shaped by the area's elevation, as one might expect in a mountainous region. At the bottom of the valley—which is wet and green, forested with plane trees, poplars, and rushes—human activities are concentrated on a small arable expanse of barely ten hectares, including natural and cultivated terraces. The place-names evoke the former cultivation of gardens (Kepoi or Kepia) and vineyards (Ambelia) on minuscule parcels of land. Above the cultivated areas, the remains of a settlement are visible at Chalospities ("ruined houses") and, on the opposite side of the river, at Pera

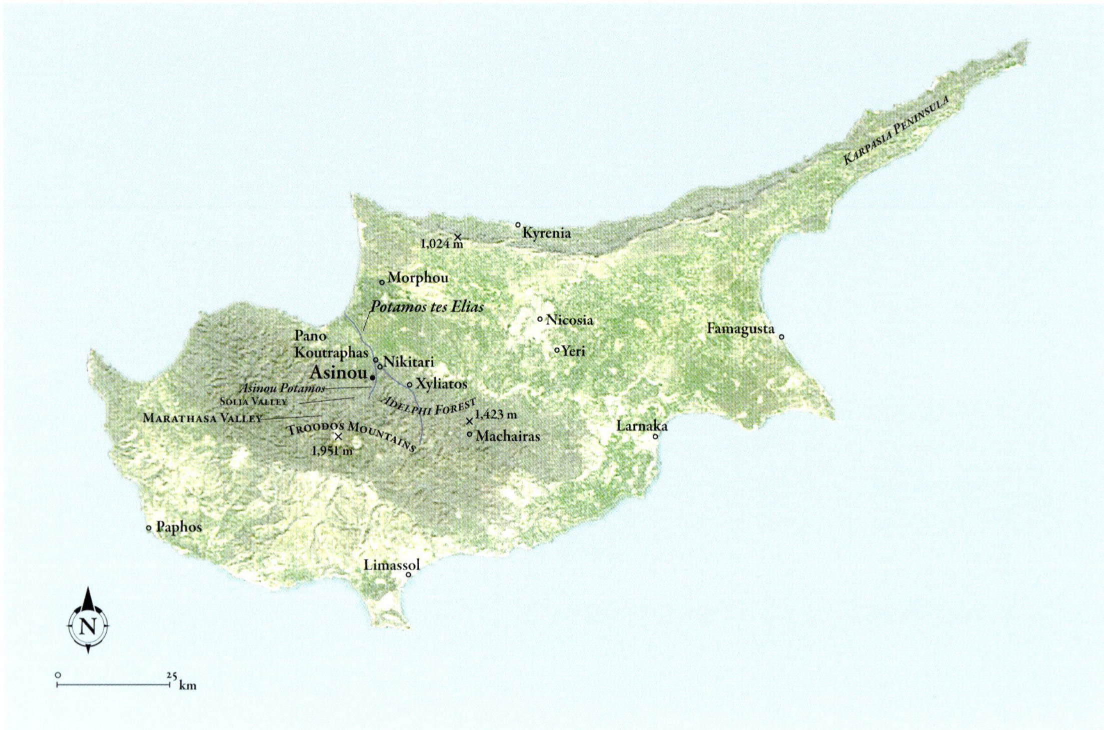

FIG. 1.1 Map of Cyprus showing the location of the Asinou Valley. After a drawing by Benoît Devillers.

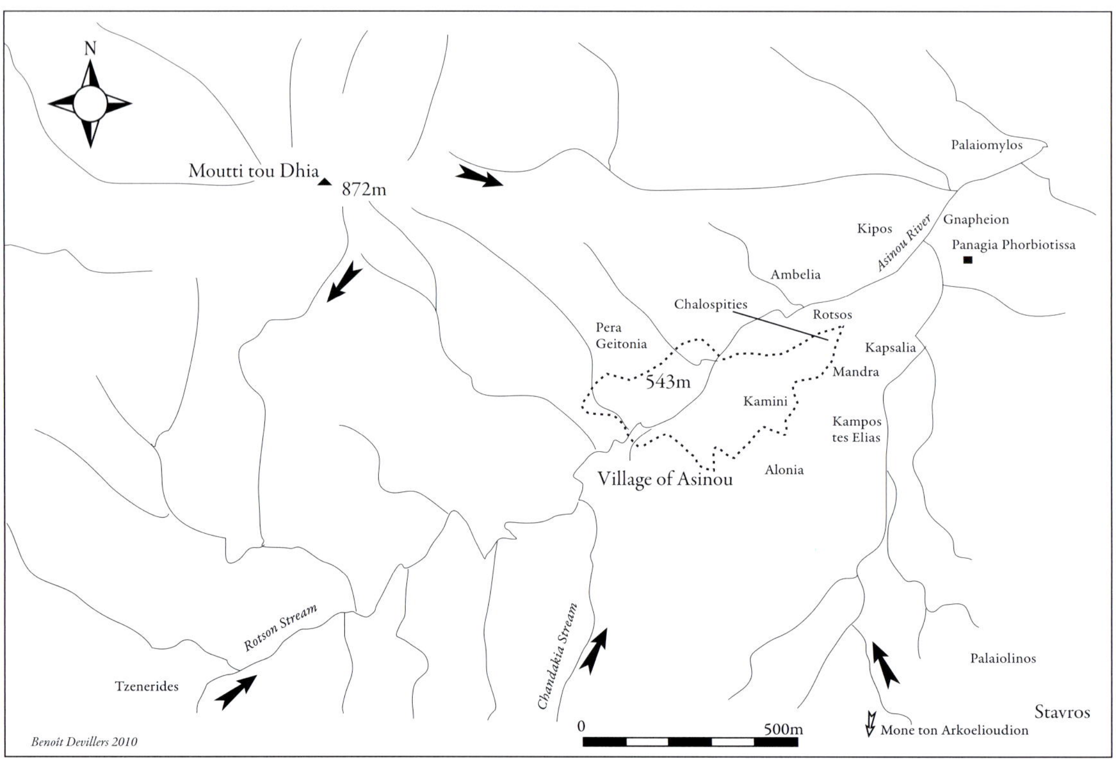

FIG. 1.2 Map of the Asinou region showing the toponyms mentioned in the text. Drawing by Benoît Devillers.

Geitonia ("the facing quarter"), a hamlet of three houses marked on Lord Kitchener's 1882 map of Cyprus. Remains of threshing grounds (Alonia), a sheepfold (Mandra), and a kiln (Kamini) are located near Chalospities; on the slope that once separated the settlement from the monastery of the Panagia Phorbiotissa, the place-names call to mind the cultivation of olives (Kampos tes Elias), a wine press (Palaiolinos), and land cleared by burning (Kapsalia). Further down, below the site of the monastery and within the gorge, the place-names recall the practice of two crafts: a tannery (Gnapheion) and a mill (Palaiomylos), whose millrace survives. When originally in use, these two operations would have required water resources exceeding those that exist today, which they would undoubtedly have drawn from two sources, one above the monastery, the other in the gorge.[1] In their former state, the lands surrounding the houses could have supported a small farming community with subsistence cultivation (vegetable plots, vineyards, grains, and olives), processed on-site, as attested by the threshing ground and the wine press, the surpluses from which could have been sold.[2] The rural economy supplied other products as well—cheese, meat, wool, and hides—from flocks whose pasturage extended over the valley floor, probably beyond Tzenerides, a hamlet that in 1882 comprised some ten buildings.[3]

The remains of occupation attest to the presence of a permanent settlement at the bottom of the valley. The modern toponym Chalospities undoubtedly corresponds to the old village of Asinou, whose name appears in sixteenth-century records. On the map of Leonida Attar (1542), the village is represented under the label "assino" by a church with a pitched roof (Fig. 1.3).[4] Toward the middle of the century, the settlement is mentioned in several lists of villages, including a 1565 census of free peasants (*francomati*); it enumerates forty-five at "casale Asinu," which suggests that some thirty families lived there permanently, undoubtedly divided between the main settlement and scattered hamlets.[5] The dispersed state of the population is corroborated by a register recording a *cizye* (the poll tax on non-Muslims) in 1612 that names three settlements: nineteen Christian households are recorded at "Qāto Āsīnū," twenty-one at "Pāno Āsīnū," and four at "Li[nou] Āsīnū."[6] These data attest to ongoing economic capacity in the valley during the seventeenth century, as recent surveys of the ancient settlement have confirmed.[7] Afterward, the settlement vanishes from published Ottoman sources and from nineteenth-century registers.

Popular tradition maintains that the village and its dependent hamlets were brutally laid waste during the Ottoman period by the "bishop" of Asinou, in retaliation for allegations by his parishioners that he had entered into a compromising relationship with a Turkish woman.[8] Collective

1. See the maps of the Department of Land and Surveys, *Cyprus, 1925–1996,* sheets 28/55, 28/56 (scale 1:5000), Asinou (1:1250); and Kitchener, *Trigonometrical Survey*, sheet 9. The etymology of the toponym "Gnapheion" is confirmed by Sakellarios, *Τὰ Κυπριακά*, 2:512.

2. See the surveys carried out in the context of the Troodos Archaeological and Environmental Survey Project: www.taesp.arts.gla.ac.uk/Landscape/SIA/TS12.htm, accessed July 2011.

3. More or less concurring findings (albeit extremely imprecise) are published in the preliminary reports of the Troodos Archaeological and Environmental Survey Project. Hadjisavvas, "Chronique des fouilles . . . en 2002," 678.

4. Cavazzana Romanelli and Grivaud, *Great Map*, 49, 140.

5. Archivio di Stato di Venezia, Avogaria di Comun, Miscellanea civile 179/3; Grivaud, *Villages désertés à Chypre*, 200, 215, 469.

6. Başbakanlık Osmanlı Arşivi, Istanbul, *Maliyeden Müdevver,* defter 5084, fol. 10. I am grateful to Vera Costantini for having brought this document to my attention and for her assistance in its transcription.

7. *ARDAC* for 2003, 88.

8. Kasiere and Koumparidou, "Λαογραφικά," provide the most detailed version of a tradition circulating during the 1920s and 1930s; Peristianes, *Μονογραφία*, 6, 17; Cyprus American Archaeological Research Institute (Nicosia), Archives, letter from Margaret Eleanor Dray to her daughter Eve, ca. 1938, 3.

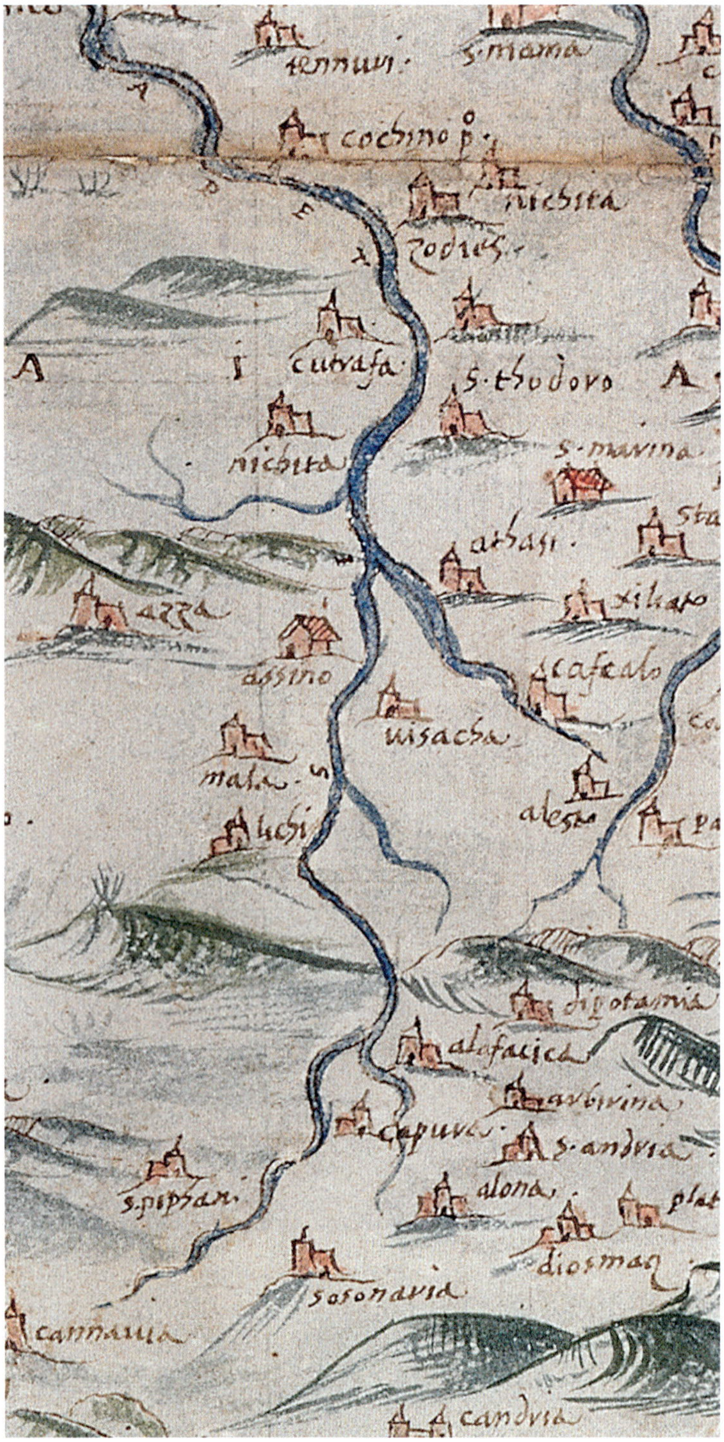

FIG. 1.3 Detail of the region of Asinou on Leonida Attar's 1542 map (Venice, Civico Museo Correr, *Mappe sciolte*, cart. 28 bis/21, n. ant. 71)

memory thus pinpoints an abrupt break in the area's settlement within an entirely plausible chronological framework, notwithstanding the complex processes involved in the abandonment of villages. It is to archaeologists that we must look to disentangle the legend, but the village's disappearance (undoubtedly after the sweeping plague epidemics that struck Cyprus between the end of the seventeenth century and the end of the eighteenth) would surely have been a leading cause of the monastery's decline. Extinction came slowly to the valley of Asinou, and only a few rural activities survived, unlike the neighboring valley of Marathassa, which enjoyed more ample water and was thus better able to weather the catastrophic chain of events that drove men and women to leave the Troodos Mountains during modern times.[9]

In Asinou's environs, sacred spaces also attest to the presence of humans. A hundred meters above the monastery of the Panagia Phorbiotissa, the remains of a church dedicated to St. Auxibius are still visible; higher up, on the hill, are the vestiges of the leveled chapel of the Cross (Stavros). At the bottom of the valley, the foundations of the church of St. John Lampadistes break the surface; Tzenerides' chapel, dedicated to St. George, survives, albeit in ruins.[10] The positioning of these cult sites placed the valley under the protection of powerful symbols of Orthodox Christianity, with the Cross downstream and St. George at the headwaters, leaving the veneration of the Virgin and local saints—Auxibius and John Lampadistes—to develop in settled areas. The absence of archaeological surveys, however, militates against a better understanding of these monuments' history and of how Asinou's sacred geography took form.

The microcosm formed by the valley of Asinou, similar to that of nearby valleys in the Troodos Mountains, has attributes that might explain why a Byzantine dignitary reserved the site for his

9. Grivaud, *Villages désertés à Chypre*, 293–301.
10. In addition to the map surveys listed above, church dedications are documented by Peristianes, *Μονογραφία*, 6, 16–17.

pious foundation. From the vantage of the island as a whole, the valley of Asinou stands apart from Cyprus's thoroughfares and its coastline; nonetheless, it could be integrated into an expansive communications network, both military and strategic, by means of the hill of the Cross, the summit of which is a mere quarter-hour's climb from the monastery. Despite its low elevation (568 meters), the hill provides an exceptional observation post, commanding views of Mount Olympus (1,951 meters) to the southwest and of Prophetes Elias (888 meters)—the summit of the Pentadaktylos Range—to the northeast. No remains of military battlements are visible on the hill, but a watch post, from which warnings could have been broadcast by smoke signals, might easily have sent messages to Olympus and Prophetes Elias, where traces of medieval stonework attest to the presence of watchtowers, certainly from the Byzantine period forward.[11] A natural relay station, the hill of the Cross connected the disparate elements of the valley of Asinou to a system of defenses still in operation when the Ottomans took the island in 1570.[12] Thus, peasants of the Troodos Mountains would quickly have learned of events taking place on the island's shores. The sense of loneliness that might strike a visitor to Asinou is misleading; during the Middle Ages, a Cypriot would not have felt it.

The Monastery of the Panagia ton Phorbion ("τῶν Φορβίων")

In this physical environment, befitting a life of contemplation, the monastery of the Panagia ton Phorbion ("τῶν Φορβίων"), or Panagia Phorbiotissa, was founded at the beginning of the twelfth century. The circumstances of the monastery's founding and its history have so eluded documentary records that our understanding of the first three centuries of its existence can be based only on dedicatory inscriptions, donor portraits, its church's iconographic program, and notes in the margins of the only manuscript known to have been used by the monastic community there: a synaxarion for the first six months of the ecclesiastical year, Parisinus Graecus 1590, in the collection of the Bibliothèque Nationale de France.[13] From the fifteenth century forward, documentation can be enriched by sparse, oblique references; nonetheless, written accounts pass over the monastery, an indication of its weak influence in medieval and modern Cypriot society. One is thus reduced to parsing sparse information, whose ambiguities cannot be conclusively resolved by studying the historical context.

The Foundation

Absent the monastery's foundation documents, the founder's (κτήτωρ) name has been preserved in an obituary in Paris. gr. 1590 recording his death on 16 November 1115: Ἐκυμηθ(η) ο (μον)αχ(ὸς) κυρ νικόλαος ὁ ισ(ὴν) [*or* ισ(χ)] και κτη[τωρ] (Fig. 1.4).[14] From this reference we may gather that Nikolaos founded a monastery in which he became a monk. Was he also its hegumen? Nothing allows us to conclude he was, insofar as the manuscript's obituaries for other individuals of high status clearly name the office they held.[15] On the other hand,

11. The medieval tower of Prophetes Elias is documented on the map of the Department of Military Survey, Ministry of Defence, United Kingdom (1973), sheet 2, WE 21 07; Karageorghis, "Chronique des fouilles," 298–99, provides indirect confirmation. Regarding the defensive installations on Olympus's summit, see the report of A. Beltram, in 1910: State Archives of Cyprus (Nicosia), 1:1711/1910. See also Jeffery, *Historic Monuments*, 289–90.

12. The communications network was apparently still operating in 1468. Richard, *Livre des remembrances*, no. 38; Grivaud, "*Strateia* à Chypre," 38–44.

13. A recent description of Paris. gr. 1590, by Constantinides and Browning, *Dated Greek Manuscripts*, 49–54 and pl. 1, includes a complete bibliography of studies bearing on the manuscript.

14. Note dated 16 November 66[2]4, indiction 9, in the transcription by J. Darrouzès, "Notes [1]," 93, which advances arguments for completing the year as 6624 (1115 CE) rather than 6654 (1145/46 CE). This dating is also followed by Constantinides and Browning, *Dated Greek Manuscripts,* 51.

15. See Demetrios: 12 December 6630, indiction 15; Dometios: 5 December, 665[4], indiction 9. Darrouzès,

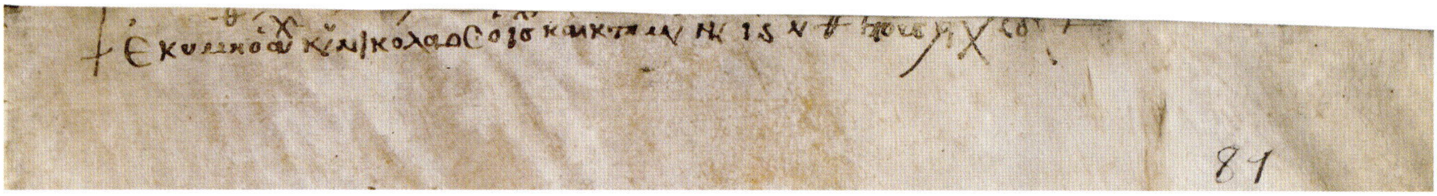

FIG. 1.4 Paris. gr. 1590, fol. 81v, upper margin. Notice of the death of the monk Nicholas (photo courtesy of the Bibliothèque nationale de France)

Nikolaos's title of *kyr,* which elevates him to the higher ranks of society, implies his ability to dedicate some of his assets to founding a religious institution, and as founder he would undoubtedly have drawn up a *ktetorikon typikon* that defined the institution's disciplinary rules and specified the arrangements for his interment and for the funerary services to be carried out in his memory.[16] As to the patronym "ισ(ήν)," undocumented in Byzantine sources relating to Cyprus, one can make out the first letters of the name (ισ) inscribed on the upper margin of folio 81 of Paris. gr. 1590, but the rest of the name is truncated, due to trimming at the margin's edge.[17] An unequivocal restoration of the name is thus not feasible, since the ην generally advanced might equally correspond to the downstrokes of a χ. The latter suggests the name "Ischyrios," a proposed reading that, while uncertain, might be in accord with art historians' conclusions.

The date of the church's founding, undocumented in texts, is generally accepted as 6614 (1105/6 CE) on the basis of the dedicatory inscription beneath the portraits of Helena and Constantine, where the donor's name appears: Magistros Nikephoros Ischyrios (Fig. 2.19); his portrait, offering the church and directing a long prayer to the Virgin, appears above the church's southern door (Fig. 3.8). His name appears a third time in the prayer inscribed on the central register of the apse (Fig. 3.7).[18] There is no uncertainty as to the benefactor responsible for the church's construction: he was an imperial dignitary, as confirmed by the reference to the reign of Alexios Komnenos in the dedicatory inscription. Sources are silent, however, on Nikephoros Ischyrios's position in local society and his specific responsibilities.[19] The fact that the bema's decoration accords a relatively important position to Barnabas and Epiphanios, the saints credited with the island's evangelization, might indicate that he belonged to a local aristocratic circle.

Historians and art historians tend to blur the distinction between Nikephoros the magistros and Nikolaos the ktetor for any number of reasons, such as the likeness of the first letters of their civil and monastic names, the closeness of their dates, the social status of ktetores and magistroi, and the juxtaposition of panels depicting SS. Nikephoros and

---

"Notes [1]," 94; Constantinides and Browning, *Dated Greek Manuscripts,* 51. On the title *kyr* see Kyritzes, "Byzantine Aristocracy"; in the case of Kyr Leon Authentes at Lagoudera, Nicolaïdès, "Panagia Arakiotissa à Lagoudéra" [1993], 13 n. 57.

16. Such concerns are generally addressed in typika, whatever their legal character. See Herman, "Istituzioni monastiche," 302–5; Janin, "Monachisme byzantin," 15–44; Konidaris, *Νομική θεωρήση*, 29–34; Galatariotou, "Byzantine Ktetorika Typika"; *BMFD*, esp. 4:1295–1302.

17. The intrusions of the modern bookbinders are even more extreme in the instance of the note that appears on the upper margin of folio 220, which is rendered unintelligible as a result.

18. Winfield, *Asinou: A Guide*, 18.

19. After the 10th century the title of magistros no longer entailed specific duties, having been relegated to the status of an honorific. See Guilland, "L'histoire administrative," 25. The title disappeared after 1118, see also Kazhdan and Ronchey, *L'aristocrazia bizantina*, 100–101; according to Georgiou, "Περί του κτίτορος," 194–95. Malamut (*Les îles*, 512) deemed Nikephoros Ischyrios to have been a local official.

Nicholas on the naos's northern wall (pp. 242–45).[20] Nonetheless, Nikephoros is never titled "ktetor" in the inscriptions.[21] The ambiguity of the data thus leaves two crucial questions unresolved: the identity of the monastery's founder and the sequence of the institution's development.

Three hypotheses may be advanced regarding the founder's identity. The first (and most plausible) posits that Nikephoros and Nikolaos are the same person and identifies the dignitary as the founder both of Asinou's church, in 1105/6, and of its monastery, in 1115 at the latest. The second hypothesis, which disassociates the two individuals, situates the founding of the church and the monastery in the context of a family foundation, with a blood relationship between Nikephoros and Nikolaos. Finally, one might advance a third hypothesis, that the monastery founded by Nikolaos enjoyed the patronage of Nikephoros the magistros, following a custom found in other regions of the empire.[22] The custom is specifically documented in Cyprus, where, about 1099, the doux Eumathios Philokales commissioned the decoration of the chapel of the Holy Trinity in the monastery of St. John Chrysostom at Koutsovendis, founded by the ktetor Georgios in 1090. It was at the turn of the eleventh century (between 1093 and 1111/12) that the monastery of the Virgin of Kykkos enjoyed the patronage of the strategos Manuel Boutomites.[23] Nothing in these three hypotheses proves that the church of the Panagia ton Phorbion was intended at that point to serve as the monastery's *katholikon*, and the gap of ten years between the church's completion (in 1105/6) and the first explicit reference to the monastery (1115) leaves the question unanswered. We know only that at some point the church's layout was reconfigured, and a narthex was subsequently added to celebrate rites specific to the prayers for the dead that were at the heart of monastic communities.

Whether or not the magistros and the ktetor were the same person, we know that both the church and the monastery were founded by a member of the laity. The choice of the site—a secluded valley—indicates a regard for the contemplative life rather than a defensive intent, for Cyprus had at that point escaped hostile invasion.[24] The magistros's motives are articulated in his prayer to the Virgin, from whom Nikephoros seeks intercession at the Last Judgment. The prayer suggests that the monastery's founding was part of a larger movement among private foundations that energized the empire during the eleventh and twelfth centuries, put into motion by members of the imperial family or by high dignitaries. In Cyprus, several monasteries were founded during the reign of Alexios Komnenos: in addition to the privately supported monastery of St. John Chrysostom and that of the Virgin of Kykkos mentioned above, there was also the church of the Panagia Alypou, founded in Yeri before 1091 by the magistros Epiphanios Paschales.[25] In this context, the founding of the

20. Among those positing an identity between the two are Papageorgiou, "Ασίνου"; Wharton, *Art of Empire*, 76; Englezakis, *Church of Cyprus*, 58; Papacostas, "Byzantine Cyprus," 2:70. A more guarded view is taken by Darrouzès, "Mouvement de fondations," 168; Malamut, *Les îles*, 512; and Constantinides and Browning, *Dated Greek Manuscripts,* 51, n. 10.

21. In contrast, the notice recording the donation of a gospel to the monastery of the Panagia Alypou, at Yeri, in October 1091, explicitly describes the making of the gift by "Ἐπιφανίου μαγίστρου τοῦ Πασχάλη καὶ κτήτορος τής τοιαύτης μονῆς. . . .": Darrouzès, "Notes [2]," 44.

22. Several examples of the various possible permutations involved in the founding of monasteries are cited by Janin, "Monachisme byzantin," 18–21; Darrouzès, "Mouvement des fondations," 160–71; Thomas, *Private Religious Foundations*, chaps. 4–9; Talbot, "Family and the Monastery"; and Dagron, "Hériter de soi-même."

23. Mango and Hawkins, "Field Work in Istanbul and Cyprus," 334–37; Darrouzès, "Mouvement des fondations," 167–68; Wharton, *Art of Empire,* 74; Constantinides, *Διήγησις της θαυματουργής εικόνας*, 143–44; Papacostas, "Koutsovendis," 61–75.

24. Malamut, *Les îles,* 89–96; Galatariotou, *Making of a Saint,* 40–67; and Asdracha, "Κύπρος ὑπὸ τοὺς Κομνηνούς," 1:317–47.

25. Darrouzès, "Mouvement des fondations," 168; Galatariotou, *Making of a Saint,* 57–58 (with a complete list of monasteries founded and churches decorated in

monastery of the Panagia ton Phorbion accords with a well-established tradition. In the absence of the *ktetorikon typikon*, the monastery's legal status cannot be ascertained; surely it was independent, as were many dignitaries' private foundations during this period.[26] It might have been a family foundation, although the necrology in Paris. gr. 1590 does not mention the burial of members of the ktetor's family. The portrait of Gephyra, next to that of Nikephoros, suggests that this relative of the magistros (spouse or daughter) was entitled to a tomb in the church or in the monastery's enclosure.[27]

Given the dearth of written records, the conditions leading to the monastery's foundation are shrouded in obscurity. Its very name is the subject of uncertainty: an obituary dated 5 December 1145 calls it the monastery of "θεοτόκου τῶν φορβίων," a name that also appears in the dedicatory inscription of Nikephoros the veterinarian (Fig. 3.10; "μονῆ τῶν Φορβίω(ν)"); it appears again in a derivative form above the lunette of the door leading to the nave (Fig. 3.11; "Μ[ή]τηρ Θ(εο)ῦ ἡ Φορβιότισσα"), but the date of this inscription is unclear.[28]

Numerous etymologies have been advanced, deriving the name from φορβή (fodder), φορβαῖος (he who procures fodder), φορβόν (medicine), φορβεία (halter or harness), and εὐφόρβιον (euphorbia, or spurges);[29] the last derivation is the most plausible in that it conforms to the Cypriot custom of naming monasteries dedicated to the Virgin after plants.[30] To this day, the valley of Asinou preserves the toponym Μονὴ τῶν Ἀρκοελιουδιῶν; it should come as no surprise, then, to find at a short distance from the "monastery of the Oleasters," that of the "Virgin of the Spurges."[31] The specific choice of the plant name alludes to the therapeutic powers of the oil extracted from spurges, first described by Dioscorides (ca. 40–ca. 90 CE), and used in traditional pharmacopeias for its purgative and anti-asthmatic properties. Quickly—perhaps at the time of its foundation but certainly by 1145 at the latest—the monastery was associated with healing; the panels of St. Anastasia and the healing saints, in the narthex, like the dedicatory inscription of Nikephoros the veterinarian, attest to the salutary atmosphere that surrounded the foundation (Figs. 5.2, 5.19; discussion on pp. 83, 116–17).

Whatever the reasons that drew Nikolaos the ktetor to locate his religious foundation in the valley of Asinou, the monastery of the Panagia ton Phorbion attracted the devotions of Christians seeking to improve their physical and spiritual well-being. Popular tradition does not preserve

---

the eleventh and twelfth centuries); Englezakis, *Church of Cyprus*, 58–59; Papacostas, "Koutsovendis," 26, 30–32.

26. Herman, "Istituzioni monastiche bizantine," 361–63; Janin, "Monachisme byzantin," 34–36; Darrouzès, "Mouvement des fondations," 175; Konidaris, *Νομική θεωρήση*, 171–81; Thomas, *Private Religious Foundations*, 214–43; *BMFD*, 4: nos. 41–44.

27. Even if burying women in male monasteries was prohibited by law, exceptions appear beginning in the 11th century, when typika of members of the imperial family or *archontes* assert a right of burial for all members of the family. Konidaris, *Νομική θεωρήση*, 119–25; Talbot, "Family and the Monastery," 124.

28. On the obituary of 1145, see Darrouzès, "Notes [1]," 94; Constantinides and Browning, *Dated Greek Manuscripts*, 51. I exclude a reference to the monastery's name that appears in Leontios's obituary, placed opposite the entry for 21 December 66[..]; the year was completed by Darrouzès ("Notes [1]," 86, with a typographical error) as 1118/19, but thirteen alternative dates might be advanced. Constantinides and Browning, *Dated Greek Manuscripts*, 51. The inscription in the lunette of the narthex door will be examined in a forthcoming publication.

29. Stylianou and Stylianou, "Παναγία Φορβιώτισσα Ασίνου," 151; Klerides, *Χωριά καὶ πολιτείες*, 175; Sacopoulo, *Asinou en 1106*, 13–14; Frigerio-Zeniou, "Μονὴ τῶν Φορβίων," 192. It bears mentioning that G. Buckler derived the name from that of the duke of Cyprus, Constantine Euphorbenos Katakalon (Buxton et al., "Church of Asinou," 346–49), but this hypothesis was rebutted by Sacopoulo, *Asinou en 1106*, 13–16, and more recently by Georgiou, "Περί του κτίτορος," 192–97.

30. See Nicolaïdès, "Étude iconographique," 110 n. 978.

31. This etymology is accepted by the Stylianous, Klerides (see the preceding note), and Papageorgiou, "Η Μονὴ Ἀψινθιωτίσσης," 73.

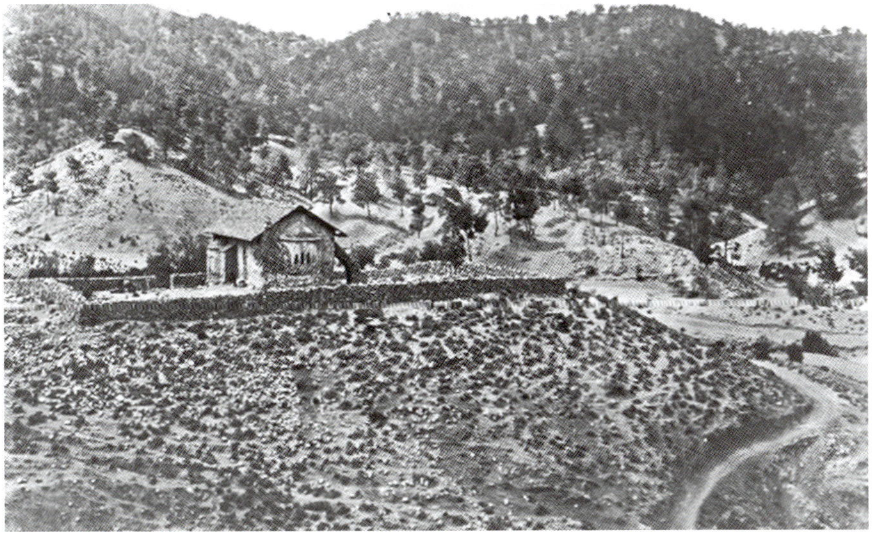

FIG. 1.5
Photograph of the site of the church of Panagia Phorbiotissa in the early 1940s (Department of Antiquities, Nicosia, no. B 86290)

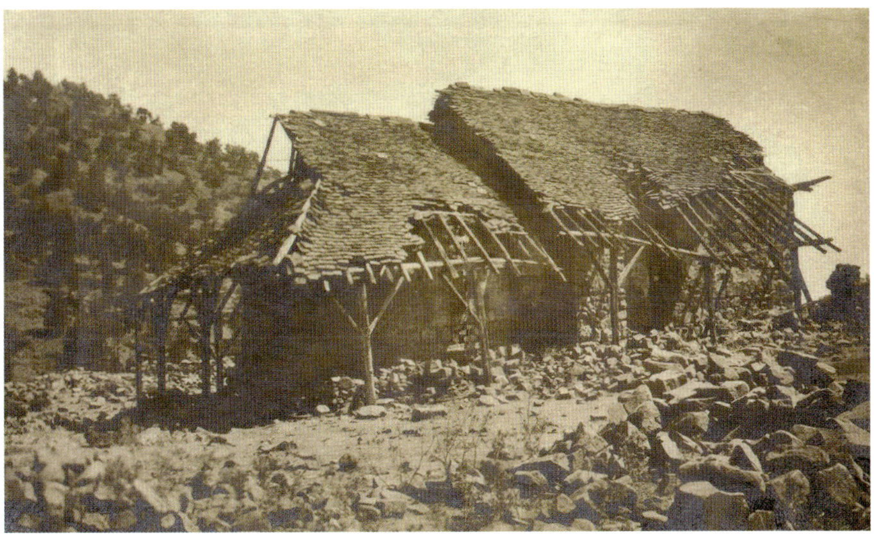

FIG. 1.6
Photograph of the church of Panagia Phorbiotissa in 1909 (Nicosia, State Archives of Cyprus, SA 1:767/1919)

the memory of a sacred spring (ἁγίασμα),[32] and the marginalia of Paris. gr. 1590 make no mention of a hospice (ξενών) for pilgrims or the infirm.[33] The leveling of the monastic complex, moreover, has made it impossible to grasp the scope of its buildings, their arrangement, or their functions. Photographs taken in the 1940s (Fig. 1.5) show sizable clusters of stones around the church, the last traces of monastic buildings whose ground plans were never recorded.[34] Other indications of the original state are suggested by a photograph from 1909 that shows the church with a shingled roof, with extensive losses that reveal the wooden girders, rafters, and columns supporting it (Fig. 1.6), similar to those that still surround the

32. Peristianes's monograph does not mention it, nor do the residents of Nikitari recall such a tradition, as Father Kyriakos has confirmed. Conversation of 5 July 2000, for which I thank him.

33. The meagerness of these data contrasts with the extensive information provided by the typikon of the monastery of St. John Chrysostom. Papacostas, "Koutsovendis," 32.

34. George Jeffery noted in 1908, "around the church are traces of the usual monastery, but now level with the ground." State Archives of Cyprus, SA 1:161/08, no. 14.

church of the Panagia Arakiotissa at Lagoudera. It is not known whether the monastery was endowed with significant relics when it was founded, unlike that of St. John Chrysostom, where relics of holy martyrs' bodies were laid at the end of the eleventh century;[35] no relics cache or receptacle has been preserved in the sanctuary of the church of the Panagia ton Phorbion, and the site does not figure among Leontios Machairas's popular pilgrimage destinations.[36] To be sure, the modest church of the present day no longer evokes its larger setting, which comprised several buildings, drawing the faithful to venerate the Virgin, healing saints, or other saints of the Orthodox Church, in the hope of intercession for their salvation, on earth as in heaven.

The Byzantine Period

During the twelfth century, the monastery developed at a pace that corresponds to the deaths of those who had been affiliated with the institution. Gephyra, spouse or daughter of Nikephoros the magistros, died on 17 December 1106, soon after the completion of the church's decoration;[37] her unusual name has suggested to some scholars a Semitic provenance that is difficult to corroborate, given the possibility that errors might have been introduced when the inscription was copied in the fourteenth century. Gephyra, a name undocumented in Byzantine sources, might be associated with Safira, a mysterious praenomen that appears in the lists of villagers in the region of Asinou and Marathassa drawn up during the sixteenth century.[38] The name's origins and its relationship with the Near East (or, in contrast, with local tradition) are potentially rich areas of research for understanding the cultural environment of Nikephoros the magistros. One yearns for evidence of Gephyra's burial within the church, for her relation to the donor would have warranted it.[39]

The marginal notes in Paris. gr. 1590 record the later deaths of hegumens: Demetrios on 12 December 1121; Dometios on Wednesday, 5 December 1145; and Leontios on Sunday, 21 December 66[..];[40] the deaths of three monks are also mentioned: Euphrosynos, on Thursday, 1 November 1173;[41] Sophronios Petraseon on 8 October 1188;[42] and Theodoulos, on 18 September of an unknown year.[43] Was the narthex built to accommodate their tombs

35. Mango and Hawkins, "Field Work in Istanbul and Cyprus," 334; Papacostas, "Koutsovendis," 32, 43.
36. Leontios Machairas, *Χρονικό της Κύπρου,* 82–88. Machairas's testimony may contain lacunae: to cite one example, he does not mention the relics at the monastery of St. John Chrysostom at Koutsovendis.
37. Generally given as 15 December 1099 (see Sacopoulo, *Asinou*, 10–11), the date of Gephyra's death was corrected by Cyril Mango, "Chypre, carrefour," 7 n. 14. The 14th-century painter undoubtedly introduced an error in copying the inscription, associating the year 6608 with indiction 15, whereas indiction 15 corresponds to 6615 (1 September 1106/31 August 1107), and indiction 7 to the year 6608. The corrected text of the inscription appears in Papacostas, "Byzantine Cyprus," 2:95. See also below, p. 54.
38. Mango, "Chypre, carrefour," 7 n. 14, was the first to deduce the Semitic origin of "Gephyra." On the frequency of Safira as a praenomen in the 16th century, see Archivio di Stato di Venezia, Consiglio dei Dieci, *Dispacci di rettori,* b. 288, c. 80 (*pratico* of the village of Kato Koutrafas, 1512); Imhaus, "Document démographique et fiscal," 384 and passim (nearly forty-five occurrences, including women of all ages). The comparative frequency of the name "Safira" might also confirm the suspicion that errors were introduced in transcribing the dates of the dedicatory inscription when it was copied in the 14th century.
39. Emmanouelides, *Δίκαιο της ταφής,* 200–201, cites numerous examples of family tombs in monasteries, mainly in Constantinople.
40. Demetrios: 12 December 6630, indiction 15; Dometios: 5 December, 665[4], indiction 9. Darrouzès, "Notes [1]," 94; Constantinides and Browning, *Dated Greek Manuscripts,* 51. On Leontios, see the discussion above, note 28, regarding the difficulties in completing the date.
41. Darrouzès, "Notes [1]," 92, correctly completes the date as 1 November 6682, indiction 7; it is given, without explanation, as 1 November 1171 by Constantinides and Browning, *Dated Greek Manuscripts,* 51.
42. Date: 8 October 6697, indiction 9: Darrouzès, "Notes [1]," 92; Constantinides and Browning, *Dated Greek Manuscripts,* 51–52, associate the year 6697 with indiction 7.
43. Darrouzès, "Notes [1]," 92; Constantinides and Browning, *Dated Greek Manuscripts,* 52.

and those of other monks?[44] Its construction provided additional space to bury members of the community, but the extent of burials in the church or the narthex remains exceedingly difficult to gauge, since no traces of a cemetery or ossuary have been found in the environs.[45]

Neither the church's inscriptions nor the marginalia of Paris. gr. 1590 shed light on the monastery's relations with the island's ecclesiastical hierarchy. The fact that prelates' names are not mentioned might be construed as an indication of the monastery's independence from formal lines of authority, although there is no certain basis for that conclusion. The manuscript contains references to St. Sabas in quatrains below the obituaries of the hegumens Leontios and Dometios.[46] Do they indicate a spiritual kinship with or an institutional dependence on the Palestinian lavra of St. Sabas?[47] The latter hypothesis seems rather speculative, even if the possibility of relations with Palestine remains an open question. Several facts suggest such ties: the allusions to St. Sabas, the Semitic praenomen Gephyra, and the provenance of the synaxarion, elements of whose paleography resemble those of Laurentianus San Marco 787, copied at the monastery τοῦ Καλαμίου—undoubtedly Kalamon in Judea—in 1049/50, before its transfer to Cyprus a century later.[48] At the same time, clear evidence is lacking, and no argument can unequivocally settle the question. The monastery of the Panagia ton Phorbion could easily have had contacts with foundations in Palestine; contacts between Cyprus and the continent were frequent before and during the Crusades. Manuscripts made their way across the sea, and several monasteries (among them, those of St. John Chrysostom and Our Lady of Machairas) were founded by monks from Syria-Palestine.[49] At present, however, the role of kyr Nikolaos's foundation in the context of these exchanges cannot be ascertained.

The monastery's financial resources during the first century of its existence are likewise a matter for speculation. The patronage of the powerful made possible both the monastery's construction and the church's decoration, calling in talented artists who used costly pigments (lapis lazuli, gold, silver, and cinnabar) to paint its frescoes and icons.[50] The same patronage would account for the monastery's acquisition of the synaxarion Paris. gr. 1590, copied in Cyprus or Palestine in 1062/63.[51] The gift would surely have included other manuscripts—if nothing else, a synaxarion for the months from March to August—but the fact that no other manuscript owned by the monastery has survived might suggest that it was not well endowed.[52]

44. Peristianes, *Μονογραφία,* 8, notes that two tombs in the narthex were looted in the 1870s.
45. On the use of narthexes as monastic cemeteries, see the examples cited by Emmanouilidès, *Δίκαιο της ταφής,* 199–200, as well as those cited below by Kalopissi-Verti, p. 207. On the Asinou narthex see below, pp. 54, 56–57, and 93–95.
46. The inscription is given in its entirety by Constantinides and Browning, *Dated Greek Manuscripts,* 51.
47. Richard, "Monastère grec de Palestine," 2:66, maintains that the monastery at Asinou was a *metochion* of St. Sabas, a claim based on no solid evidence and rightly questioned by Papacostas, "Byzantine Cyprus," 2:70.
48. Darrouzès, "Notes [1]," 85–86; idem, "Autres manuscrits," 132–33, 144–45; Constantinides and Browning, *Dated Greek Manuscripts,* 49–50; Gamillscheg, "Zypern oder nicht Zypern?" 240; Papacostas, "Byzantine Cyprus," 2:70.
49. Darrouzès, "Autres manuscrits," 132–33; Englezakis, *Church of Cyprus,* 6, 94–95; Papacostas, "Koutsovendis," 29–50.
50. On the pigments, see Chapter 7. A single icon dating to the 12th century survives, that of St. John the Baptist. Hadjichristodoulou and Myrianthefs, *Ναός,* 42, 44–45; Papageorgiou, *Icons of Cyprus,* 12 and no. 6; Sophocleous, *Icons of Cyprus,* 77 and no. 5. See also n. 86 below. The high aesthetic quality of the doors of sculpted wood, now lost, is noteworthy; these might be the original doors. G. Soteriou, *Βυζαντινὰ μνημεῖα,* pl. 142 A (detail drawn by Th. Mogabgab), pl. 142 B.
51. Regarding the manuscript's Palestinian / Cypriot provenance, see Delehaye, *Synaxarium,* cols. xx–xxii; Darrouzès, "Notes [1]," 85–86; Constantinides and Browning, *Dated Greek Manuscripts,* 49–50.
52. This conclusion warrants some caution for two reasons: on the one hand, the inventory of 1773 mentions the presence of a gospel (see p. 34 below); on the other,

Soon thereafter, the monastery seems to have stagnated, as Jean Darrouzès observed.[53] While the obituaries in the marginal notes name three hegumens, there is no mention of the presence of *oikonomoi* or other officials at the monastery. Even bearing in mind that other manuscripts may have been lost, what data we have on the size of the community suggest that it was rather small. The most plausible hypothesis regarding the foundation's assets is that they consisted of the land that forms the valley of Asinou, although it is uncertain whether the rural settlement preceded the foundation. In either case, had the endowment been limited to land immediately adjacent to the monastery, it could not have supported a community of significant size. Nonetheless, revenues derived from diverse rents, together with a regular flow of donations, might have sustained some ambitious undertakings, notably the construction of the narthex, for which stone was brought in from other parts of the island (p. 57). Ultimately, however, both the extent and the composition of the monastery's assets are quite beyond our reckoning.

The Frankish Period

The change of political regime that followed the capture of Cyprus by Richard the Lionheart in May and June 1191 did not call into question the existence or the status of Byzantine monastic foundations.[54] As did all the Greek monasteries of the Lusignan kingdom, with the sole exception of Stavrovouni, the activities of the monastery of the Panagia ton Phorbion continued under the Byzantine rite. When the naos was restored during the fourteenth century, the paintings commemorating the foundation of Nikephoros Ischyrios the magistros were copied—a sign of respect for the earlier provisions. The monastery continued to function as it had, and the faithful still came to offer their devotions, whatever their confession, as attested by the variety of portraits painted in the narthex at the end of the thirteenth century and during the course of the fourteenth.[55]

This institutional permanence, based on respect for custom, masks changes that documentary evidence strives to clarify. The main question remains: Could the private foundation survive in adhering to the provisions of the *ketorikon typikon*? In the case of a family foundation, the continued presence of a descendant at the head of the foundation is unlikely, as much for political reasons (the family might have left Cyprus after 1191) as biological ones: lineages beyond six or seven generations are rare during the medieval period.[56] After 1220, moreover, the foundation would have been under the dual control of the Latin Church and Frankish political authority, which oversaw the recruitment of monks, as much to limit the influence of Greek monasticism in the kingdom as to stave off the flight of serfs into monasteries.[57] The Bulla Cypria of 1260 moderated these constraints by reinstating the authority of Orthodox bishops over monasteries on the condition that the hegumens swear an oath of fealty to the Latin Church; at the same time, novitiation remained subject to the approval of either the fief's master or the king.[58]

The effects of these new disciplinary constraints on daily life in the monastery of the Panagia ton Phorbion are difficult to grasp. The community of monks, apparently considerably

---

the recent discovery of an inventory of thirty books at the church of St. John the Baptist in Argaki, a village 20 km north of Asinou, proves that, in 1363, small establishments could own substantial libraries. Couroupou and Géhin, "Nouveaux documents chypriotes," 147–64.

53. Darrouzès, "Notes [1]," 85.

54. On the high regard for Byzantine religious foundations in the kingdom of Cyprus, see Richard, "Monastère grec," 65–74; Schabel, "Religion," 184–90.

55. See below, pp. 179–90.

56. The exodus of archontes' families is reported by Neophytos the Recluse: Galatariotou, *Making of a Saint,* 201–3.

57. Coureas and Schabel, *Cartulary*, nos. 82–86; Papadopoullos, "Ἐκκλησία Κύπρου," 4:558–62; Coureas, *Latin Church in Cyprus*, 259–74; Schabel, "Religion," 190–92.

58. This concern informs Byzantine legislation from the beginnings of monasticism in the 4th century onward. See Konidaris, *Νομική θεωρήση*, 77–79.

diminished over the course of the Byzantine period, seems scarcely to have grown thereafter, if we can rely on the evidence provided by the necrology of Paris. gr. 1590: twelve monks' names are inscribed there for the period extending from the thirteenth to the fifteenth century. Moreover, the community would have needed to resolve the problem of its spiritual direction; logically, the monks would have participated in the election of their superior, an election subject to the approval of the bishop of Soli (Nicosia), but none of the notes in Paris. gr. 1590 names a hegumen, and the portraits in the narthex do not include those of the community's superiors.

The paradox of this omission is clarified by other marginalia, the series of portraits in the narthex, and the inscription above the lintel of the door that leads from the narthex to the naos, dated 1332/33. Despite its lacunae, the inscription describes the restoration of the paintings in the monastery at the behest of Theophilos and a group of laypersons (κοινὸς λαός, Figs. 3.11, 5.37; transcription on p. 176). It is evident, on the basis of this reference, that Theophilos was a member of the monastic community; this makes it possible to identify him with the portrait of Theophilos the monk above the lintel in the narthex. The narthex contains a total of twelve donor portraits, including those of seven monks (Barnabas, Theophilos, Germanos, Laurentios, Baylas, Leontios, and Kallinikos) and five laypersons: two men (Georgios and Basilios Drako[cheres]) and three women (Anastasia Saramalina, Anna Lachana, and the Latin lady); these portraits belong to the campaign of 1332–33 with the exception of those of Anastasia Saramalina and the Frankish female donor, depicted with her two sons in the apse, which date from an earlier program of decoration.[59]

None of these names appears in the synaxarion's necrology,[60] although the obituaries confirm the evidence of the frescoes in documenting the participation of both secular clerics and laypersons in the life of the institution. This process is illustrated by the notices recording the deaths of some ten individuals outside the community. In two instances, the subjects are relatives of monks: on 13 October of an unknown year, the deacon Gregorios died, "του πασχαλι του στραβοννικολα (μον)αχ(οῦ)";[61] Leon Romopoulos, brother of the monk Theodoulos, died in an unknown year on 17 January.[62] No other obituary defines the relationship between the deceased and the monastery. The deaths were undoubtedly recorded after the donations were conveyed to the monastery, but perhaps before the construction of a tomb in or near the church. Nonetheless, no donation of property is explicitly described as such, a striking contrast with the marginal notes in two other manuscripts used in Cypriot monasteries, Paris. gr. 280 and 1588, in which even the most modest gifts are carefully recorded.[63]

Among the dead recorded in the synaxarion of the Panagia ton Phorbion are three secular clerics: kyr priest Leontios του κουφα[...], nomikos of Zotokatokopia (undoubtedly the present-day village of Katokopia) on 31 August 1318;[64] Leontios, priest τοῦ νομικοῦ, who practiced in the diocese of Soli, on 23 November 1320;[65] and Michael, son of the former and an active *hierodiakonos* in the same

59. Regarding these inscriptions, see below, pp. 179–90.

60. The sole instance of a possible identity between one of the donors depicted in the narthex and an obit in the synaxarion is that of the layman Georgios and Geo[rgios] Koutrapheotes, who died on 22 December of an unrecorded year. Darrouzès, "Notes [1]," 94; Constantinides and Browning, *Dated Greek Manuscripts*, 53.

61. Darrouzès, "Notes [1]," 92; Constantinides and Browning, *Dated Greek Manuscripts*, 52.

62. Darrouzès, "Notes [1]," 95; Constantinides and Browning, *Dated Greek Manuscripts*, 53.

63. Darrouzès, "Obituaire chypriote"; idem, "Notes [3]," 223–25, 227–40.

64. Precise date: 31 August [6]826: Darrouzès, "Notes [1]," 95; Constantinides and Browning, *Dated Greek Manuscripts*, 52 (with a typographical error in the Julian year).

65. Precise date: 23 November [6]829: Darrouzès, "Notes [1]," 93; Constantinides and Browning, *Dated Greek Manuscripts*, 52.

district as his father, on 27 November 1320.[66] The accord in the dates, the juridical functions of the two Leontioses, and the references to the diocese of Soli suggest that the ecclesiastical hierarchy's control of the monastery was effected through priests or notaries from the environs of Asinou during a period only slightly predating the restoration of the paintings. We cannot infer from this evidence, however, that these priests acted as stewards of the monastery's property (*epitropoi*); but if the foundation document stipulated the institution's complete independence, the monastery would surely have found itself in a difficult position because of the application of the Bulla Cypria, which placed all monasteries under the authority of the Orthodox hierarchy. Another note in the synaxarion, written in an early fourteenth-century hand, confirms the continuity of the liturgical and juridical-legal framework: the account of a ceremony held on 13 September, the eve of the feast of the Exaltation of the Holy Cross, contains acclamations of the ecumenical patriarch, the basileus, the bishop of the diocese, the primate, the hegumen (or archpriest), and the Orthodox Christian people.[67] These invocations might well attest to a formal liturgical tradition during the Byzantine period, but in the context of the Lusignan kingdom, they implied a respect for precedent.

Beyond the canonical obligations governing its relations with ecclesiastical authorities, the monastery of the Panagia ton Phorbion saw its influence broadcast by the development of practices of Byzantine origin. An undated note placed opposite the entry for 4 February of an unrecorded year attributes the quality of "συναδελφος ημ(ων)" to the monk Nikolaos Voioannes and promises him prayers, as it does to the nun Xaine, "συντροφη(αν) αυτ(ου)."[68] One might conclude from this that Nikolaos Voioannes (the patronym is documented in the Troodos Mountains as late as 1549),[69] had married Xaine; both took religious orders, he in the monastery of the Panagia ton Phorbion, she undoubtedly in another establishment. Nikolaos Voioannes was connected to the monastery by a form of affiliation derived from the Byzantine *adelphaton*, better documented at the monastery of the Priests (in the region of Paphos) during the first half of the fourteenth century, and later at the church of the Panagia Polyeleotissa in the Marathassa Valley.[70]

The isolated reference to an adelphaton, undoubtedly from the fourteenth century, does not lend itself to firm conclusions about the character of this affiliation or how it functioned in the monastery at Asinou. The Byzantine adelphaton, attested from the middle of the eleventh century onward and common practice in the larger monasteries of the empire by the fourteenth century, took the form of a contract under which a donor granted an institution a sum of money or property; in exchange, the monastery agreed to pay the donor a fixed annuity and to admit him into the community at the end of his life, with his dependents, should he wish to take holy orders.[71] In Cyprus this type of affiliation is more amply documented with respect to the sanctuary of the Panagia Polyeleotissa between 1393 and 1431, where the "ἀδελφᾶτον" was obtained on the same day that the faithful made their gifts, in cash or in kind, to the church, "διὰ ψυχικὴν ὀφαίλαιαν"; in exchange, the donor or members of his family (or both) were granted the benefit of prayers or commemorative masses. None of the marginal notes explicitly specifies that the

66. Precise date: 27 November [6]829: Darrouzès, "Notes [1]," 94; Constantinides and Browning, *Dated Greek Manuscripts,* 52.
67. Darrouzès, "Notes [1]," 86; Constantinides and Browning, *Dated Greek Manuscripts,* 53.
68. Darrouzès, "Notes [1]," 95; Constantinides and Browning, *Dated Greek Manuscripts,* 53.

69. Imhaus, "Document démographique et fiscal," 396–98, 401, 409, 416, 418, 508 (at the village of San Zuan de Rames), 420 (at Prodromos), 422–23 (at Ano Plati), 467 (at Treis Elies).
70. See the notes published by Darrouzès, "Obituaire chypriote," 25–62, and "Notes [3]," 227–40; Grivaud, *Grecs et Francs*, 290–91, 312.
71. Herman, "Regelung der Armut," 444–50; Evangelatou-Notara, "ΑΔΕΛΦΑΤΟΝ ΨΥΧΙΚΟΝ"; Smyrlis, *Fortune des grands monastères*, 138–45.

synadelphos would receive an annuity or an entitlement to a tomb in the sanctuary in exchange; on the other hand, nothing defines the obligations incumbent on the *synadelphoi* with regard to participation in other forms of collective devotion.[72]

Nor does the presence of a single "συνάδελφος" at the monastery of the Panagia ton Phorbion prove that all the laity mentioned in the obituaries or that all the donors depicted in the narthex held this status. Nonetheless, the participation of secular clerics and the laity in the life of the monastery seems a given; an open question is whether they participated in the monastery's administration, in the form of a standing committee composed of ordinary and secular clergy and laypersons, empowered to administer the monastery's property. The patronyms of the secular clergy and the laity affiliated with the monastery all attest to their local origins; in addition to the two priests or notaries and the deacon mentioned above, along with Nikolaos Voioannes, an obituary refers to a villager from Kato Koutraphas (Georgios Koutraphiotes). Finally, it seems opportune to draw a connection between the patronym of Anastasia Saramalina, a donor depicted in the narthex, and the toponym Cαραμάλι in the neighboring valley of Xyliatos.[73] Clearly the sanctuary drew its audience on a local level; none of the chronicles, Greek or Frankish, of the kingdom of Lusignan mentions its name. Neither Leontios Machairas nor Étienne de Lusignan includes it in his lists of pilgrimage centers.[74] Bereft of significant relics, the monastery of the Panagia ton Phorbion could not compete with the great island sanctuaries, although the portrait of Anna Lachana might belie this assertion, if she is related to the Nestorian family of Famagusta.[75]

The known assets of the monastery were, by the same token, limited to properties within the region. A note records a violent tornado on 16 July 1319 that destroyed grain and barley harvests left on the threshing grounds. The monastery's land at Katokopia, planted with flax, was left to dry out, and the harvest of five "*misadia*" sold at the village of Filia brought in a mere hundred *nomismata*.[76] In the absence of records documenting donations by the faithful to the monastery, one might presume that the property of the monks would not have amounted to more than a few cultivated parcels of land. From this perspective, the hypothesis that the monastery bred horses, based on the analysis of inscriptions (see below, pp. 83, 184–85) and of the clothing of several donors depicted in the narthex, is plausible, since the village of Asinou, tucked away as it is, would have had the requisite pasturage for grazing.[77] Nonetheless, one should not be too quick to draw conclusions, since no source from the Frankish period mentions the practice of horse breeding outside of the king's stables.[78]

Bearing in mind that a lack of data frustrates any attempt to determine the extent of the monastery's landholdings, it seems unlikely that monks would have owned the valley and village of Asinou, since Byzantine foundations under Frankish dominion rarely had assets comprising entire villages.

72. Darrouzès, "Notes [3]," 227–40; for examples consistent with these at the monastery of the Priests, see idem, "Obituaire chypriote," 25–62; Evangelatou-Notara, "ΑΔΕΛΦΑΤΟΝ ΨΥΧΙΚΟΝ," 166–70.

73. Christodoulou and Constantinidis, *Complete Gazetteer of Cyprus*, s. v. (WD.03.76); this is the sole instance of this toponym in Cyprus.

74. Machairas, *Χρονικό της Κύπρου,* 81–88; Étienne de Lusignan, *Description de toute l'isle de Chypre*, 37r–v, 64r–65r.

75. Machairas (*Χρονικό της Κύπρου,* 112–15) documents the Nestorian Lacha family (λαχανεστούρεις) at Famagusta during the years 1360–70.

76. Darrouzès, "Notes [1]," 92; Constantinides and Browning, *Dated Greek Manuscripts,* 50.

77. Frigerio-Zeniou, "Μονὴ τῶν Φορβίων," 192–93.

78. Because of their military function, horses were always subject to stringent control by officers of the royal constabulary. For the limited information available on the royal stables, see Machairas, *Χρονικό της Κύπρου,* 357 (Peter I owned two hundred horses), or, with respect to accounting documents, Grivaud, "État des comptes," 399. The control on horses appears in juridical literature, which emphasizes the practice of *restor*. Greilsammer, *Le livre au Roi*, chap. 49; John of Ibelin, *Le Livre des Assises*, chap. 223, 584–87.

Valuations of the holdings of religious institutions at the beginning of the sixteenth century document only two monasteries—that of St. George of Mangana and the abbey of Apsinthiotissa—receiving ground rents from villages; other foundations would have derived their revenues from scattered properties, as did the church of the Virgin of Kykkos.[79] Archives dating to the period of Frankish rule provide no information whatsoever on the settlement of Asinou; on that basis, one might reasonably conclude that the valley and any hamlets therein constituted part of the fiefdom of Nikitari. As a result, its lords would have owned the land and the monastery de jure and consequently would have been entitled to name the community's superior.[80] In most cases, it would have been sufficient for the lord to ratify the monks' selection, and the Byzantine foundation would have kept to its rules without his intervention. From this perspective, the portrait of the Frankish female donor with her two sons (Fig. 5.1) might indicate the veneration of a local cult by a family of Frankish lords, extending even to their choosing the monastery as their resting place. By way of comparison, it is noteworthy that during the fourteenth and fifteenth centuries, the monastery of the Priests surrounded itself with Frankish, Greek, or Armenian protectors by means of the synadelphoi. Perrin, the son of the "lady" of Lapithos, was apparently buried there in 1400.[81]

Manifestations of Latin devotion to Greek sanctuaries should come as no surprise given the number of examples among the churches of the Troodos Mountains. Later, under the reign of John II (1432–58), the leap from private devotion to official protection was made when the king placed two serfs conscripted from hamlets in the Troodos Mountains at the "abaie d'Asnie." This measure—a benefit granted to other Greek monasteries as well—illustrates the religious politics of the Lusignan kings, eager to defend the Cypriot cults by offering them material aid, demonstrated in the provision of servile labor during a period when manpower was scarce. On 2 March 1440, John II authorized the count of Jaffa, Jacques de Fleury, to buy back, for the sum of four hundred *besants*, the two serfs that he had loaned to the abbey.[82] The archival documents do not specify whether the king replaced the serfs, or whether the monastery derived additional benefit from regular gifts from the royal treasury, its status closer to that of an institution answerable to a *ius patronato*.[83]

This royal protection, documented at a late stage in the monastery's history, does not mask the likely loss of patronage by those wielding power and influence after 1191.[84] Founded by kyr Nikolaos, the Byzantine monastery relied on charity during the Frankish period. These donations would have been sufficient to shore up the church, perhaps after the violent earthquake of 8 August 1303, which shook the island's center region.[85] Donations made it possible to repaint the narthex and a portion of the naos, around 1332/33, but they seem to have been the result of a coalescence of "popular" initiatives, undoubtedly through the associations—confraternities, perhaps—that brought the laity together. It is difficult, however, to attribute to such an undertaking the commissioning of several fine icons, painted probably in the fourteenth century, whose association with the church (where they were housed until 1974) is not clearly understood at present.[86]

79. Mas-Latrie, *Histoire de l'île de Chypre*, 3:503–4; Grivaud, "Monastère de Kykkos."
80. Pursuant to rules established under the agreements of 1222. Coureas and Schabel, *Cartulary*, no. 95; Schabel, *Synodicum Nicosiense*, 294; Richard, "Monastère grec," 72–73.
81. Darrouzès, "Un obituaire chypriote," 28–29.
82. Richard, *Documents chypriotes*, 146–47.
83. Grivaud, *Grecs et Francs,* 286–95.
84. It was a source of concern to Neophytos the Recluse: Galatariotou, *Making of a Saint,* 175–76.
85. Schreiner, *Byzantinischen Kleinchroniken*, 1:203; Constantinides and Browning, *Dated Greek Manuscripts,* 161. Earlier earthquakes might have damaged the structure. Grivaud, *Villages désertés à Chypre*, 431; see also below, pp. 64–65.
86. When these icons were given remains unknown, as does their function, insofar as the church's small templon could not have accommodated them. These

Other changes might have informed daily life in the institution. Three fourteenth-century obituaries of female religious figures raise several questions.[87] Are they notes recorded by a priest officiating on behalf of convents in the region? Or might one conclude that the Byzantine foundation had been transformed into a double monastery, enlarged with an annex for nuns, situated near the original buildings (and within the enclosure of the monastery at the nearby Μονὴ τῶν Ἀρκοελιουδιῶν)? Surprising though it is, this situation arose during the same period in Constantinople and Crete, despite regularly repeated prohibitions mandating the separation of the sexes within foundations.[88] One might infer that the monastery at Asinou grew through the construction of new buildings, perhaps funded by the generosity of the three female donors depicted in the narthex.[89] In the century following, this female presence is no longer evident, but the only information of substance for the period concerns the death of the hieromonk Neophytos on 8 November 1452.[90] During this time the church and the narthex seem to have been used regularly for funerals, as attested by graffiti on the frames of the northern and southern doors of the church bearing the dates 1446 and 1450 (Figs. 6.31, 6.33).[91] The faithful were laid to rest at the monastery of the Virgin of Asinou, as they were at other Cypriot monasteries,[92] but if juridical and disciplinary prohibitions were respected, only Christians adhering to the Greek rite could be buried in an Orthodox monastery.[93]

During the period of Frankish rule, it is difficult to trace the history of the foundation with all the detail needed to capture the complexity of an institution and a religious life in which the faithful often challenged rules laid down by the ecclesiastical hierarchy. At the same time, a noteworthy aspect endures: that of a popular devotion to the monastery that drew in people from the environs of Asinou, people who might equally have favored the monasteries of the Morphou Basin or the valleys of the Troodos Mountains (St. Mamas, St. John the Baptist at Argaki, St. Nicholas of the Roof [τῆς Στέγης], and Lagoudera, to name but a few). Despite this competition, the little monastery dedicated to the Virgin at Asinou did attract the faithful, for reasons that we can only guess at. The desire for a place to bury and to commemorate

are reproduced in color in Hadjichristodoulou and Myrianthefs, *Ναός,* 44–45. In addition to the thirteen icons associated with Asinou listed in ibid., 41–45, one can add the icon of the Mother of God dated 1638 cited on p. 33 below; a fifteenth-century icon of St. John the Baptist now in the church of the Baptist in Nikitari; and bema doors of about 1680 and a number of other late seventeenth-century icons that Rupert Gunnis reported seeing in the same church (*Historic Cyprus,* 354).

87. Obituary of the nun Anthouse, Saturday, 23 November [6]907/1398. Without indication of the year, but inscribed in a 14th-century hand: obits of the nun Euphemia (20 October) and the nun Marina Teroukina (7 January); Darrouzès, "Notes [1]," 92, 95; Constantinides and Browning, *Dated Greek Manuscripts,* 52, 53. Darrouzès's hypothesis, accepted by Constantinides and Browning, on the Frankish origin of Marina Teroukina (the feminine form of the patronym De Rocca) is unconvincing; the de la Roche family, the titulary of the count of Karpase, is rendered "τε Λα Ρότζε" by Machairas, *Χρονικό της Κύπρου,* 136; no mention of the Italian eponym Roccia or Rocca, moreover, appears in known Frankish or Italian sources, nor in the genealogical literature.

88. Janin, "Monachisme byzantin," 42–44; Konidaris, *Νομική θεωρήση,* 121–25.

89. See below, p. 367.

90. Darrouzès, "Notes [1]," 92; Constantinides and Browning, *Dated Greek Manuscripts,* 52.

91. Winfield, *Asinou: A Guide,* 20.

92. Regarding burials inside monastery churches, one might take as an example the unpublished report of surveys carried out in the katholikon of St. Mamas of Morphou by A. H. S. Megaw in 1958. Department of Antiquities, file 46/5, 45–65. For other explicit evidence regarding the burial of laypersons at the entrance to the porch of the church (called "monastery" in 1393) of the Panagia Polyeleotissa, see Darrouzès, "Notes [3]," 228, 238, 240.

93. The difficulties in obtaining dispensations for burial in churches of a different rite are mentioned in the case of individuals belonging to social elites: Rudt de Collenberg, "Les premiers Podocataro," 130–82.

the dead, conditioned on donations, is a trait common to all the faiths of the medieval kingdoms, whether Greek or Frankish. It cannot have been a decisive factor in the daily life of the monastery of the Panagia ton Phorbion, which fulfilled the same funerary functions as other religious institutions on the island.

The monastery's distinction seems to have been its status as the main sanctuary dedicated to the Virgin in the region of the Morphou Basin. The votive panel of the Frankish lady with her two sons at the foot of the Virgin of Mercy (Fig. 5.1) illustrates the powerful attraction of a cult that, at the end of the thirteenth century, drew believers who adhered to different rites; certainly we might also look to Marian devotion as the motive for the commissioning the icon of the Panagia "Kykkotissa" currently housed in the Byzantine Museum of Nicosia.[94] In drawing closer to "Greek" forms of devotion, the Franks thus challenged the prohibitions imposed by the hierarchy of the Church of Rome; in 1368 both the archbishop of Nicosia and King Peter I deplored women of the Latin rite patronizing Greek or schismatic churches.[95] The veneration of the Cross, observed at several churches of the Troodos Mountains, represents another of these cults, although we do not know whether it was particular to the monastery.[96] The account of the ceremony of 13 September mentioned above attests to widespread attendance by the faithful, who answered the invocations of the dignitaries with a response; afterward the congregation entered the church, offered their devotions to the Holy Wood, and chanted *stichera*.[97] The text does not describe the sacred object toward which their devotions were directed; but it was not likely a fragment of the True Cross, if the lists of Leontios Machairas and Étienne de Lusignan are reliable.[98] It seems more plausible that the ceremony's focus was the panel in the naos in which SS. Helena and Constantine flank the Cross (Figs. 2.19, 6.15), although the possibility of a local tradition founded on another relic cannot be excluded, since the 1773 inventory of the monastery's property (see below) mentions the presence of a relic of the Cross from the church τοῦ Πυργάτη (at Kakopetria). Moreover, the chapel of the Cross, situated above the monastery, might have played a role unknown to us today. One important component of the devotion to the monastery of the Panagia Phorbiotissa was the healing environment associated with the sanctuary's name, corroborated by the votive panel of Anastasia Saramalina accompanied by her patron saint. These similarities between Christian cults, Greek and Latin, attest to the fact that the monastery at Asinou followed the mainstream of the kingdom's religious life, especially after 1291, when the Lusignan rulers transformed their kingdom into an outpost of militant Christianity, ostensibly gathering relics and miracle-working icons rescued from sanctuaries in countries under Muslim domination.[99]

The Venetian Period

The extinction of the Lusignans in 1474 and the island's annexation in Venice's *dominio del mar* did not significantly change daily life in the monastery. Eager to preserve the social and religious equilibriums it had inherited, Venice maintained the institutions of the past,[100] and the monastery, it stands to reason, was spared the prospect of new obstacles in its relations with ecclesiastical or temporal hierarchies.

Daily life in the monastery would have been minimally affected by improvements in living conditions, both demographic and economic, evident in all regions of the island between the end of the fifteenth century and 1570. No campaign to restore

94. Papageorghiou, *Icons of Cyprus* [1992], pl. 35, dated to the 13th century; Carr, "Art," 298–99 and fig. 8, dated to the last quarter of the 13th century.

95. Coureas and Schabel, *Cartulary*, no. 131; Schabel, *Synodicum Nicosiense*, X, no. 60.

96. Connor, "Female Saints," 215.

97. Darrouzès, "Notes [1]," 86; Constantinides and Browning, *Dated Greek Manuscripts*, 53.

98. Machairas, *Χρονικό της Κύπρου*, 88; de Lusignan, *Description*, 61r, 64r–65r.

99. Grivaud, *Grecs et Francs*, 323–39.

100. Arbel, "Κύπρος ὑπὸ ἐνετικὴ κυριαρχία," 4:460–66.

the paintings was undertaken—not, at least, on the ambitious scale of that of 1332/33; no donor portrait was added to those of preceding periods, although two panels were painted on the northern wall of the naos, representing saints Symeon Stylites and Onouphrios, and the panel of St. Nikephoros was repainted (Fig. 6.20).[101] The marginal notes of Paris. gr. 1590, for their part, are silent on the monastery's activities during the sixteenth century, as are any Venetian archives.

This meager evidence suggests that the monastery barely continued to survive, especially when its resources are compared with those of several churches in nearby valleys, monastic or otherwise, graced by new embellishments during the course of the sixteenth century: the monastery of the Panagia Podithou and the churches of the Archangel and St. Sozomenos in Galata; the "Latin" chapel of St. John Lampadistes at Kalopanayiotis; and the monastery of the Panagia Kourdaliotissa.[102] On that evidence, might one conclude that new centers of devotion—in particular, those dedicated to the Virgin—competed with the cult of the Panagia Phorbiotissa? That the patronage of the powerful was directed toward foundations better able to satisfy their spiritual needs? These questions do not elicit unequivocal answers, but all evidence suggests that the monasteries associated with Byzantine foundations struggled to draw the faithful and to reap the gifts on which their survival depended. The appeals filed in the 1550s by the hegumens of St. Nicholas of the Roof, the Virgin of Kykkos, and the Virgin of Elikon show that the meagerness of these institutions' assets compelled them to seek tax relief, as charity of sorts, from the Venetian senate.[103] Only the monastery of St. John Lampadistes sailed through the centuries, endowed with new decorations or the addition of a side chapel; its prosperity would explain the renown of its patron saint, clearly attested from the fourteenth through the sixteenth century.[104]

While evidence regarding the monastery of the Panagia Phorbiotissa is even sketchier during the Venetian period of the sixteenth century than it is in prior or subsequent centuries (another curious paradox), the foundation of kyr Nikolaos would probably have needed to address the fact that the faithful were redirecting their charity toward new sanctuaries. Given the present state of documentary evidence, however, this question, like that of the monastery's assets, remains unanswered. The only evidence, albeit indirect, which might suggest the possibility that the monastic community enjoyed some measure of prosperity derives from the significant number of male peasants eligible to bear arms at "casale Assinu" in 1565 (see above). Whether or not these peasants were dependents of the monastery, they would surely have cultivated land, pastured their flocks, or perhaps worked in the tannery, the winepress, or the mill at the bottom of the valley. In the absence of archaeological evidence, however, caution remains the byword in determining how the monastery fared when Venice controlled the island.

The Ottoman Period

Physically isolated from areas of battle, the religious foundation did not suffer materially during the war that took place during the summer of 1570. The monastery's situation, moreover, seems to have been entirely unexceptional when Ottoman officers undertook the 1572 census (*tahrir*), which provides the earliest substantive information on the monastery and its property.[105] Unexpectedly, the register overlooks one settlement in the valley, suggesting that the serfs counted in 1565 did not fall under the jurisdiction of the village of Asinou this time,

101. Winfield, *Asinou: A Guide*, 13, and personal communication with A. W. Carr on their revised dating.
102. Stylianou and Stylianou, *Painted Churches*, 84–96, 141–50, 312–20; Frigiero-Zenou, *L'art "italo-byzantin,"* 9–203.
103. Ploumides, "Έγγραφα"; Grivaud, "Monastère de Kykkos."
104. Machairas, *Χρονικό της Κύπρου*, 85–86; de Lusignan, *Description*, 58v.
105. Ankara, Tapu ve Kadastro Müdürlüğü Arşivleri, *Kuyudu kadime*, no. 506/64, 57.

but elsewhere—probably Nikitari, since the 1572 register suggests that the serf population there was substantially larger than it had been in 1565.[106] This could be attributable either to tabulation errors by Venetian officers or to the difficulty of determining which jurisdiction held sway over those populations that earned their livelihood from the rural economy.

The tahrir of 1572 does not enumerate the monks residing in the monastery ("Manāstır-i Āsīnū"), combining all data under a single entry—that of the institution's fiscal revenues, determined on the basis of a universal tax that combined the milling rights, the customary tax on sheep, one-fifth of the grain harvest, and other revenues.[107] The tax equaled 315 aspers, from which one may deduce the monastery's revenues at approximately 1,500 aspers. No taxes directed specifically at Christians were imposed on the monastery, pursuant to the exemption for clerics,[108] whereas Nikitari's twenty-seven heads of household and three unmarried males paid 900 aspers pursuant to the land tax assessed on Christians (*ispence*); thus, the total tax bill of the monastery of Asinou constitutes barely 14 percent of the taxes collected from Nikitari (2,304 aspers).[109] There is no question that the foundation of the Panagia Phorbiotissa was not wealthy, either in land or in revenues; that, at best, its revenues met the needs of a community of four or five monks; and that the institution remained dependent on contributions from the faithful for the maintenance or restoration of its buildings.

The monastery's poverty once again forced the community to seek the protection of the ecclesiastical hierarchy, certainly after 1585, when, pursuant to Selim II's decree of 1565, Cyprus was obligated to buy back its monasteries.[110] At the end of the century, the foundation of the Panagia Phorbiotissa was surely in the same straits as other small institutions facing the hopeless task of finding independent means to repurchase their land and buildings so as to acquire the rights inherent in assets of pious foundations (*waqf*s). Until the 1630s, letters and deputations of Cypriot clergymen to the princes of Russia and Moldavia-Wallachia increased, more often than not at the instigation of archbishops seeking charitable donations.[111] It is in this context that we must understand the list of fifteen names, placed under those of Archbishop Christodoulos (1606–1640) and Makarios, from Soli, that encircle the chalice of Christ Emmanuel in the niche carved out in the bema's southern wall (Fig. 1.7).[112]

This patronage, granted between 1620 and 1630, made it possible for the monastery of the Panagia Phorbiotissa to remain solvent. Thus, the church was given a portable icon depicting the Virgin, described in 1922 by Hieronymos Peristianes: the Virgin, facing front, holds the Christ Child in her left hand and gazes at him. A sculpted and gilded nimbus, decorated with flowers carved in relief, surrounds her face; her robe is rendered in black and gilded lines. An inscription at the foot of the icon names her Panagia Eleousa and records the dedication:

> Δέησις τοῦ δούλου τοῦ Θεοῦ Μελετίου Ἱερομονάχου καὶ τοῦ δούλου τοῦ Θεοῦ Μανουὴλ Ἀναγνώστου.

On the back, traces of an older icon of Helena and Constantine are visible, with another two-line

106. For Nikitari, two *francomati* are enumerated in 1565, corresponding to a single family; the 1572 census records twenty-seven heads of households and three unmarried males. Grivaud, *Villages désertés à Chypre,* 469; Ankara, Tapu ve Kadastro Müdürlüğü Arşivleri, *Kuyudu kadime,* no. 506/64, 57.

107. Ankara, loc. cit.: "ḳısm mine-l-hums ʿan ḥubūbāt ve resm-i āsyāb ve ʿādet-i āġnām ve sāʾir maḥṣūlāt." I am grateful to Elias Kolovos for the transcription and translation.

108. Jennings, *Christians and Muslims,* 154–55.

109. Ankara, loc. cit.

110. For the broader context, see Fotić, "Official Explanations." For Cyprus in particular, see Archimandrite Kyprianos, *Ἱστορία χρονολογική,* 458; Chasiotes, *Ισπανικά έγγραφα,* 22; Theocharides, *Οθωμανικά έγγραφα,* vol. 1 (1572–1719): nos. 7, 10–12; Grivaud, *Villages désertés à Chypre,* 391–92.

111. Englezakis, *Church of Cyprus,* 223–27.

112. Winfield, *Asinou: A Guide,* 13.

inscription at the base, partly erased, completing the preceding dedication:

> [. . . . .] + [.]᾿Ιλυ ἱστορογραφήθισαν αἱ παροῦσαι σο[υ] ᾿Ικόνες [24 letters missing] προστασίᾳ [. . . . . .] διὰ [ἐξό]δου καὶ πόθου τοῦ δούλου τοῦ Θεοῦ Μελετίου Ἱερομονάχου καὶ Ἡγουμένου τῆς Σεβασμίας Μονῆς ταύτης καὶ [οἱ] ἀγαπόντες τὸν εὔ[χεσθε ὑπὲρ αὐτοῦ].

In 1935, Georgios Soteriou, who published the icon (as Panagia Hodegetria), noted the same date that Peristianes had: 1638 (,ΑΧΛΗʹ).[113]

The intercession of the ecclesiastical hierarchy thus apparently reenergized the monastery during the first third of the seventeenth century. In 1638, the community was under the direction of the hegumen Meletios, seconded by the *anagnostes* (lector) Manuel. Finally, it is noteworthy that an icon of St. John Lampadistes, which may have been placed in the iconostasis that had been installed in the prior century,[114] revived the old Byzantine foundation in associating it with the cult of a widely popular saint from Kalopanayiotis. An inventory of the property of the Panagia Phorbiotissa taken in 1773 records the presence of the saint's relics, but whether they were laid in the 1630s or earlier (when the saint's icon was placed in the iconostasis) remains unknown; nonetheless these data, viewed collectively, suggest that, after a sluggish period, the monastery saw a renewal of activity, the result of a revival of cults organized with the prelates' consent. The monastery's deference to the jurisdiction of the Cypriot Church is verified by the transfer of Paris. gr. 1590 to Archbishop Nikephoros (r. 1641–1674); soon thereafter, the manuscript left the island, having been sold to antiquaries acting on behalf of the

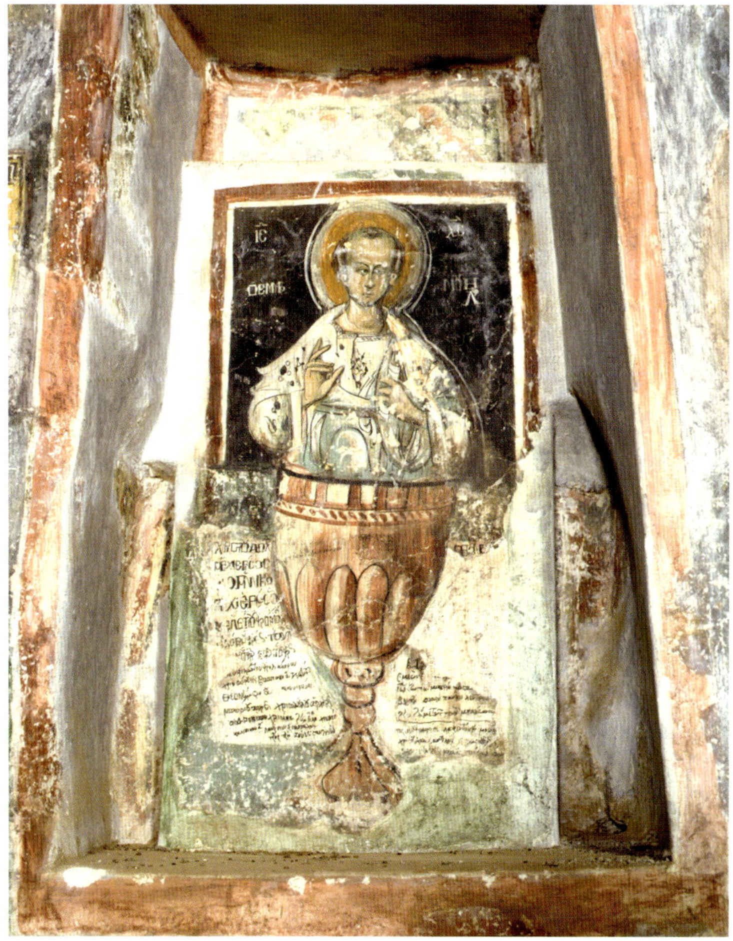

FIG. 1.7 Image of Christ in a chalice, with the signatures of Archbishop Christodoulos and others. Painted originally on the reinforcing masonry on the south side of the apse, the image was detached in 1953, when the masonry was removed, and was moved to the niche on the south side of the bema (photo courtesy of the Leventis Foundation and the Archaeological Research Unit, University of Cyprus, no. 006257)

113. Peristianes, *Μονογραφία,* 7; Soteriou, *Βυζαντινὰ μνημεῖα,* pl. 123B.
114. For the icon, see Hadjichristodoulou and Myrianthefs, *Ναός,* 41 and unnumbered figure on 45, and in Soteriou, *Βυζαντινὰ μνημεῖα,* fig. 120b. On the sixteenth-century iconostasis see Hadjichristodoulou and Myrianthefs, *Church*, 41.

comte de Colbert; in 1736 the synaxarion entered the French royal collections.[115]

The small victories that made possible the monastery's survival during the first century of Ottoman domination slowly evaporated, for the foundation, like many small rural institutions, was slipping into decline. The Ukrainian monk Basil Barsky, who made an extended visit to Cypriot holy places between 1734 and 1736, did not stop at Asinou; the name itself was unknown to him.[116] Barsky's silence points to the monastery's weak presence in Cypriot society during the first half of the eighteenth century.[117] Nonetheless, the monastery continued to find a source of patronage in more powerful institutions. In 1765 the hegumen of Kykkos donated two icons, which were placed in the church: one depicts Christ, the other a Virgin and Child in a Veneto-Byzantine style, according to Rupert Gunnis.[118] In accepting gifts from a monastery that had become particularly influential in Cyprus during the Ottoman period, the monastery of the Panagia Phorbiotissa undoubtedly sought to remain solvent, hoping for little from its own meager assets.

The records of the bishopric of Kyrenia—inaccessible since 1974—in fact contain valuable information on the monastery's property in 1773. Among the sacred objects listed there are the relics of the body of St. John Lampadistes, a cross from the church τοῦ Πυργάτη (at Kakopetria), and a gospel decorated with a scene of the crucifixion. An oil mill was operated in the monastery, in which nine *pithoi* were stored; the landholdings comprised 175 *skales* (approximately forty-four hectares): eighty surrounding the monastery and forty opposite the houses (ἀντίπερα τῶν ὀσπητιῶν), with the remainder consisting of eighteen small scattered lots. Its property included seventy-eight olive trees (including thirty-five surrounding the monastery), four vineyards at Kakopetria, a flock of fifty goats, a pair of mules, and a pair of oxen. Finally, at Nikitari, a *metochion* of eight houses was associated with the monastery, which produced oil and halloumi.[119]

As in the Middle Ages, the landholdings were concentrated in the nearby region of Asinou, both in the valley and the environs of Nikitari, with the exception of the vineyards at Kakopetria. On the surface, it seems a meager endowment, producing oil and cheese; there is no mention whatsoever of grain harvests or of hides; at this point, apparently, neither the mill nor the tannery was operating. The property, moreover, was widely dispersed, since in all likelihood it had been donated by peasants in the region. Once again, the monastery faced the problem of its financial survival. Its spiritual influence was renewed by relics borrowed from the neighboring valleys of Marathassa and Solia, but the foundation's decline in the last third of the eighteenth century seems to have been inexorable.

The monastery collapsed at the turn of the century. In 1788, Archimandrite Kyprianos mentions it among the eleven monasteries that were under the jurisdiction of the metropolitan of Kyrenia, but by 1825 the name no longer appears in the bishopric's registers.[120] This extinction was not sudden, as local traditions would have us believe, for it was the consequence of a slow transformation

115. Darrouzès, "Notes [1]," 94; Constantinides and Browning, *Dated Greek Manuscripts,* 53–54. One might hazard a guess that the manuscript was purchased by Athanasios the rhetor in 1643 or by Johannes Wansleben in 1671: Omont, *Missions archéologiques*, 1:14–15, 65, 78–80.

116. In the list of monasteries that he did not visit, Barsky names "ἡ Ἀμιρή," which the account's modern editor identifies with Asinou. *Barsky's Travels in Cyprus*, 101. In fact, as Papageorgiou has noted, the reference is to the monastery of the Panagia "τῆς Ἀμιροῦς": see "Αμιροὺς Παναγίας μοναστήρι."

117. This is not proof of the monastery's extinction, as noted by Klerides, *25 μοναστήρια στὴν Κύπρο*, 2:84.

118. According to a local tradition, the two icons were stolen by a Turkish woman who, seized with remorse, subsequently left them at the church of the Transfiguration at Petra, where they remained during the 1930s. Gunnis, *Historic Cyprus*, 379–80.

119. Kyriazes, *Τὰ μοναστήρια ἐν Κύπρῳ*, 110.

120. Archimandrite Kyprianos, *Ἱστορία χρονολογική*, 585; Kokkinoftas and Theocharides, "Μοναστηριακά δεδομένα."

of the rural economy following a long demographic decline. Many villages and monasteries were stricken from maps in the course of the eighteenth century.[121] The extinction of the foundation of the Panagia Phorbiotissa had already been looming for many years, for the institution's survival was due to the generosity and financial backing of the island's powerbrokers. Larger institutions displaced smaller ones as centers of pilgrimage; during the Ottoman period, Kykkos became one of the main sanctuaries dedicated to the Virgin, undoubtedly siphoning off the faithful who earlier had offered their devotions to the Panagia Phorbiotissa.

The Historic Monument in the Monastery's Shadow

After the closing of the monastery of Asinou, the estates and the buildings, under the control of the metropolitan of Kyrenia, quickly fell into ruin; only the church managed to survive on the proceeds from a few olive trees leased to peasants from Nikitari. The church, known as Asinou, appears in the *Tahrīr Emlāk* of 1867 as number 7918; in 1875 the *Emlāk Yoklama* records its landed property, consisting of six olive trees cultivated by Hadji Yacoumi on the church's behalf.[122] A contract dated 21 August 1909 records that the church's twenty-five olive trees were leased in exchange for sixty-eight *okes* of oil during the years 1909–12 (seventeen okes annually) to a group of five villagers from Nikitari (Christodoulos Hadji Solomou, Haralambo Christodoulou, Ioanni Apostoli, Christothea Franzi, and Myrophora Kypri).[123] With the extinction of the monastery, what little remained of the church's endowment was insufficient to maintain it. By July 1879, Mondry Baudouin and Edmond Potter noted that, despite the high quality of the paintings that remained visible, the monument was entirely in ruins.[124] Once again the funds necessary to restore the church had to be raised; numerous appeals to the British authorities were made before the work was finally undertaken.

The monument's rediscovery seems to be due to Major Tankerville J. Chamberlayne and the architect George Jeffery, who, starting in 1907, called it to the attention of the Museum Council. On 30 October of that year, Chamberlayne presented three photographs of the church (now lost) in support of the request of Nikitari's inhabitants that the roof be restored; the metropolitan of Kyrenia offered funds for that purpose on the condition that the government provide, at no cost, the necessary timber and qualified personnel to supervise the work.[125] Jeffery lent his support to the request, after a visit in early 1908, when he confirmed that the church was in stable condition despite the holes in the roof and recommended that it be repaired, the roof tiles replaced, and the lattice of decaying and useless wood removed (see Fig. 1.6).[126]

The failure of these early reports to elicit a response from the Museum Council's management prompted a new petition by the *muhtar* of Nikitari, Costi Hadji Haralambo, on 23 May 1912; the muhtar's correspondence mentions that M. A. Carletti had drawn up a plan of the church, which, owned by the metropolitan of Kyrenia, was falling into ruin. Donations collected on the occasion of the church's feast day, each Easter Tuesday, totaled a mere five to ten pounds, although between fifty and a hundred people attended the services. Over the course of three or four years, the individual in charge of the church, Christodoulos Hadji Solomou, raised no more than thirty pounds.[127] Without the intervention of public authorities, the church was in danger of collapse.

121. Grivaud, *Villages désertés à Chypre,* 416–19.
122. State Archives of Cyprus, SA 1:767/19, no. 7.
123. Ibid., no. 6 (contract prepared by Chariton Ierodiakonos).
124. École française d'Athènes, Archives, *Chypre I*, 1, 49.
125. State Archives of Cyprus, SA 1: 3591/07. Cf. below, p. 36, and n. 130.
126. Ibid., SA 1:161/08, no. 14.
127. Ibid., SA 1:767/19, no. 6.

Some time elapsed before these initiatives led to action. On 13 May 1919, A. K. Bovill, principal forest officer, documenting his findings with photographs, reported that the roof of Asinou's church was by now nearly destroyed. Informed of this, the bishop of Kyrenia announced that he was prepared to underwrite the costs, while Bovill offered the requisite timber on condition that the government provide a master carpenter.[128] A few days later, on 18 May, Jeffery, expressing disappointment that the recommendations he had presented in 1907 had come to naught, reiterated his proposals for the restoration, and requested that the church be classified as an "ancient monument," as he had earlier proposed.[129] A decision finally came in 1922, leading to the complete restoration of the church's roof and the removal of its structural supports. The monument was now restored, ready to be studied by historians, among the earliest of whom were Hieronymos Peristianes in 1922 and, ten years later, W. H. Buckler. Thanks to their studies, the monument gained growing renown among Byzantine art historians.[130]

Although isolated from any settlement, the church did not entirely lose its liturgical functions. In 1932 it continued to attract pilgrims who came to pray at the church; a few feast days were celebrated there, but the altar's condition suggests that the Divine Liturgy was rarely held.[131] In 1949, the parish priest for Nikitari, Anastasios Savvas, was appointed the church's guardian by the metropolitan of Kyrenia; in his capacity as the church's *ephemerios*, he maintained its property, which at the end of the 1950s consisted of a few almond trees.[132] During more than thirty years, he celebrated five Divine Liturgies annually. In addition to celebrating the Feast of the Virgin, he bestowed blessings (baptism, betrothal, and marriage) on Cypriots attracted by the monument's beauty and welcomed pilgrims and tourists.[133]

Meanwhile, several significant events increased the renown of the church of Asinou toward the end of the twentieth century. The restoration of the paintings under the aegis of Dumbarton Oaks, coinciding with the Republic of Cyprus's independence in 1960, returned the monument to its rightful place in the history of Byzantine art. After northern Cyprus was occupied by the Turkish army in the summer of 1974, access to numerous pilgrimage sites was barred, and the church at Asinou reaped the benefit of the redirection of pilgrimage sites southward. A decade later, in 1985, it was inscribed on UNESCO's World Heritage List (see above, p. 1). In 1989, some twenty thousand pilgrims joined in the feast of the church, which started on Easter Sunday and ended on Easter Tuesday.[134] By the same token, the development of tourism led several agencies to include a stop at Asinou in their tour of the island. Today, large crowds flock to the little church, stirring up dust, brushing against the walls, and lighting tapers and oil lamps, thus endangering its frescoes.[135]

Nearly a thousand years after its founding, the church of the Panagia Phorbiotissa seems still in search of protectors, a curious leitmotif of its history.

128. Ibid., SA 1:767/19, nos. 1–2.
129. Ibid., SA 1:767/19, no. 1, indicating that Jeffery questioned the date of 1100, deeming the church's plan typical of late medieval (16th-century) churches.
130 For an account of the events from 1907 onward, but focused on the architectural history of Asinou, see below, pp. 65–66.
131. Buxton et al., "Church of Asinou," 328.
132. Department of Antiquities, Nicosia, file N2/5/2, nos. 4–5, 7.
133. Ibid., nos. 60, 99.
134. Letter from Chrysanthos, metropolitan of Morphou, dated 2 October 1989: Department of Antiquities, Nicosia, file N2/5/3, no. 51.
135. The crowds were a source of concern to the director of the department of antiquities, Vassos Karageorghis: Department of Antiquities, Nicosia, file N2/5/2, no. 155 (21 October 1985).

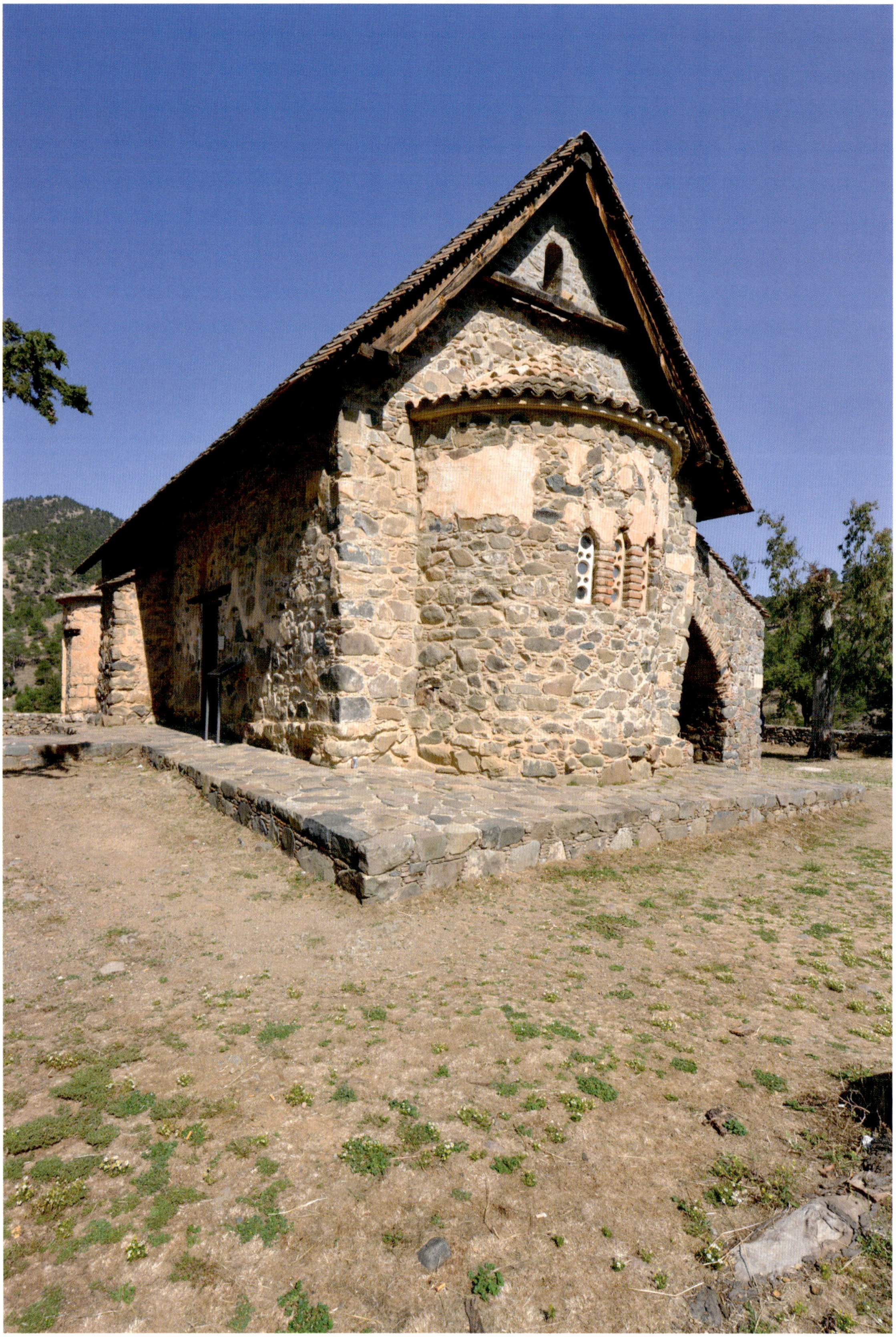

The church of Panagia Phorbiotissa, exterior from the east
(photo courtesy of G. L. Carr)

CHAPTER TWO

The Architecture of the Church of the Panagia Phorbiotissa

Athanasios Papageorgiou

The church of the Panagia at Asinou is the only remnant of the Monastery of the "Panagia ton Phorbion (τῶν Φορβίων)" or "Phorbiotissa." Evidence of the original monastery survives in the epithet of the Virgin, "Μ(ήτ)ηρ Θ(εο)ῦ ἡ Φορβιώτισσα," inscribed in the wall painting in the blind arch over the entrance to the naos from the narthex (the original west door of the church; Figs. 3.11, 5.37) and in the invocation accompanying the mural icon of St. George in the south apse of the narthex (Figs. 3.10, 4.1). This chapter is devoted to the architecture of the church: the background and development of its architectural type, the features of its fabric and construction, and its successive modifications over time (Intro. Fig. 3).

Architectural Typology of the Church of the Panagia at Asinou

The church building is a small rectangular hall with a stone vault and an apsidal end in the east side (Fig. 2.1). This simple architectural plan was already in use in Egypt, Syria, Mesopotamia, and Asia Minor in the fourth century CE. In Egypt, where several such chapels from the fourth to the seventh century still survive in the Monastery and Necropolis of Bawit,[1] the walls and vaults are built of mud brick. In Syria, single-aisled churches are not vaulted. Those in the south, largely dated to the fourth century by their inscriptions, have flat roofs constructed with stone slabs laid

1. Clédat, *Le monastère et la nécropole de Baouît* [1904], 13–14, Chapel III, rectangular hall without an apse, covered with a vault; 69, fig. 38, Chapel XVI, a rectangular hall of 4 × 4 m with a rectangular niche in the east wall; 73, Figs. 44–45, Chapel XVII, rectangle of 4.60 × 4.60 m covered with a blind dome; 87, fig. 49, chapel XVIII, 12.60 × 4.65 m covered with a vault; 133, fig. 61, Chapel XXVI, hall 3.60 × 3.60 m covered with a vault, with a rectangular niche in the southern half of the east wall; 153, fig. 64, Chapel XXVIII, a rectangular room 10.70 × 4.60 m separated by two engaged responds on the south and north walls into two equal parts. See also Clédat, *Le monastère et la nécropole* [1916], 1–4, pls. 1–17.

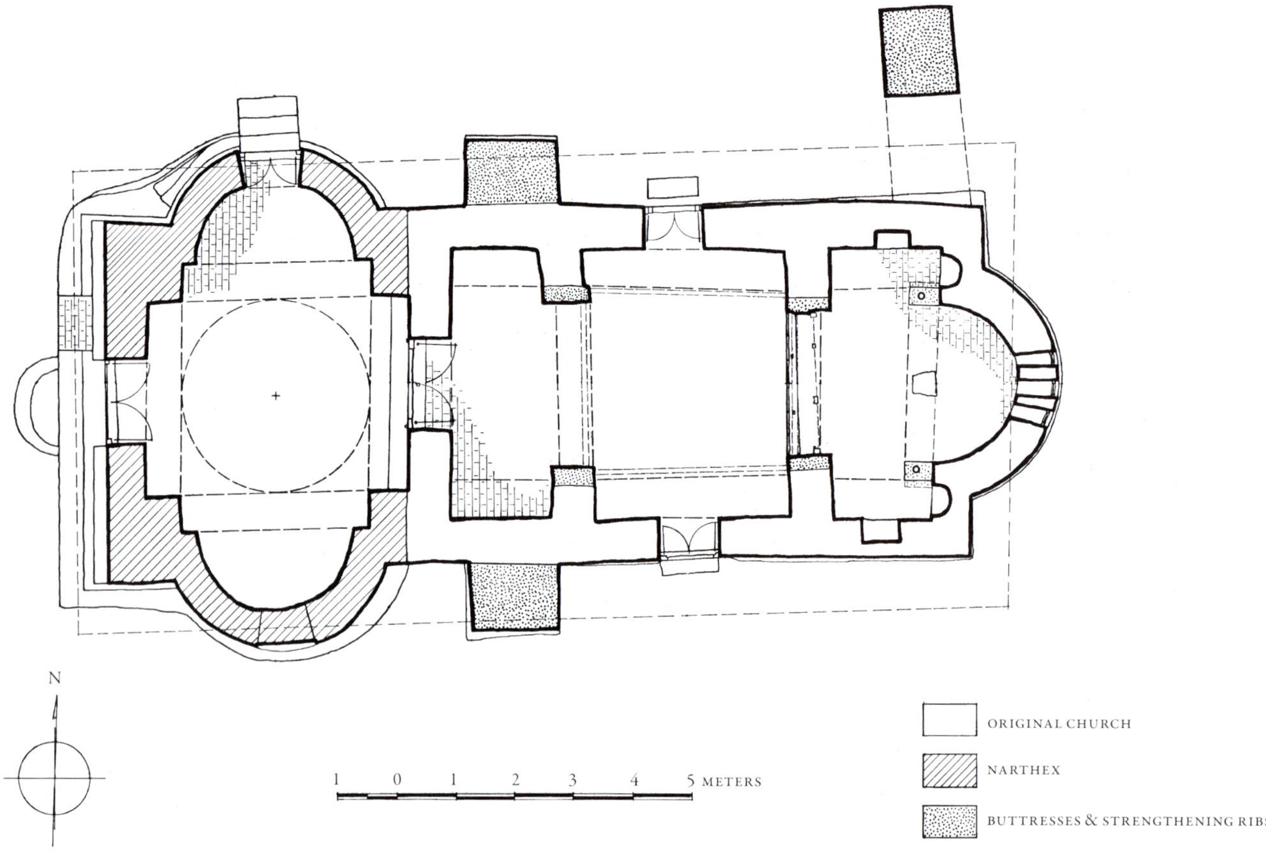

FIG. 2.1 Ground plan of the church of Asinou. Drawing by Richard Anderson, Dumbarton Oaks BF.F.1993. F0908

on transverse arches and covered with beaten clay.[2] Those in the north, on the other hand, are covered with wooden pitched roofs.[3] The walls of these churches were built with dressed stones and were richly decorated.[4]

In Mesopotamia, according to Richard Krautheimer, "Church buildings are known only from very few excavations, and none of the buildings can be safely dated. . . . They are, as a rule, longitudinal halls terminated by a tripartite sanctuary—a square chancel flanked by corresponding rooms, all three accessible from the nave through narrow doors. Supports, either low columns or piers, project from the side walls into the nave and form

2. Butler, *Early Churches in Syria*, 178. Butler classified these churches according to the number of transverse arches and the appearance of the sanctuary. Type A: the church at Anz near Shaqqa (19, ill. 12); the chapel inside the fortress of Deir al-Kahf (19–20, ill. 13). Type B: Umm el-Jimal, east church (21, ill. 16). The churches cited here are of the 4th century. Those of the 5th century differ principally in their proportions, being shorter and wider: e.g., Lubben, Agraina church of 417 CE (41, ill. 40), Umm el-Jimal (42, ill. 41–42).

3. Butler, *Early Churches*, 74.

4. Ibid., 74–77. Type A: Sergible (75, ill. 76), Banakfur (75, ill. 77). Type B: Srir (76, ill. 78), chapel of convent near Brad (76). Type C: Nuriye (76, ill. 79), Kfer in the Djebel al-Ala (76, ill. 80). Type D: Djebel Riha (77, ill. 81). For the single-aisle churches of northern Syria, see also Tchalenko, *Villages antiques de la Syrie*, 1: 325–39, 2: pls. 13–14, 193. The walls of these churches are built with rectangular stones and have rich, decorative carvings around the doors.

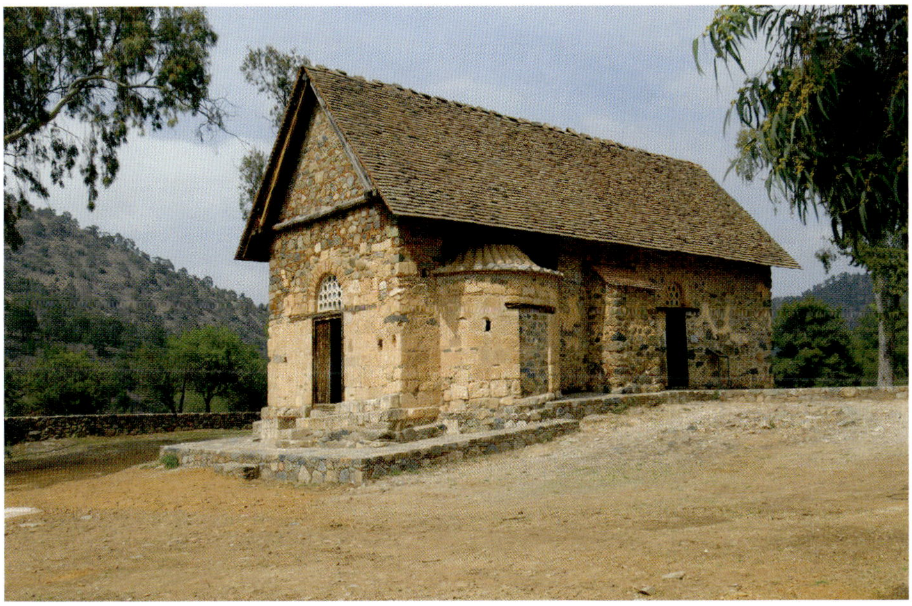

FIG. 2.2
Exterior, south side of the church of Asinou (photo courtesy of G. L. Carr)

a series of niches, covered by short transverse barrel-vaults."[5] In the Anatolian Plateau, several such churches were still standing in the early years of the twentieth century, but they have since been completely destroyed. Many of them were small vaulted chapels with an apse to the east and, sometimes, a narthex to the west. The apses and arches were usually horseshoe-shaped. Some were built with well-cut stones, but others were built with rubble.[6]

A large group of village churches, monastic churches, and martyria still survives in the Tur Abdin, some of them dated by inscription or other historical evidence. Because Tur Abdin is located between Mesopotamia (south), Syria (west), and the Anatolian Plateau (north), its architecture was influenced by that of these three provinces. The churches comprise a longitudinal barrel-vaulted hall with a stilted semicircular apse. The walls are built with small stones.[7]

The simple barrel-vaulted church is also found in Greece and on the Greek islands.[8] This style had

5. Krautheimer, *Early Christian and Byzantine Architecture*, 302.

6. Ramsay and Bell, *Thousand and One Churches*, 9: "The fact that so many doorways with their monolithic side-posts and lintels remain standing, while the walls have almost or quite disappeared, suggests that structures of which the doorways formed part were humble and unpretentious architecture." Chapel 17 has a horseshoe-shaped apse (145, fig. 110); arches in Chapel 36 were horseshoe-shaped (177); the apse of Chapel 46 is horseshoe-shaped (229, fig. 187); the vaults of the naos and narthex of the chapel at Sarigül to the east of Viran Sheher were horseshoe shaped (232, fig. 268). Other vaulted chapels are no. 26, 27, 28 (147); chapels at Asamadi (258, fig. 213), at Gelvere (324–39, fig. 352–53), at Yedi Kapulu (325–26, fig. 254, ground plan, 255, 257), at Ana Tepesi (332, fig. 260, ground plan, 261, 264), and at Sarigül (332, fig. 265, ground plan).

7. Krautheimer, *Early Christian and Byzantine Architecture*, 302.

8. Lasithiotakis, "Κυριαρχοῦντες τύποι χριστιανικῶν ναῶν"; Vocotopoulos, *Ἡ ἐκκλησιαστικὴ ἀρχιτεκτονική*, 105–6; Nikonanos, *Βυζαντινοὶ ναοὶ τῆς Θεσσαλίας*, 43–49, 86–90 (English summary, 177–90). In Drandakes, *Βυζαντινὲς τοιχογραφίες τῆς Μέσα Μάνης*, see St. Theodore at Tsopaka, 12th–13th c. (29, figs. 1–3); St. Petros at Palaichori, 10th c. (64, fig. on p. 66); St. John at Kaphiona, before 1300 (p. 69, fig. on p. 66); the SS. Theodore near Kaphiona of 1144/45 (72, fig. 3); St. George at Mina, 13th c. (133); St. Nicholas at Polemita, 14th c. (150); St. Prokopios near Episkope, 9th c. (22); St. Peter near Gardenitsa, 12th–13th c. (259, fig. on p. 260); Holy Anargyroi at Kepoula, 1265 (307–9, fig. on p. 308); St. Niketas at Kepoula, 10th c. (347, fig. on p. 341); St. George Kerias, 13th c. (354 ff.,

already appeared in Mani in the ninth to tenth century, and resurfaced somewhat later elsewhere. Single-aisle, barrel-vaulted churches also appeared in the Balkans and in south Italy.[9]

In Cyprus, single-aisle, wooden-roofed basilicas appeared at the end of the early Christian period. A small one was located near Alassa,[10] while a larger one was excavated at "Kalogeroi," near Germasogeia.[11] The current understanding of the single-aisle vaulted church of the seventh and eighth centuries is complicated by the violent disruptions of the Arab raids.[12] These occurred under Muʿawiya in 649[13] and 653–54;[14] under al-Walid II in 726 and 743;[15] under Marwan II in 747, when the Arab navy was destroyed in the port of Keramaia in Asia Minor,[16] again according to Theophanes in

fig. on p. 356); St. George at Kato Boularioi, 13th c. (362). In Bouras, Kalogeropoulou, and Andreade, *Εκκλησίες της Αττικής*, see the churches of St. Peter at Koropi (9–10, fig. 1), St. Athanasios at Koropi (11–12, fig. 3), St. Kyriake at Keratea, 12th–13th c. (93–95, fig. 14), St. Paraskeve at Panakto, 15th c. (?) (288–90, fig. 32, 2), Panagitsa at Villia, 14th–15th c. (291–92, fig. 34). Usually the small vaulted churches are not referred to, as in Demetrokalles, *Βυζαντινή ναοδομία στη Νάξο*, 42; or Pennas, *Η βυζαντινή Αίγινα*, who mentions only one church, the Omorphe Ekklesia (dedicated to the SS. Theodore), which was built at the end of the 12th century, while there are in fact several small vaulted chapels. See Moutsopoulos, *Ἡ Παληαχώρα τῆς Αἰγίνης*, 59–61, St. Barbara; 61–62, SS. Theodore; 63, St. Nicholas; 63–64, St. Eleutherios; 64, St. Nicholas; and others (65 ff and Figs. 14–45). It is clear that most authors dedicate few lines to these humble structures, like Gkioles, *Βυζαντινή ναοδομία*, 62–63. Bouras and Boura, *Η Ελλαδική ναοδομία*, mention only some of the vaulted chapels, e.g., Omorphe Ekklesia in Aigina (55–57, Figs. 34–35), St. John at Gardenitsa (102–3, Figs. 91–92), St. Peter at Gardenitsa (104–5), St. Nicholas Glezoy (Mani) (112–41, Figs. 107–9), etc. Bouras, *Βυζαντινή και μεταβυζαντινή αρχιτεκτονική*, writes only very briefly about the small vaulted chapels for a later period, e.g., St. John Chrysostom at Geraki (188, fig. 222).

9. On Bulgaria, see Mavrodinof, *L'église à nef unique* (not available to me); Mijatev, *Die mittelalterliche Baukunst in Bulgarien*, 19 and fig. 13 (Sofia), 111–13, figs. 133, 134 (two churches in Pliska), 168 and fig. 201 (church no. 4 in Trapazica, Tarnovo), and 184ff. He dates Sofia in the 4th–6th centuries and Trapazica in the 12th, but offers no dates for the remaining examples, some of which are wood roofed. On southern Italy, see Venditti, *Architettura bizantina nell'Italia meridionale*, 2: 850–52, Figs. 465–92. The examples he dates are 12th century; most of these churches are wood-roofed.

10. *ARDAC* for 1996, 48–49.

11. Hadjisavvas, "Chronique des fouilles … en 2001," 710.

12. Hill, *History of Cyprus*, 1:285–93; Chatzipsaltes, "Ἡ Κύπρος, τὸ Βυζάντιον καὶ τὸ Ἰσλάμ," 21ff.; idem, "Ἡ Κύπρος κατὰ τὸ δεύτερον ἥμισυ"; Dikigoropoulos, "Political Status of Cyprus"; Papageorgiou, "Les premières incursions Arabes à Chypre"; idem, "Μία σύγχρονη πηγή"; Kyrris, "Nature of the Arab-Byzantine Relations"; idem, "Ἡ Κύπρος, τὸ Βυζάντιον καὶ οἱ Ἄραβες"; Beihammer, "Audiatur et altera pars"; idem, "Zypern und die byzantinisch-arabische See-Politik vom 8. zu Beginn des 10. Jahrhunderts"; Oikonomakes, "Η Κύπρος και οι Άραβες"; Christides, *The Image of Cyprus*; Browning, "Ἡ Κύπρος καὶ οἱ Ἄραβες"; idem, "Byzantium and Islam in Cyprus."

13. It seems that only Salamis and its surrounding area were sacked in 649. The Arabs left Cyprus hurriedly because they were informed of the approach of the Byzantine fleet. That the first Arab raid was limited to the area of Salamis-Constantia is confirmed by the life of St. Therapon (*AASS*, Mai 6:684–85), and the inscription found during the excavation of the atrium of the basilica of Soloi: see Gagniers and Tinh, *Soloi: Dix campagnes des fouilles*, 115–25; Papageorgiou, "Μιὰ σύγχρονη πηγή," and the more complete publication of Papageorgiou, "Ἡ Ἐπισκοπὴ τῶν Σόλων," esp. 18–19. Thus neither the information of Theophanes that Muʿawiya, the head of the Arab forces, "has taken Constantia and the whole island and looted it" (Theophanes, *Chronographia*, ed. C. De Boor, 1:343) nor the information of the Arab sources that he signed a treaty with the Cypriots is correct. See Christides, *The Image of Cyprus*, 2, n. 44; Papageorgiou, "Les premières incursions Arabes"; and Browning, "Ἡ Κύπρος καὶ οἱ Ἄραβες" and "Byzantium and Islam."

14. In this raid Cyprus was completely sacked and conquered: see Baladhuri, *Kitab Futuh al-Buldan*, 209, who reports that the second Arab invasion of Cyprus was in the year 33 (2 August 653–21 July 654); Christides, *Image of Cyprus*, 21.

15. Theophanes, *Chronographia*, 417. He transferred many prisoners to Syria, who were returned to Cyprus in 750. See Christides, *Image of Cyprus,* 44.

16. Theophanes, *Chronographia*, 424; Paul the Deacon, "Historia Miscella," in PL 95:1095; Philippou,

773;[17] and under Harun al-Rashid in 790 and 805.[18] Our knowledge of this type of architecture is also limited by the destruction of the majestic wooden-roofed basilicas of Salamis, Paphos, Kourion, Amathous, Soloi, and Lapithos; by the displacements of population caused both by Emperor Justinian II's forcible settlement of many Cypriots, along with their archbishop John, in the area of Cyzicus in 691;[19] and by recurrent Arab deportation of prisoners.[20]

Two factors stand out. First, the early Arab raids clearly did not systematically devastate all churches. Thus, Theodore, bishop of Paphos, speaking in the church of Tremithous on the feast day of St. Spyridon, 14 December 655—in the presence of Sergios the archbishop of Cyprus, Paul the archbishop of Crete, Theodore the bishop of Tremithous, Theodore the bishop of Kition, and Eusebios the bishop of Lapithos—narrated a miracle of St. Spyridon that was depicted on the wall "above the middle gate, i.e., the main entrance to the church."[21] The two archbishops and the other bishops witnessed this old painting.[22] The church cited here was destroyed later in the eighth century and was replaced by another wooden-roofed basilica, which was subsequently rebuilt, again as a vaulted basilica, after it had been destroyed for a second time.[23]

Second, the displacements of population exposed Cypriots to the building types customary on the mainland. These movements included not only the deportation and eventual repatriation of Cypriots conscripted by Justinian II or taken prisoner in the Arab raids but also the movement of monastic figures to and from the mainland. Cypriot monks could be found in the famous monastic centers of Asia Minor, such as Latros.[24]

In turn, a movement of monks and nuns to Cyprus followed the imposition of Iconoclasm in the eighth century. Because of the treaty between Byzantium and the Arabs in 688,[25] Cyprus was outside the jurisdiction of the Byzantine emperors, and for this reason St. Stephen the Younger advised his disciples to seek refuge from Iconoclast persecution in Cyprus.[26] On the other hand, Lachanodrakon, general of the Thracesian theme, is said to have exiled thousands of iconophile religious to the

"Η ναυμαχία τῆς Κεραμαίας"; Christides, *Image of Cyprus,* 47–49.

17. Theophanes, *Chronographia*, 446; Christides, *Image of Cyprus,* 70.

18. Theophanes, *Chronographia*, 482; Makin, *Historia saracenica*, 152. Al-Tabari reports that he took 16,000 prisoners, as quoted in Brooks, "Byzantines and Arabs," 746.

19. Theophanes, *Chronographia*, 365; Michael the Syrian, *Chronique*, 2:470; Stratos, *Τὸ Βυζάντιο στὸν Ζ' αἰώνα*, 42, 69.

20. See preceding six notes. ʿAbd al-Malik reacted to Justinian II's deportation of Cypriots by raiding the island, taking many prisoners, and transferring them to Syria. See Papageorgiou, "Η Κύπρος κατὰ τοὺς βυζαντινοὺς χρόνους," 44; Christides, *Image of Cyprus*, 42–43.

21. Ven, *La Légende de S. Spyridon*, 88–89: "Τούτου δὲ τοῦ παραδόξου θαύματος μνημόσυνόν ἐστιν ἔτι καὶ νῦν ἐν τῇ πόλει τοῦ σεβασμίου πατρὸς Τριμιθοῦντι ἐπάνω τοῦ μέσου πυλεῶνος ἤγουν τῆς ἀρχοντικῆς θύρας τοῦ ναοῦ ἔνθα κεῖται τὸ τίμιον λείψανον τοῦ ἁγίου πατρὸς ἡμῶν Σπυρίδωνος, εἰκὼν πᾶσαν τὴν διήγησιν ταύτην γεγραμμένην ἔχουσα μετὰ καὶ ἄλλων τινῶν τῶν μὴ γεγραμμένων ἐνταῦθα."

22. Ibid., 90.

23. Papageorgiou, "Ἔρευνα ἐν τῷ ναῷ τοῦ Ἁγίου Σπυρίδωνος."

24. The best known were George of Cyprus, who lived in a monastery at Latros after his condemnation by the Iconoclastic Synod of 754, and Paul, the patriarch of Constantinople, who advised the empress Eirene to convene the Second Ecumenical Council of Nicaea in 787. See Mitsides, *Ἡ παρουσία τῆς Ἐκκλησίας τῆς Κύπρου*, 55ff. on George and 52–54 on Paul.

25. Theophanes, *Chronographia*, 363. Cyprus was also included in the treaty, which was signed by Justinian II and the Caliph ʿAbd al-Malik. Theophanes gives no details about Cyprus except that it was to remain neutral between the two powers and was to pay equal taxes to both. Further terms emerge from other sources: see Papageorgiou, "Η Κύπρος κατὰ τοὺς βυζαντινοὺς χρόνους," 43–44; Christides, *Image of Cyprus*, 34–37.

26. Auzépy, *La vie d'Etienne le Jeune*, 125 §28, 219–20; "Vita Stephani Junioris," in PG 100:117.

island on the orders of Constantine V.[27] The Vita of St. Romanos the Neomartyr (11 May 780) confirms such exile: "In his [Abbasid caliph Mahdi's] first year they carried off to him five other monks, who had been taken captive on Cyprus. Three of them were from Amorium but two from other places. They had been consigned to Cyprus by the iconoclastic emperor Constantine."[28]

The eighth century, in sum, was a period of upheaval and fermentation for the population of Cyprus, which had been diminished by slaughter and captivity. But at the same time, this population was augmented by immigrants fleeing Arab persecution in Syria and Palestine and by iconophiles leaving Asia Minor. The island's cities certainly bore the brunt of Arab destruction. But, with few exceptions, they were not abandoned. Churches in towns burned and destroyed by the Arabs were rebuilt, at first with wooden roofs, as at the basilicas of Soloi,[29] St. Herakleidios,[30] Kanakaria,[31] and others, but soon thereafter in smaller scale with stone-built vaults and domes, as in the basilicas at Aphendrika and Syka near Rizokarpasso,[32] the church of Panagia Kanakaria at Lythrankomi,[33] and the church built in the corridor leading from the destroyed basilica of St. Epiphanios at Salamis to its baptistery.[34]

By the second half of the eighth century, the diminished population of Cyprus was already accustomed to the smaller churches of the newly introduced architectural types with their stone-built vaults and domes. At the basilica of the Holy Trinity east of Yialousa, the chapel built in the corridor leading from the narthex to the baptistery was narrower than the south aisle of the basilica.[35] This chapel is ruinous; the earliest preserved example of the smaller stone churches is the chapel of St. Solomone near Komi tou Yialou.[36] Its vault is divided into two bays by an arch supported on engaged responds on the north and south walls. The existing layer of wall paintings in this church, dated to the ninth century on the basis of their style and iconography, has been proved to cover a yet earlier layer of imagery. After the occupation of the area by the Turkish Army in 1974 and the expulsion of the Greeks from the area, smugglers removed the bust of one of the Maries at the tomb of Christ, the early Christian iconography of the resurrection of Christ.[37] When they did so, an earlier fresco of much higher quality was found, showing that the building must antedate the ninth century.[38] Unfortunately, this painting was also removed.

This simple form of vaulted chapel continued to be built in later centuries, as exemplified by SS. Andronikos and Athanasia at Rizokarpasso of the tenth century,[39] St. Marina at Pyrgos east of Yialousa from the twelfth century,[40] St. George Sakkas near Yialousa of the eleventh or twelfth

27. Theophanes, *Chronographia*, 445.
28. Peeters, "St. Romain le Néomartyr," 419: "Eius (= Mahdi) anno primo abduxerunt ad eum alios quinque monachos, qui a Cypro captivi abducti fuerant. Tres eorum Amorienses erant duo autem aliunde orti. Qui in Cyprus a Constantino imperatore iconomacho relegati fuerant."
29. Gagniers and Tinh, *Soloi*, 124. The author does not say that the basilica was re-roofed with wood.
30. Papageorgiou, *Ἡ παλαιοχριστιανικὴ καὶ βυζαντινὴ ἀρχαιολογία*, 8.
31. Megaw and Hawkins, *Church of the Panagia Kanakariá*, 30–32.
32. Ibid., 31; A. H. S. Megaw, "Three Vaulted Basilicas in Cyprus"; idem, "Byzantine Architecture and Decoration in Cyprus," 76–78.
33. As in two preceding notes.
34. Megaw, "Three Vaulted Basilicas," 48–56.
35. Papageorgiou, *Η παλαιοχριστιανική . . . κατὰ τὸ 1963*, 4–7; idem, *Η παλαιοχριστιανική . . . κατὰ τὸ 1965–1966*, 4–9.
36. Papageorgiou, *Ἡ παλαιοχριστιανική . . . κατὰ τὰ ἔτη 1967–1968*, 38–46.
37. Papageorgiou, "Ἡ Παλαιοχριστιανικὴ τέχνη στὴν Κύπρο," 324–26.
38. I saw a photograph (transparency) of this painting in the house of a freelance archaeologist-art historian in a European country in 1990.
39. *ARDAC* 1973, 15–16, Figs. 21–22; Chotzakoglou, "Βυζαντινή αρχιτεκτονική και τέχνη," 1:521; Papageorgiou, *Christian Art*, 335–37, figs. 1–2.
40. *ARDAC* 1970, 11, Figs. 25–26; Chotzakoglou, "Βυζαντινή αρχιτεκτονική και τέχνη," 1:651; Papageorgiou, *Christian Art*, 457, fig. 1.

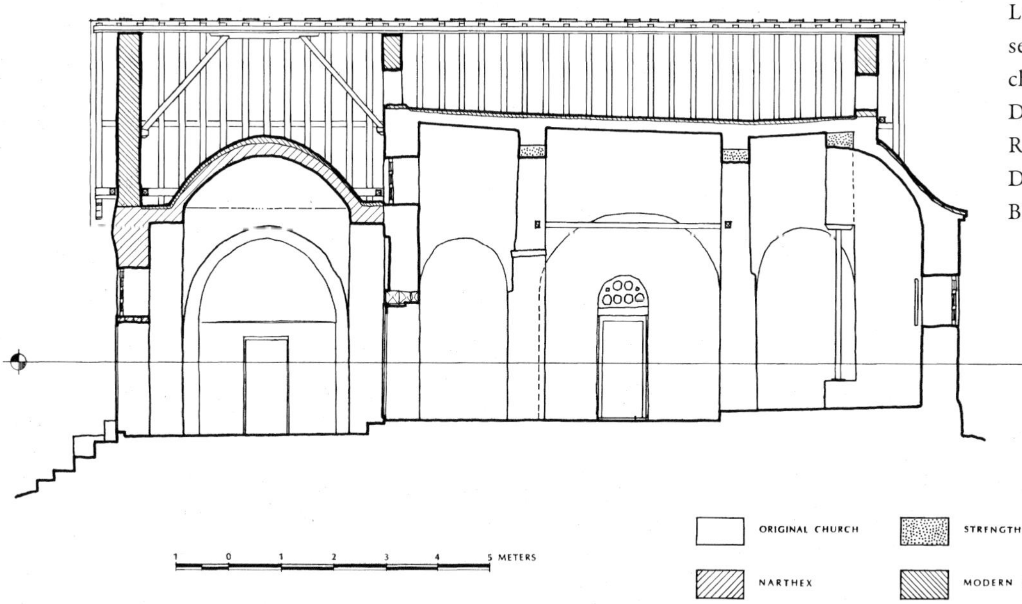

FIG. 2.3
Longitudinal section of the church of Asinou. Drawing by Richard Anderson, Dumbarton Oaks BF.F.1993. F0913

century,[41] St. Nicholas near Oikos from the twelfth century,[42] the chapel of St. George at "Ktiri" of St. Ambrosios (Limassol district), and the ruined chapel of St. Nicholas at Akamas, near the Baths of Aphrodite, from the twelfth century.[43]

In the twelfth century this architectural type became more elaborate. Engaged responds supporting a second transverse arch were attached to the north and south walls, thus dividing the naos into three bays, as in the original phase of the church of St. Menas at Ygramis in the Akamas;[44] the church of St. George near St. Konon at Akamas;[45] the church of Asinou itself (Figs. 2.1, 2.3); the church of the Panagia Amasgou, Monagri, from around 1200;[46] and the church of SS. Sergios and Bakkhos near Neta, also of the twelfth century.[47] At the same time the responds support three blind arches along each wall, of which the middle one is wider and higher than the two others, emphasizing the central bay in a way reminiscent of the domed hall churches. This is the case at Asinou (Fig. 2.1), the Panagia Amasgou, St. Basil near Xylotympou,[48] and the church of SS. Sergios and Bakkhos near Neta.[49] In other examples, including the twelfth-century churches of St. Philon at Agridia east of Rizokarpasso[50] and St. Mavra in Rizokarpasso,[51] there are again three blind arches on the north and

41. *ARDAC* 1973, 16, Figs. 25–26; Chotzakoglou, "Βυζαντινή αρχιτεκτονική και τέχνη," 1:520.
42. Papacostas, "Byzantine Cyprus," fig. 203.
43. Unpublished.
44. *ARDAC* for 1986, 25, and Figs. 28–29; Chotzakoglou, "Βυζαντινή αρχιτεκτονική και τέχνη," 1:520.
45. Ibid.
46. Boyd, "Church of the Panagia Amasgou," 277, 285.
47. Chotzakoglou, "Βυζαντινή αρχιτεκτονική και τέχνη," 1:520.
48. *ARDAC* for 1973, 17, Figs. 30–31; Chotzakoglou, "Βυζαντινή αρχιτεκτονική και τέχνη," 1:627.
49. Ibid., 1:520.
50. Soteriou, *Βυζαντινὰ μνημεῖα*, pl. 29; Papageorgiou, *Ἡ παλαιοχριστιανικὴ . . . κατὰ τὰ ἔτη 1967–1968*, 83, fig. 84; Papageorgiou, *Christian Art*, 347, 350 fig. 1, 351 fig. 1; Chotzakoglou, "Βυζαντινή αρχιτεκτονική και τέχνη," fig. 183.
51. Papageorgiou, *Ἡ παλαιοχριστιανικὴ . . . κατὰ τὰ ἔτη 1967–1968*, 81–83; idem, *Christian Art*, 343–44

south walls, but they are of equal width and height. The western blind arch of the south wall of the church of St. Philon at Agridia is wider than the other two because there is a tomb beneath it (perhaps the donor's tomb).

The Plan of the Church of Panagia at Asinou

The plan of the church of Panagia at Asinou is similar to the plan of the domed-hall churches, except for the dome (Intro. Fig. 1, Fig. 2.1).[52] It is a rectangular hall, 8.43 × 4.39 m inside, ending at the east in a semicircular apse. The chord of the present apse is 2.61 m and its radius is 1.32 m. The walls are 0.69 m thick and are built with gabbros diabase stones and lime mortar. The stones are gabbros, melagabbros, pyroxenetic gabbros, and microgabbros up to a height of two meters from the foundations, and diabase mixed with basalts and microgabbros above that.[53] Only in the higher courses of the north wall are ashlar blocks used (Figs. 2.4, 2.5). The stones are irregular, and fragments of tiles and bricks are used to keep them in place. The north and south walls each have two responds supporting three blind arches of unequal proportions. Thus the span of the eastern blind arch of the south wall measures 1.60 m, the central one 3.325 m, and the west one 1.735 m. The span of those on the north wall measures 1.815 m in the east, 3.345 m in the center, and 1.50 m in the west. Since these arches are semicircular, their height is also unequal, the central ones being higher and almost segmental. Those of the south wall rise to 3.31 m in the east, 3.86 m in the center, and 3.40 m in the west. On the north wall they rise to 3.30 m in the east, 3.86 in the center, and 3.29 in the west. The blind arches add to the thickness of the north and south walls, making them strong enough to counterbalance the thrust of the vault covering the church.

In the east wall, flanking the apse, are two semicircular niches: the one on the north is 0.50 m wide and 0.755 m high, and the one on the south 0.445 m wide and 0.695 m high (Figs. 2.1, 2.6). They are both 0.325 m deep, and the one on the north serves as a prothesis. Rectangular niches 0.90 to 0.975 m above the floor open into the eastern part of the north and south walls, that on the south measuring 0.54 × 0.38 × 0.975 m, and that on the north measuring 0.513 × 0.53 × 0.575 m. As noted, the walls are subdivided by engaged responds that support the blind arches of the north and south walls.

Three doors, almost in the middle of the north, the south, and the west walls, provide access to the church. The south door is 0.985 m wide (Figs. 2.2, 2.7, 2.8), the west door is 1.445 m wide (Fig. 2.21), and the north door is 0.92 m wide (Figs. 2.5, 2.18). Slight differences are also observed in their height: the west door rises to 2.20 m, the south door to 2.035 m, and the north door to 1.93 m. The leaves of the north door of the church were decorated with wood carvings.[54] This door was transferred to the bishop's palace in Kyrenia for safekeeping in the 1930s and was lost after the occupation of Kyrenia by Turkish forces in 1974. It seems to have been somewhat later and of less clearly Byzantine character than the door of the katholikon of the monastery of St. John Chrysostom of Koutsovendis, which was still in place in 1989.[55] Further examples of carved wooden doors akin to those from Asinou survive from later periods.[56] Above the wooden lintels of these doors

fig. 1, 345 figs. 1–2. The blind arches of the church are horseshoe-shaped.

52. Ćurčić, *Middle Byzantine Architecture on Cyprus*, 14 and 29; see also Nicolaïdès, "Étude iconographique," 9–10.

53. I thank the Director of the Geological Department of Cyprus, Dr. P. Michaelides, who allowed the geologist Mr. Eustathios Tsolakes to visit the church of Asinou to examine the stones built into the walls and to take the samples used by the first geological officer, Mr. Yiannakis Panagides, in identifying their provenance. I express my gratitude to both of them.

54. Soteriou, *Βυζαντινὰ μνημεῖα*, pl. 142, 1–2.

55. Ibid., pl. 144a; Tsiknopoullos, *Ἡ Ἱερὰ Μονὴ τοῦ Χρυσοστόμου*, Figs. on pp. 103, 104.

56. Some are still in place, like the north door of the church of the Panagia at Moutoullas (Soteriou, *Βυζαντινὰ μνημεῖα*, pl. 143b) and the west door of the

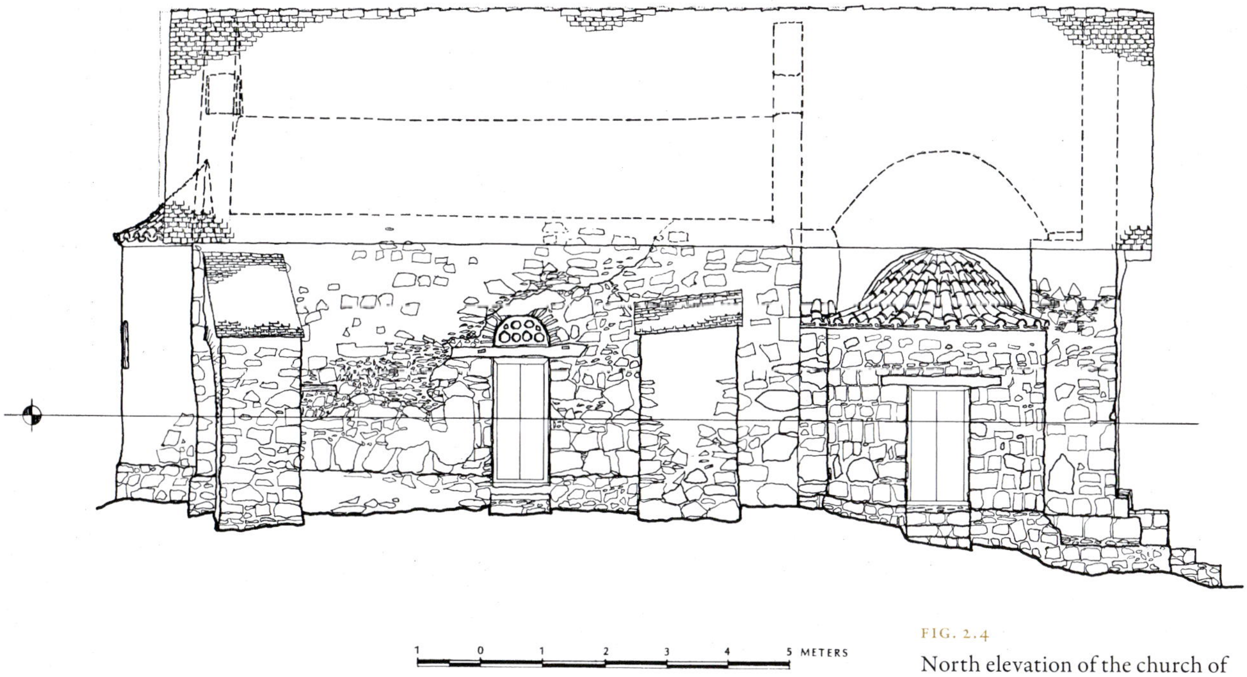

FIG. 2.4
North elevation of the church of Asinou. Drawing by Richard Anderson, Dumbarton Oaks BF.F.1993. F0911

are semicircular openings admitting some light into the interior of the church (Fig. 2.9). Further light was originally shed by a single window (0.42 × 0.82 m) 4.03 m above the present floor on the west wall (Figs. 2.10, 2.11, 6.35), and by the triple window of the apse (Figs. 2.12, 2.13). The semicircular arches of these openings are built of brick in the recessed technique. The bricks are 0.045 to 0.064 m thick and the mortar 0.055 to 0.065 m. The recessed bricks are 0.023 to 0.045 m thick. This technique is clearly evident in the arches above the south door of the church and the west door of the narthex (Figs. 2.9, 2.22).[57] Bricks

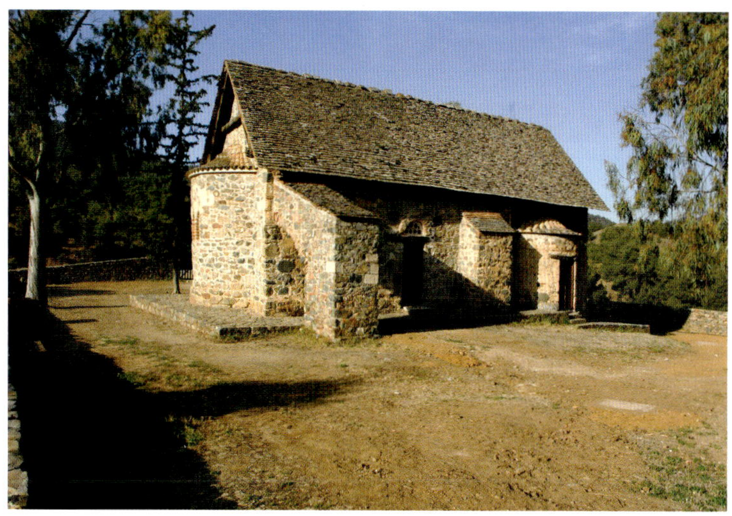

FIG. 2.5 Exterior, north side of the church of Asinou (photo courtesy of G. L. Carr)

chapel of the Akathistos Hymn in the monastery of St. John Lampadistes at Kalopanayiotis (ibid., pl. 143a). The north door of the same chapel, however, was removed to the "narthex" of the chapel for display; the west door of the Archangel church at Pedoulas has been removed and put in the narthex because of its fragile condition; and the door of the chapel of SS. Andronikos and Athanasia at Kalopanayiotis has been removed for protection.

57. This is the only confirmed example of recessed brick technique in Cyprus. In the other cases (chapel of the Holy Trinity at the monastery of St. John Chrysostom,

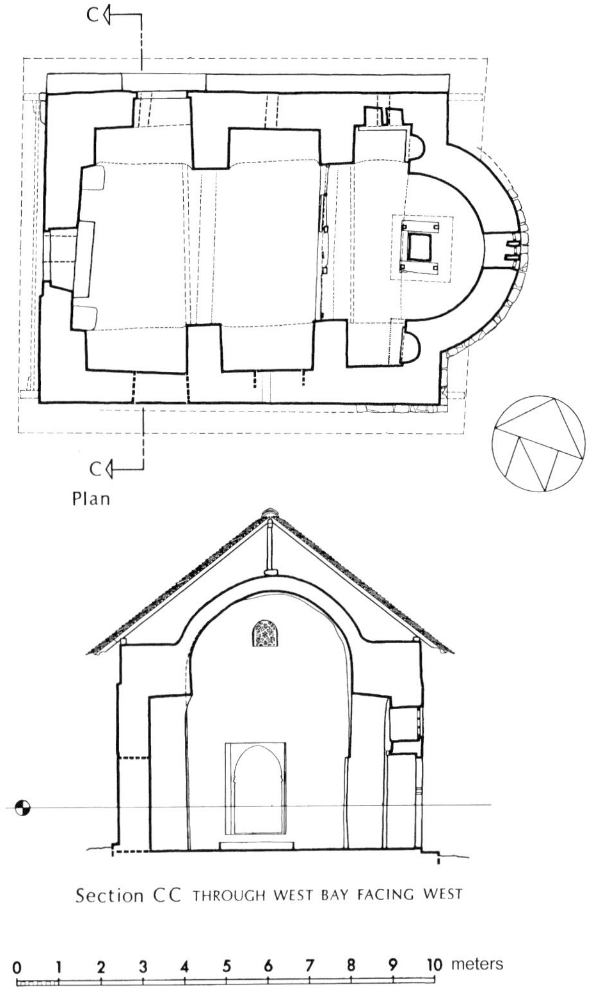

FIG. 2.6 Plan and section of the naos of the church of Asinou. Drawing by Richard Anderson, Dumbarton Oaks BF.F.1993. F0916

are also used for the construction of the triple window of the apse (Figs. 2.13, 2.14).

The triple windows are 0.18, 0.19, and 0.20 m wide on the inside and 0.26, 0.26, and 0.245 m on the outside. A slight variation is also evident in their height, both inside (0.80–0.815 m) and outside (0.82–0.85 m). Originally, the windows of the apse, the west wall, and the semicircular openings above the north and south doors were closed with gypsum panels with glass roundels. Only the window on the west wall still preserves its glass panel (Figs. 2.10, 2.11).[58]

The church is covered by a stone-built vault (Fig. 2.15). The central bay of the vault is deformed on the interior (Fig. 2.16, top), and the original semicircular transverse arches were underpinned with pointed arches. There is no information on how the vault was covered. If we take for granted that the later dedicatory wall painting on the south wall of the church reproduced an original one (Fig. 6.50), then the vault was covered with tiles (*tegulae* and *imbrices* in Latin; στρωτῆρες and καλυπτῆρες in Greek), as were the vaults of the church of St. Nicholas of the Roof (τῆς Στέγης) near Kakopetria (eleventh century), Panagia Kanakaria at Lythrankomi (ninth to twelfth centuries), and Panagia Apsinthiotissa (around 1100). However, the roof of the model of the church as depicted in the painting, offered by the founder to the Virgin, is pitched rather than round. Whether this implies a wooden second roof is discussed below.

The external walls of the church were unarticulated, but the masonry was covered with colored mortar imitating ashlar revetment (Fig. 2.17).[59] Cloisonné ashlar blocks are almost unknown in Cyprus. The only example is found in the dome of the

---

the katholikon and trapeza [refectory] of the monastery of Panagia Apsinthiotissa, and the church of St. Hilarion in the castle of St. Hilarion), although the thickness of the mortar is more than the thickness of the bricks, the recessed brick technique has not been confirmed. This technique, however, is not a criterion for dating, since the recessed brick technique was used from the 11th to the 14th century. Vocotopoulos, "Concealed Course Technique"; Ousterhout, "Observations on the 'Recessed Brick' Technique"; idem, "Some Notes on the Construction," 49–50. In Cyprus, brick construction is limited to the late 11th and 12th centuries: Papageorgiou, "Constantinopolitan Influence." In Cyprus after the 12th century, the joints of the bricks are thinner than the bricks, thus excluding any suspicion of recessed brick technique.

58. The three main glass panels are one above the other. The middle one, which was missing, was replaced during repairs to the church in 1954. Similar glass panels are preserved in a window of the dome of the church of the Panagia at Trikomo, as observed during the repairs of the church in 1966.

59. Ćurčić, *Middle Byzantine Architecture,* 30.

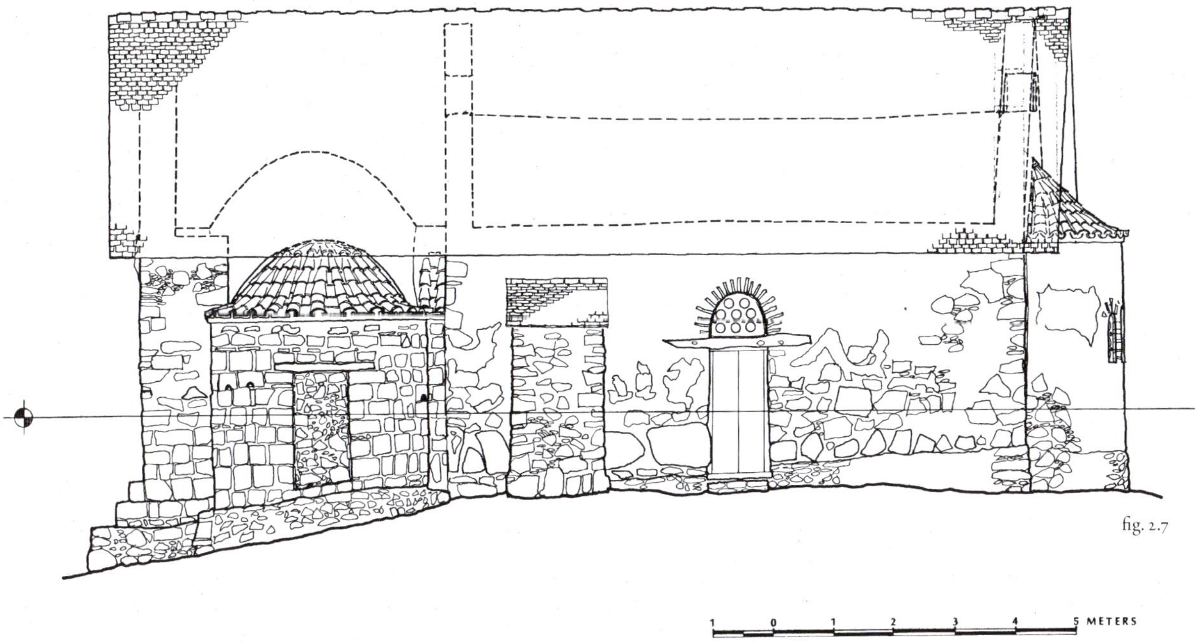

fig. 2.7

FIG. 2.7
South elevation of the church of Asinou. Drawing by Richard Anderson, Dumbarton Oaks BF.F.1993. F0910

FIG. 2.8
South door of the church of Asinou (photo courtesy of Athanasios Papageorgiou)

FIG. 2.9
The arch above the south door of the naos of the church of Asinou (photo courtesy of Athanasios Papageorgiou)

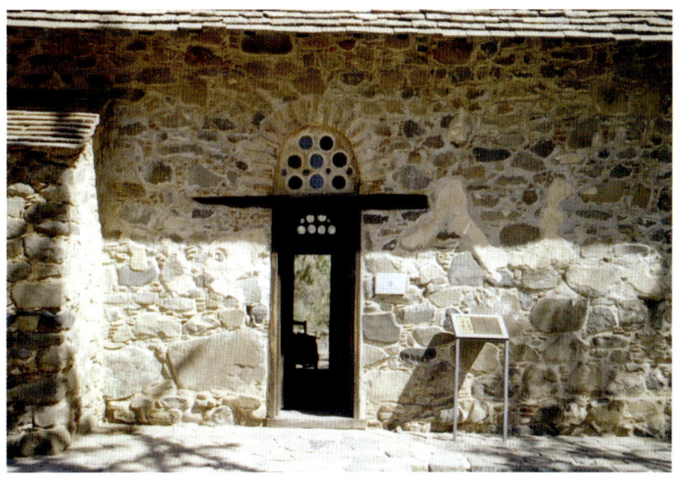

fig. 2.8

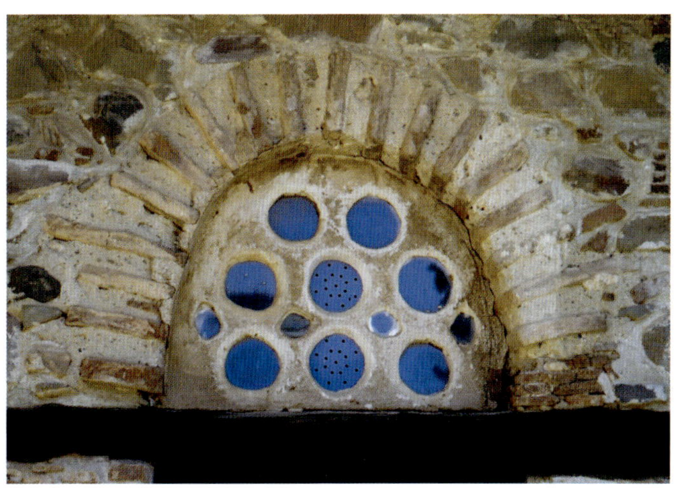

fig. 2.9

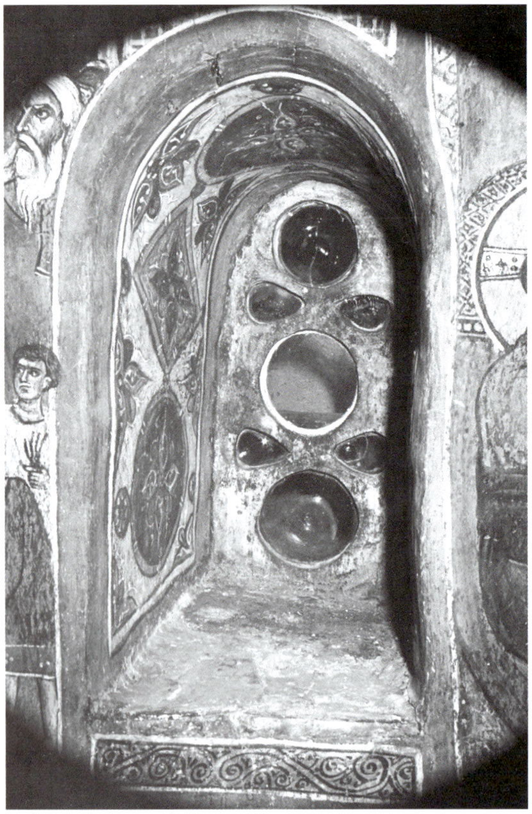

fig. 2.10

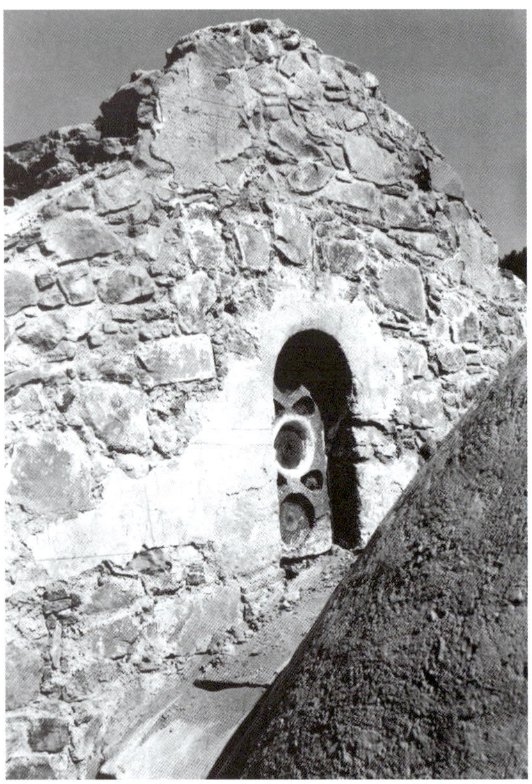

fig. 2.11

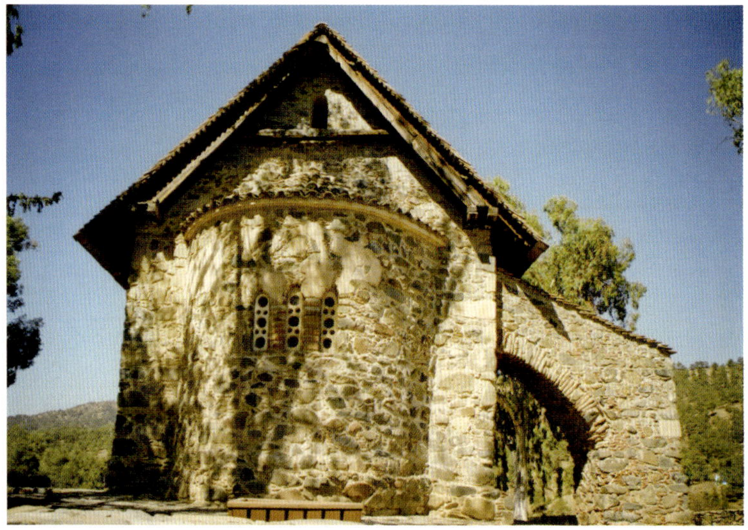

fig. 2.12

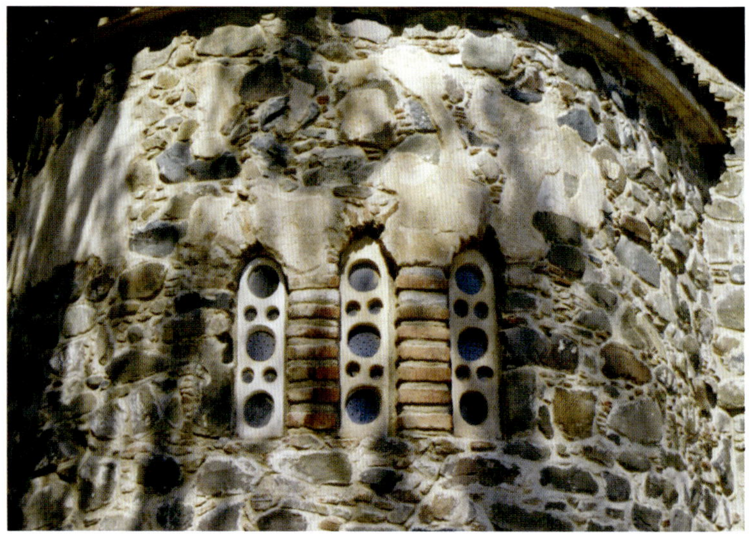

fig. 2.13

FIG. 2.10

The window on the west wall of the church of Asinou, interior view (photo courtesy of Dumbarton Oaks, Winfield 841A)

FIG. 2.11

The window on the west wall of the church of Asinou, exterior view during the repairs of the church in 1953 (photo courtesy of Athanasios Papageorgiou)

FIG. 2.12

The apse of the church of Asinou (photo courtesy of Athanasios Papageorgiou)

FIG. 2.13

The triple window of the apse of the church of Asinou (photo courtesy of Athanasios Papageorgiou)

parekklesion of the Holy Trinity at the monastery of St. John Chrysostom at Koutsovendis, a contemporary building unlikely to have influenced the imitation revetment at the church of Asinou. Indeed, there is a zigzag line in the large joints of the rectangular panels at Asinou that is not used in the cloisonné ashlar construction of the dome of the Holy Trinity. Remnants of this imitation still survive on the pediment of the west wall, on the north wall of the narthex, and on the apse itself (Figs. 2.13, 2.17, 2.23). Whether this imitation of revetment was used also on the north wall of the church is not known. The north wall retains some wall paintings: a fragmentary Deesis above the north door and a fragment of the Anastasis below, to its east (Fig. 2.18). The extent of this figural decoration is not known. Usually external decoration in Cyprus is limited. So far as I know, external decoration at the church of St. Nicholas of the Roof was restricted to a half figure of St. Nicholas, painted in the blind arch above the west door before the erection of the narthex of the church. The same is observed at Asinou itself, where the Virgin Phorbiotissa was painted above the west entrance to the church before the erection of the narthex (Fig. 5.37). The patron saint in each case was painted in the blind arch over the entrance to the church. In somewhat later churches—e.g., at the Panagia Arakiotissa near Lagoudera (1192) and the west wall of the Panagia at Moutoullas (1280)—the external decoration is also limited. Only around 1500 does such decoration expand. The western wall of the Holy Cross of Agiasmati near Platanistassa (1494), the north wall of the church of the Panagia at Moutoullas around 1500, and the west wall of the church of the Panagia Podithou (1502) were wholly painted.[60] At Asinou, a small fragment of mortar covering the masonry still remains high up at the east end of the north wall, but it is too small to indicate whether it is a remnant of a wall painting or a bit of imitation revetment. The same is true of another fragment in the intrados of the later flying

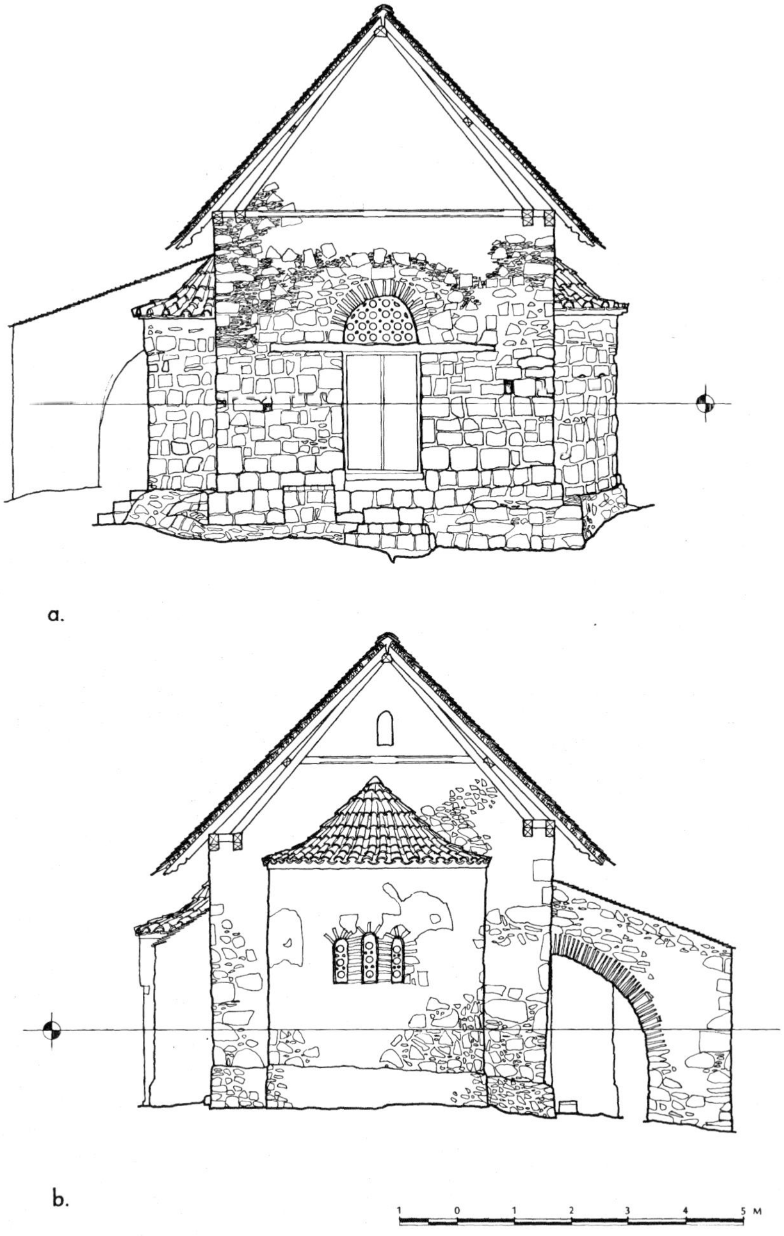

FIG. 2.14 West elevation (a) and east elevation (b) of the church of Asinou. Drawing by Richard Anderson, Dumbarton Oaks BF.F.1993. F0909

60. Stylianou and Stylianou, *Painted Churches*, 218 (Holy Cross of Agiasmati), 330 (Panagia of Moutoullas), 98 (Podithou).

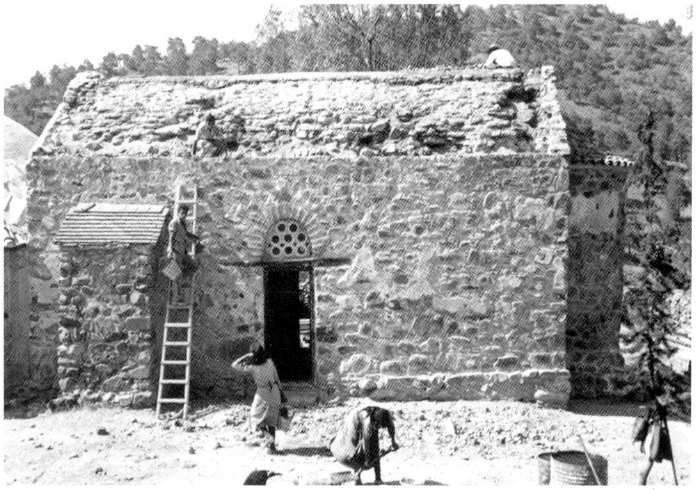

fig. 2.15

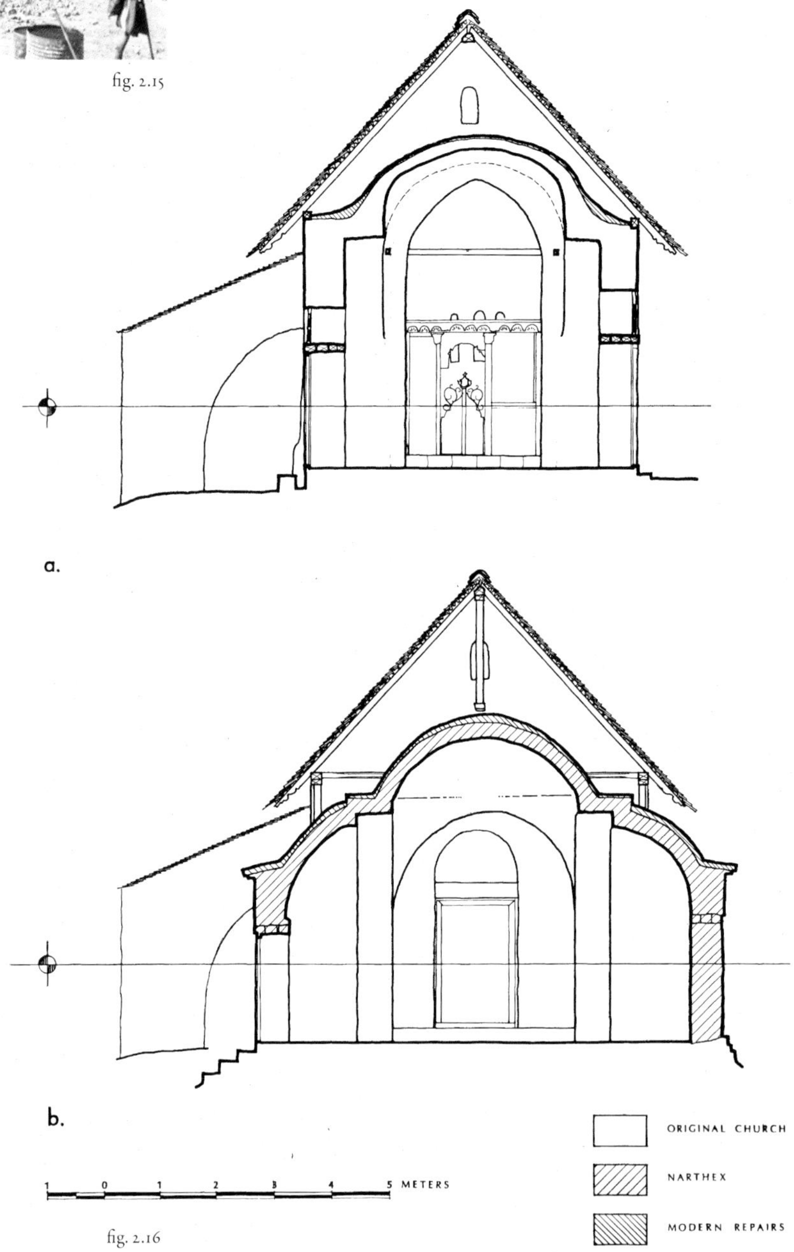

fig. 2.16

FIG. 2.15

The external surface of the south half of the vault during the repairs of the church of Asinou in 1953 (photo courtesy of Athanasios Papageorgiou)

FIG. 2.16

a. Deformation of the central bay of the church of Asinou; b. Section of the narthex of the church of Asinou. Drawing by Richard Anderson, Dumbarton Oaks BF.F.1993. F0912

buttress on the north wall. Whatever these paintings were, they show that the external appearance of the church was originally different.

The exact date of the foundation of the church is not known. The beginning of the dedicatory inscription giving the date of 1105/6 under the painting of SS. Constantine and Helena is masked by a later respond, so it is not known whether the inscription starts with ἀνηγέρθη (was built) ὁ πάνσεπτος ναὸς διὰ συνδρομης . . . or ἱστοριογραφήθη (was adorned with images) ὁ πάνσεπτος ναὸς διὰ συνδρομῆς . . . Today one can see only . . . συνδρομῆς κ(αὶ) πολλου πόθου Νικ/ηφόρου Μαγίστρου του Υσχιρίου · βασιλευων[το]ς Αλεξίου του Κομνηνου · έτους ςχιδ · ιν(δικτιῶνος) ιδ: ". . . support and great effort of Nikephoros Ischyrios the magistros, in the reign of Alexios Komnenos, the year 6614, indiction fourteen" (Fig. 2.19).[61]

Another inscription is given in the votive panel on the south wall (Figs. 3.8, 6.50, 6.51). Here Magistros Nikephoros, represented offering the church to the Virgin and being presented by her to Christ, is accompanied by a woman, in much smaller scale, whose date of death is given. It reads: Μηνῖ Δηκ(εμ)βρίο ϊζ / ιν(δικτιῶνος) ϊε ἔτους ,ςχη ἐκυ/μήθη ἡ δουλι του Θ(εο)υ Γέφυ/ρα: "On December 17 of the fifteenth indiction of the year 6608 died Gephyra, the servant of God." Unfortunately, the indiction does not correspond with the *annus mundi*: the year, 6608, or 1099, was not a fifteenth indiction.[62] The error was pointed

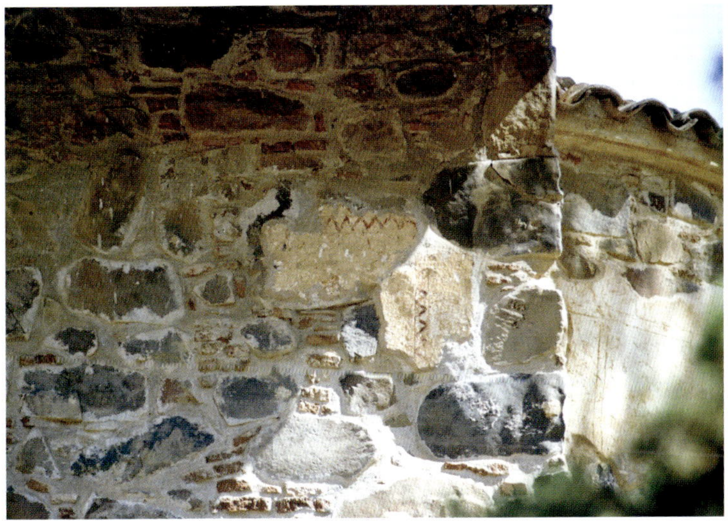

FIG. 2.17 Remnants of marble imitation of cloisonné ashlar revetment (photo courtesy of Athanasios Papageorgiou)

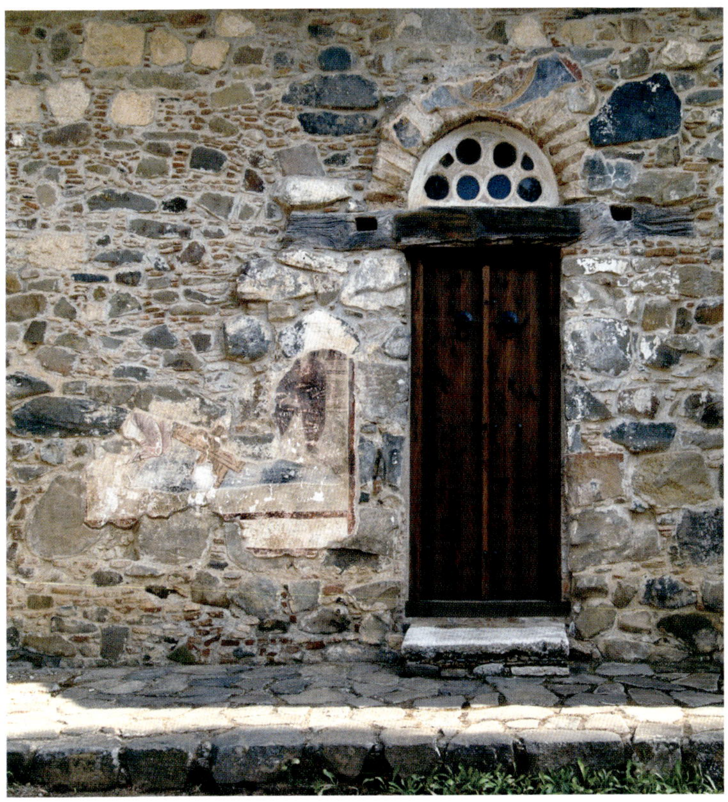

FIG. 2.18 Remnants of wall paintings of the Deesis and Anastasis around the north door of the church of Asinou (photo courtesy of G. L. Carr)

61. The inscription is discussed in a forthcoming publication by A. Nicolaïdès on Asinou's 12th-century frescoes.

62. In Buxton et al., "Church of Asinou," 343, W. H. Buckler tried to reconcile the indiction and the *annus mundi* by emendation of the inscription: Μηνὶ Δεκεβρίο ἰ[νδικτίωνος] ζ' ἡμ[έρα] ιε' έτους ,ςχη' ἐκυμήθην ἡ δούλη τοῦ θ[εο]ῦ Γέφυρα. Buckler was followed by Sacopoulo, *Asinou*, 10–11. The inscription is clear and, therefore, the emendation is unacceptable. On donor inscriptions in Cyprus, see Nicolaïdès, "Étude iconographique," 6 n. 37; Frigerio-Zeniou, "Οι δωρητές στην εκκλησία της Παναγίας Ποδίθου"; Stylianou and Stylianou, "Donors and Dedicatory Inscriptions"; Papageorgiou, "Βυζαντινή επιγραφική στην Κύπρο."

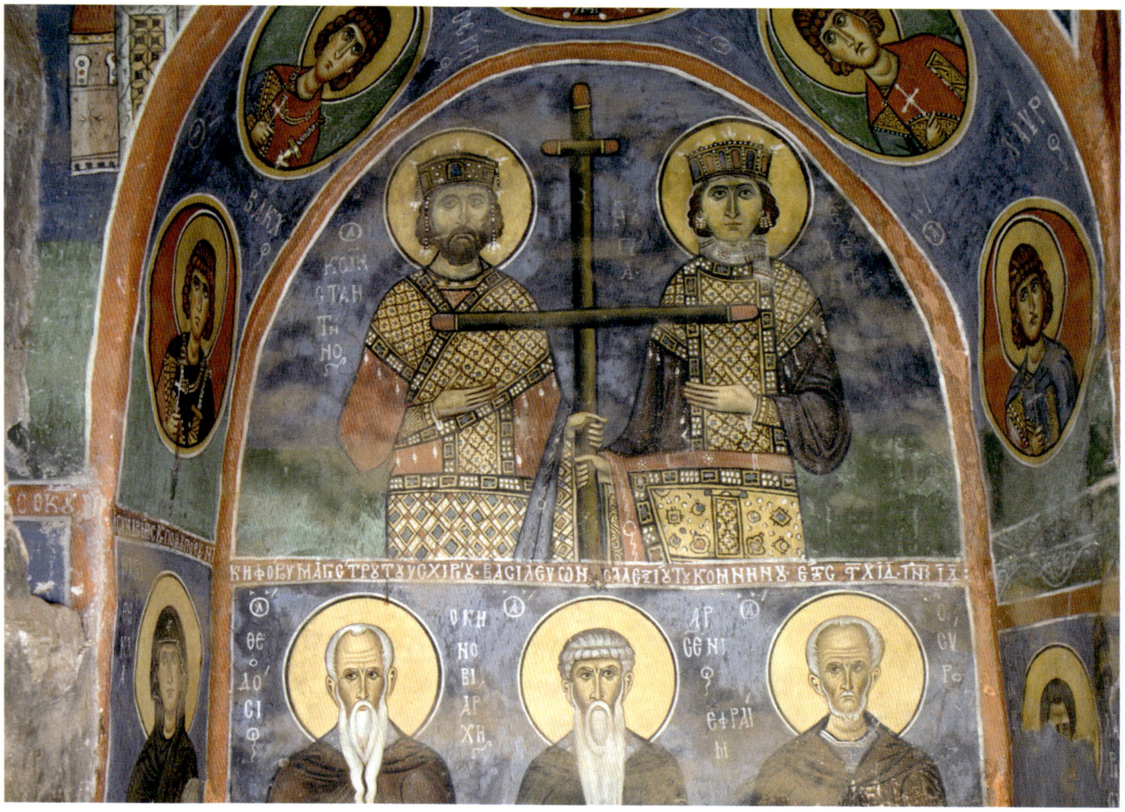

FIG. 2.19 The inscription recording the foundation of the church by the magistros Nikephoros in the period of Alexios I Komnenos (photo courtesy of the Leventis Foundation and the Archaeological Research Unit, University of Cyprus, no. 006285)

out in a publication of 1965, where it was suggested that the indiction was wrongly written by the fourteenth-century painter, who misread the original date when he copied the twelfth-century dedicatory painting.[63] In 1976 Cyril Mango suggested that the actual year of death of the woman accompanying the donor was the date recorded for the decoration of the church, i.e., 1105/6.[64] Under these circumstances, though, the fourteenth-century painter would have incorrectly copied both the indiction and the *annus mundi*. Although not impossible, such an error would be unusual. The possibility that a relative of Nikephoros was associated with or already buried in the church in 1099 complicates the exact dating of its construction, but for architectural purposes, it makes no difference whether the construction was in 1099 or in 1105/6.

Sometime in the twelfth century a narthex was added abutting the west wall of the church (Figs. 2.1, 2.2, 2.20). It is built on a lower level (0.40 m) owing to the inclination of the ground. This is not usual, since at other eleventh- and twelfth-century churches the narthex was built on the same

63. Papageorgiou, *Masterpieces of the Byzantine Art of Cyprus*, 17.

64. Mango, "Chypre, carrefour du monde byzantin," 7, n. 14. On these inscriptions and their complications, see Grivaud above, p. 22. The problem is complicated by the fact that Darrouzès, "Notes pour servir à l'histoire de Chypre" [1953], 93—in editing the marginal notes of Paris. gr. 1590, which belonged to the monastery of the Panagia ton Phorbion—found that the name of the founder was recorded as Νικόλαος IC(...) with an abbreviation

usually denoting HN. The problems posed by this inscription are discussed by Grivaud above, pp. 17–19.

level as the naos: see St. Nicholas of the Roof near Kakopetria, chapel of the Holy Trinity at the monastery of St. John Chrysostom in Koutsovendis, Panagia Aphendrika at Koutsovendis, Panagia Apsinthiotissa near Sychari, St. George Chortakion, St. Theodore Chortakion near Sotera in the Famagusta District, St. Hilarion in the homonymous castle, St. George in the castle of Kyrenia, Acheiropoietos near Karavas, and Panagia Kanakaria at Lythrankomi. The narthex is cruciform in plan with very short crossarms ending to the north and south in semicircular apses.[65] Both apses have the same radius of 1.30 m but a slightly different chord. The chord of the south apse is 2.67 m and that of the north is 2.64 m. The central part of the narthex is covered by a blind dome on pendentives, like the narthex of the church of St. Nicholas of the Roof near Kakopetria, the

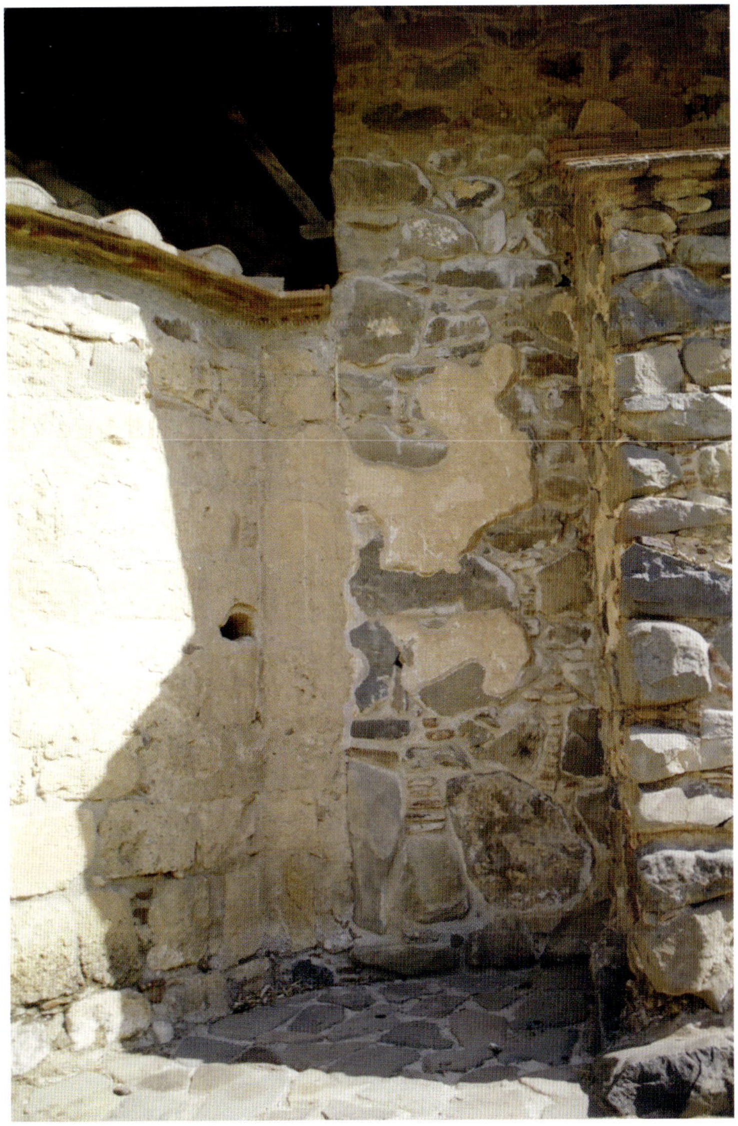

FIG. 2.20 Perpendicular junction of the walls of the church and narthex of the church of Asinou (photo courtesy of Athanasios Papageorgiou)

65. Narthexes with apsidal ends to the north and south are not uncommon in Cyprus during the late 11th and 12th centuries. Papageorgiou, "Narthex of the Churches," cites the following examples. The katholikon of the monastery of St. John Chrysostom at Koutsoventis was consecrated on 9 December 1090: Dmitrievskij, *Opisanie liturgitseskich rukopsej*, 3:121; Mango and Hawkins, "Report on Field Work," 333–39; Mango, "Monastery of St. Chrysostomos," Figs. 6–7. The katholikon of the monastery of Panagia Apsinthiotissa of around 1100: Papageorgiou, "Η Μονή Αψινθιώτισσας," 77, fig. 1. The ruined church of St. Paul at Gomaristra, Kyrenia mountains, 12th century: Prokopiou, "Άγιος Παύλος, Κυπαρισσόβουνου"; see also Prokopiou, Ο *συνεπτυγμένος σταυροειδής εγγεγραμμένος ναός*, 136–38; and Papageorgiou, *Christian Art*, 123–24. The church of St. George at Aphendrika, east of Rizokarpasso, dated 10th–12th century: Soteriou, *Βυζαντινὰ μνημεῖα*, fig. 7 and pl. 13b (dated as early Byzantine); Papageorgiou, *Η παλαιοχριστιανική . . . κατὰ τὸ 1964*, 15; Demetrokalles, *Οἱ δίκογχοι χριστιανικοὶ ναοί*, 61–62, fig. 77; Megaw, "Byzantine Architecture and Decoration," 78. The earlier katholikon of the monastery of Hiereon or Agia Moni: Papageorgiou, *Η παλαιοχριστιανική και βυζαντινή αρχαιολογία* [1964], 15. Nicolaïdès, "Étude iconographique," 11, pl. 1, suggests (pers. comm. with A. H. S. Megaw) that the narthex of the church of the Panagia tou Arakos originally had apses to the north and south. A church in ruins, of unknown dedication, southwest of the monastery of St. John Chrysostom at Koutsovendis, also had a narthex with apsidal ends (personal notes of the author). Although the narthex with apsidal ends was already known in the early Christian period (narthex of the basilica of Kampanopetra in Salamis of the 6th century and in all probability also the narthex of the basilica of St. Epiphanios also in Salamis from around 400 CE), it seems that, in the middle Byzantine period, the narthex with apsidal ends was reintroduced to Cyprus from Constantinople at the end of the 11th century. See Papageorgiou, "Narthex of the Churches," 444.

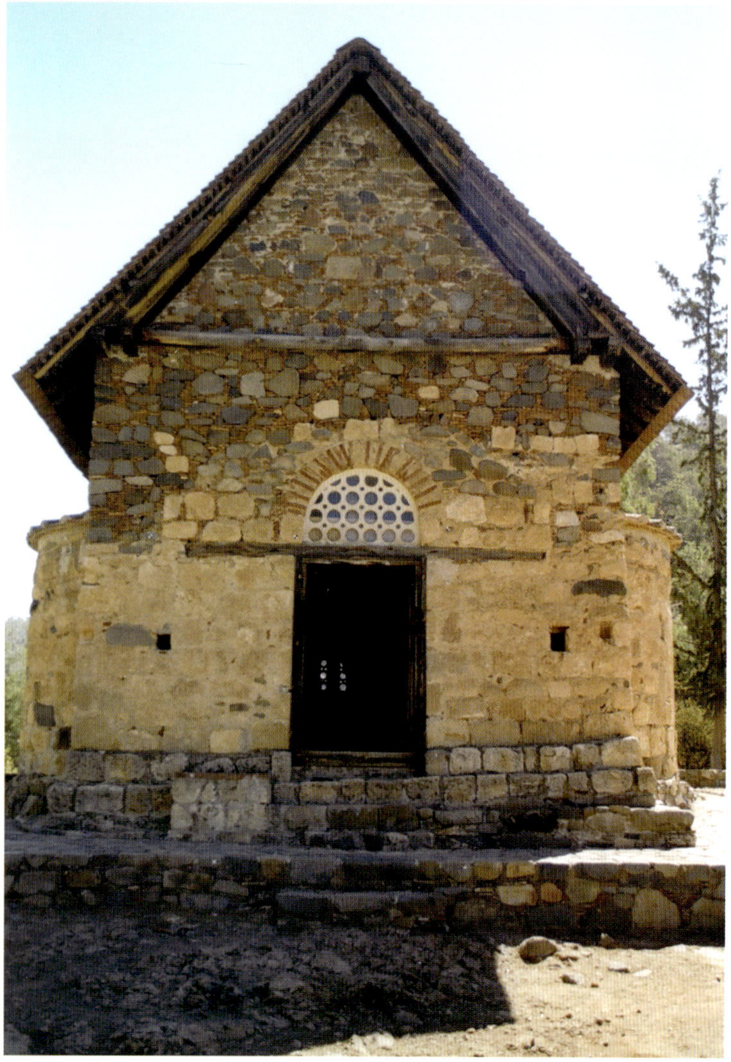

fig. 2.21

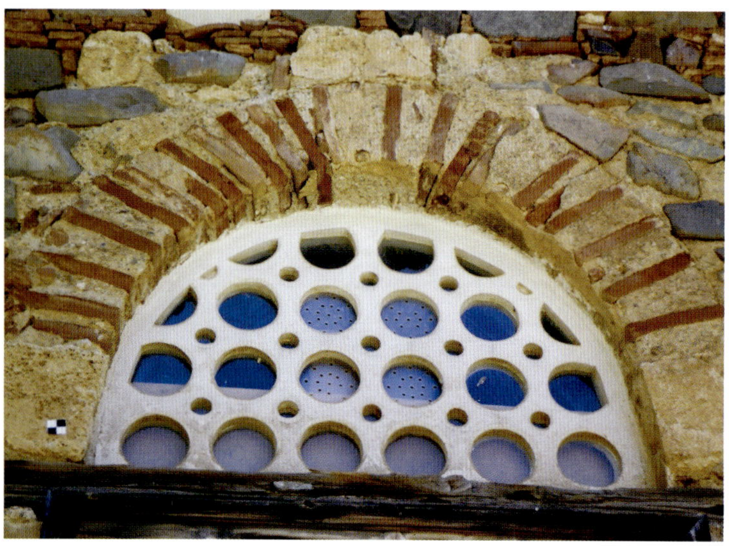

fig. 2.22

FIG. 2.21
The west façade of the church of Asinou (photo courtesy of Athanasios Papageorgiou)

FIG. 2.22
The arch above the west door of the narthex of the church of Asinou (photo courtesy of Athanasios Papageorgiou)

ruined church of St. Theodore Chortakion near Sotera in the Famagusta District, the church of Panagia Galoktiste at Pano Pyrgos, and the later narthex of the church of St. George Sakkas near Yialousa.[66] The internal dimensions of the narthex, including the apses, are 7.05 m from north to south and 4.45 m from east to west.

Three doors provided access to the narthex, as in the katholikon of St. Nicholas of the Roof, the demolished katholikon of St. John Chrysostom at Koutsovendis, and the katholikon of Apsinthiotissa. The main door is in the west wall and stands 1.355 m wide and 2.14 m high (Fig. 2.21). Above it is an arched opening 1.30 m wide with a radius of 0.85 m (Fig. 2.22). The door in the north apse is 0.85 m wide and 1.80 m high (Fig. 2.23). The door in the south apse is now visible only on the external face of the apse (Fig. 2.24). This door was evidently walled up very shortly after the narthex was constructed, when the interior decoration was painted.

Remnants of decoration are visible in the apse beneath the wall painting of St. George (Fig. 4.1). The date of this decoration, which I believe to be contemporary with the closure of the door, and its relation to the St. George and other remnants of early painting in the narthex are discussed in Chapters 4, 5, and 7. Attention has focused on it because of the insight it might yield into the dating of the narthex, significant for our understanding of the church's function. Since the arches of the narthex are slightly pointed, like those of the church of the Panagia tou Arakos near Lagoudera and the church of St. Basil near Xylotympou, the

66. Ibid., 446.

narthex must have been erected after the middle of the twelfth century.[67] I believe this date is supported by the earlier layer of wall paintings in the narthex, visible in different parts of its walls where the paintings of 1332/33 have been destroyed.

For the construction of the walls of the narthex, ashlar was used extensively. It is primarily made of reef stones: different kinds of psammites (bioclastic, fossiliferous sandstones) and gypsum. These stones are not found near Asinou. The reefs of Koroneia (area of Koutraphas, 7 km from Asinou) are friable and therefore not suitable for building. Another area where reefs are found is in the river by the village of Potami (10 km from Asinou), but here there is no gypsum. Good quality reef stones and gypsum are found around Mitsero, 14 km distant as the crow flies, or 18–20 km by modern roads. The stones used for the walls of the narthex are of different sizes and shapes with variable dressing and quality. They were not, therefore, from a particular quarry, but were instead taken from earlier buildings. They are used in the south apse to a height of 2.50 m and in the southwest corner of the narthex to a height of 3.57 m, while on the northwest they are used to the level of the lintel. On the west wall of the narthex only two courses are built over the lintel of the door. The wall of the north apse is built with ashlar up to the eaves (Figs. 2.1, 2.4, 2.7, 2.14 top, 2.21, 2.23).

On the south apse of the narthex are three arched holes, one with a recessed arch on the east side and two with plain arches on the west side of the closed door (Figs. 2.2, 2.24). These holes are not remnants of windows, because they are at different heights from the foundations and are unequal in size. Also, if opened to the interior, they would have affected the southeast and southwest angle supports of the vaulting of the narthex. The arched stones are reused, and therefore they may have been used, like the rectangular holes on the west wall and in the north apse, as scaffolding holes. The upper section of the walls of the narthex is built with diabase stones and extensive use of brick fragments. The thickness of the west wall is 0.66–0.69 m, while that of the north apse is 0.63 m. There is no

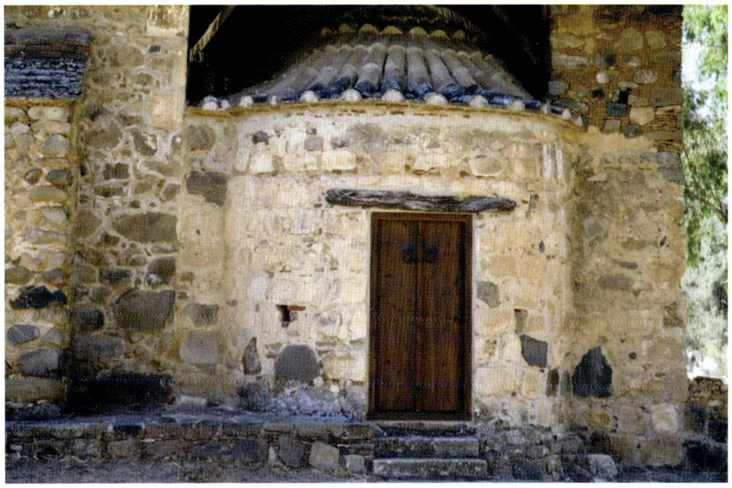

FIG. 2.23 The north apse of the narthex of Asinou (photo courtesy of Athanasios Papageorgiou)

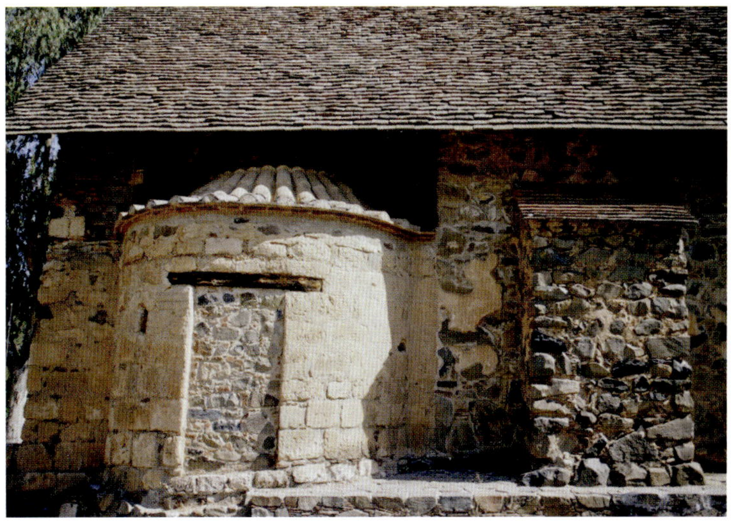

FIG. 2.24 The closed south door of the narthex of Asinou (photo courtesy of Athanasios Papageorgiou)

67. The pointed arch was in use in Cyprus for aqueducts from the 4th century CE: see Last, "Kourion: The Ancient Water Supply," 53, 54. It was used in the 7th century in the aqueduct of Salamis, as is evident from the standing arches near the village of St. Sergios. After a lapse of some centuries the pointed vault reappeared at the beginning of the 12th century in the ossuaries of the funeral chapel of St. Savvas of the monastery of Apsinthiotissa.

evidence that the walls of the narthex were externally plastered like those of the church proper.

Was the decoration of the external surfaces of the walls of the church protected, or was it exposed to the weather? Until 1920 a steeply pitched wooden roof extended about six feet beyond the south, west, and north walls of the church (Fig. 1.6).[68] It was supported on wooden poles and formed an open gallery on three sides of the building. There is no information concerning the date of the addition of the steeply pitched wooden roof above the vaults of the church and its narthex. There are, rather, two conflicting pieces of evidence: the picture of the church donated by Nikephoros to the Virgin (Fig. 6.50), and the oral information of the foreman and chief foreman of the Department of Antiquities who supervised the works of 1954 and 1959. They testify that the extrados of the vault of the church was uneven (Fig. 2.15). A. H. S. Megaw, the director of the Department of Antiquities who inspected the works on the church in 1954 and 1959, stated that the vault of the church was unbroken, thus countering the opinion of the authors of the 1933 monographic article on Asinou in *Archaeologia*, that the vault of the central bay of the church had been destroyed and rebuilt.[69] The Annual Report of the Director of Antiquities for the year 1959 states explicitly, "The top of the vault was repaired and its exterior covered with lime concrete."[70] This means that the exterior of the vault was not covered with either lime concrete or tiles. There is no doubt that the painter of the fourteenth-century donor image also painted the image of a church, the vault of which was covered with tiles. Could this be a convention for the representation of churches? Of course, there is a representation of a church with a steep, pitched wooden roof covered with flat tiles late in the thirteenth century (1280) in the church of the Panagia at Moutoullas.[71] More persuasively rendered examples appear later, in the representation of the church of the Archangel Michael of Pedoulas (1474),[72] or the church of Holy Cross of Agiasmati near Platanistassa.[73]

The use of a second, pitched roof covered with flat tiles is not uncommon in Cyprus. In the period under discussion, a second roof covers the domes and vaults of the churches of St. Nicholas of the Roof near Kakopetria, the Panagia tou Arakos near Lagoudera, St. Mavra near Koilani, the Panagia Amasgou near Monagri, and the Holy Cross, Pelendri. But when was such a second roof used for the first time? There is no concrete evidence about this. It is notable, however, that the church of St. Nicholas of the Roof is the only church in Cyprus that is named for its roof. Clearly, it had such a roof. The church of St. Nicholas is of the cross-in-square type with a dome, and it has a narthex with a blind dome like Asinou's, albeit without the lateral apses—though it is not unlikely that an apse was originally located on the north side of the narthex. There is no information about the exact date of its second roof, but it cannot be later than the second half of the twelfth century. This is indicated by the large icon of the patron saint that is now in the Byzantine Museum in Nicosia.[74] The icon, painted in the second half of the thirteenth century, identifies the saint as Ἅγιος Νικόλαος τῆς Στέγις, "St. Nicholas of the Roof," labeling him with what must have been the name of the church. Enough time must have passed since the roof was added that the church had come to be known as "of the roof." To support the new roof, the tops of the north and south walls were raised and gables were constructed above the east and west walls; the apse was not included. On the north wall there is an arched opening. The arch is more pointed than

68. Jeffery, *Description of the Historic Monuments*, 284.
69. Buxton et al., "Church of Asinou," pl. 93, fig. 1.
70. *ARDAC* for 1959, 13; Megaw and Hawkins, "Church of the Holy Apostles," 284, n. 22. Unfortunately, no photograph of the surface of the vault exists. The two photographs in the archives of the Department of Antiquities present the remaking of the lime concrete (hydraulic) over the dome of the narthex and the vault of the church.
71. Soteriou, *Βυζαντινὰ μνημεῖα*, pl. 90.
72. Ibid., pl. 100c.
73. Papageorgiou, *Οἱ ξυλόστεγοι ναοί της Κύπρου*, 83, fig. 22.
74. Papageorgiou, *Icons of Cyprus* [1992], pl. 32.

the arches and vaults of the narthex of the church at Asinou and the church of the Panagia tou Arakos, constructed earlier than the 1192 date of its paintings. However, this arch is not unlike the arches of the church of St. Basil near Xylotympou, dated by the style and iconography of its earliest paintings to the late twelfth century.[75] Therefore, a similar date, the second half of the twelfth century, is plausible also for the construction of the steep, pitched wooden roof with flat tiles over the original vaults and domes of the church of St. Nicholas. A link between the church of St. Nicholas and that of Asinou is offered by a remnant of the imitation cloisonné or marble revetment on the west gable of the second roof at St. Nicholas of the Roof, which resembles that in Asinou's narthex. Is it possible, therefore, that the second, steep, pitched wooden roof over the vault of Asinou was installed after the addition of the narthex, in the second half of the twelfth century? There is no information as to how the external surfaces of the vaults of the narthex were covered. Owing to the complexity of the surfaces, though, the pitched roof would have been a simple and relatively inexpensive solution. The second, pitched roof of the church was in poor condition by the time it attracted informed attention in 1918, when H. Peristianes gave a lecture on the "Ancient Town and the Church of Asinis (now 'Asinou')."[76] The photograph of the church published by Peristianes testifies to the fact that the wooden roof of the church was extended westward on a lower level to cover the narthex, as well. Further information about that roof is probably irretrievable: between the time of Peristianes's lecture and its publication in 1922, the roof was repaired by the Metropolis of Kyrenia under the supervision of George Jeffery (see below). It seems that the repair of the roof changed its appearance by removing the open gallery around the church. Indeed the photograph taken in 1931 and published in *Archaeologia* in 1933 presents the steeply pitched, wooden roof as it is today.[77]

Even the initial fabric of the church of Asinou has not been preserved in its original form. Like many other churches of Cyprus it has suffered from the frequent earthquakes and other vicissitudes that have struck the island during the past nine centuries.[78] Two areas of damage stand out. First, evidence of destruction is clear on the external face of the north wall of the church, around the north entrance (Fig. 2.18). A slight deformation is also evident on the vault of the central bay of the church (Figs. 2.16, 2.25). The repaired outer face of the upper part of the north wall is recessed in comparison with the original one, which leans outward. To strengthen the north wall, buttresses were constructed at each of its two ends. The buttress at the west end of the wall is rectangular, with dimensions of 1.04 m on the east side, 1.55 m on the north side, and 1.12 on the west (Fig. 2.5). At the eastern end of the wall is a flying buttress of 1.30 × 1.46 m, spanning a distance of 3.10 m including the buttress itself (Figs. 2.5, 2.26). The intrados of the arch is built of brick and tiles (*tegulae* and *imbrices*; Figs. 2.27, 2.28). The tiles of this buttress are 0.028 to 0.036 m thick. The mortar joints are similar. Another buttress is built at the west end of the south wall, measuring 1.07 m on its east side, 1.57 on the south, and 1.07 on the west (Fig. 2.2). There is no evidence regarding the date of the repairs of the north wall and the construction of the buttresses. It must have been later than the twelfth century, since the bricks used for the construction of the flying buttress are thinner by 0.060 to 0.070 m than

75. Spanou, "Η τέχνη στη μητροπολιτική περιφέρεια Κιτίου," 29–32, Figs. 12, 13; Chotzakoglou, "Βυζαντινή αρχιτεκτονική και τέχνη" (as in note 39 above), Figs. 494, 495.
76. Peristianes, *Μονογραφία τῆς ἀρχαίας πόλεως καὶ ἐκκλησίας τῆς Ἀσίνης (νῦν Ἀσίνους).*

77. Buxton et al., "Church of Asinou," pl. 93, fig. 1.
78. For the seismicity of Cyprus, see Abraseys, *Seismicity of Cyprus*. The author gives a bibliography on the earthquakes that affected Cyprus in the past and, on the basis of modern methods, examines all earthquakes that were felt in Cyprus from 1894 to 1991, even if the epicenter was in a neighboring country. Grivaud, in *Villages désertés à Chypre*, 431–33, gives a catalogue of earthquakes from 1181 to 1870 CE.

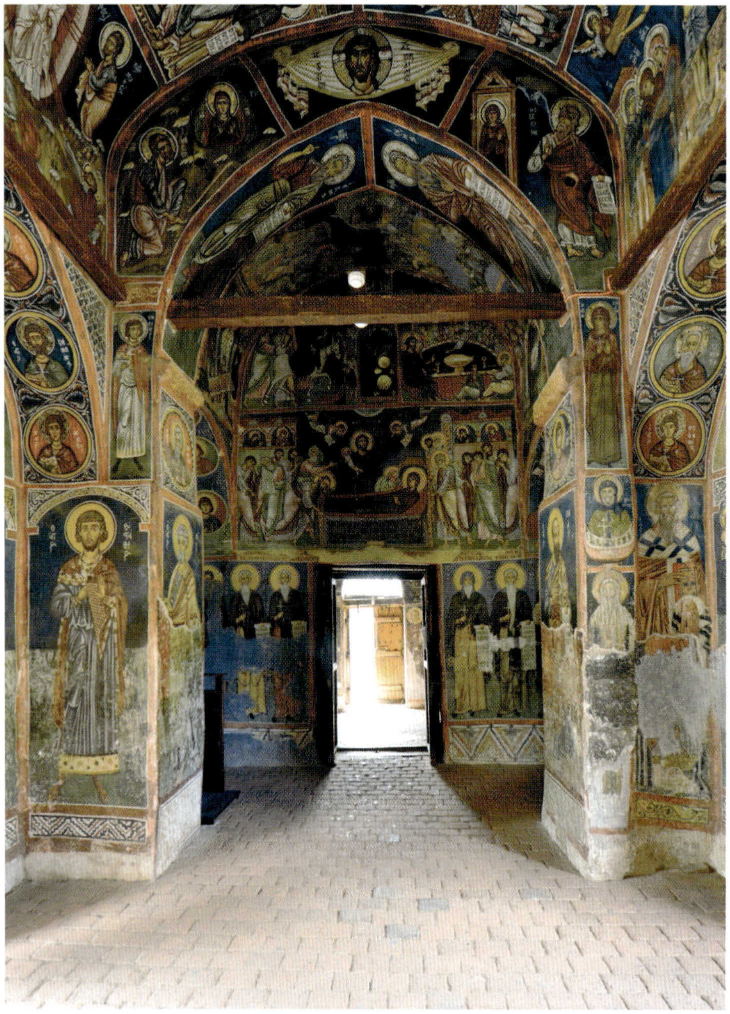

FIG. 2.25 The interior of the naos of the church of Asinou, looking west (photo courtesy of G. L. Carr)

those used for the arches of the church and the narthex. At the same time, four engaged responds were constructed against the existing ones inside the church, supporting two strongly pointed arches under the original, semicircular transverses that divide the vault into three bays. The responds inside the church seem to have been built in haste. They are not rectangular and the western respond of the north wall protrudes to the east by 0.12 to 0.18 m, forming an irregular angle where it joins the original one (Fig. 2.1).

A second major area of damage is the semidome of the apse. The original semidome collapsed, and was reconstructed and enlarged by adding two responds on either side of the apse.[79] The new semidome is pointed and extends inward to cover a portion of the painting of the Ascension on the eastern part of the vault of the church (Fig. 2.29). The responds supporting the new semidome masked the original paintings of the Annunciation and the Communion of St. Mary of Egypt (Figs. 2.30–32).[80] These paintings were revealed again after two iron pipes replaced the responds during the repairs of the church in 1953–54 by the Department of Antiquities (Fig. 6.4, 6.5).

Was the damage to the apse contemporary with that to the central bay of the naos? There is no information about the date of the damage to these two areas. The materials used for the repairs of the central part of the north wall, the construction of the internal responds and the two arches they support, and the construction of the responds used for the extension of the apse are all similar. This is quite clear. The west face of the two responds supporting the western arch of the central bay of the church (Fig. 2.19, at left), as well as the western face of that arch, remain undecorated (Fig. 6.1). The same is true of the east face of the two eastern responds and the east face of the arch they support, as well as part of the south face of the east respond of the north wall and the north face of the east respond of the south wall, above the existing iconostasis and up to the paintings of David and Solomon adorning the upper parts of the two responds (Figs. 2.29, 6.37, 6.42 [at right]). Also undecorated were the two responds added to the east wall of the church to support the extension of the apse (Figs. 2.30, 2.31). The masonry of the responds on the north and south walls is similar to the masonry of the two responds of the east wall removed in 1954.

There is, however, a problem. The paintings in the extended semidome of the apse are not contemporary with those that adorn the central bay of the naos, the added responds of the north and

79. Buxton et al., "Church of Asinou," 330 and plans on 334–35; *ARDAC* for 1954, 10.
80. *ARDAC* for 1954, 10.

FIG. 2.26
The flying buttress on the north side of the church of Asinou (photo courtesy of Athanasios Papageorgiou)

FIG. 2.27
The intrados of the flying buttress on the north side of the church of Asinou (photo courtesy of Athanasios Papageorgiou)

FIG. 2.28
The intrados of the flying buttress on the north side of the church of Asinou: detail of bricks (photo courtesy of Athanasios Papageorgiou)

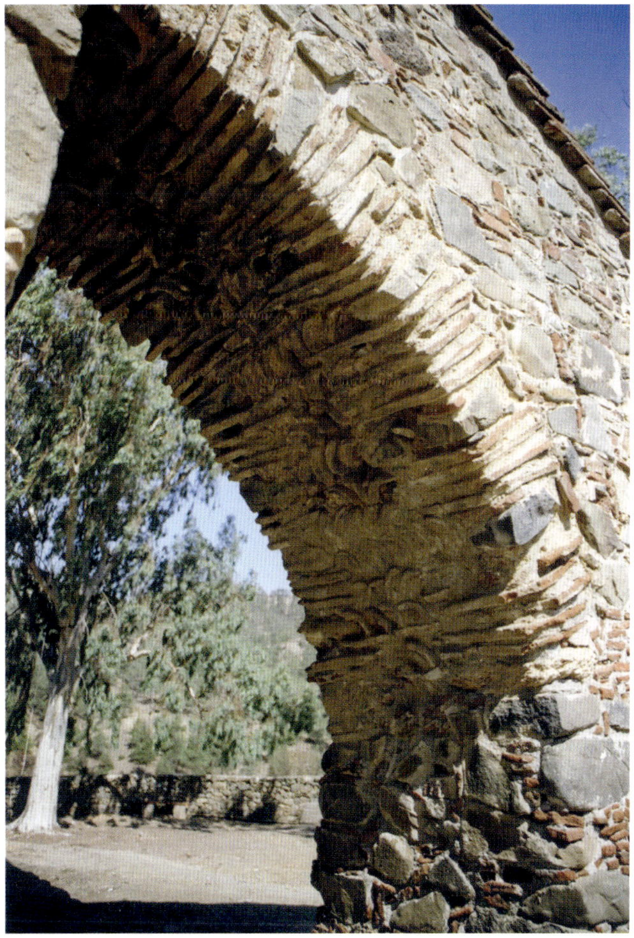

fig. 2.27

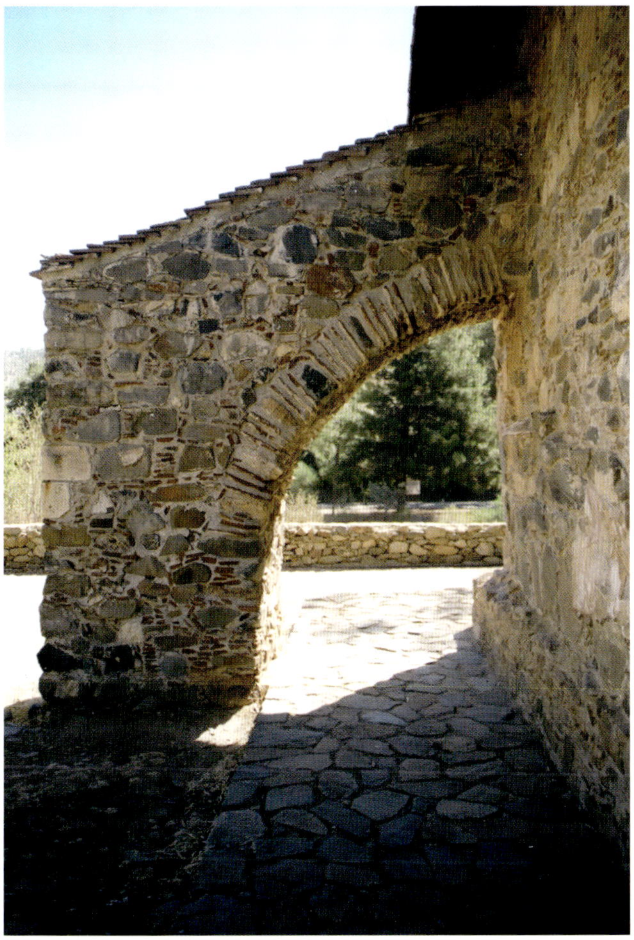

fig. 2.26

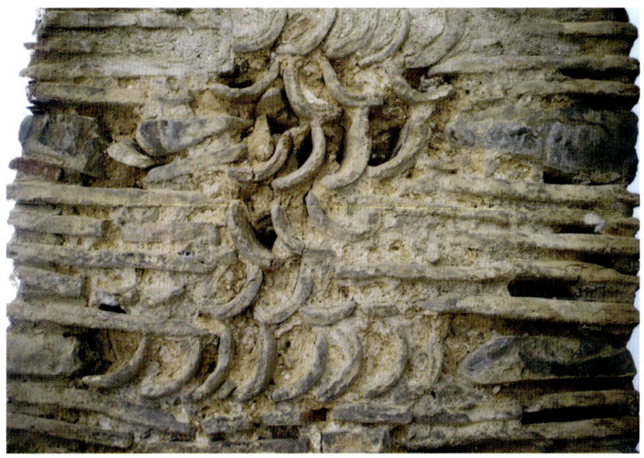

fig. 2.28

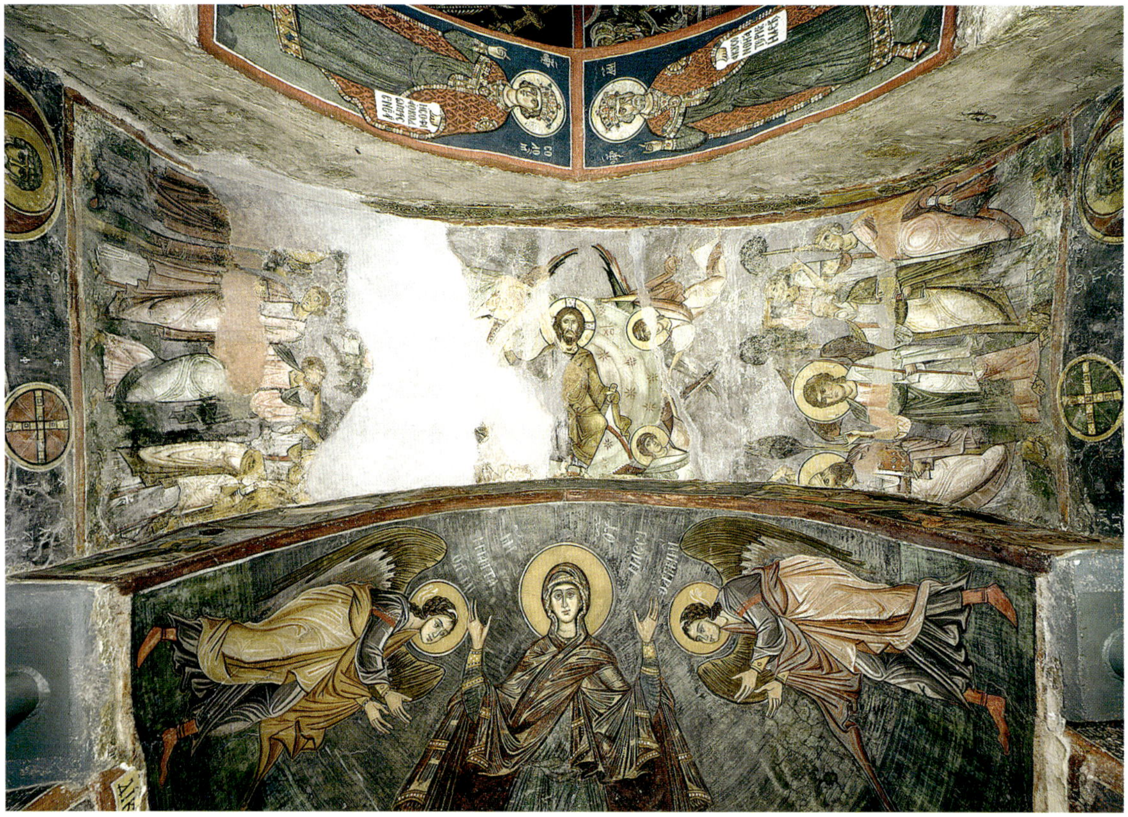

fig. 2.29

FIG. 2.29
Bema vault of Asinou, showing the bare east face of the added transverse arch (photo courtesy of Dumbarton Oaks, B.T.As.F.1.1)

FIG. 2.30
Respond constructed on the east wall, south of the apse of Asinou, to support the extended semidome, before its removal (photo courtesy of Athanasios Papageorgiou)

FIG. 2.31
Respond constructed on the east wall, north of the apse of Asinou, to support the extended semidome, before its removal (photo courtesy of Athanasios Papageorgiou)

FIG. 2.32
East wall, north side of apse. St. Mary of Egypt, revealed after a respond was replaced by a metal pipe (photo courtesy of G. L. Carr)

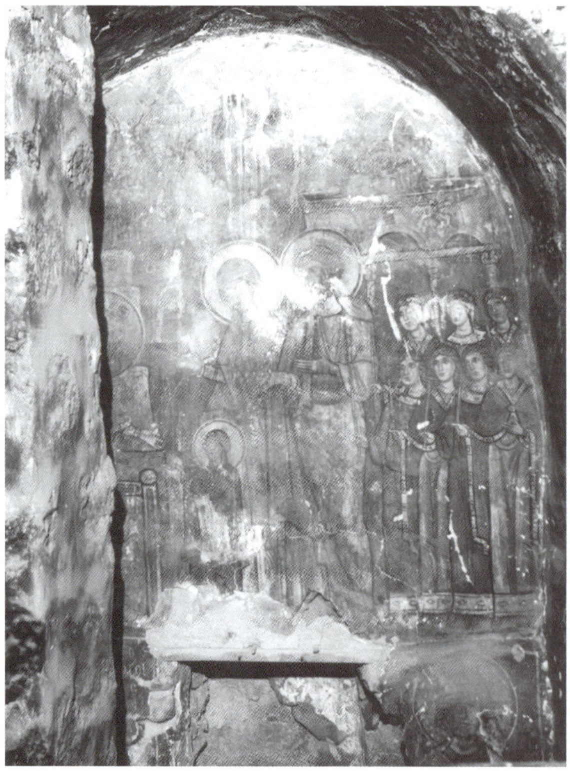

fig. 2.30

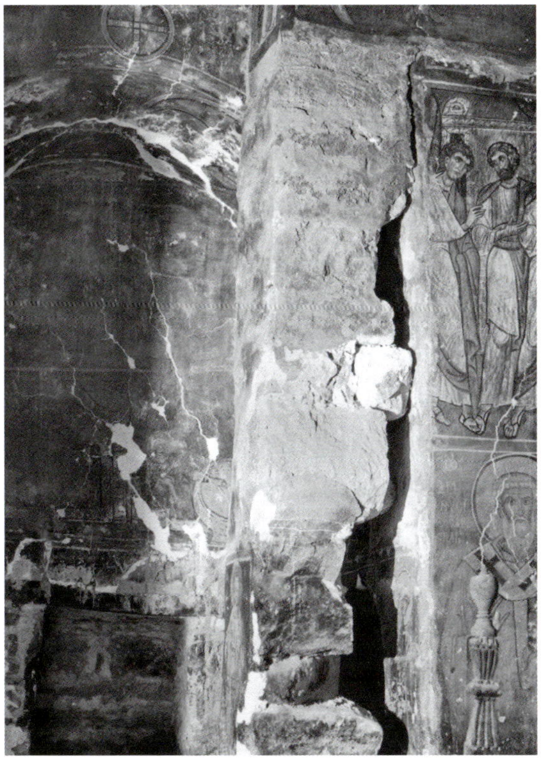

fig. 2.31

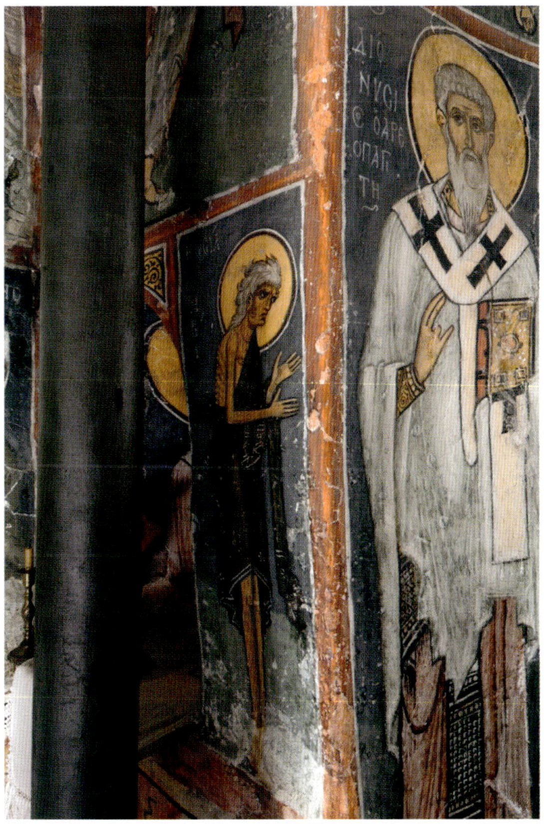

fig. 2.32

south walls, and the arches they support. The Virgin orant between the archangels Michael and Gabriel painted in the semidome of the extended apse has been dated to the thirteenth century,[81] while the paintings decorating the added responds and arches supporting the central bay of the church look later. Should, therefore, the damage to these areas also be assigned to two different periods? Although no date is preserved, the reconstruction of the apse conch must have occurred in the thirteenth century, as the dating of its paintings to the thirteenth century is now generally accepted. Did the repairs to the central part of the north wall and the addition of the four responds to the arches in the central bay also take place in the thirteenth century? If so, only the two western responds received adornment in the thirteenth century, and both the arches and the central part of the vault remained unadorned until the redecoration of the central bay. This is not impossible, for portions of the responds and the arches they support remain undecorated still today. Moreover, much of the original painting on the north and south walls must have remained, for the lower parts can still be seen under the later paintings. However, no evidence is preserved on the central part of the vault of any paintings of 1105/6.[82] Could the central part of the vault have remained without decoration for a long period? It is this part of the church that the faithful see when entering through the north and south doors.

81. Young, in "Byzantine Painting," 329–34, suggested that, because the wall paintings in the enlarged semidome of the apse were painted in the 13th century, the semidome of the apse must have collapsed in the 13th century. We have information about two earthquakes in the area of Paphos during the 13th century, but not in the area of Asinou. However, information about seismic activity in Cyprus is not complete. Thus, if the wall paintings of the semidome of the enlarged apse of Asinou are of the 13th century (see also Chapters 5–6), then the destruction of the apse and the deformation of the central part of the vault could have been caused by an earthquake in the 13th century.
82. David Winfield found insignificant remnants of earlier wall paintings under the existing ones, which cannot be dated.

But there is another possibility. The damage to the central part of the north wall and the deformation of the central part of the vault may have happened later. Indeed, several earthquakes struck Cyprus during the thirteenth and early fourteenth centuries. Thus an earthquake in 1222 is reported by scribe C in Vatican, Palat. gr. 367: "On Wednesday, May 11, at the sixth hour occurred the divinely caused wrath of the great earthquake in the year 6730."[83] This earthquake destroyed the castle of Saranda Kolones in Paphos, according to Oliver Scholasticus.[84] Another disastrous earthquake struck Cyprus on 12 May 1227. This earthquake is reported on folio 217 of Paris. gr. 1588:

> And on the same day occurred a great earthquake on this island of Cyprus, and many churches and many villages and the kastron of Paphos were destroyed, and many people were killed, men and women and children, and the earthquake lasted four years [sic]... of the year 673[5] on Wednesday at the third hour of the day.[85]

Florio Bustron reports that in 1267 "Cyprus was visited by plague, locusts, and *many earthquakes*."[86] Scribe A recorded on folio 172r of Vatican, Palat. gr. 367 yet another earthquake on 8 August 1303: "In the month of August of the year [6]811 on the fifth day at the first hour of the day a big earthquake happened in the city of Nicosia."[87] Though this earthquake was "big" (μέγας), it caused no damage in Cyprus according to Florio Bustron.[88] It is possible therefore that the semidome of Asinou's apse was destroyed by one of the thirteenth-century earthquakes, more plausibly that of either 1222 or 1227, which were very destructive, than that of 1267, for which Bustron gave no report of damage. Thus the reconstruction and accompanying enlargement of the apse would have taken place after 1227.

The repairs to the external face of the central part of the north wall are not dated (Fig. 2.18). We have no information concerning the redecoration of the central area around the north door. Today the Deesis above the door is badly damaged. Since it now leans outward, it is probable that an earthquake caused the damage to the north wall. No remnants of any repainting survive, which is curious, since it was usual in medieval Cyprus to fill in damaged parts or to undertake a complete repainting. However, one must bear in mind that this painting and the adjacent wall painting of the Anastasis were exposed to the weather as the overhang of the second, wooden roof gave way to damage. It must not therefore be ruled out that the area around the north door was refurbished, and that this was destroyed when it was exposed to the weather. Since these wall paintings are earlier than the thirteenth century, however, they are not useful in dating the damage to the wall.

83. Constantinides and Browning, *Dated Greek Manuscripts*, 161; Schreiner, *Die byzantinischen Kleinchroniken*, 1:199: Μηνὶ Μαίω ῑᾱ ἡμέρ(α) τετράδ(η) ὅρ(α) ἕκτη γέγον(εν) ἡ θεόηλατ(ος) ὀργὴ τοῦ μ(εγάλ)ου σεισμοῦ εις τὴν ͵ςψλ ἐχρονί(αν). See also Komodikes, "Θεομηνίες και Θεοσημίες στην Κύπρο," 126–27.

84. Megaw, "Supplementary Excavations on a Castle Site," 327, n. 15.

85. Darrouzès, "Un obituaire chypriote," 44: καὶ τῇ αὐτῇ ἡμέρᾳ ἐγένετο σεισμὸς μέγας ἐν τῇδε τῇ νίσσῳ τῇ Κύπρῳ καὶ ἐχάλασαν ἐκκλησίαι πολλαὶ καὶ χωρία πολλὰ καὶ τὸ κάστρο ἡ Πάφος καὶ ἐφονεύθησαν λαὸς πολλὺς ἄνδρες τε καὶ γυναῖκες καὶ νίπια καὶ ἐκράτισεν ὁ σεισμὸς χρόνους τέσσαρες.... καθολ.... ἡμέραν, ἔτους ͵ςψλ[ε], ἡμέρᾳ τετάρτῃ, ὥρᾳ τρίτῃ τῆς ἡμέρας. See also Schreiner, *Die byzantinischen Kleinchroniken*, 2:607; Constantinides and Browning, *Dated Greek Manuscripts*, 77.

86. Bustron, *Historia overo commentarii de Cipro*, 112: "venne in Cipro la peste le cavalette e *molti terremoti*."

87. Constantinides and Browning, *Dated Greek Manuscripts*, 161; Schreiner, *Die byzantinischen Kleinchroniken*, 1:203: "+ Μηνὶ αὐγούστω η̄ τ(ῆς) ω̄ῑᾱ εγχρ(ο)ν(ίας) ἡμέρ(ᾳ) ε' ὥρ(α) α τ(ῆς) ἡμέρ(ας) γέγονε σεισμὸ(ς) μ(έ)γ(ας) ἐν τῇ πόλ(ει) λευκουσία."

88. Bustron, *Historia*, 134: "Del 1303 alli 8 agosto, in l'isola di Cipro, fu un' gram terremoto, e duro assai, il cale fu sentito in molti loci del mondo, et in Candia e Rhodi, fece gran danno con molte de piu persone. In Cipro per merse del Nostro Signor Iddio non la fatto danno alcuno di momentos." See also Hill, *History of Cyprus*, 2:216 and note 4, where other sources are mentioned.

If we take the damage to the apse as a terminus post quem and the fourteenth-century date of the overpainting in the central bay as a terminus ante quem, we must seek a date for the damage to the north wall in the later thirteenth or fourteenth centuries. The written sources have cited two earthquakes, those of 1267 and 1303, not to mention the possibility of further, unrecorded earthquakes during the first half of the fourteenth century. As 1267 is early for our purposes, we must settle upon the earthquake of 1303, or some other unrecorded during the first half of the fourteenth century. It is true that Florio Bustron discounted the destructiveness of this earthquake, but it struck Nicosia and was qualified as "great" in the relevant note in Vatican, Palat. gr. 367. Yet another hypothesis must not be excluded completely. A tornado is usually accompanied by heavy rainfall, lightning, and thunder. Such a tornado struck the lands belonging to the monastery of the Panagia Phorbiotissa itself in the area of Zodia-Katokopia on 16 July 1319.[89] Damage from this tornado or the accompanying lightning might have struck the central part of the north wall, although this cannot be proved. At any rate, the repairs to the central part of the north wall and the hasty construction of the buttresses, responds, and transverse arches might have taken place in the first half of the fourteenth century, and the central bay of the church, including the responds and arches, might have been redecorated soon thereafter.

Toward the end of the eighteenth century the monastery was abandoned, like many other monasteries in Cyprus. Since then the monastic buildings have been destroyed and only the church has survived. The debris of the monastic buildings seen at the beginning of the twentieth century by George Jeffery, of which there is a photograph in the State Archives (Fig. 1.6), had disappeared before the 1940s. The church was left without any maintenance for a long period. The doors, except the west door of the narthex and the north door of the main church, were destroyed and walled up.

By this time, the steeply pitched wooden roof was badly damaged and most of its tiles were lost.[90] The penetration of rainwater through the vault caused damage to some of the original wall paintings: the Pentecost, the Washing of the Feet, the Ascension, and the paintings in the two eastern blind arches of the church. Already at the beginning of the twentieth century, the church's need for repairs was urgent. In 1907 the Commissioner of Kyrenia, Major J. Tankerville Chamberlayne, author of the book *Lacrimae Nicossienses*, sent the committee of the Cyprus Museum three photographs and a letter describing the deplorable state of the church. The secretary of the committee forwarded the three photographs to the then-curator of antiquities. These photographs, unfortunately, were lost.[91]

In 1908 Professor Simos Menardos, a member of the committee of the Cyprus Museum, drew the attention of the committee members to the great number of Byzantine churches and their great antiquarian interest and urged the committee to take steps for the preservation—insofar as might be possible—of the structures themselves and of the fresco paintings contained in many of them. The secretary of the committee addressed a request to George Jeffery, who was interested in the church of Asinou. On 25 March 1908, Jeffery sent his report on the church to the committee of the Cyprus Museum.[92] As of 1919, however, nothing had been done. In that year Principal Forest Officer Bovill addressed a letter to the chief secretary asking for a chief carpenter from the Public Works Department to supervise the repairs of the second, steeply pitched roof of the church of Asinou. Attached to his letter was a photograph of the church, which is still preserved.[93] In his letter, Bovill stated that he intended to provide the necessary wood, while the Metropolis of Kyrenia

89. Constantinides and Browning, *Dated Greek Manuscripts*, 50; Darrouzès, "Notes pour servir" [1953], 92.

90. Report of G. Jeffery. SA file 1:3591/ 1907, red 11.
91. SA file 1:3591/ 1907, reds 1–2.
92. SA file 1:3591/ 1907, reds 14–17.
93. SA file 767/ 1919, red 2.

agreed to undertake the expenses. The church of Asinou was declared an Ancient Monument in 1920 as the result of a letter from the curator of the Cyprus Museum, M. Markides, to the chief secretary, dated 30 October 1919.[94] After that the repair of the church took place, as described by Peristianes.[95]

In 1954 the church was again in bad condition. The north and south walls had each split into two leaves with a cavity in between, and the pitched roof was badly damaged. "The cavities were grouted and to bind the structure together and resist the thrust of the roof-timbers, which being laid in the vaulting have no cross-ties, the whole church (the narthex alone excepted) was ringed with a reinforced concrete collar concealed in the masonry."[96]

In 1959 the top of the vault of the church was repaired and its exterior covered with lime concrete. The wooden supports of the tile roof were renewed and damaged tiles were replaced.[97] In December 1985 the ninth ordinary session of the UNESCO World Heritage Committee added the church of the Panagia Phorbiotissa Asinou to the list of world heritage monuments.[98]

94. SA file: 767/ 1919, r. 4.
95. Peristianes, *Μονογραφία*.
96. *ARDAC* for 1954, 10.
97. *ARDAC* for 1959, 13.
98. Report Maison de l'UNESCO, SC-85/CONF.008/9.

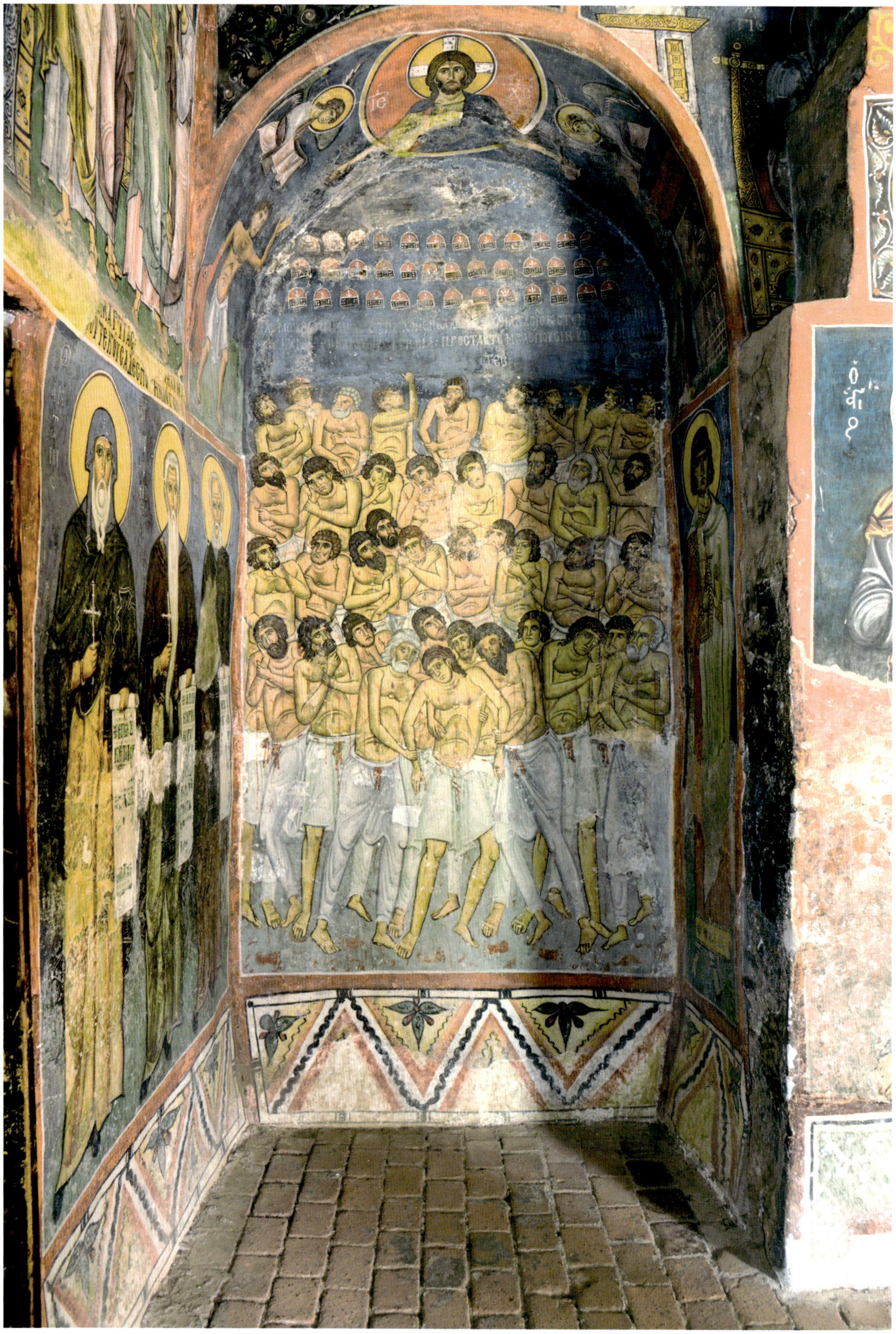

The church of Panagia Phorbiotissa, naos, western bay, north wall: The Forty Martyrs of Sebaste (photo courtesy of G.L. Carr)

CHAPTER THREE

The Metrical Inscriptions in the Murals of the Panagia Phorbiotissa

Nancy Patterson Ševčenko

Every fresco in the church of Asinou, regardless of period, is accompanied by some kind of writing—most often a caption identifying a holy portrait or a narrative scene, or a Biblical citation. In some cases, however, the writing is more extensive and may include a poem in twelve-syllable verse. It is to these latter inscriptions that this chapter is devoted.[1]

In twelve-syllable verse, a favored poetic form in the middle Byzantine period, each line has two parts, one consisting of five syllables and one of seven. The sequence of these two parts can be altered at will, but there is regularly a stress on the penultimate—that is, the eleventh—syllable. The poems that appear on the frescoes at Asinou comprise anywhere between two and eight lines of verse. Although the lines are sometimes written out continuously, the ends of many individual lines are

1. Many inscriptions in the church were transcribed by W. H. Buckler in Buxton et al., "Church of Asinou," 335–45; by Stylianou and Stylianou, "Donors and Dedicatory Inscriptions," 98–99; and by Sacopoulo, *Asinou en 1106*, esp. 9–13. Fresh transcriptions made to confirm or to correct those done by Buckler were undertaken by Ihor Ševčenko in 1966, when the cleaning of the frescoes was still in progress. The entire Asinou team owes a debt of gratitude to Professor Ševčenko for his invaluable assistance. For a preliminary report on the metrical inscriptions at Asinou, see N. P. Ševčenko, "Painted Metrical Inscriptions at Asinou." Since this chapter was written in 2002, two masterly studies of Byzantine epigrams have been published, which deal with the issues raised here in a somewhat more philological context: Lauxtermann, *Byzantine Poetry from Pisides to Geometres*, and Rhoby, *Byzantinische Epigramme auf Fresken und Mosaiken*. In the latter publication an entire section (pp. 341–52) is devoted to the transcription (with previous readings noted) and analysis of the epigrams on the frescoes at Asinou. I have adopted or adapted Rhoby's transcriptions in most cases, and tried to incorporate references to both these important studies wherever possible. Additional articles on epigrams are contained in the acts of a workshop on the subject held in Vienna in 2006: Hörandner and Rhoby, *Die Kulturhistorische Bedeutung Byzantinischer Epigramme*. I also wish to thank the three anonymous reviewers for their careful reading of this text, and for their invaluable suggestions and rectifications.

marked with a pair or more of vertically arranged painted dots, a feature that greatly helps the scholar to reconstruct these poems.[2]

The poems at Asinou, although all in twelve-syllable verse, are of several different types and periods. Among the twelfth-century ones is the six-verse dedicatory inscription that accompanies the portrait of the donor Nikephoros the magistros and his wife on the south wall of the naos; though the fresco was painted in the fourteenth century, the inscription appears to be a faithful copy of the twelfth-century original. There is Nikephoros's appeal to the Virgin Pantanassa written around the base of the conch of the apse, and yet another poem addressed to the Virgin written under the scene of the Dormition on the west wall of the naos. In addition, there are the short poems written on the fresco of the Forty Martyrs, located on the north wall of the naos (four verses); on the scenes of the Birth and Presentation of the Virgin in the bema (two verses each); and on the responds of the apse, accompanying the scene of the Ascension in the vault above.

The other poems attached to frescoes at Asinou include a dedicatory inscription written to accompany the late twelfth-century mounted figure of St. George in the narthex, and a poem written around the image of the Virgin Phorbiotissa in the lunette over the door from the narthex into the naos (four verses?). There are also two variants of a familiar poem, the Virgin's appeal to Christ for mercy on mankind, written on scrolls held by two different figures of the Virgin, one of 1332/33 located near the entrance from narthex to naos (two verses) and the other a slightly later, fourteenth-century figure located near the entrance to the bema from the naos (five verses).

Although twelve-syllable verses were composed for every sort of Byzantine occasion, they are known today primarily from Byzantine literary anthologies, where they are shorn of their original context, or from inscribed works of art found primarily in stone, metal, ivory, manuscripts, and textiles—but rarely, except for dedicatory verses, in monumental painting.[3] The metrical inscriptions in the church at Asinou provide us with a rare opportunity to examine the use of such poetry in the context of church decoration. Do the twelfth-century verses at Asinou represent what was once common practice, or is the church an aberration, a reflection of the special concerns of a specific patron?

The texts of the Asinou poems are presented here in roughly chronological order, beginning with the poems written on frescoes dating from the campaign of 1106.

A. The Twelfth-Century Poems

1. Poems Accompanying the Narrative Scenes

The fresco of the Forty Martyrs of Sebaste in the northwest corner of the naos at Asinou is divided into two tiers: in the lower half of the composition, the martyrs shiver in the freezing lake; in the upper half, Christ lowers their crowns of martyrdom. Between the two tiers, running across the whole width of the fresco, a poem has been inscribed on the blue background in two long lines. Two

2. On Byzantine twelve-syllable (dodecasyllable) verse, see Maas, "Der byzantinische Zwölfsilber."

3. The complex relationship of the epigrams transcribed in Byzantine literary anthologies to surviving works of art in other media has received considerable scholarly attention in recent times. The list that follows names only those studies that have been published since 1992: Hörandner, "Ein Zyklus von Epigrammen" and "Cycle of Epigrams"; Olster, "Byzantine Hermeneutics"; Lauxtermann, "Byzantine Epigram"; Talbot, "Epigrams of Manuel Philes"; Maguire, *Image and Imagination*, 1–25; Papamastorakes, "Επιτύμβιες παράστασεις," with English summary; I. Ševčenko, "Lost Panels of the North Door"; Talbot, "Epigrams in Context"; Grossmann, "Zur nicht erhaltenen Nordtür der Dornbuschkapelle"; I. Ševčenko, "Captions to a David Cycle"; Hörandner, "Randbemerkungen zum Thema Epigramme und Kunstwerke"; Lauxtermann, *Byzantine Poetry*; Kepetzi, "Autour d'une inscription métrique"; and Rhoby, *Byzantinische Epigramme*. A corpus of opening lines has been assembled by Vassis, *Initia carminum Byzantinorum*.

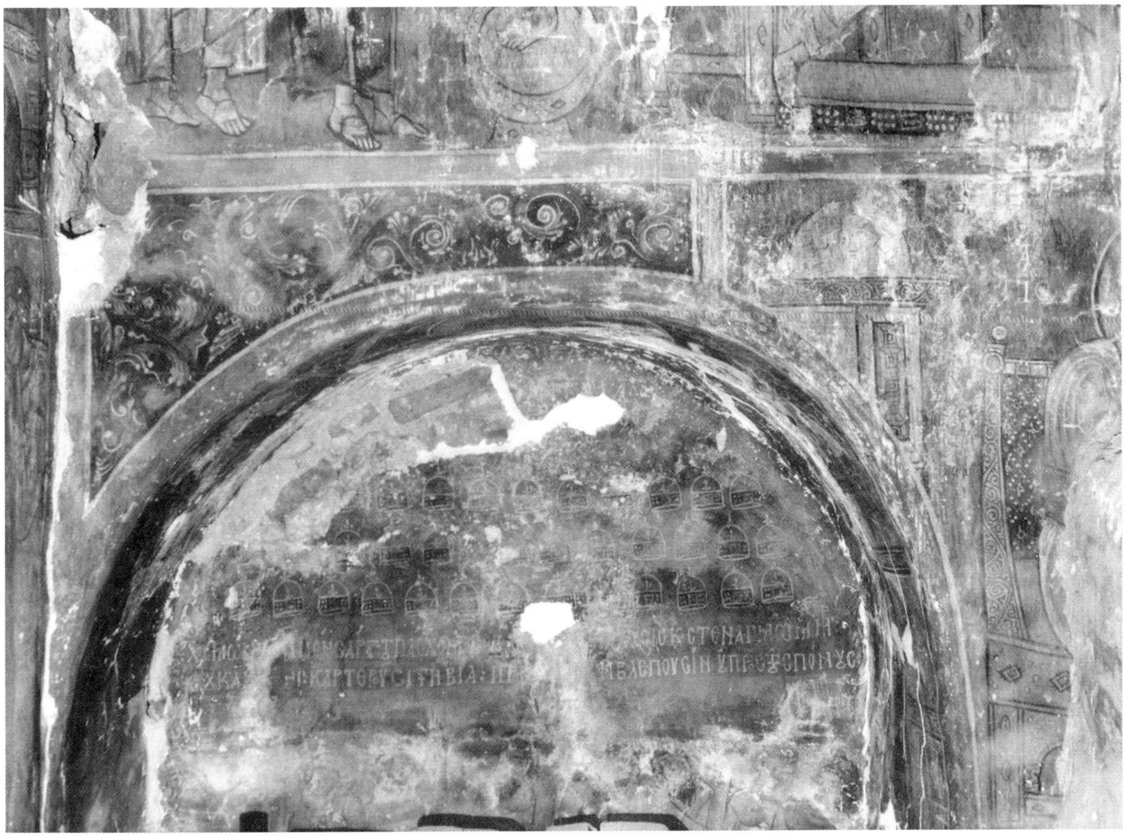

FIG. 3.1 Naos, western bay, north wall. Forty Martyrs of Sebaste: verse inscription (photo courtesy of Dumbarton Oaks, Cyprus, Department of Antiquities, No. C 2983)

twelve-syllable verses are contained in each line of writing (Fig. 3.1):[4]

> \+ Χιμῶν [. . .]πόν σάρξ το πάσχον ενθάδε:
> [. . .]σχόν ακουσὶς κ(αὶ) στεναγμω[.] μ(α)ρ(τύρων): /
> [. . .] ουκ ακο[υσ]ης καρτερούσι τη βία:
> προς τα στέφι βλέπουσιν· οὐ πρὸς τοὺς πόνους [+]

As scholars have already noted, this epigram, however well suited to the fresco it accompanies, was not invented for the Asinou composition itself, but rather is a version of a poem composed at a considerably earlier date by John Geometres (tenth century). It is known from Byzantine literary anthologies.

> \+ Χειμὼν τὸ λυποῦν, σὰρξ τὸ πάσχον ἐνθάδε·
> προσσχὼν ἀκούσεις καὶ στεναγμὸν μαρτύρων·
> εἰ δ' οὐκ ἀκούσεις, καρτεροῦσι τὴν βίαν,
> πρὸς τὰ στέφη βλέποντες, οὐ πρὸς τοὺς πόνους. +[5]

4. Rhoby, *Byzantinische Epigramme*, 350–52, no. 237.

5. Published from Paris. suppl. gr. 690, fol. 118v by Sternbach, *Methodii patriarchae et Ignatii patriarchae carmina inedita*, 156–57, who attributes the poem to Mauropous, and by Sajdak, "Spicilegium Geometreum," [*Eos* 32] 197 (# 8), who attributes it to Geometres (pp. 193–95). The poem is one of a group of five poems to the Forty Martyrs contained in this manuscript. See also Lauxtermann, "Byzantine Epigram," 59, 141–44, and now his *Byzantine Poetry*, 149–50; Maguire, *Image and Imagination*, 12–13, and his earlier "Depiction of Sorrow," 152. Lauxtermann has introduced convincing evidence for the attribution to Geometres, noting that the 10th-century "Anonymous Patrician" plagiarizes phrases of the poem in one of his own (Ἄνθρωπε πρόσχες . . . εἰ δ' οὐκ ἀκούσεις, τὴν τέχνην μὴ φαυλίσῃς;

Winter (brings) the pain, flesh the suffering here.
If you pay attention, you will even hear the groans of the martyrs;
But if you do not listen, they will (still) endure the violence (of the cold),
Looking to the crowns, not to the toils.[6]

This poem enjoyed a certain success, and with varying attributions was copied in a number of different Byzantine manuscripts.[7]

Despite its venerable origin, the poem fits nicely with the twelfth-century composition at Asinou. All the imagery of the poem is visible: the ice-blue lake, the suffering bodies and melancholy faces of the martyrs, and their upward glances or gestures directed toward the hovering crowns.[8] The word ἐνθάδε in the first line indicates that the poem was intended to refer to an actual image.[9] Its language suggests that the reader stands before a representation so vivid as to make audible the very groans of the martyrs. Even if they are not heard, the Forty still endure the pain of the bitter cold and concentrate upon the arrival of their martyrs' crowns. The poem dwells on this moment of transition and transcendence, and is located appropriately between the representation of the bodily trials of the martyrs and the vision of their heavenly reward.

Though the contemporary images of the Forty Martyrs in the Cypriot churches of St. Nicholas of the Roof (τῆς Στέγης) at Kakopetria and SS. Joachim and Anna at Kalliana are both extremely similar to that at Asinou, neither incorporates a poem into the composition.[10] Nor do we know of any surviving Forty Martyrs composition—regardless of medium—accompanied by this or any other poem, despite the poem's success in literary circles and the existence of images of the Forty Martyrs in this very form from the tenth century on.[11]

Lampros, "Τὰ ὑπ' ἀριθμὸν ΡΙΖ' καὶ ΡΓ' κατάλοιπα," 49, ll. 5, 9), which he could scarcely have done with any work of Mauropous. See Lauxtermann, *Byzantine Poetry*, 169, 298–99, Rhoby, *Byzantinische Epigramme*, 350–51, and Opstall, "Verses on Paper," 55 and fig. 1.

6. This translation slightly modifies those provided by Maguire, *Image and Imagination*, 12, Lauxtermann, *Byzantine Poetry*, 149, and Opstall, "Verses on Paper," 55, to accord more precisely with the version inscribed on the fresco. The Geometres poem uses βλέποντες instead of βλέπουσιν in the last line, and τὴν βίαν instead of τῃ βίᾳ at the end of the previous line. The letter between the omega of στεναγμω and μαρτύρων should by rights be a N, but it looks instead like the abbreviation of the first half of the word megalomartyr, often abbreviated to μγμρ, which, however, would not work with the meter of the poem.

7. It appears with slight variations under the name of Manuel Philes in the Florence collection of his poems (Bibl. Laurenziana, Plut. XXXII: 19, fol. 288v), Miller, *Manuelis Philae Carmina*, 1:438 (Florence no. 241). See Lauxtermann, "Byzantine Epigram," 142; *Byzantine Poetry*, 298 note 10; 301. Two anonymous poems on the Forty Martyrs from a 10th-century manuscript in Oxford (Bodl. Barocci 50) have been published by Browning, "Unpublished Corpus," 304 (nos. 26–27). There are also two poems by Christopher of Mitylene (11th century): Kurtz, *Die Gedichte des Christophoros Mitylenaios*, 68 (no. 106), 90–91 (no. 133); another is attributed to Philes in Miller, *Manuelis Philae Carmina*, 1:35 (Escorial no. 79).

8. The poem does not, however, include all the elements found in the painted composition at Asinou: it leaves out, except by implication, the figure of Christ, as well as the subplot of the flight of one of the Forty to the warm bath on the shore, and the eager bath attendant who hastens to take his place. These elements at Asinou, it should be said, are relegated to the vault framing the lunette with the main composition. For the relation of the iconography to Byzantine rhetoric on the Forty Martyrs, see Maguire, *Art and Eloquence in Byzantium*, 34–42.

9. Lauxtermann, *Byzantine Poetry*, 151; I. Ševčenko, "Captions to a David Cycle," 336; Follieri, "Un carmine giambico," 103–5.

10. Stylianou and Stylianou, *Painted Churches*, Figs. 22, 50. For a color plate of the Kakopetria fresco, see Hein et al., *Cyprus*, fig. 47.

11. For the iconography of the composition of the Forty Martyrs, see the entry "Forty Martyrs of Sebasteia" in *ODB* 2:799–800, with references.

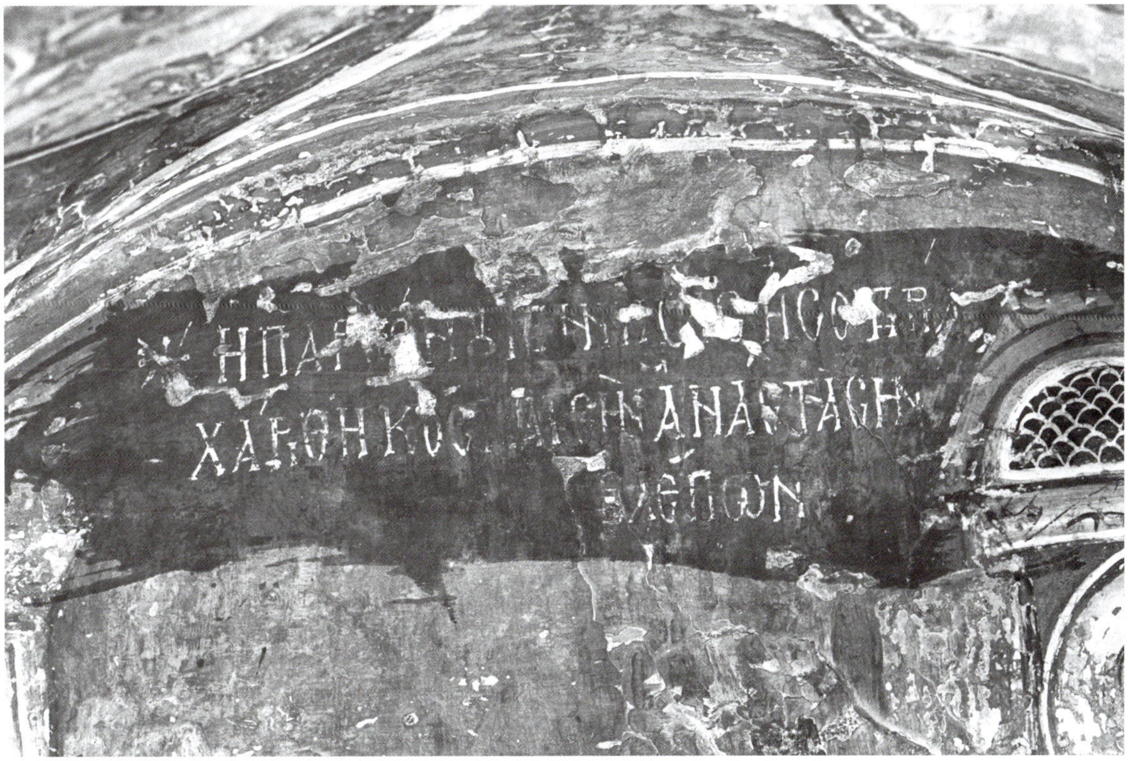

FIG. 3.2 Bema, north wall. Birth of the Virgin: verse inscription (photo courtesy of Dumbarton Oaks # L 67.985 [IŠ])

The epigram accompanying the scene of the Birth of the Virgin on the north wall of the bema is shorter, being just two verses long (Fig. 3.2).[12]

+ ἡ παρθένου γεννησις ἡ σοτηρία /
χάριθη κόσμαι σὴν ἀνάστασην / βλέπων [+]

corrected as:

+ ἡ παρθένου γέννησις, ἡ σωτηρία.
χάρηθι, κόσμε, σὴν ἀνάστασιν βλέπων. +

The birth of the Virgin (means) salvation.
Rejoice, O world, seeing your resurrection.

The poem is written across the top of the fresco. It emphasizes how the Virgin's birth constitutes the beginning of the story of salvation, a theme encountered in the day's homiletics and hymnography as well.[13] Though the poem does not directly refer to

12. Rhoby, *Byzantinische Epigramme*, 352, no. 238. For a color plate, see Hadjichristodoulou and Myrianthefs, *Church of Our Lady of Asinou*, 17.

13. Cf. the homily of John of Damascus on the Birth of the Virgin: Σήμερον ἀρχὴ σωτηρίας τῷ κόσμῳ. Ἀλαλάξατε τῷ κυρίῳ, πᾶσα ἡ γῆ, ᾄσατε καὶ ἀγαλλιᾶσθε, καὶ ψάλλετε (PG 96:669B). Cf. also the troparia of the feast (September 8): Ἰωακεὶμ καὶ ἡ Ἄννα πανηγυρίζουσι, τὴν ἀπαρχὴν τεκόντες τῆς ἡμῶν σωτηρίας (*Μηναῖον τοῦ Σεπτεμβρίου*, 100: for Little Vespers); Σήμερον τῆς παγκοσμίου χαρᾶς τὰ προοίμια· σήμερον ἔπνευσαν αὖραι, σωτηρίας προάγγελοι (102: for Great Vespers); Ἡ γέννησίς σου Θεοτόκε, χαρὰν ἐμήνυσε πάσῃ τῇ οἰκουμένῃ . . . Χριστός . . . καταργήσας τὸν θάνατον, ἐδωρήσατο ἡμῖν ζωὴν τὴν αἰώνιον (105: for Great Vespers), etc. For translations of these troparia, see Mary and Ware, *Festal Menaion*, 98–130. See also Schirò, *Analecta Hymnica Graeca, Canones Septembris*, canons 8–12, pp. 108–57, esp. 110.55, 120.111, 122.173–74, 149.90–91, etc. Further parallels can be found in the hymnography of July 25, the feast of the dormition of Anna: Τὴν ἀπαρχὴν τῆς ἡμῶν σωτηρίας, φαιδρῶς ἡ γεννήσασα (*Μηναῖον τοῦ*

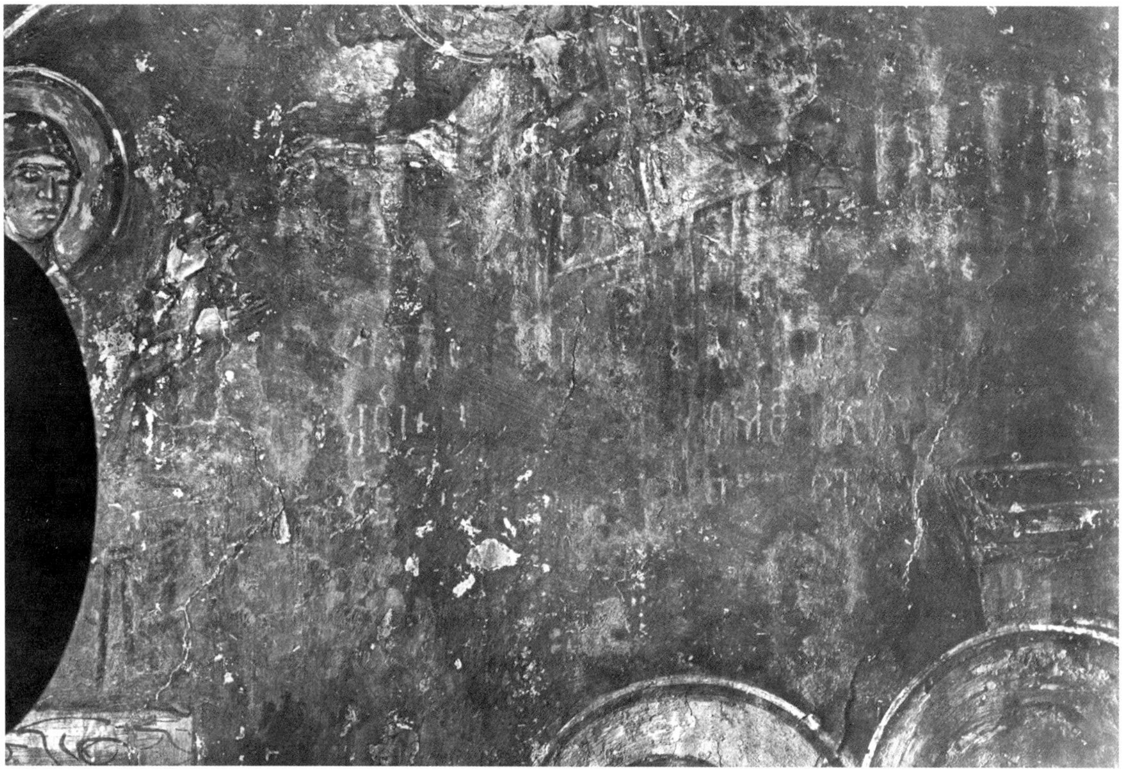

FIG. 3.3 Bema, south wall. Presentation of the Virgin in the Temple: inscription (photo courtesy of Dumbarton Oaks # L 67. 933 [IŠ])

any image, the "world" is counseled to "see" its own resurrection in this event. There is nothing specific in the iconography of the Asinou composition that would visually reinforce the message of the poem, though the figure of Joachim in an upstairs window, overlooking the birth, does seem to be deliberately included as a witness.[14]

There are several other Byzantine poems devoted to the Birth of the Virgin, but they dwell primarily on the miracle of the birth, not on the theological significance of the event, as here.[15]

The contemporary fresco of the Birth of the Virgin at Trikomo on Cyprus, though fragmentary, is similar in iconography (including the figure of Joachim as witness), but neither it nor the fresco of the scene at Kalliana includes the poetic inscription.[16]

There must have been a comparable poem inscribed on the scene of the Presentation of the Virgin in the Temple, which is located opposite that of her Birth, on the south wall of the bema (Fig. 3.3). Unfortunately, this inscription is now almost entirely destroyed, and all that can be read is:

Ἰουλίου, 218: Idiomelon for the Lite). See also Rhoby, *Byzantinische Epigramme*, 352, for a parallel from the writings of St. Neophytos.

14. On the iconography of the scene of the Birth of the Virgin, see *ODB* 1:291.

15. The poems include a 10th-century anonymous one: Browning, "Unpublished Corpus," 297 (no. 10); one by Geometres: Sajdak, "Spicilegium," 197 (no. 9) and Lauxtermann, *Byzantine Poetry*, 299; two by Theodore Prodromos: Papagiannis, *Theodoros Prodromos*, 2:193–94 (nos. 184a, 184b = PG 133:1175–77), and one by Philes: Miller, *Manuelis Philae Carmina*, 1:129–30 (Escorial no. 255).

16. The fresco at Kalliana is also located on the north wall of the bema, behind the iconostasis.

την [. . .] αγ[. . .] π̣α̣ν̣α̣γ̣ι̣[. . .]
[. . .]σιξ̣ιν [. . .]ομένι κόρι[.]
κ [. . .]ξ̣ [.] χ̣ β̣ [. . .] ετα
ὁ
Ζαχαρι

The words are written below the figure of the angel, to the right of the figure of the Virgin seated in the sanctuary, just above the heads of her parents. If this poem reflects the troparia for the feast as much as does the poem for the Birth of the Virgin, one can attempt to fill out some words by incorporating in some way certain phrases that occur frequently in the troparia:[17]

to line 1: τὰ ἅγια τῶν ἁγίων
to line 2: [προσαγ]ομένη / [εἰσερχ]ομένη / [εἰσαγ]-ομένη / [κεκλει]ομένη κόρη
to lines 3–5: [εὐφραίν]εται ὁ Ζαχαρί[ας]

Other Byzantine poems on the Presentation of the Virgin (including one by Geometres, one by Michael Psellos, two by Theodore Prodromos, and an anonymous one) focus either on the lights held by the maidens escorting the Virgin (representing the light of the New Law versus the shadows of the Old) or on the Virgin (representing a gate for the holy, as she passes through the holy gates of the sanctuary).[18] We have no way of determining which, if indeed either, of these themes was addressed in the poem at Asinou.

One other metrical inscription accompanies a narrative fresco in the bema area: it is located on the western faces of the two apse responds (Figs. 3.4, 3.5). Although the inscription is placed directly over the divided scene of the Annunciation, it apparently relates instead to the Ascension in the vault above. The two halves, both written on narrow framed upright panels, probably form one epigram, although the upper parts of each half are hidden behind the present plaster and the metal supporting column. The texts run as follows with the divisions between the verses being somewhat hypothetical where no punctuation or divider dots have survived:

North panel (Fig. 3.4):
[. . .] δεξηόθεν:
ηξιτ̣[. . .] μετα δοξις του κηριε:
καὶ ἀπο ση [. . .] σκιά στου[. . .] ξ λ̣
εν τõ μεσω̃ τ[. . .] / εν τη κρίση / μη κρίνης / +

South panel (Fig. 3.5):
στων + μα[. . .]οστόδοτη σελας: ταυγισεκοταμενοι τ[.]ν α/νο προς τον̣
κ(αὶ) νύν βλε/πουσίν ἐρρό/μενὸν τόν / κτήστην:
όν / συνήθος ἔχου/σιν αγγελοῖ βλέ/πιν.[19]

Only two phrases are comprehensible: the ἐν τῷ μέσῳ τ(ῶν) ἐν τῇ κρίσει μὴ κρίνης at the end of the north panel ("At the judgment, do not condemn [me] to their midst"), and the final two lines of the text on the south panel:

καὶ νῦν βλέπουσιν αἰρόμενον τὸν κτίστην
ὃν συνήθως ἔχουσιν ἄγγελοι βλέπειν

And now they see the creator being taken up,
He whom [only] the angels are accustomed to see.

A troparion for the feast may help in the reconstruction of the end of the first line: [. . . τοῦ πατρὸς] δεξιόθεν.[20]

17. *Μηναῖον τοῦ Νοεμβρίου*, 258, 263, 270, 275, 276, etc. The feast is celebrated on 21 November. For translations of the troparia, see Mary and Ware, *Festal Menaion*, 164–98.
18. Cramer, *Anecdota Graeca*, 304; Westerink, *Michael Psellus*, 457 (no. 79); Hörandner, "Cycle of Epigrams," 118 (no. 1) = Lampros, "Ὁ Μαρκιανὸς κῶδιξ 524," 143 (no. 183); Papagiannis, *Theodoros Prodromos* 2:194–96 (no. 185a, 185b = PG 133:1177–78). See also Lauxtermann, *Byzantine Poetry*, 300 (MS. Athos, Lavra B 43, fol. 67v: 3).
19. The reason for the insertion of the cross in line 1 is unclear to me.
20. *Πεντηκοστάριον*, 176: ἀνῆλθες καὶ ἐκάθισας τοῦ Πατρὸς δεξιόθεν. There are also parallels for the penultimate verse of this poem, e.g., Ἐσκίρτησαν Ἀπόστολοι, ὁρῶντες μετάρσιον σήμερον τὸν κτίστην αἰρόμενον (first

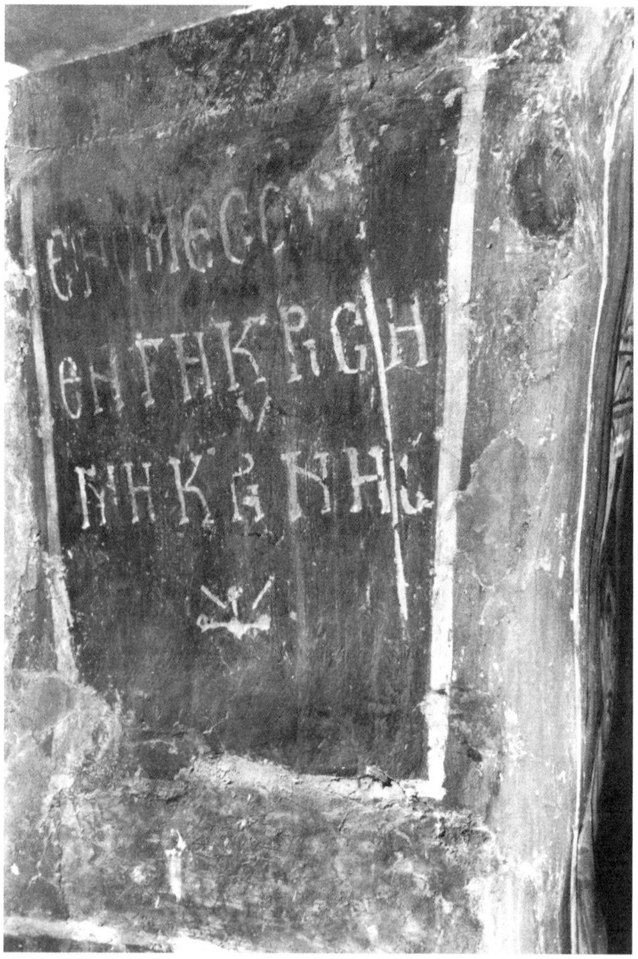

FIG. 3.4 Bema, northern apse respond: inscription, detail (photo courtesy of Dumbarton Oaks # As/L.67.248)

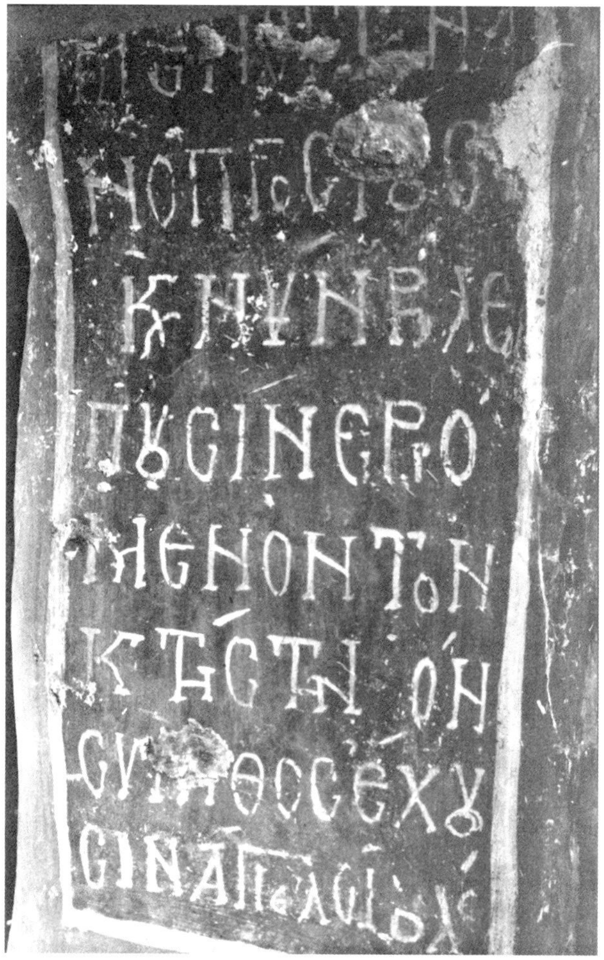

FIG. 3.5 Bema, southern apse respond: inscription, detail (photo courtesy of Dumbarton Oaks # As/L.67.244)

A number of middle Byzantine poems on the Ascension survive: three by Christopher of Mitylene, one by Mauropous, one by Psellos, three among the anonymous poems dedicated to Christological feasts edited by Wolfram Hörandner, two by Theodore Prodromos, one by Gregory of Corinth, and one found in the Pentekostarion.[21] None of these seems to bear any particular resemblance to the poem at Asinou.

The words μὴ κρίνῃς are written on the open book that lies on the throne of the Hetoimasia in the dome at Trikomo.[22] The image of Christ in the

troparion of the 7th ode of the Ascension canon by Joseph the hymnographer: *Πεντηκοστάριον*, 177).

21. Christopher of Mitylene: Follieri, "Il calendario giambico," 300 (no. 53); Kurtz, *Die Gedichte*, 87 (no. 126) = Lampros, "Ὁ Μαρκιανὸς κῶδιξ," 175 (no. 326); Lampros, 141 (no. 171); Mauropous: Lagarde, *Ioannis Euchaitorum metropolitae*, 7–8 (no. 10); cf. Lauxtermann, "Byzantine Epigram," 143 (a shortened version from MS. Athos, Lavra B 43); Psellos: Westerink, *Michael Psellus*, 457 (no. 77); Anonymous: Hörandner, "Ein Zyklus," 109 (no. 16 a–c); Prodromos: Papagiannis, *Theodoros Prodromos*, 2:247–49 (nos. 236a, 236b = PG 133:1197–98); Gregory of Corinth (Gregory Pardos): Hunger, "Gregorios von Korinth," 645 (no. 11); *Πεντηκοστάριον*, 178 (preceding Synaxarion reading).

22. Carr and Morrocco, *Byzantine Masterpiece*, fig. 16; Hein et al., *Cyprus*, fig. 169. Cf. the final phrase

center of this dome at Trikomo has overtones of the Last Judgment, both in its iconography and in its surrounding inscription.[23] The severity of the visage of Christ in the Ascension at Asinou may suggest that a comparable association between the ascending and the returning Christ was intended.

2. The Dedicatory Poems

A metrical inscription consisting of two long lines of text runs around the base of the conch in the apse (Figs. 3.6, 3.7; see also Fig. 6.4).[24] It addresses the Virgin Pantanassa; mentions the (Day of) Judgment; and includes the name of the donor, the magistros (Nikephoros) Ischyrios (ὁ Ισχυρίων). This individual's name occurs twice elsewhere in the church: in the prose inscription running along the west end of the south wall of the naos and providing the date of 1106 for the fresco decoration (Fig. 2.19), and (without the family name Ischyrios) in the dedicatory poem over the south door of the naos (Fig. 3.8, discussed below).[25] The apse inscription is transcribed as follows:

> \+ ω παντανασσα κ(αὶ) πα[. . .]
> [. . . νη]ς ψυχῆς μου:
> καὶ γενοῦ μοι μεσήτης ἓν ὧρα / δίκης:
> ὅπος ἐκφύγω μ[. . .]ω
> [. . . ο]ς μαγιστρὸς ὁ ὑσχυρίων: +

The inscription is followed by two units of pseudo-Cufic design. It was written in black letters on a narrow yellow band. At a later time, the original poem was plastered over and then recopied in white on a blue ground, the second inscription preserving the same text but running a few letters behind the original. Traces of this second inscription are visible on the back of the plaster that was removed to uncover the original, black-on-yellow one.

The poem closely echoes a poem found in the exact same location in the apse at Trikomo.[26] The Trikomo poem is slightly better preserved, enabling us to reconstruct and correct the one at Asinou in the following manner:

> \+ ὦ παντάνασσα καὶ πά[ντων ὑπερτέρα:
> δέσποινα ἁγνὴ καὶ μῆτερ τοῦ κυρίου:
> ἴδε τὸν πόθον τῆς ταλαίνη]ς ψ[υ]χῆς μου:
> καὶ γενοῦ μοι μεσῖτις ἐν ὥρα δίκης:
> ὅπως ἐκφύγω μ[έρος τῶν . . .]ω[. . .
> Νικηφόρο]ς μάγιστρος ὁ Ἰσχυρίων: +[27]

> O Pantanassa, and all-[surpassing
> chaste lady and mother of the Lord,
> see the desire of my miserable] soul
> and become my intercessor in the hour of judgment
> that I may be spared the lot of [. . .
> Nikephoros] magistros, of the (family of the) Ischyrioi.

Although the Trikomo version also contains a personal appeal to the Virgin, presumably in the voice of a donor ("See the desire . . . of my miserable soul, and be my intercessor in the hour of judgment"), the poem there apparently does not include

---

in the metrical inscription painted on the back of an 11th/12th-century icon of the Last Judgment on Mount Sinai: οἰκτίρμονος μάλιστα μὴ κριτοῦ τότε: Soteriou and Soteriou, *Εἰκόνες τῆς Μονῆς Σινᾶ*, 130, fig. 150.

23. Papageorgiou, "Paintings in the Dome," esp. 149–51; Carr and Morrocco, *Byzantine Masterpiece*, 47–54; Velmans, "Quelques programmes iconographiques," 137–45 and fig. 6.

24. Cf. Rhoby, *Byzantinische Epigramme*, 379.

25. Nicolaïdès, "Les *ktitores* dans la peinture."

26. For the text of the Trikomo inscription see Rhoby, *Byzantinische Epigramme*, 377–80, no. 360. See also Stylianou and Stylianou, *Painted Churches*, 488; Carr and Morrocco, *Byzantine Masterpiece*, 47 and fig. 15; Maguire, "*Abaton* and *Oikonomia*," 104, fig. 15.

27. For parallels to the opening line, see the troparion for Lauds for November 21: ἡ Θεοτόκος ὄντως, ἀνεδείχθη τῷ κόσμῳ ὡς πάντων ὑπερτέρα (*Μηναῖον τοῦ Νοεμβρίου*, 276). See also χαῖρε ἁπάντων κτισμάτων ὑπερτέρα, or σὺ γὰρ ὑπερτέρα πάσης κτίσεως; and, for line 2, Ἁγνὴ παναγία Δέσποινα in various canons to the Virgin: Eustratiades, *Θεοτοκάριον*, 81, 135, 253. It is interesting to note that the word μάγιστρος is accented three different ways at Asinou, perhaps evidence of different hands at work.

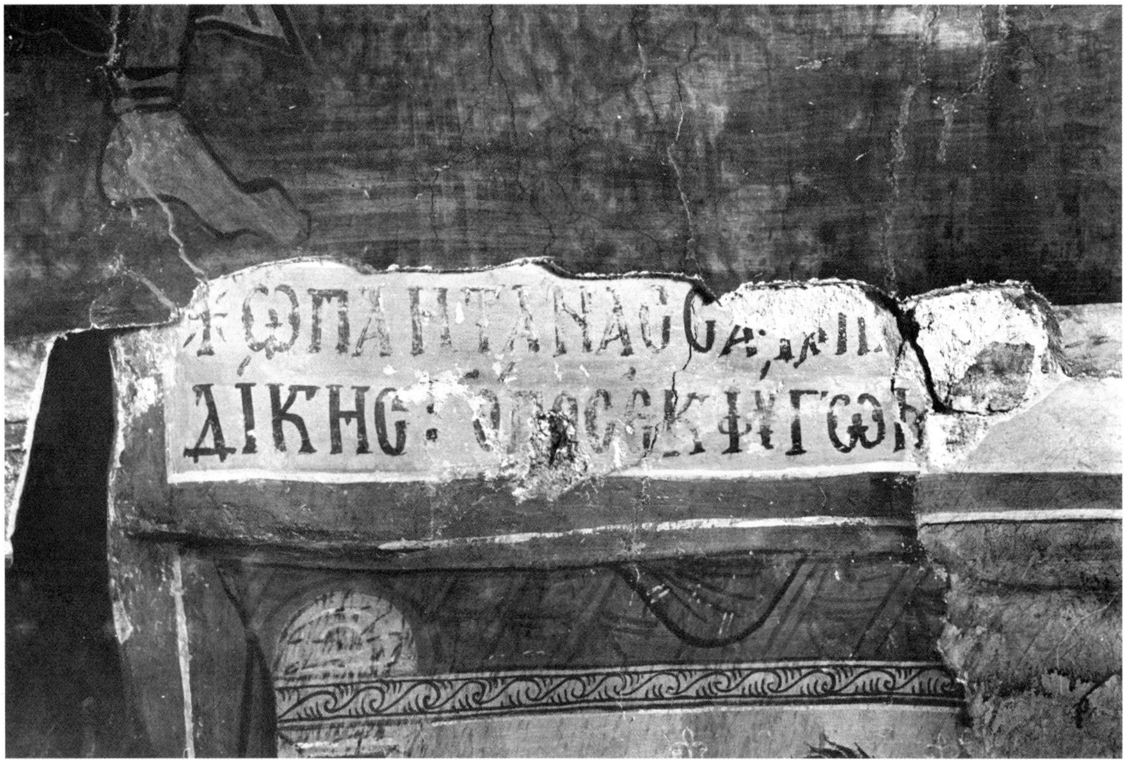

fig. 3.6

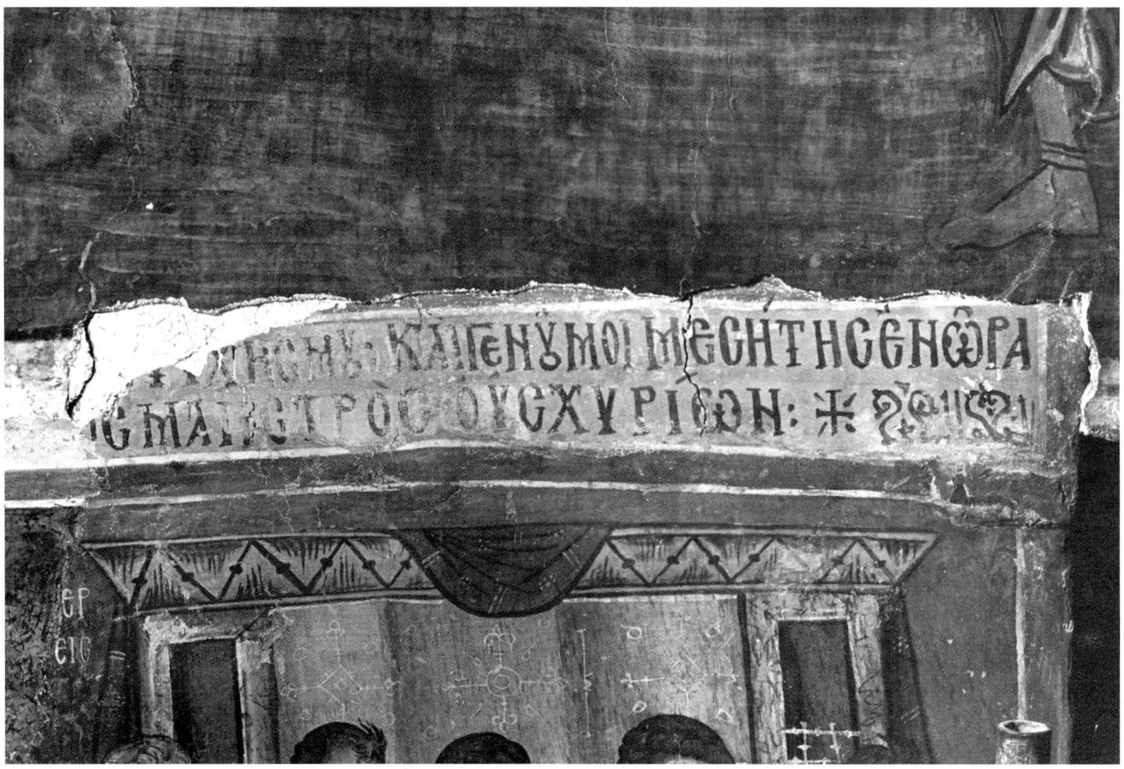

fig.3.7

FIGS. 3.6 AND 3.7 Apse: Verse inscription (photos courtesy Dumbarton Oaks # As/L.67.951 [IŠ] and As/L.67.948 [IŠ])

the name of the individual. It is restricted to five verses, whereas the poem at Asinou adds a sixth verse naming the magistros. The near-identity of the two apse poems, however, suggests that the original figure of the Virgin in the apse at Asinou may have looked like the surviving image at Trikomo and not like the thirteenth-century Virgin that occupies the apse at Asinou today.[28]

There is no evidence for a donor portrait alongside the apse Virgin in either church. At Asinou, the portrait of Nikephoros appears elsewhere, in conjunction with a dedicatory inscription on the south wall of the naos, painted in the fourteenth century but presumably repeating the words of the original twelfth-century poem (Fig. 3.8).[29] It reads:

Πολλοῖς τεθηλῶς / ἀγαθοῖς ἐν τω βίο
ών/περ χοριγõς οράθης συ / παρθένε
Νικηφόρος μάγιστρος εἰκτρος ή/κ(αί)της
ἤγιρα τωνδε τῶ ναον μετα πόθου
ἀνθου/περ ετο προστάτυν εὑρικ(αί)νε
ἐν ημέ/ρα σε τι φρικώδη τῆς δίκης

and normalized as:

Πολλοῖς τεθηλὼς ἀγαθοῖς ἐν τῷ βίῳ
ὧνπερ χορηγὸς ὠράθης σύ, παρθένε,
Νικηφόρος μάγιστρος οἰκτρὸς ἱκέτης
ἤγειρα τόνδε τὸν ναὸν μετὰ πόθου
ἀνθ' οὗπερ αἰτῶ προστάτιν εὑρηκέναι
ἐν ἡμέρᾳ σε τῇ φρικώδει τῆς δίκης

Having been blessed in life with many good things
Of which thou, O Virgin, wast seen to be the provider,
I, Nikephoros magistros, a pitiable supplicant,
Erected this church with devotion,
In return for which I beg to find thee my protectress
On the terrible day of judgment.[30]

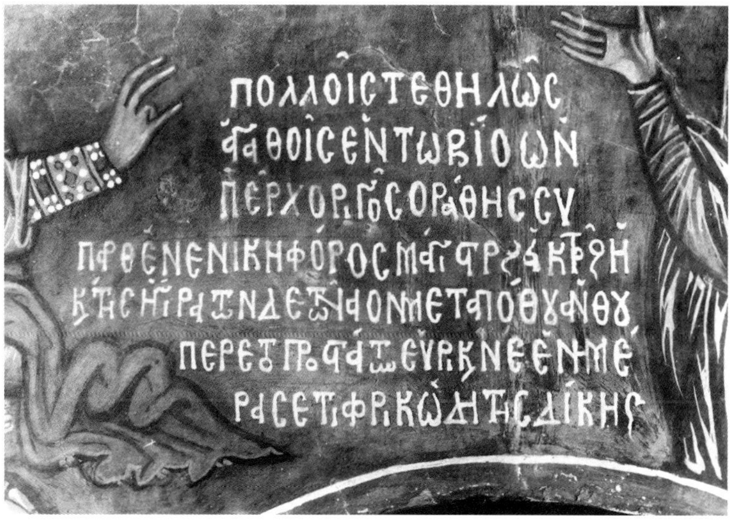

FIG. 3.8 Naos, central bay, south wall: verse inscription of the donor Nikephoros magistros (photo courtesy of Dumbarton Oaks, As.L.67.203)

There is no linguistic difficulty involved in assigning this poem to the original twelfth-century decoration. A close parallel in content is found in the late twelfth-century verse dedicatory inscription of another magistros Nikephoros, this one Nikephoros Kasnitzes in Kastoria.[31] The reference to the Day of Judgment as φρικώδης (terrible) has twelfth-century counterparts. Alternate forms of this word are found in the Dormition inscription at Asinou itself (see below) and in a similar dedicatory context on the pier fresco of St. Nicholas in his church at Kakopetria.[32]

28. The 12th-century fresco of the Virgin over the door from the narthex into the naos at Asinou closely resembles the Virgin in the apse at Trikomo.

29. Rhoby, *Byzantinische Epigramme*, 348–50, no. 236.

30. Ibid., 350 reconstructs ή κ(αί)της in line 3 as οἰκέτης rather than ἱκέτης, translating the word then as "servant," rather than as "supplicant" as I have done here.

31. Ibid., 176. See also Gerstel, *Beholding the Sacred Mysteries*, 90 (Appendix, no. 9), with translation. This poem lacks the Asinou donor's appeal for aid at the Last Judgment.

32. For the inscription at Kakopetria, see Rhoby, *Byzantinische Epigramme*, 318. See also Stylianou and Stylianou, *Painted Churches*, fig. 25; Hein et al., *Cyprus*,

Although they presumably had to be composed ad hoc, so that the donor's name could fit smoothly into the meter, there is no shortage of metrical dedicatory inscriptions surviving in fresco; they are more common than those that accompany narrative scenes, even though the latter poems could presumably have been quite easily borrowed from literary collections without poetic effort or need for alteration.[33] The poem here addresses the Virgin and outlines a mutual exchange of favors: the Virgin has awarded Nikephoros many benefits during his lifetime, in return for which he has erected a church dedicated to her, for which, in turn, she will—he hopes—reward him, by acting as his defender on the Day of Judgment. The evidence for these transactions is offered in the fresco as well: the worldly blessings that Nikephoros attributes to the Virgin are reflected in the fine clothes worn by the magistros and the smaller figure of Gephyra beside him;[34] he holds forth the church he has erected; the Virgin, a large-scale figure, acknowledges his donation by resting her hand on the roof of the church; and Christ's recognition of his mother and of the donor's gift is conveyed through his raised and blessing hand. Rumblings of the coming Day of Judgment are conveyed by the mass of angels clustered behind his throne (see Fig. 6.50).

The words here are written on the background of the fresco, between the standing Virgin, who presents the donor Nikephoros to Christ, and Christ, who is enthroned. Despite the gestures indicating an active verbal exchange between Christ and the Virgin, the words of the poem are those of Nikephoros alone, directed only to the Virgin. A similar composition, though in this case incorporating the spoken words of Christ, is found over a tomb in the church of the Savior at Spas-Nereditsa near Novgorod. There Christ, enthroned at the left, addresses the donor (a prince) directly; his hand is extended in speech or blessing and his words are written out on the fresco between him and the prince.[35] The location of the dedicatory composition at Asinou, directly over the south door to the church, assuming this to be the original placement, could possibly prove significant for determining the site of the tomb of the magistros Nikephoros.

It is worth noting that the inscription alongside the figure of Gephyra (Fig. 6.51) is not in verse, and offers no more than the day of her death.

The last of the twelfth-century metrical inscriptions at Asinou runs under the Dormition fresco, on the west wall of the naos (Fig. 3.9).[36] It is quite damaged, and only the beginnings and the ends of the two long lines of writing have been preserved. Originally the poem probably had five or six verses. As with the apse inscription, there are two layers, but here the original text seems to have been written in black letters on a narrow red band of fresco that is continuous with the Dormition fresco; on top of that comes the poem written in black letters on yellow, in the same hand as the *lower* layer of the apse inscription. The red layer is visible only in two small patches below the two ends of the Virgin's bier, in the damaged central section of the yellow-ground inscription. On the left patch, only the tips of six or seven letters can be seen, possibly starting with *να*, but otherwise unidentifiable; on the right, one can read [. . .]ήτρ[. .] αμ[. . .]. These letters presumably belong to the first line or lines of the original poem, which must have been written first upon a

fig. 44. Φρικώδη is also used in connection with judgment in the poem on the Sinai Last Judgment icon (see note 22, above): ὡς Δανιὴλ πρόειδε φρικώδη κρίσιν (Soteriou and Soteriou, *Εἰκόνες τῆς Μονῆς Σινᾶ*, 130; fig. 150).

33. Kalopissi-Verti, *Dedicatory Inscriptions*, 25, note 27, lists the metrical ones in her corpus. For examples on Cyprus, see Stylianou and Stylianou, "Donors and Dedicatory Inscriptions," nos. 5, 12; Nicolaïdès, "Étude iconographique," 5. For examples of the 12th century at Kastoria, see Drakopoulou, *Η πόλη τῆς Καστοριάς*, esp. 41–49. See also Gerstel, *Beholding the Sacred Mysteries*, Appendix, no. 8, and from later periods, nos. 21, 22. See also Lauxtermann, *Byzantine Poetry*, 151.

34. On the question of this figure's identity, see pp. 20, 22–23, 53–54, 234, 291, 293, 296.

35. Lazarev, *Old Russian Murals and Mosaics*, Appendix, fig. 57. Cf. N. P. Ševčenko, "Close Encounters," 275 and note 22. The fresco may date to the late 12th century.

36. Rhoby, *Byzantinische Epigramme*, 347–48, no. 235.

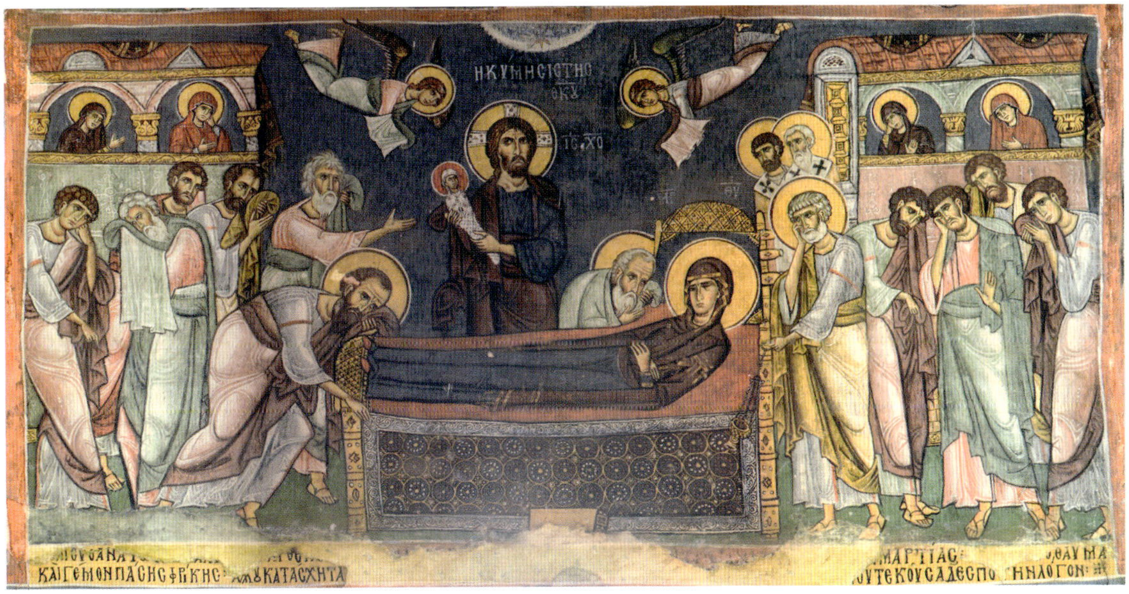

FIG. 3.9 Naos, west wall. Dormition: inscription (photo courtesy of G. L. Carr)

red ground, then reinscribed on the yellow ground that covers the red. The yellow-ground poem reads:

[+ κ]αὶ συ θανάτω[...]αν[... Π]αρθένε[...]
[...] ἁμαρτίας:
[...] το θαῦμα / καὶ γέμον πάσης φρίκης:
ἀλλ' οὐ κατάσχη τα [...]
[...]του τεκοῦσα δεσπότην Λόγον: +

And you, (O) Virgin, in death [...]
redemption of sin [...]
[is] the miracle, and full of every (kind of) fright
But (it/he/she) will not possess/restrain the [...]
[she who] bears the Lord the Logos

The patch of letters located between Π]αρθένε and ἁμαρτίας ([...]ήτρ[..] αμ[...]) suggests that the poem may have originally read: λ]ύτρον [...] ἁμαρτίας.

The fragmentary state of this inscription renders any reconstruction impossible.[37] This poem addresses the Virgin directly, as does the one in the apse; it may again refer to the Day of Judgment, and it mentions the "redemption of sin," presumably the donor's. As it is written on the same sort of narrow band and starts with the word καί ("and"), it may have been designed to invite the reader to link it with the apse inscription. If this inscription addresses the Virgin through the representation of her death, as is suggested by the reference to (her?) death in its opening words, this would be unusual. Such prayers are usually addressed to a standing or seated image of the Virgin.

3. The St. George Dedicatory Inscription

The earliest of the various metrical inscriptions in the narthex accompanies the mounted figure of St. George in the south conch (Figs. 3.10, 4.1, 4.6, 4.8).[38] The poem consists of eight lines of verse, to which a ninth, seemingly nonmetrical, line has

37. Ibid., 347, reconstructs the poem with eight verses (Rhoby adds two between the first and second lines transcribed here), and cites parallels from Symeon the New Theologian. One fragmentary inscription, not even surely metrical, uses some of the same words: it is carved under an image of the Dormition on a wooden panel in the Hermitage: Piatnitsky et al., *Sinai, Byzantium, Russia*, no. B 119. Modifications to the transcription of the Greek are proposed by Chotzakoglou in his review of that exhibition catalogue, *JÖB* 53 (2003): 347.

38. Rhoby, *Byzantinische Epigramme*, 342–44, no. 232.

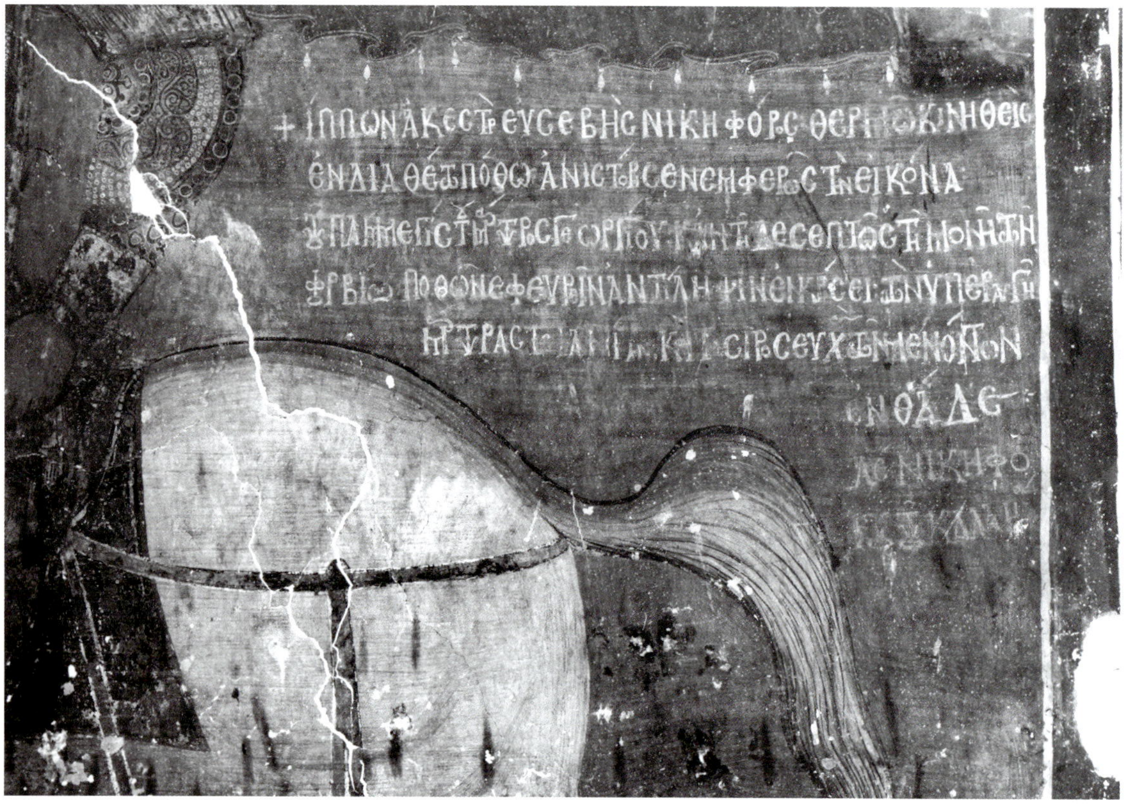

FIG. 3.10 Narthex, south apse. St. George: verse inscription (photo courtesy of Dumbarton Oaks # L63.208 [CM])

been added. The poem, written above the horse's rump and tail and under George's flying red cloak, runs as follows:

+ ἵππων ἀκεστὴρ εὐσεβὴς Νικηφόρος:
θερμῶ κινηθεὶς / ἐνδιαθέτω πόθω
ἀνιστόρησεν ἐμφερῶς τὴν εἰκόνα: /
τοῦ παμμεγίστου μάρτυρος Γεωργίου
κἀν τῇδε σεπτῶς τῇ μονῇ τῶν / Φορβίω(ν)
ποθῶν ἐφευρεῖν ἀντίληψιν ἐν κρίσει·
τὼν ὑπὲραυγῆ / μ(ά)ρτυρα στεφανίτην
καὶ τὰς προσευχ(ὰς) τῶν μενόντων / ἐνθάδε. /

δέ(ησις) Νικηφορ/ου τοῦ Καλληά

A healer of horses, Nikephoros the pious,
moved by warm heartfelt desire
with like feeling painted the image
of the very great martyr George;
and reverently in this monastery of the Phorbia,
desirous of finding help at [the] Judgment
from that most brilliant crowned martyr,
and the prayers of those dwelling here.

Prayer of Nikephoros the farrier (?).[39]

In content, this inscription is similar to that of many a church founder, except that here the donation is not an entire structure, but only an isolated fresco.[40] The words record the pious deed of the

39. The translation is based on that of Buckler (Buxton et al., "Church of Asinou," 338). The language of the poem remains slightly ambiguous, in that the phrase κἀν could be taken to imply that an image of St. George was painted *also* in the church of the Phorbia.

40. A similar appeal to a painted image of St. George can be found near the image of this saint and his miracles in the north aisle of the church of the Anargyroi

horse-healer Nikephoros (no apparent relation to the founder of the church of Asinou, the magistros Nikephoros Ischyrios). It is a straightforward statement of his offering, and of the reward he hopes to reap from it, written on the offering itself: that, at the Last Judgment, he will have as aid in his defense both St. George himself and the prayers of the monks dwelling in the monastery. Such an expectation lies behind the foundation of many Byzantine monastic institutions and pious gifts. This poem is not written in the voice of Nikephoros, and is not a direct appeal to St. George, but is rather a simple statement of gift and expected recompense.

The phrase ἵππων ἀκεστήρ, the healer of horses, must refer to a veterinary doctor.[41] The presence of a veterinarian makes sense given Grivaud's suggestion that the monastery of Asinou was involved in raising horses (above, p. 27) and the association of the name of the institution with a medicinal plant (p. 20).[42] In this context, the image of a mounted St. George would also have had a special resonance.

The final line of the inscription, "Prayer of Nikephoros the farrier (?)," has usually been thought to belong with the eight previous ones. But there is some evidence to suggest that these words were an afterthought. They are written in a paler, yellower color; they contain eleven syllables, not twelve; and they seem to repeat the message of the poem's first line. Hence it is likely that the poem consisted of only eight lines of verse, ending with the word ἐνθάδε, and that the ninth line is a separate inscription.

The words of this added inscription, also discussed by Nicolaïdès (p. 101), are written in a paint closely resembling that used for the shadows on the horse's rump and flank, and must have been introduced after the fresco and its accompanying poem were complete. The speaker of this added invocation is also named Nikephoros, perhaps a farrier (if Καλληάς = καλλιγᾶς) or a man whose full name was Nikephoros Καλλίας. It is not clear whether he is the same person as the veterinarian Nikephoros mentioned in the poem as donor of the fresco, or a different, somewhat later devotee.[43]

B. The Fourteenth-Century Poems

1. The Lunette Inscription in the Narthex

This inscription runs around the lunette above the door from the narthex to the naos, framing the image of the Virgin Phorbiotissa (Fig. 3.11). It is written in black letters on a yellow ground, probably in imitation of the twelfth-century apse and Dormition inscriptions.[44] It is well preserved, and although there are signs of earlier fresco layers in the lunette itself (the image of the Virgin and child is from the twelfth century) and on the lintel (the row of ornament), nothing suggests that the inscription repeats an earlier one from the twelfth century.

in Kastoria (late 12th century): Pelekanidis and Chatzidakis, *Kastoria*, 39. Another appeal to a specific holy figure for help on the Last Day is found in the Kakopetria fresco mentioned earlier (note 32). In both cases the donor believes that the image of the saint that he has had painted will earn him the support of the saint on Judgment Day. In the dedicatory inscription at Lagoudera, Leon claims the aid of the Virgin because he has commissioned her image: for the text, see Nicolaïdès, "Étude iconographique," 5 and figs. 4–5.

41. The word ἀκεστορία is used in the context of veterinary medicine in a poem in the Planudean Anthology (Book 16, no. 271): see McCabe, *A Byzantine Encyclopaedia of Horse Medicine*, 290–91. I wish to thank Dr. McCabe for her help in interpreting this poem. The Stylianous translate Ἵππων ἀκεστήρ as "tamer (trainer) of horses": Stylianou and Stylianou, "Donors," 105. The translation of ἀκεστήρ is discussed by Rhoby, *Byzantinische Epigramme*, 343–44; he translates the phrase as "healer of horses".

42. On horse-rearing at Asinou, see Frigerio-Zeniou, "Μονὴ τῶν Φορβίων."

43. For Nikephoros as a farrier, see McCabe, *A Byzantine Encyclopaedia*, 290–91. It is just conceivable that this Nikephoros was the painter of the fresco, who appended an invocation of his own at the end of his commission. Rhoby, *Byzantinische Epigramme*, 342, believes Καλληά to be a proper surname, Kallias.

44. The same writing and ground is used for the Biblical citation that runs around the northern conch of the naos.

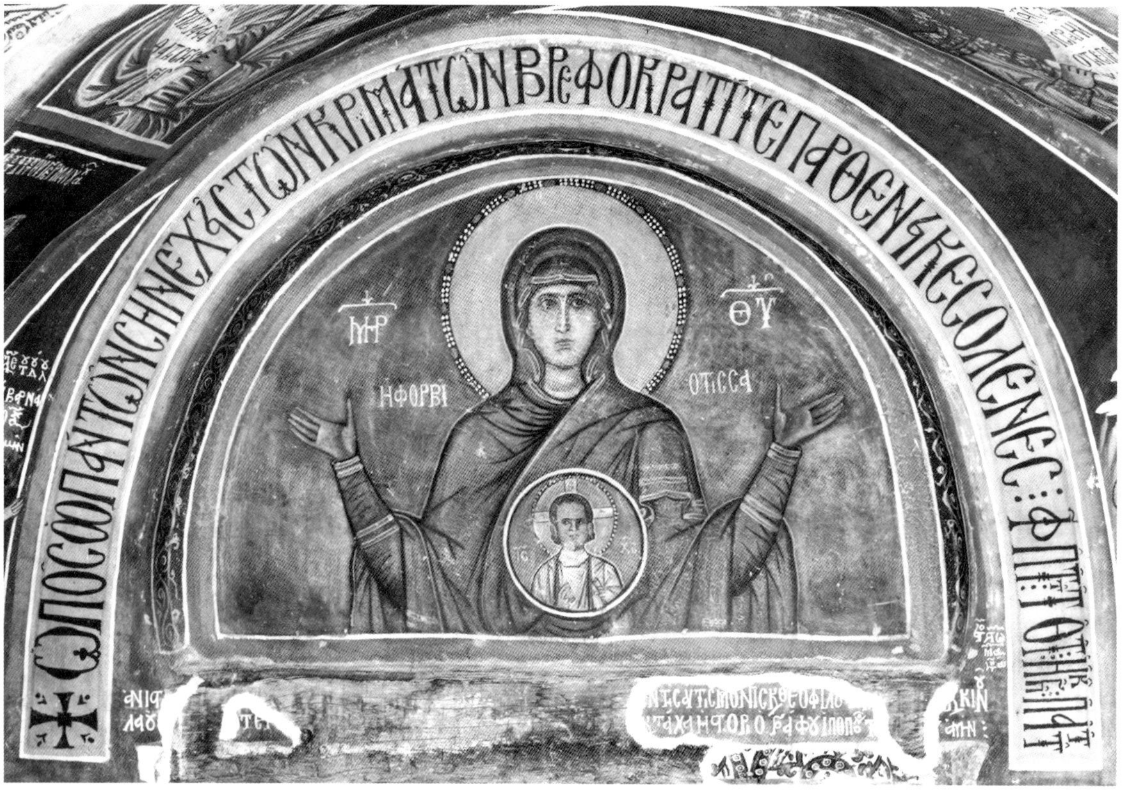

FIG. 3.11 Narthex, east wall. Verse inscription around the Mother of God Phorbiotissa (photo courtesy of Dumbarton Oaks #As.B.67.25)

The inscription, though perfectly legible, is enigmatic.[45] It begins as follows:

> + Ω πõς ὡ πάντῶν σηνεχεῖς τῶν κριμάτῶν
> βρεφοκρατίτε παρθενεικες ὀλένες ⁝

It then concludes with what appears to be a series of cryptograms or acrostics. Thanks to the division signs, one can presume that, compressed within these cryptic letters, are either four lines of verse or just two. Since there are four dots after the Τ Θ Τ phrase and only three after the others, the latter could be merely dividing the five and seven syllables that make up a single line.

Φ Π Τ Τ ⁝
Τ Θ Τ ⁞
Η Κ Γ Π ⁝
Π Α Τ Τ

The first text, as corrected, reads:

> + Ὦ πῶς ὁ πάντων συνεχὴς τῶν κριμάτων
> βρεφοκρατεῖται παρθενικαῖς ὠλέναις;

O how is He who holds together all judgments held as a babe in a virgin's arms?[46]

45. Rhoby, *Byzantinische Epigramme*, 344–46, no. 233. On this inscription, see also Savage, "Interrelationship of Text, Imagery and Architecture," 101 and fig. 1.

46. Translation based upon that of Maguire, *Art and Eloquence*, 57, and his *Image and Imagination*, 13. Rhoby, *Byzantinische Epigramme*, 345–46 suggests that the word κτισμάτων would make better sense here than the chosen κριμάτων. An alternative to συνεχής could be συνοχεύς, as was suggested by an anonymous reader.

This verse meditates on the exquisite paradox of the Virgin holding the omnipotent Christ in her arms. The Byzantine topos is subtly colored with a reference to the Last Judgment depicted nearby.[47] Here, though, the text does not at all suit the image it accompanies, which shows the Virgin with her arms outstretched and Christ enclosed in a medallion on her chest. Such a discrepancy between poem and image is without parallel in the church, and can be explained by the fact that the image is two centuries older than the surrounding inscription: by the fourteenth century, when the latter was painted, inscriptions and frescoes had already begun to go their separate ways.

The acrostics have been rather arbitrarily reconstructed, but they still have not been satisfactorily deciphered.[48] The church of Asinou is full of cryptograms. There are four surviving sets flanking crosses painted on the door jambs, and two sets flanking star patterns at the apex of the prothesis and diakonikon arches. On one door jamb (the east jamb of the north entrance to the naos) there is a Φ Π combination, but whether the opening letters of the lunette cryptogram are related in any way to the common formula Φ Χ Φ Π is unknown. The cryptograms next to the crosses serve primarily to mark entrances or protect vaults, and they evidently have an apotropaic function (see Figs. 5.49, 5.50, 6.30, 6.32, 6.34, and accompanying discussion).[49] Thus, though they follow two lines of verse, the enigmatic letters around the lunette of the Virgin Phorbiotissa in the narthex may have a purpose quite separate from that of the poem, and should be viewed in connection with their location over a portal.

2. The Two Virgin Paraklesis Scrolls

At Asinou there are two different images of the Virgin standing, holding a scroll, and petitioning Christ for mercy upon mankind. One is in the narthex and the other is in the naos. Both figures stand to the left of doorways, across from a standing figure of Christ.

The Virgin in the narthex bears the epithet "Eleousa," the merciful; the Christ to the right of the doorway has the masculine version of the same epithet, "Eleemon" (Figs. 3.12, 5.30). The fresco has been painted over an earlier one. A short two-verse poem is written on the Virgin's scroll, miserably spelled and lacking any markings to divide the verses. It is written in black letters on a white scroll; the letters are fitted exactly between horizontal guidelines that have been incised into the plaster:[50]

> + λητὰς / προσάγει / μητρικὰς / ἡ Παρθαί/νος,
> τõ / αὐτὸ καμ/πὶ προς βρο/τῶν σοτιρήαν

This can be reconstructed as:

> + λιτὰς προσάγει μητρικὰς ἡ Παρθένος,
> τὸν αὐτὸν κάμπτει πρὸς βροτῶν σωτηρίαν

47. Maguire, *Art and Eloquence*, 56–59. In *Image and Imagination* (13–14), Maguire compares the verse to an anonymous poem of the 10th century edited by Robert Browning in his "Unpublished Corpus," 297. For further parallels, see Rhoby, *Byzantinische Epigramme*, 345. The sentiment can be traced at least as far back as the famous homily of the patriarch Photios on the apse mosaic of St. Sophia: *Homily* 17, tr. Mango, *Art of the Byzantine Empire*, 187. See also the Theotokion that follows the 6th ode of a canon to St. Nicholas by John the Monk (Mauropous): PG 96:1388A.

48. Peristianes suggested φύλαττε τῆς Θεοτόκου ἡκεσίαις παντοκράτωρ (*Μονογραφία*, 10); Buckler suggested φ(ύλαξον) π(ιστεύοντας) τ(ούτου) τ(οῦ) τ(όπου)· Θ(εο)τ(όκῳ) ἡκ(έτα)ς τ(ῇ) πα(ν)τ(ο)τ(ρόφῳ) (Buckler et al., "Church of Asinou," 336). There is no basis for either reconstruction. I would prefer to see the first word as Φ(ῶς) and the ΤΘΤ as τ(ῆς) Θ(εο)τ(όκου), but this, too, is speculation. It should be noted that the opening Φ has a flourish over it as an abbreviation mark that differs from the simple round abbreviation marks over the other letters, and that the H may have a rough breathing, while the A has no breathing at all. On these various resolutions to the acrostics, see Rhoby, *Byzantinische Epigramme*, 345.

49. Cf. the doorjambs at Lagoudera: Nicolaïdès, "Panagia Arakiotissa à Lagoudèra," [1993], 132–34. On cryptograms such as these, see Walter, "IC XC NI KA"; Babić, "Les croix à cryptogrammes."

50. Rhoby, *Byzantinische Epigramme*, 346–47, no. 234.

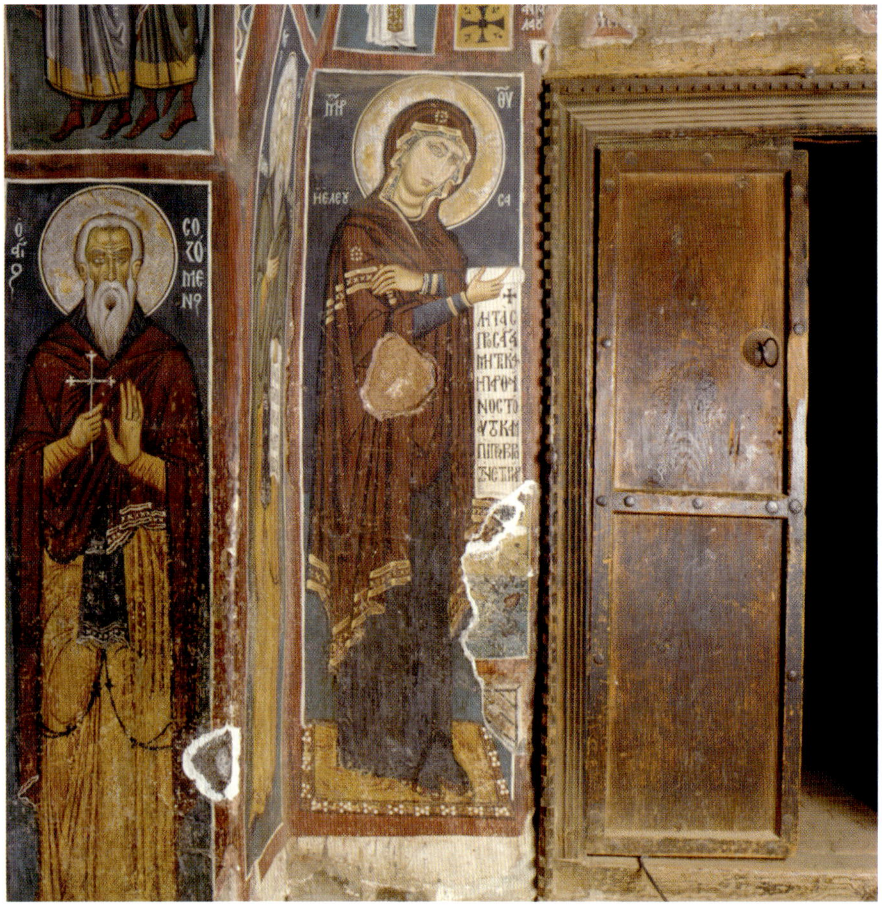

FIG 3.12

Narthex, east wall. Virgin Paraklesis: verse inscription (photo courtesy of Dumbarton Oaks, Winfield 110.18a)

The Virgin offers her motherly entreaties,
she steers him toward the salvation of mortals.

This poem has no precise parallel.[51] The Virgin here is not in fact speaking at all: the poem she holds on her scroll merely states what is taking place at the meeting between her and Christ.

The image of the Virgin in the naos is to the left of the entrance into the bema. On her scroll is written a complete dialogue, with the Virgin's words painted in black and Christ's responses in red (Figs. 3.13, 6.16).[52] The words on the scroll are:

Δέξε / δεισυν τεις τε/κούσις σε Λόγε
Τη μ[η]/τερ ἐτεῖς των βρο/τῶν σοτειριάν
Παρο/ργισάν με συμπα/θισο(ν) ηέ μου
ἀλλ οῦ/κ (ἐ)πειστρέφουσῦν και / σόσ(ον) [χ]αρην /
εξουσυ(ν) λιτρον εὐχαριστό σι Λόγ(ε)

With the spelling corrected, the inscription reads:

51. Ibid., 346, lists some comparable phrases that appear on works of art. The reading offered here of the first words of the second line of verse (τὸν αὐτὸν κάμπτει) is discussed by Rhoby, ibid., 347; he prefers τῶ αὐτοκαμπεῖ. See also the verse written above a representation of the Deesis in a lost Psalter of ca. 1100 that was once in Berlin (Universität, Abteilung für Christliche Archäologie und kirchliche Kunst, cod. 3807, fol. 2r): λιτὰς προσάγει παρθένος σὺν προδρόμῳ (Cutler, *Aristocratic Psalters*, 33; fig. 101). An anonymous reader kindly brought this verse to my attention. See also below, pp. 87, 248, on the relationship between this poem and the similar one displayed by the Virgin Paraklesis in the naos.

52. Rhoby, *Byzantinische Epigramme*, 352, no. 240.

Δέξαι δέησιν τῆς τεκούσης σε, Λόγε.
Τί, μ[ῆ]τερ, αἰτεῖς; Τῶν βροτῶν σωτηρίαν.
Παρώργισάν με. Συμπάθησον, υἱέ μου.
Ἀλλ᾽ οὐκ ἐπιστρέφουσιν. Καὶ σῶσον [χ]άριν.
ἕξουσι λύτρον. Εὐχαριστῶ σοι, Λόγε.

"Receive the entreaty of the one who bore you, O Logos."
"What is it you seek, mother?" "The salvation of mortals."
"They have angered me." "Have compassion, my son."
"But they do not repent." "And save [them out of your] charity."
"They shall be redeemed." "I thank you, O Logos."

The figure of the scroll-bearing Virgin is widely-known, as Kalopissi-Verti shows (pp. 155–57), and the text that she bears is an old one. Versions of it can be seen throughout the Byzantine world from at least the eleventh century onward. Almost identical versions are held by the Virgin elsewhere on Cyprus, characteristically on the north pier of the iconostasis: one sees it at Lagoudera, Kalliana, Moutoullas, Kalopanayiotis, and Galata.[53] The first verse (Δέξαι δέησιν...) of the version at Asinou is not usually included in these other

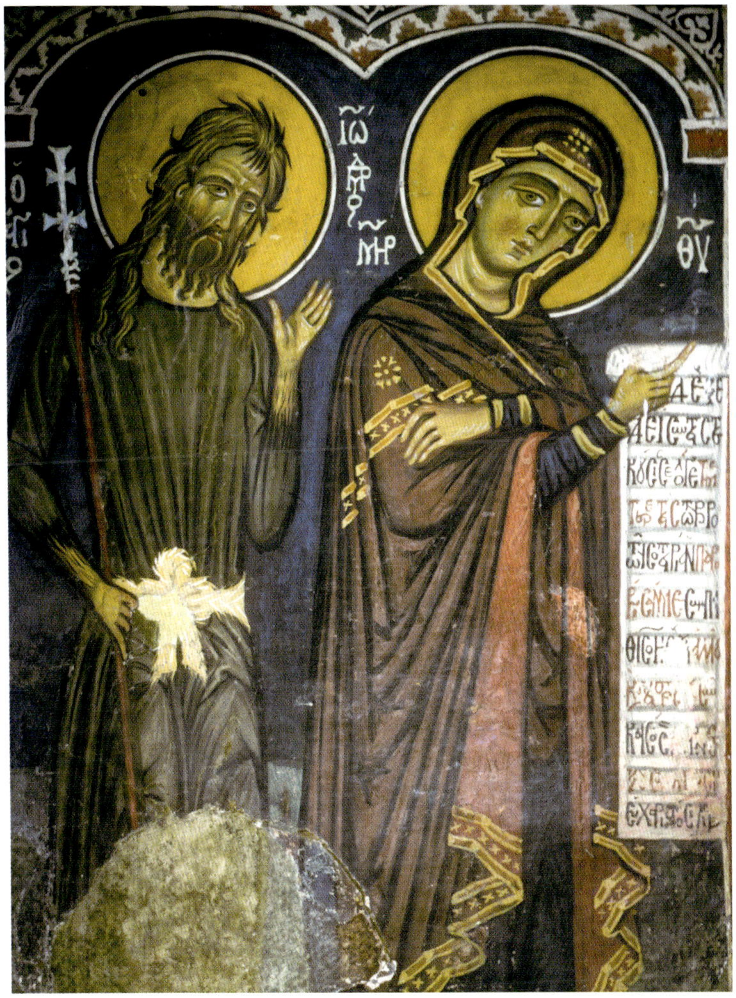

FIG. 3.13 Naos, north bema respond. Virgin Paraklesis: verse inscription (photo courtesy of Dumbarton Oaks # As.B67.12)

examples, although it does appear at Moutoullas (1280).[54] The technique of differentiating the two voices with alternating colors of paint first appears in the very late twelfth century.[55]

53. On the text of this poem, see, with earlier bibliography and a long list of examples, ibid., 329–41. A canon by Theodore of Stoudios (9th century) already contains a dialogue between Christ and the Virgin, though on behalf of an individual petitioner—not, as here, on behalf of mankind in general. See also Lauxtermann, *Byzantine Poetry*, 166–70. The Virgin's scroll at Kalliana reads σωτηρια(ν) / (Πα)ρωργισαν με συμπάθ(η)σο(ν) (υ)ιέ μου· / αλλ οὐκ επιστρέφουσι· κ(αὶ) σῶσον χάρην·/ ἐξουσιν λυ(τρον)...... εὔχ(αριστω...). The Kalliana image is reproduced in Chotzakoglou, "Βυζαντινή αρχιτεκτονική και τέχνη," 2: fig. 425. For the Cypriot examples, see Rhoby, *Byzantinische Epigramme*, 334–38; Mouriki, "Wall Paintings of the Church of the Panagia," 189–90, fig. 7; and Young, "Byzantine Painting in Cyprus," 197, fig. 15. The Galata frescoes remain unpublished. See also Der Nersessian, "Two Images of the Virgin," 81–85; Figs. 10–11.

54. Rhoby, *Byzantinische Epigramme*, 334. The verse appears in a slightly different form in the Painter's Manual by Dionysios of Fourna: *Ἑρμηνεία*, 280. See Lauxtermann, *Byzantine Poetry*, 167, note 47.

55. At Lagoudera and at Kurbinovo: Hadermann-Misguich, *Kurbinovo*, 1:229–30; 2: Figs. 116–18.

The figure of the Virgin extending her petition to Christ is usually known as the Virgin Paraklesis (the Virgin of Intercession), but in Byzantine iconography the epithet may vary: she is also called the Eleousa, as she is here in the narthex at Asinou, at Lagoudera, and in certain other churches on Cyprus.[56]

General Remarks

The poems of the twelfth-century fresco campaign at Asinou fall into several different categories: donor inscriptions, supplicatory prayers, and poems accompanying the narrative representations.

Although there was apparently no Last Judgment composition included in the original twelfth-century program of decoration at Asinou, the fear of final judgment underlies all the donor inscriptions, and perhaps others as well. On the south wall and again in the apse, the magistros Nikephoros directly addresses the Virgin and voices his hope that she will act as his defender on the terrible Day of Judgment. A similar appeal may be contained in the inscription under the scene of the Dormition. If so, this poem would constitute the third appeal in the church by the same individual, painted on three of the four walls of the church. The appeals are all attached to images of the Virgin: around her (standing?) figure in the apse, near her audience with Christ, and under her lifeless body on the west wall. Though there is no evidence that any appeal was ever inscribed on the north wall, the Virgin images and the poems directed toward her can be said together to form a sort of protective shield around the naos.

The focus on the intercessory role of the Virgin that we encounter in the twelfth-century inscriptions is reiterated in the later decoration, in the poems on the scrolls held by the two images of the standing Virgin. Here her appeal—now not just on behalf of Nikephoros but for mankind in general—is shown in the process of being transmitted to Christ. Christ's positive verbal response ("They shall be redeemed"), inscribed on one of the Virgin's scrolls, is a counterpart to the welcoming gesture he extends to Nikephoros, who approaches Christ's throne on the panel on the south wall.

The other metrical inscriptions from the twelfth century are all written in close contact with narrative compositions: the Birth and Presentation of the Virgin, the Ascension of Christ, and the Forty Martyrs. With the exception of the Ascension poem, all these verses are inscribed directly on the blue background.

The poem attached to the Birth of the Virgin fresco succinctly draws out the importance of this event in the story of salvation: "The Birth of the Virgin [is] salvation," it says in the first verse; and in the second, the world is told to rejoice, "seeing" its resurrection. Henry Maguire has proposed that the scene of the Presentation of the Virgin in the Temple was viewed as a lesson in "oikonomia," a reassurance to a monk that if God could allow the Virgin to enter the prohibited Holy of Holies, then the law could, in the end, be stretched for him as well.[57] The Presentation scene at Asinou would also have carried overtones of salvation. The Ascension poem seems to relate Christ's ascent to his ultimate return, as in the Biblical text ("This same Jesus, which is taken up from you into heaven, shall so come in like manner as ye have seen him go into heaven"; Acts 1:11) and thus connects the soteriological themes of the narratives with the eschatological theme of the donor inscriptions.

The poems attached to the twelfth-century narrative compositions, then, are more exegesis than ekphrasis. They guide the viewer in reading the images, revealing the implications of the depicted events in the context of the church program as a whole.[58]

56. Nicolaïdès, "Étude iconographique," 107, with examples. The Virgin in the naos has no epithet other than Mother of God.

57. Maguire, "*Abaton* and *Oikonomia*," 95–105.

58. For epigrams as guides to the reading of images during the Hellenistic period, see Goldhill, "Naive and Knowing Eye." See also Hörandner, "Cycle of Epigrams," 123; Lauxtermann, *Byzantine Poetry*, 195–96. Of special

The Forty Martyrs poem differs somewhat—it refers directly to the image it accompanies—but the purpose is essentially the same. Where other poems devoted to the Forty Martyrs compare the cold weather to the warmth of the martyr's devotion, or dwell on other aspects of the story, the Asinou verses take the familiar image of the shivering Forty and highlight their triumph over the demands of the flesh, a theme certainly appropriate to the monastic context. It is possible that, in this particular Forty Martyrs image at Asinou, its unusual preoccupation with their physical suffering, especially their bleeding bodies and bloody footprints, is meant to emphasize the painful trials involved in a monk's progress in triumphing over the flesh, with the temptation of the warm bath suggesting the lure of the everyday world that must be renounced. It is no accident that the fresco is adjacent to the sequence of scenes devoted to the Passion of Christ.

Not all the narrative compositions in the church are accompanied by epigrams, and some explanation for this should be sought. Of course, many of the original compositions have been lost, and there is no way to assess just how many scenes once had poems attached. But from the evidence of those that survive, it appears that epigrams were chosen to accompany those scenes that might need to be elucidated or drawn into the overall scheme. Thus the poem chosen for the Forty Martyrs serves to draw the scene into Asinou's monastic atmosphere by downplaying the military aspect of the story and emphasizing instead the martyrs' bodily suffering and its reward, as a metaphor for the monastic experience. The placement of the early Virgin scenes behind the iconostasis, in the bema where no woman was allowed to enter, might also have required some form of explanation.[59] So, where other surviving epigrams on the subject of the Birth of the Virgin dwell on its miraculous aspects, the poem in the bema at Asinou stresses the importance of the event in initiating the whole process of salvation.

The wedding of picture and poem that we find at Asinou may be an early indication of the thrust toward programmatic cohesion that would increasingly characterize Byzantine church decoration over the course of the twelfth century. Here the cohesion is still in its infancy; as it developed further, such explanatory inscriptions were needed less, and they would soon disappear entirely.

What can the poems tell us about Asinou in general? Until their sources can be determined exactly, it would be risky to draw any conclusions about the level of culture they reveal. All that can be said with any assurance regarding the sources of the poems is that: (1) The Forty Martyrs poem derives from one that existed in poetry collections made considerably earlier than 1106 and outside of Cyprus; it may have traveled with the iconography; (2) the Birth of the Virgin poem seems to be a verse "summary" of homiletic and liturgical interpretations of the event; and (3) the poem written on the Virgin's scroll in the naos was so widely used in Byzantium as to be quasi-liturgical. As for the apse poem addressed to the Virgin Pantanassa, its recurrence at Trikomo (without the donor's name) may indicate that both churches were painted by the same workshop, or that the poem was used more widely than we might imagine. The other poems either derive from literary collections that have yet to be identified, or—like the poem on the south wall—were composed ad hoc for the donor.

The poem attached to the fresco of the Birth of the Virgin is fairly unpretentious; it, too, could conceivably have been composed locally on the basis of

interest here is Rhoby's section devoted to "Interaktion von Wort und Bild" (67–70), in the introduction to his *Byzantinische Epigramme* (37–73). A contemporary (10th-century) marginal note in the Leo Bible (MS Vat. Reg. gr. 1, fol. 1v) speaks of the epigrams written around the Old Testament scenes in that manuscript as summaries of the content of the images: ". . . metric iambic verses run around on the four sides of the frame explaining the meaning of the historiated scenes clearly and concisely" (trans. Lauxtermann, *Byzantine Poetry*, 191). See Mathews, "Epigrams of Leo Sacellarios," 99.

59. The scene of the Birth of the Virgin is located in exactly the same position at Kalliana. At Trikomo and at Kakopetria, the scenes of the life of the Virgin are placed in the south part of the naos.

familiar liturgical texts. The poems are remarkably pure in meter, but the spelling is generally phonetic and inaccurate, a discrepancy that might result from oral transmission. On only one fresco, the St. George panel, is the spelling nearly perfect; whether this indicates a rise in local literary culture in the later twelfth century, or merely a different and higher level of patronage, is hard to say.

The presence of these metrical inscriptions on Asinou's frescoes confirms that in the middle Byzantine period epigrams were incorporated into monumental painting as well as manuscripts, icons, and ivories. But how common this may have been remains an open question. Documented examples of middle Byzantine epigrams in the context of monumental painting—outside the realm of donor or dedicatory inscriptions—are relatively rare. We know that some poems of Theodore of Stoudios were used; one anonymous poem referring to apse compositions appears twice, once in a church of the tenth century and again in one of the eleventh; and a poem written on the fresco of the Annunciation at the Mavriotissa at Kastoria has been identified as a version of an anonymous epigram found in the Marciana manuscript.[60] Yet almost none of the epigrams on church feasts composed by such prolific middle-Byzantine poets as John Geometres, Christopher of Mitylene, John Mauropous, Nicholas Kallikles, and Theodore Prodromos have been found inscribed on frescoes.[61] The eleventh-century metrical calendar of Christopher of Mitylene appears on frescoes of the Palaiologan period, but the poem in this case was taken surely not from any literary collection but from the Synaxarion of Constantinople, where these verses had been inserted sometime during the twelfth century.[62]

Neither a mere aberration nor a lone survivor of a long-established tradition, Asinou can be best explained by its character as a private foundation. While the grander and more public churches of the middle-Byzantine period tended to cite well-known Biblical or liturgical passages, this little church uses less-familiar texts, texts that fall somewhere between liturgy and literary culture, texts that reflect the donor's taste, his own reading, or perhaps even his literary talents. This church decoration is more like an inscribed object offered privately to God than a work that addresses a large community. The Asinou inscriptions, at least those from the twelfth century—which at first glance appear to derive from a variety of sources and traditions—may in fact resonate with the voice of a single individual addressing in a variety of ways the issues of his own death and salvation.

60. An epigram of Theodore of Stoudios, ten lines of dodecasyllable verse, was apparently written (or perhaps carved) over the entrance to the naos of Nea Mone on Chios, according to a 17th-century visitor; another poem by this author was used at Grottaferrata and at the Great Lavra on Athos, and one by Prodromos was seen in the now-destroyed Cappadocian church of St. Stephen at Nis, in Lake Eğridir. For references to these and other examples, see Lauxtermann, *Byzantine Poetry*, 32, 71, 81, 92–93, 186 note 90, 339–40, 352; Rhoby, *Byzantinische Epigramme*, passim. On the Chios epigram, see now Barber, "Mimesis and Memory," 327–32. On the poem found at both St. Achilleios at Prespa and at the Panagia ton Chalkeon in Thessalonike, see now Gerstel, *Beholding the Sacred Mysteries*, 81 (Appendix, no. 1); fig. 3; Rhoby, *Byzantinische Epigramme*, 187–92. For the Mavriotissa poem, see Hörandner, "Cycle of Epigrams," 118, no. 2 (= Lampros, "Ὁ Μαρκιανὸς κῶδιξ," no. 184). The clusters of epigrams devoted to the church feasts may indicate a connection with feast cycles in monumental art, but even this is not entirely clear.

61. But see Kepetzi, "Autour d'une inscription," 177, for the role of Mauropous, and for the story of a priest asking around for epigrams on the Aspasmos of the apostles Peter and Paul. On epigrams concerning works of art, see Lauxtermann, *Byzantine Poetry*, 149–96.

62. Delehaye, *Synaxarium*, Class M (cols. xxxviii–xlvi). See Follieri, "Il calendario giambico"; eadem, *I calendari in metro innografico*, esp. 1:8–15; Gligorijević-Maksimović, "Slikani kalendar," with French summary; Mitsakis, "Byzantine and Modern Greek Parahymnography." See also Rhoby, *Byzantinische Epigramme*, 204–6, nos. 114–17, on the epigrams of Christopher of Mitylene inscribed on the calendar frescoes at St. Nicholas Orphanos, Thessalonike. The Oxford "Picture-Book" Menologion has Synaxarion verses by Nikephoros Kallistos Xanthopoulos: Hutter, *El Menologio de Oxford*, 163–64.

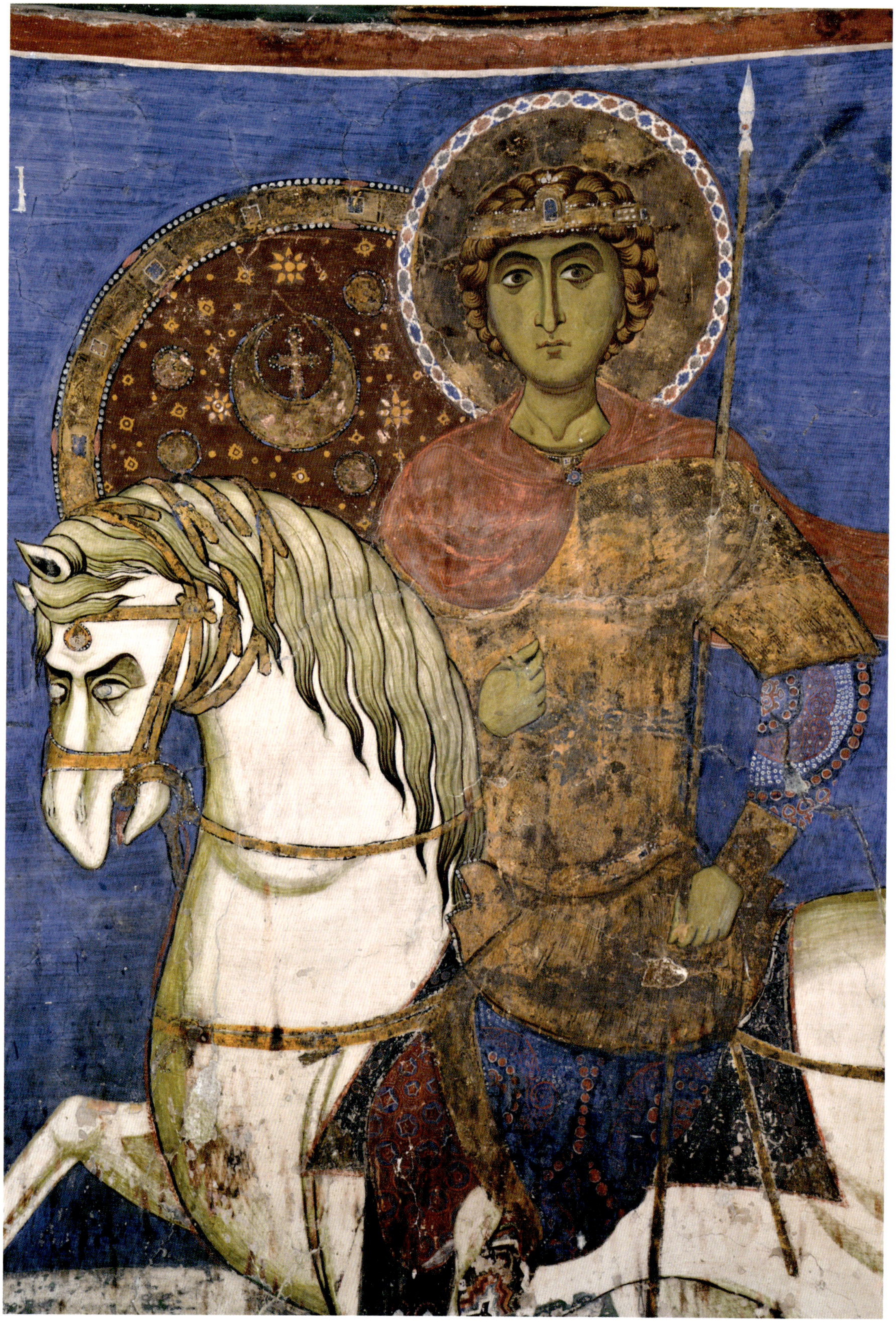

The church of Panagia Phorbiotissa, narthex, south apse: mural icon of St. George, detail (photo courtesy of G. L. Carr)

CHAPTER FOUR

The Murals of the Narthex

The Paintings of the Twelfth Century

Part One: Date and Iconography

Andréas Nicolaïdès

THE FIRST PAINTINGS AT ASINOU AFTER THOSE OF 1105/6 were installed in the narthex. They were painted there before the comprehensive campaign of 1332/33 covered all surfaces except the image of the Mother of God Phorbiotissa over the door to the naos and the murals in the southern apse,[1] but they survive only in fragments and pose many questions. The most visible of them is the brilliant mural icon of St. George on the wall of the southern apse, to which the bulk of this chapter is devoted (Fig. 4.1; see also Fig. 5.1). Otherwise we retain only small fragments, exposed where the plaster of 1332/33 has been abraded. These are inventoried by Sophia Kalopissi-Verti in Chapter 5, and include the following: (1) fragments of an archangel beneath the mural icon of the archangel Michael on the wall of the north apse (Fig. 5.35); (2) a fragment of a painted ornament with a split-palmette pattern on the lintel of the door to the narthex, beneath the Mother of God Phorbiotissa (Figs. 3.11, 5.37); (3) a segment of green ground with a small plant, and a white dado with red and black wavy lines beneath the Virgin Paraklesis to the left of this door (Fig. 5.30); (4) traces of a dado with a pattern resembling opus sectile that runs from the right jamb of the same door to the area below the St. George (Figs. 5.1, 5.30); (5) a trace of the split-palmette pattern on a plaster layer below the figure of the patron Georgios on the jamb of the south apse (Fig. 5.44). The date(s) of these paintings, their relation to the icon of St. George, whether any of them coincide with the inauguration of the narthex, and whether they represent a homogeneous campaign or an episodic accretion of individual votives, are all open questions.

In Chapter 2, Athanasios Papageorgiou addresses the date at which the narthex was built (pp. 54, 56–57). That date poses the following key question. The church had become a katholikon by 1115 (see p. 19 above); if it was founded as such, it is curious that it was not furnished with a narthex from the beginning, for a number of katholika

1. The overdoor with the image of the Mother of God Phorbiotissa belongs to the campaign of 1105/6 and will be discussed in conjunction with that campaign in a forthcoming publication.

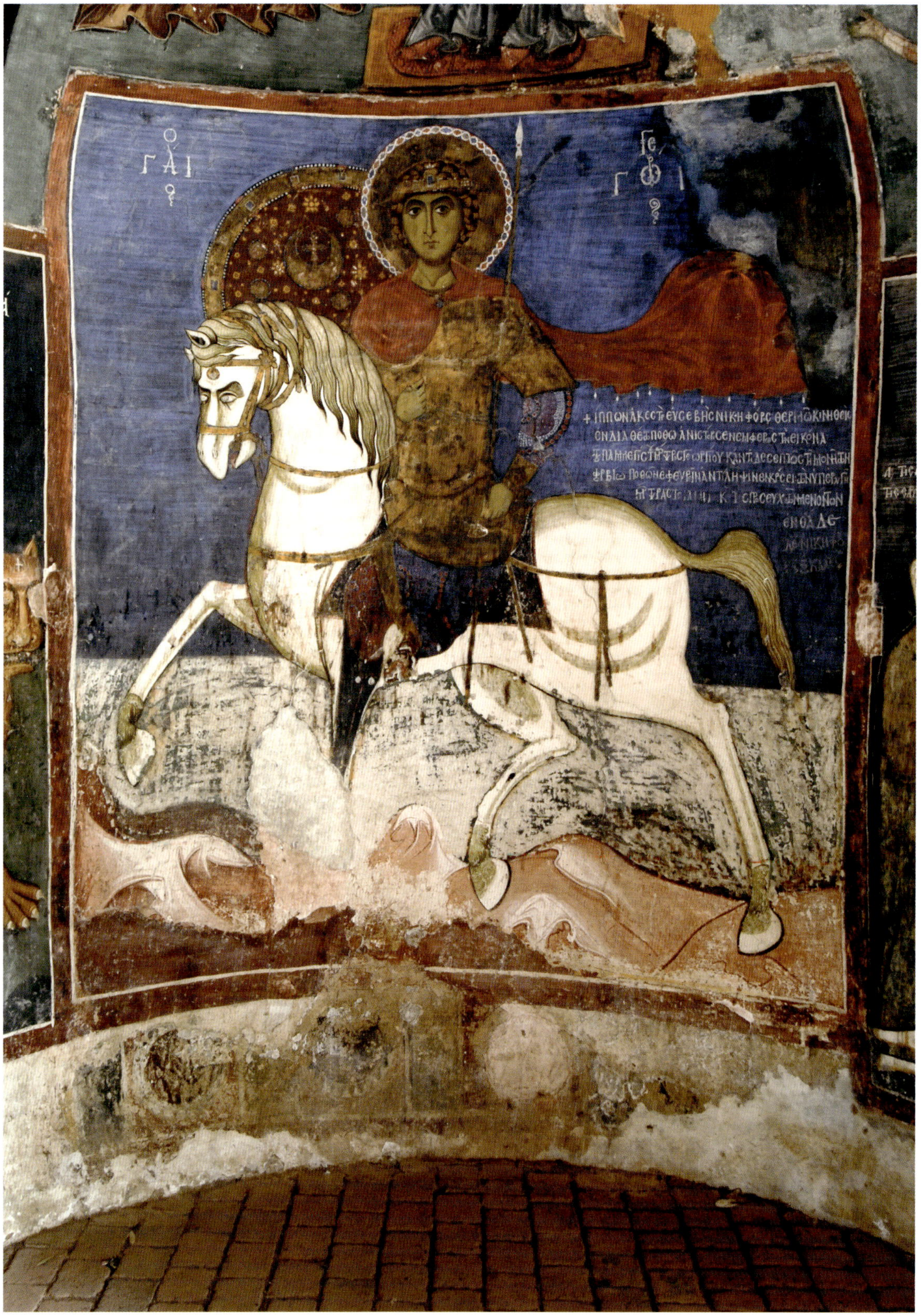

FIG. 4.1 Narthex, south conch. St. George (photo courtesy of G. L. Carr)

on Cyprus from the years around 1100—including St. John Chrysostom, Koutsovendis; the Virgin Apsinthiotissa; St. George at Aphendrika; and St. Paul at Gomaristra in Lapithos—were furnished with narthexes of the same Constantinopolitan type seen at Asinou, with apsidioles on each side (see pp. 55–56 above). In turn, given that other churches acquired a narthex when they became monastic, it is hard to explain why Asinou should have had to wait so long, i.e., fifteen to fifty years, to acquire one.[2] This question turns our attention to the paintings, to see if they throw any light on the early history of the narthex. Their evidence is meager, but three facts stand out. One is the date assigned by Sophia Kalopissi-Verti to the dado, which she places in the late twelfth century on the basis of its kinship with the Enkleistra and Lagoudera (see below, p. 206);[3] the second is the continuity observed both by David Winfield in this chapter, and by Ioanna Kakoulli in Chapter 7, between the plaster of this dado and the plaster of the St. George, thus uniting them chronologically (see pp. 102–3, 317–19, 337–40); and the third is the split-palmette motif. Persuasively associated with the final third of the twelfth century, this motif appears not only on the lintel of the eastern door and the jamb of the apse, as Kalopissi-Verti notes (p. 192), but also in the brocaded tunic of the St. George (Figs. 4.1, 4.3), in the brocaded covers of the back of the throne of the Virgin with Child in the conch of the apse at Lagoudera (before 1192), in the valance of the funerary bed of the Virgin in the Dormition at Perachorio, in the brocaded tunic and the leggings of the St. Demetrios at St. Anthony at Kellia, and in the altar in the apse of St. Panteleimon in Nerezi (1164).[4] These three observations suggest that what survives of the early painting in the narthex was produced over a limited span of time in the final quarter of the twelfth century, long after the church became monastic, unless the fragments of the archangel and the green ground with plants, seen under the paintings of 1332–33, are remnants of the original painted program that sometime after 1115 followed the construction of the narthex. Whether it constituted a coherent program or a set of episodic votives cannot be answered, but Sophia Kalopissi-Verti's observation (p. 198) and my own that the colors in the archangel coincide with none of the other phases of painting in the narthex suggests that this, like the St. George, was an independent icon. The magnificent image of St. George dominates the rest of this chapter.

The mural icon—so identified in its dedicatory poem: ἀνιστόρησεν ἐμφερῶς τὴν εἰκόνα—in the south apse is labeled with a cruciform inscription as St. George: ὁ ἅγιος Γεώργιος (Figs. 4.1, 3.10; p. 110). Described as μάρτυρα στεφανίτην, the crowned martyr, George is portrayed with opulent materials—gold, silver, cinnabar, and lapis lazuli (Fig. 4.2; pp. 322, 325–26, 332–34). A fair-haired youth in jeweled armor,[5] he rides a striding white horse in a rippling pink setting that can be seen as either mountains or waves. His golden saddle, rimmed with pearls and gems, lies on a large, richly embroidered *epochon* (the trapezoidal second saddle; Fig. 4.3). He rides eastward toward the bema of the church. No dragon, princess, or pillion rider intrudes;[6] in their absence it seems likely

2. Papageorgiou, "Narthex of the Churches," 446–47. According to D. Winfield (in conversation), the cracks observed on the painting of the Virgin Phorbiotissa of 1105/6 over the western door of the church proves that it was an exterior image for a long time, about fifty years. In my opinion fifteen or fifty years may not make a substantial difference, considering the rain, hail, snow, and other rude climatic conditions of the Troodos to which the painting would have been exposed.

3. See also Nicolaïdès, "Arakiotissa à Lagoudéra" [1993], 1:139, j; 2:5, 8, b (respectively).

4. Respectively, ibid., 1:168; Megaw and Hawkins, "Church of the Holy Apostles," 333, fig. 42; Perdiki, "Peintures Murales," 224 fig. 107; Sinkević, *The Church of St. Panteleimon at Nerezi,* fig. XVI.

5. Thus St. Theodore of Sykeon in the late 6th century called him λαμπρὸν τῇ ἐσθῆτι, ταῖς δὲ θριξὶν οὖλον, as quoted by Walter, "Origins of the Cult," 319.

6. These themes appear on a large number of icons from the 13th century onward at Sinai, and in Georgian manuscripts and mural paintings from the 11th century onward. Thus I see no need to link the image at Asinou with the posthumous miracles involving the capture of a youth

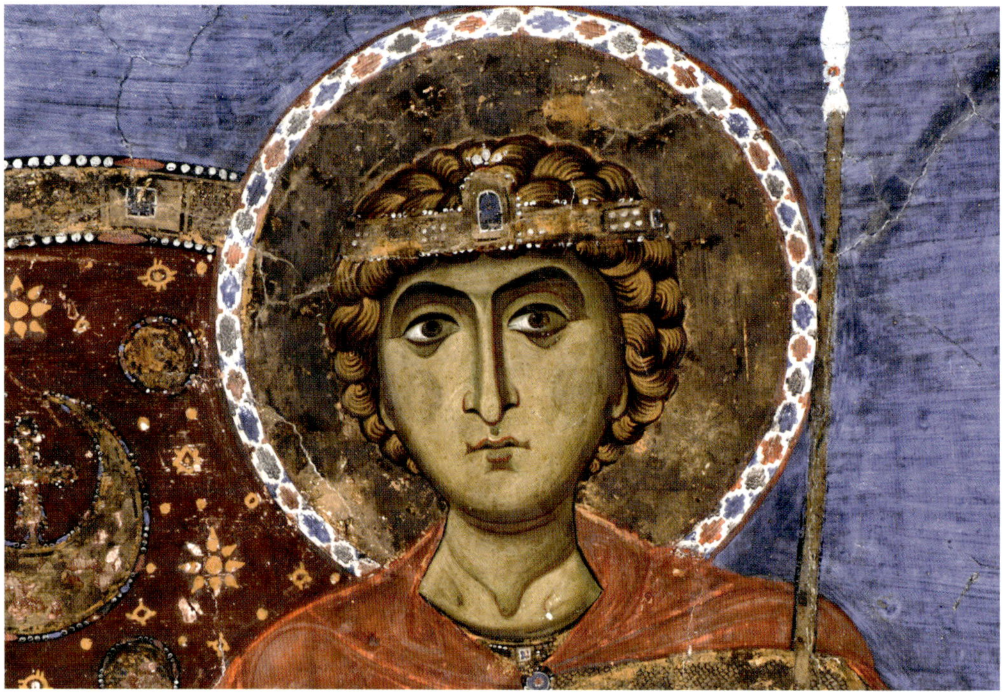

FIG. 4.2 Narthex, south conch. St. George, detail of head (photo courtesy of G. L. Carr)

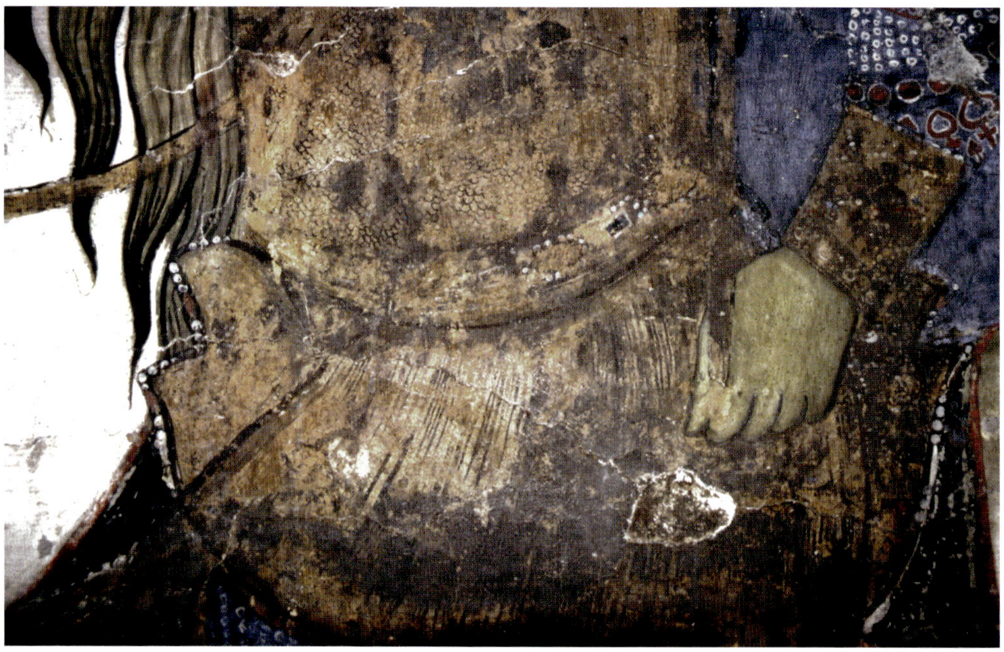

FIG. 4.3 Narthex, south conch. St. George, detail of armor and saddle (photo courtesy of A. Nicolaïdès)

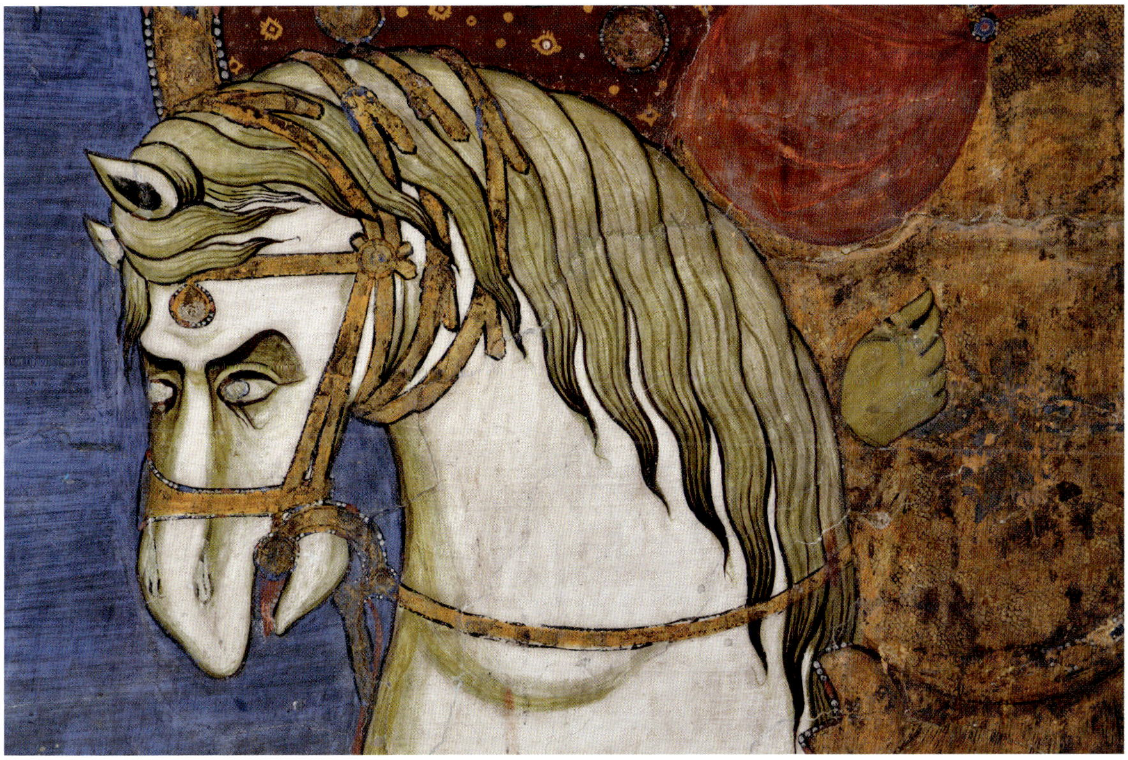

FIG. 4.4 Narthex, south conch. St. George, detail of horse's head (photo courtesy of G. L. Carr)

that George is set in a spare landscape, not on the waves as in the story of the rescued youth, and that he thus represents a newly emerging iconographic type. Chief of the elite corps of sainted *stratelatai* (generals), including Theodore, Demetrios, and Prokopios, George was renowned throughout the Christian world and was venerated with enthusiasm in both East and West.[7]

Here, George wears the *stemmatogyrion* and sumptuous military garb,[8] intricately designed and meticulously executed in accord with twelfth-century taste. To judge from pseudo-Kodinos, the *stemmatogyrion* was a crown adopted in the eleventh century in the imperial palace; under the Komnenoi it became an indispensable attribute of holy warriors, as exemplified especially by the portraits of military saints in the church of the Virgin Kosmosoteira.[9] The military costume of

of Mytilene. See Cormack and Mihalarias, "Crusader Painting of St. George?"; Walter, "Origins," 321–22.

7. Venerated as megalomartyr and *tropaiophoros*, supposed to have died around 303, commemorated on 23 April: Delehaye, *Synaxarium*, col. 623–26; Chiovaro et al., *Histoire des saints*, 11:14–15, 100; *BHG* 1:212–13. On the cult and literary tradition of George in general, see Walter, *Warrior Saints*, 109–44, with earlier bibliography; idem, "Origins"; and, above all, Kazhdan, "List of Saints," 1: no. 50 (1–8); Underwood, *Kariye Djami*, 1:252; S. Papadopoulos, G. Bekatoros, and M. Soteriou, in *ΘΗΕ* 4 (1964): coll. 429–39, s.v. Γεώργιος. One cannot fail to cite the homily of Arkadios, bishop of Cyprus (+640), dedicated to George and delivered in a church of the saint, most probably in Cyprus: see Delehaye, *Les légendes grecques*, 2–5, 45–76; Walter, "Origins."

8. See the excellent analysis of military costume in Parani, *Reconstructing the Reality*, 101–58.

9. See, above all, Bakirtzis, "Warrior Saints or Portraits," 85–86, pl. 9.1–4; Patterson [Ševčenko], "Byzantine Frescoes at Pherrai," 77–78, 80; Panayiotidi, "Wall-Paintings in the Church of the Virgin Kosmosoteira,"

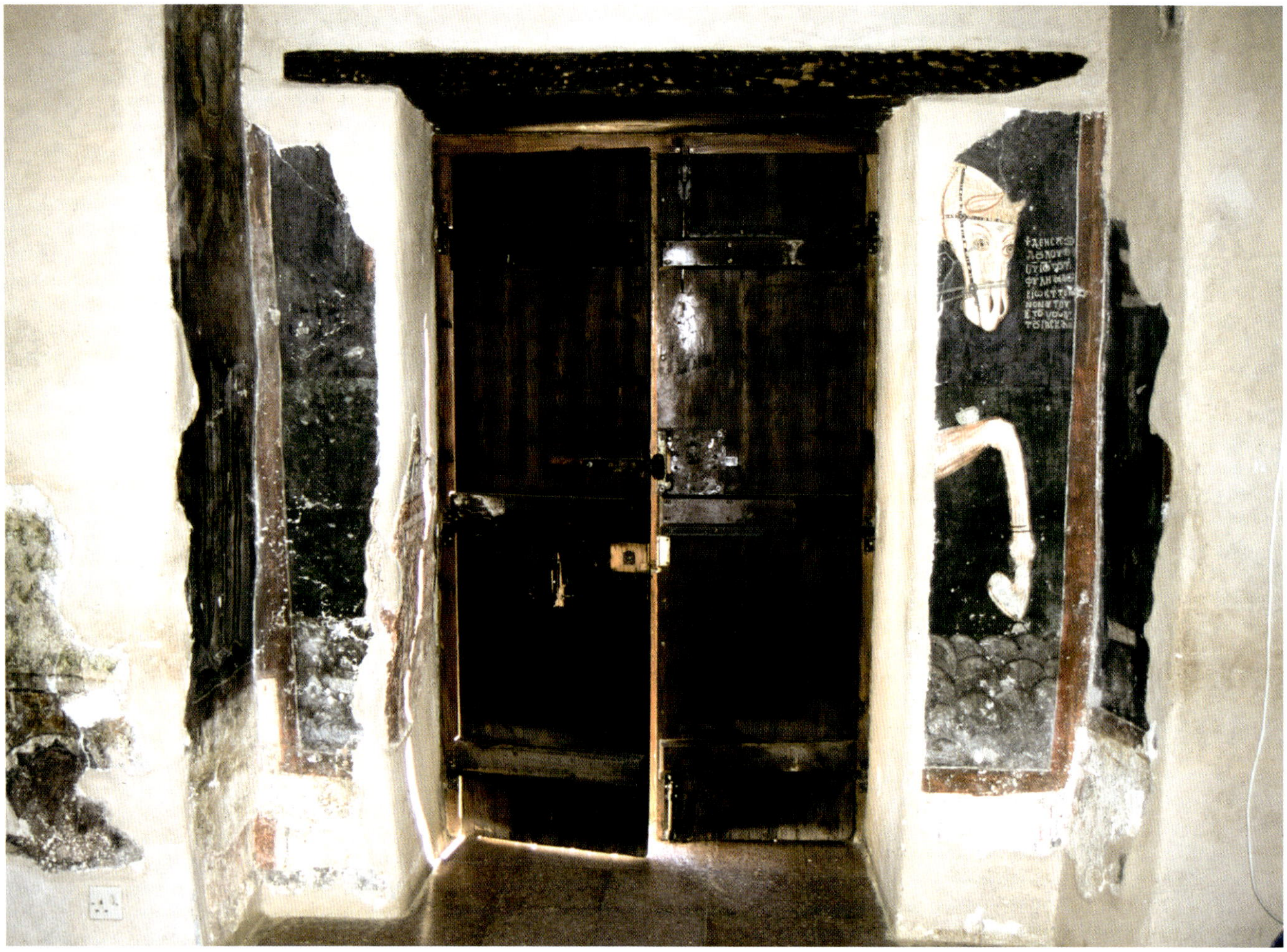

FIG. 4.5 Kakopetria, St. Nicholas of the Roof (τῆς Στέγης). West wall of the narthex, equestrian image of St. George (photo courtesy of A. Nicolaïdès)

St. George at Asinou consists of a gilded mail shirt, the *lorikion* or *alysidotos thorax*, studded with pearls and gems at the collar on the visible shoulder and above all at the waist,[10] and bound by a *cingulum* or *zonarion*, a sash of light blue knotted at mid-chest. Associated with the mail shirt are the long, leather *pteryges* that protect the hips and the upper arms to the elbow (Fig. 5.4).[11] The pteryges are worn

figs. 6–7; Papamastorakes, "Ένα εικαστικό εγκώμιο," 232. The same is true of several icons of St. George at Sinai: see Mouriki, "Icons," 183, fig. 57; G. Soteriou, *Βυζαντινὰ μνημεῖα*, 1: no. 169, 18. See also the representations of George in the Mani, for instance at St. John Chrysostom in Geraki: Moutsopoulos and Demetrokalles, *Γεράκι*, 40–41; 226, figs. 13, 14.

10. It is the same on the icons of SS. Sergios and Bakkhos on Sinai: G. Soteriou, *Βυζαντινὰ μνημεῖα*, vol. 1, nos. 185, 197; Mouriki, "Icons," 192, fig. 66. Most recently attributed to crusader Lebanon (see Nelson and Collins, *Holy Image, Hallowed Ground*, 251–53), these could have originated in Cyprus.

11. On military costume, see Mouriki, *Nea Moni*; Underwood, *Kariye Djami*, 1:254–55; and the very fine chapter on the subject in Hendy, *Catalogue of Byzantine Coins*, 4.1:143–80. Parani, *Reconstructing the Reality*, 114, believes that composite armor was an "artistic invention." Mail shirt and *pteryges* are seen as well at St. Anthony, Kellia, on the portrait of

with a short brocaded tunic that is predominantly bright blue and is bordered with pearls. The warrior saint wears sumptuously decorated, dark red leggings under black greaves that cover his leg below the knee; they have a braided red band on the side topped with two large pearls or balls. An ample chlamys painted in cinnabar (see p. 326 below), fastened over his chest with a pearled brooch, the φιβλίον, is embroidered with white crosslets and edged with fourteen pear-shaped pearls; it flows out behind him in a flourish of fabric that balances the haunch of the horse. Its dynamic curve later captured the imagination of the painter of the panel above it, and he echoed it in reverse in the Virgin's veil (Fig. 5.1) In his left hand the holy general grasps a lance, while in his right he holds the gilded reins of his horse. A magnificent round shield, supported—one assumes—on his right shoulder, is encircled with gems, decorated with stars and medallions, and embellished with pearls around a cross supported on a crescent moon: τὸ φεγγίον referred to in the *Book of Ceremonies*.[12] Similarly, a small crescent moon is attached to the golden bridle on the horse's chest (Fig. 4.6). The crescent is seen again on the bucklers of the equestrian St. George and of the standing St. Demetrios at Kellia (late twelfth century), at St. John Chrysostom and St. Athanasios in Geraki (thirteenth century), and elsewhere.[13]

The "militarized" image of the saint, according to Alexander Kazhdan, brings out his power as a thaumaturge.[14] But it surely responds, above all, to George's role as the military saint par excellence of the Komnenian empire, a role exemplified by the ἁγιογεωργάτα, coins issued by John II Komnenos on which an armed St. George accompanies the emperor.[15] Certainly, on Cyprus, George's churches far outnumbered those of other warrior saints.[16] George was also, however, a protector of cattle, surely all the more appealing to the icon's donor, the veterinarian (*hippiatros*) Nikephoros.[17]

Father Christopher Walter has studied the iconography of St. George, which has a vast bibliography.[18] Though the legends (the *Miracula*) that portray him on horseback are dated to the twelfth century, his imagery displays him this way already in the eleventh century, for instance—to cite the earliest of many dated examples—at St. Barbara, Soğanlı (1016–21), where the saint is seen armed and astride a horse to the left of the western door to the naos of the church.[19] On Cyprus there is the

St. George on the wall to the south of the north-west pier (Yerasimou, Papaioakeim, and Spanou, *Η κατά Κίτιον αγιογραφική τέχνη*, 28, fig. 9); at Nerezi, where composite armor is worn by St. Prokopios (Sinković, *Church of St. Panteleimon at Nerezi*, 148, fig. 55); and on the mural icon of St. George himself at St. George, Kurbinovo (Grozdanov and Hadermann-Misguich, *Kurbinovo*, fig. 31).

12. Constantine VII Porphyrogenitus, *Livre des cérémonies*, 2.1:103, line 11 (chap. 74 [65]); 2.2:108: a sort of scepter surmounted by a crescent moon borne by tribunes.

13. Yerasimou et al., *Η κατά Κίτιον αγιογραφική τέχνη*, 28, fig. 9; Perdiki, "Peintures Murales," 71–74, figs. 72–74, 76–77, 109. Moutsopoulos and Demetrokallis, *Γεράκι*, 40; 226, figs. 13–14; 244, fig. 80.

14. Kazhdan, "List of Saints," no. 50 (2–3).

15. These were aspra tracheia in electrum showing George in armor with drawn sword beside John II: Kazhdan, "List of Saints," no. 50 (3), and above all Hendy, *Coinage and Money*, 32, pl. 10 (1–6), 104, 437, etc.; idem, in *Catalogue of Byzantine Coins*, 57, 260–61.

16. Delehaye, "Saints de Chypre," 195, 267, 270, 284, 287. He cites 67 localities that bear the name of St. George, as compared with eight for Theodore and four for Demetrios.

17. Kazhdan, "List of Saints," 50, 3 (for his miracles, see also Festugière, *Sainte Thècle*, 257–347).

18. Walter, *Warrior Saints*, 109–44; idem, "Origins," esp. 316–22. See also *RBK*, 2:1049–59, s.v. "Heilige" (Soldaten), entry by A. Chatzinikolaou; *LCI*, vol. 6 (1974), 365–73, s.v. "Georg," entry by L. Palli; Kretzenbacher, *Griechische Reiterheilige*, 7–35; N. Thierry, "Aux limites du sacré," 240–43; Vassilaki, "Cretan Icon." See, finally, Gerstel, "Art and Identity," 267ff.

19. On the *Miracula* of St. George see *ODB* 2:834–35. On the imagery see Jerphanion, *Une nouvelle province de l'art*, 2.1: 322, pl. 187, 2; Restle, *Byzantine Wall Painting*, 3: no. 121, fig. 436. Other examples include Lembatavank in Georgia of the 7th century (Jolivet-Lévy, *Les Églises byzantines de Cappadoce*, 190, note 79); and a number in Cappadocia: St. George at Zindanönü (7th to 9th century), Karabulut kilisesi (first quarter of 11th century);

fragmentary figure of an equestrian St. George from the twelfth or thirteenth century at St. Nicholas of the Roof (τῆς Στέγης). There, as at Asinou, St. George was depicted as a mounted warrior in the narthex, in this case on the west wall. At an unspecified date, most probably after the thirteenth century, a door was cut at this place in the wall, and today one sees only the remains of the painting of the horse to either side of it (Fig. 4.5). The church of St. Anthony at Kellia retains three representations of St. George in his equestrian guise from the twelfth and thirteenth centuries, and at St. Demetrianos Andridiotes at Dali, of 1317, a monumental mounted warrior George without a dragon occupies the whole of the north wall of the central bay, his face toward the entrance door on the south side of the church.[20]

The fact that the St. George at Asinou was painted over the walled-up southern door to the narthex, standing between the eastern and western doors into the narthex and facing its northern door, is unquestionably important. Catherine Jolivet-Lévy has noted the persistence in Cappadocia of an early Christian tradition of placing warrior saints near the entrance to churches as apotropaia.[21] If this was the case at Asinou, then it would seem most probable that the patron Nikephoros knew that the wall of the south apse masked a hidden door, and so for prophylactic purposes painted his great icon over it. It is, in fact, hard to imagine why the door of a newly completed narthex would so quickly have been closed up.[22] Rather, it is more probable that the wealthy Nikephoros or his anonymous painter—the "Master of St. George"—were unable to find a space in the narthex ample enough for the magnificent icon they desired, except by walling up one of the four portals. Closing the hemicycle of the south apsidiole offered a surface large enough to accommodate a prophylactic mural icon of St. George mounted and set in a rugged natural landscape. It is also noteworthy that the choice of the south apsidiole was meaningful, if one takes into account that the monastic buildings of the Phorbiotissa monastery were located to the north of the katholikon (see below, p. 298). Hence, when the monks were entering the narthex from its northern door, they would face St. George's icon.

The iconographic type for which such ample wall space was required, with George on horseback in a spare natural setting, corresponds to a type known by the epithet "Diasorites." This epithet, which is associated with Asia Minor,[23] is not cited in either the cruciform inscription that names the St. George here, or in the poetic epigram of the patron, Nikephoros (see above, p. 77). In the thirteenth century, however, the name Diasorites was widely associated with the image of St. George on horseback in a natural setting, without the dragon, but sometimes with and sometimes without the

the church of the cistern (first half of the 11th century); St. Eustathios (Göreme 11 of the early 10th century); Göreme 18, Göreme 20, Göreme 21 (all of the second half of the 11th century); Göreme 28, Yılanlı kilise (late 11th or early 12th century); and Derin dere kilisesi (9th century): see ibid., 59, 81 note 106, 122, 113, 125, 126, 136, 190. In the second half of the 11th century, St. George also appeared on horseback on the seal of the praitor George Spanopoulos: *DOSeals* 5:28.1. More frequently, though, he appeared without the horse. Moreover, he need not be the saint in question when a dragon-slayer is shown. One appreciates Father Walter's humor when he remarks that "no saint had the monopoly of this beneficent work. . . . even women saints . . . Paraskevi, killed dragons. There is consequently no reason to identify early unnamed pictures of a saint killing a dragon with Saint George" (idem, "Origins," 320).

20. Yerasimou et al., *Η κατά Κίτιον αγιογραφική τέχνη*, 28, figs. 7, 8, 9.

21. Jolivet-Lévy, *Les Églises*, 190.

22. On p. 56, above, Athanasios Papageorgiou writes that the south door of the narthex "was evidently walled up very shortly after the completion of the construction of the narthex. . . ." I would not be so assertive, for if this was the case, why were the stones used to close the door so different from those of the rest of the narthex?

23. See Amantos, "Σύμμεικτα"; Demetrokalles, "O ναός του Αγίου Γεωργίου"; and Wassiliou, "O Άγιος Γεώργιος ο Διασορίτης." One should note that the formula "saint George de Diasora," read in Hadjichristodoulou, *Church of Our Lady of Asinou*, is an error.

young Paphlagonian pillion rider from Mytilene. The thirteenth-century icon of Phaneromene in Nicosia, the icon of 1260 at Sinai, the mid-thirteenth-century icon in the British Museum, the seals in the Numismatic Museum in Athens, and even the much later painting of 1474 at Pedoulas demonstrate this.[24] Thus, it is perhaps not too audacious to suggest that the image at Asinou is already a Diasorites in all but name. The image of St. George is a protector not merely of Nikephoros, as Nancy Ševčenko points out in Chapter 3, but of the narthex and therefore the monks of the monastery. As to the second occurrence of the name Nikephoros, now Nikephoros Kallias, I agree with Ševčenko that it is not clear whether he is the same person as the veterinarian Nikephoros, donor of the fresco, or a later devotee. Alternatively, one might identify him as the artist, based on the close kinship, noted by Ševčenko, between the paint used for his invocation and that seen on the rump of the horse. One wonders, however, whether the artist would have masked his identity so modestly, when Theodore Apseudes signed his work with such eloquence at the Enkleistra of St. Neophytos, as did the hieromonk Theodore, the "itinerant artist" who painted at Lagoudera. The question remains open.[25]

The date of the St. George at Asinou has aroused endless controversy. Buckler, who saw it still obscured with soot and smoke, assigned it—along with the images of St. Anastasia and the Latin Lady—to 1225–50;[26] the Stylianous put it first around 1200 and then in the late twelfth century;[27] Athanasios Papageorgiou prefers a date in the second half of the twelfth century for the construction of the narthex and a date in the thirteenth century for the painting of St. George;[28] Marina Sacopoulo only clouded the issue when she spoke of "l'image que Nicéphore Kallias a fait restaurer";[29] and David Winfield, whose opinion follows in this chapter, adopts the second half of the twelfth century, on the basis of kinship with the paintings of 1183 at the Enkleistra and those at Lagoudera. I share his opinion. The various iconographic elements, including what is clearly a diadem, and the military panoply of the Komnenian era, show that St. George is a warrior saint—not a "Byzantine crusader," as the Stylianous wrote—the protector par excellence of the *archontes* as he was of the emperor John II Komnenos. If one adds to this the extremely elegant stylistic features that so closely resemble the frescoes of St. Neophytos (1183) and Lagoudera (completed 1192), as well as the motif of the brocaded clothes (discussed above), the basis for controversy vanishes: the icon must be dated in the last decades of the twelfth century, most plausibly from 1164 (Nerezi) through 1180 (Perachorio) up to ca. 1192 (Lagoudera). The other images in the narthex at Asinou connected to its construction, such as the archangel and the green back round with plants, were assuredly painted in less precious colors. This is why the image studied here was not covered over in 1332/33, but left visible and venerable, a mural icon of the megalomartyr and *tropaiophoros* George.

24. On the icon from Phaneromene, see Panagi, *Ο Ιερός ναός Παναγίας Φανερωμένης*, 52. On the Sinai icon see Evans, *Byzantium: Faith and Power*, 376, no. 231; Cormack and Mihalarias, "Crusader Painting"; Cormack, "St. George," 150–51, no. 9, in Acheimastou-Potamianou, *From Byzantium to El Greco*; Wassiliou, "Ο Άγιος Γεώργιος." For Pedoulas, see Soteriou, *Βυζαντινὰ μνημεῖα*, 1: pl. 103 (right).

25. See, respectively, Mango and Hawkins, "Hermitage of St. Neophytos," 183, and Nicolaïdès, "Étude iconographique," 8.

26. Buxton et al., "Church of Asinou," 333.

27. Stylianou and Stylianou, *Painted Churches*, 137–38.

28. Personal conversation between Athanasios Papageorgiou and the author, summer 2004.

29. Sacopoulo, *Asinou*, 12–13. Manifestly, she was ill at ease with the image, passing in silence over its iconography as well as its date, and she may not have known that it did not belong to the campaign of 1105/6. I dismiss as incoherent the opinion in Hein et al., *Cyprus*, 57–59.

Part Two: The Mural of St. George: Technique and Conservation

David Winfield

We turn now to a descriptive analysis of the painting.[30] It was the first of the surviving paintings to be executed on the walls of the narthex, and it is unrelated in materials and technique to any other paintings within the church.

Panel Size, Plaster, and Preliminary Drawing

Panel Size: The panel is 2.15 m high (not including the dado pattern underneath it). The width is 1.55 m across the base and 1.45 m across the top.

The Plaster: The plaster edges are difficult to analyze in their relation to the neighboring figure of St. Anastasia Pharmakolytria (the Poison-Curer) and the figures of the Virgin of Mercy and three Latin donors that decorate the conch above St. George (fig. 7.29). The uncertainty is caused by the fact that the plaster edges of the St. George were hacked away and were not left with a tapered edge prior to an overlap of new plaster for the later paintings. It nevertheless seems certain that the panel of St. George represents the earliest layer of painted plaster in this part of the narthex.

To create the panel, the original south door into the narthex was blocked and the plaster for the St. George panel was rendered over the wall with its blocked door in a single layer. The plaster of the dado pattern beneath St. George was part of the same rendering as the panel with the saint. The plaster is a mixture of lime with a straw or chaff

30. This description of St. George has benefited greatly from a discussion about it with my wife, June Winfield. She made the fine measured drawing of St. George, and I thank her for her help. The writer was in charge of conservation at the churches of Asinou and Lagoudera in Cyprus. He was also in charge of further repair work at other churches in Cyprus where Dumbarton Oaks had worked. He followed current custom in taking microsamples of original paintwork. The analysis of these samples would have added greatly to the accuracy of the following description. Unfortunately, the then-Director of Dumbarton Oaks rejected the samples as of no interest; they were later destroyed in a fire in 1991 that destroyed most of the author's library and furniture.

binder; it was given a carefully smoothed finish. A thin wash of lime slurry may have been added to give a smoother surface for the painter to work on.

The White Horse—Plaster Additions: For the whole area of the white horse, two relatively thick layers of lime were added over the panel's lime-and-chaff plaster, thus giving a physical impression of bulkiness to the horse.[31] In the horse's right foreleg, a small area of this lime has flaked away, showing that it was rendered in two layers. The first layer is grayish and, where visible, there are no signs of preliminary color or drawing upon it. It contains small fragments of aggregate, which may be of fine sand. The upper layer is a pure white of fine texture.

On the head of the horse, some evidence can be seen that the plaster was roughly marked out for the general placing of these additional plaster layers for the horse. The rough vertical brushstrokes in the plaster, perhaps made with a plastering brush, may delineate the placing of the horse's head. There must certainly also have been more markings at an early stage in order to indicate the whole shape of the horse so that the extra lime layers for its body could be accurately rendered.[32]

Preliminary Drawing: On the extra layers of lime for the horse can be seen traces of preliminary drawing. These are visible on his right foreleg and his back left leg. In the few damaged areas where it is visible, the preliminary drawing is in red. It was made before the background colors were washed in.

A number of very thin incision lines were made so that the outline of the preliminary drawing could still be seen when the first washes of coloring would have obscured the red drawing. Incisions can be seen marking St. George's left forearm, the base of his torso, and the spear. A straight incision line running at a diagonal to the saint's body can be seen under the paint for the cloak, on the level of his shoulder. This line does not relate to the shapes and folds of the clothing and it may represent an earlier thought as to the placing of the lance. There are also incised lines marking the slightly open mouth of the horse. The lines are very shallow and unobtrusive. There are probably many more incision lines that are now covered up by layers of paint.

The Background

The original upper two-thirds of the background color consists of a gray-black ground color (charcoal black) overpainted with a thin wash of brilliant blue (ultramarine or lapis lazuli). The gray-black ground color lends increased depth and intensity to the final blue color. The use of a dark ground color also meant that only a thin wash of the expensive blue paint was needed, whereas several thick layers of blue paint would have been needed if it were painted directly over the white plaster.

The lower third of the background can be divided into two areas (Figs. 4.1, 4.6). The first area is green (green earth) painted over the same gray-black background color that was used for the blue background above it. A straight horizontal line delineates it from the upper blue background at the level of the horse's belly. An enigmatic dark area behind the right foreleg of the horse looks a bit like an object painted over the green ground. In fact it consists of burn marks and grease from votive candles that were stuck onto the paint. The second area, at the bottom of the panel, represents either sea or mountain. It is a beautiful piece of artistry, with its cresting and breaking flow

31. The use of a raised plaster surface to give added emphasis to a particular feature of a Byzantine painting has not often been remarked. This is probably due to the poor lighting in most Byzantine churches and a lack of close technical observation of them. One 13th-century example is on the north side of the apse of Hagia Sophia, Trebizond. In the scene of the gathering of the Apostles, the head of Christ is painted on a raised area of plaster. The raised area might consist of a new plaster patch for the head. The idea of raising an area of plaster to give added emphasis to the subject may well have evolved from the practice of plaster patching, which is discussed in Winfield and Winfield, *Panaghia tou Arakos.* The most obvious example of adding emphasis to a figure in Byzantine painting is seen in raised and gilded haloes. On raised haloes, see pp. 105, 344, below.

32. Plaster markings to indicate the basic elements in a composition were observed at Lagoudera, where the paintings are dated to 1192. See Winfield and Winfield, *Panaghia tou Arakos,* 279–80.

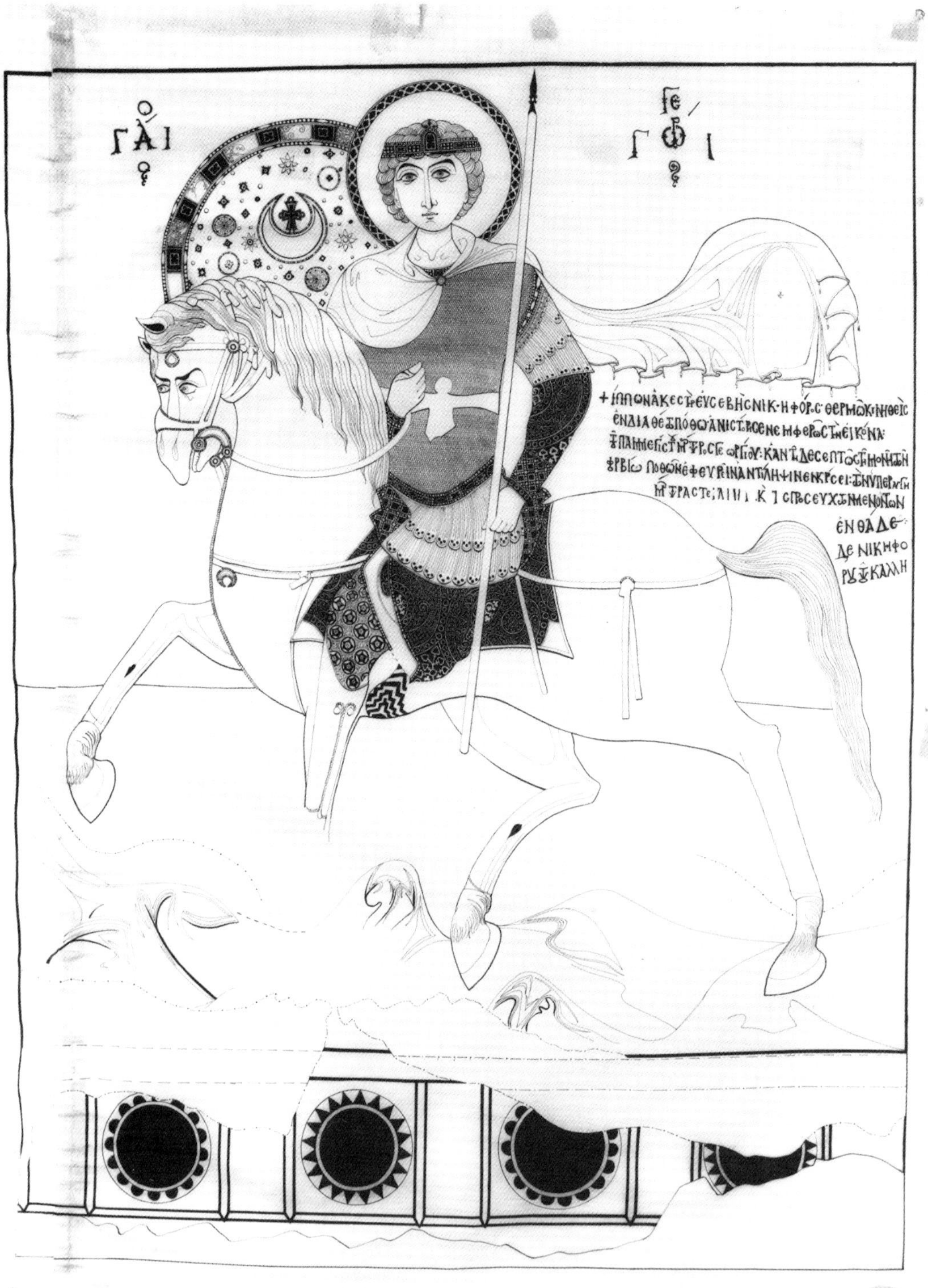

FIG. 4.6

Narthex, south conch. St. George. Drawing by June Winfield

of forms that echoes the lines of the horse and the wind-blown folds of the saint's cloak. The flowing movement of the foreground contrasts strongly with the typical Byzantine treatment of mountain backgrounds, which are made with sharp and angular rock shapes. Thus it may draw aesthetically upon the rhythmic play of waves found in images of St. George rescuing the youth, though as Nicolaïdès notes, there is no indication that the icon was intended to represent this episode.

The coloring of the foreground is built up in the same manner that Byzantine painters used for mountains. The ground color is a light pink made up of a mixture of red ocher and white lime. Over this, a darker pink was used for broad lines of shadow color. Plain, thin red ocher lines of shadow were added to establish the forms of the waves. The red ocher is a hue different from the red used elsewhere in the painting (see Chap. 7).

Since there is no sign of another background color below the pink ground, it must have been planned at the preliminary drawing phase of the painting. At the bottom right-hand edge of the panel there is a preliminary drawing line in yellow. It may mark the horizontal base of the panel or it could be connected with the foreground.

The foreground was repainted in the dull, dark-red ocher used by the 1333 painter. The repainting obscured most of the elegant shaping of the original, wavy forms. During the author's cleaning of the paintings, this overpaint was removed whenever there was original paint underneath it, but it was left intact where the original paint had been destroyed. The repainting took up a larger area than the original. Traces of the repainted outline can be seen on the left- and right-hand sides of the panel and the upper part of it extends over the original green.

The Figure of St. George

The saint's body, head, and torso are in a fully frontal vertical stance. He holds the reins of the horse in his right hand and a lance in his left. Only his left leg is visible, from ankle to mid-thigh; thereafter garments obscure it. The foot has been obliterated by damage, as has the design of the stirrup. The leg is shown in strict profile and the meeting of the torso and lower limb is concealed by the highly decorated overlaps of garments.

The Halo: The halo was drawn using a compass, but no incised outlines can be seen because of the thick white outline (Fig. 4.2). It was given a yellow ground color, which was then overlaid with a mordant and an amalgam of gold and silver leaf. Only small traces of gilding remain. The discolored greenish mordant gives a dull appearance, which is relieved by the wide white border to the halo. The white is thick and has a definite raised substance, similar to the body of the horse. Coarse brushstrokes can be seen in it. The white halo border is relieved by a continuous stepped pattern all through it, colored in alternating bright blue and red as well as grey, which may have been the mordant for silver that has flaked off.

The Buildup of the Flesh Colors: The present greenish appearance of the flesh areas of the hands and face belie the complicated buildup of the flesh colors in these areas. Though the painter used white lime of thickly textured consistency, other colors are thin in texture and opacity. It could be that a heavier saturation of the green ground layer has permeated the flesh colors that are built up on it.

Close examination of the face and hands reveals that a complex layering system of colors was applied in these areas.[33] The base color was yellow, upon which an overall green ground was applied. Features, such as the fingers, were outlined with brown lines. Several coats of flesh color in receding layers were then laid in over the green ground. At this stage, some highlighting in bright red would have been

33. At present there does not appear to exist an accurate description of the stages of buildup of coloring for Byzantine faces. June Winfield made an analysis of one face at Lagoudhera which has 11 or 12 tones or colours. This will appear in a forthcoming publication. In the meanwhile reference can be made to the descriptions of facial colouring in Winfield and Winfield, *Church of the Panaghia tou Arakos*, 308–11. The writer believes it was a painter from the Paphos school that painted both the St. George at Asinou and the 1192 Lagoudera paintings.

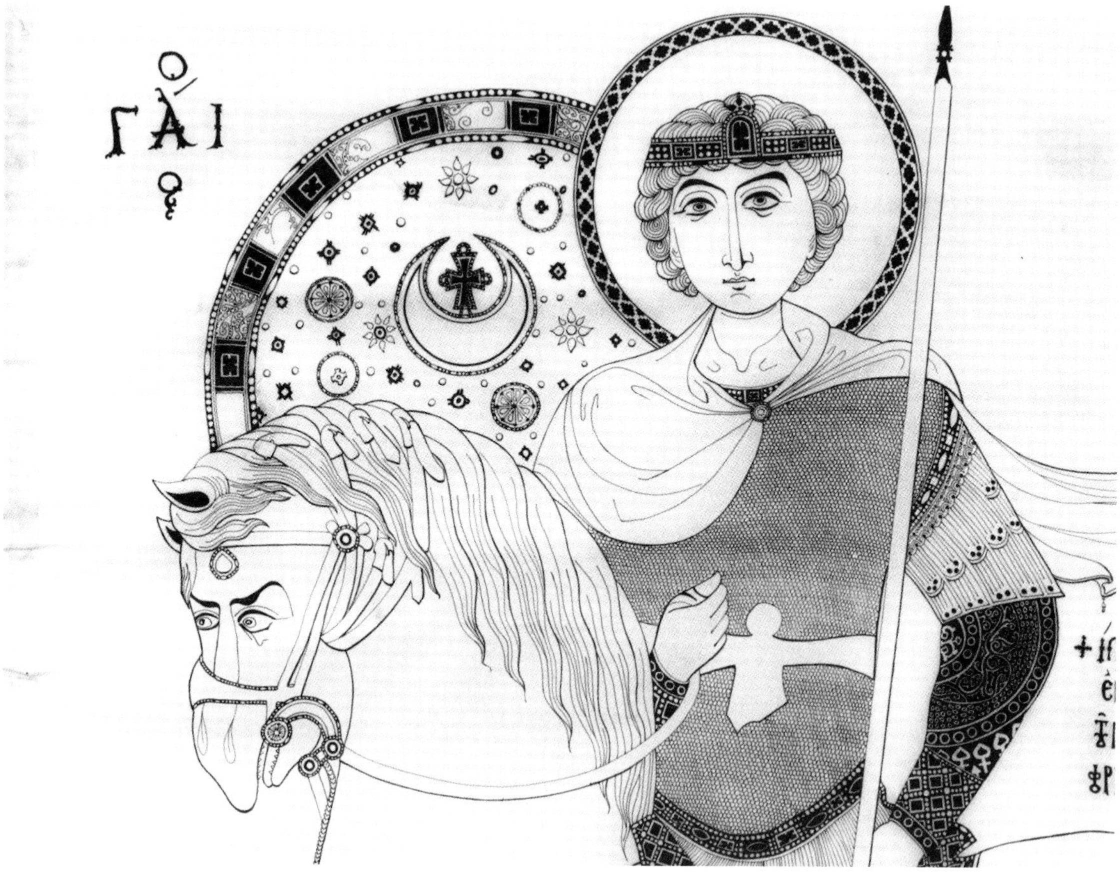

FIG. 4.7 Narthex, south conch. St. George. Drawing by June Winfield

applied over the flesh colors. This is particularly clear in the discolored red patches on the cheeks. Creamy yellow highlighting was added in lines and in blobs. This can be seen on the bridge of the nose and on the hands, where the creamy yellow is used to indicate the knuckle and the outline of the nail on the thumb of St. George's right hand. Finally, the flesh areas were defined with black lines and outlines.

The buildup of the face—with its diverse features, hollows, and reliefs—required more sophisticated treatment than the hand. Once the features were drawn in over the green ground of the face and neck, receding areas—such as the side of the nose, the deep eye sockets, and the sides of the face and neck—were painted dark green. Several layers of flesh colors were then laid in with their edges attenuated by lifting the brush. Each application of flesh color left visible areas of the previous layer, thus giving the impression of blending. These flesh colors were applied on the prominent, highlighted areas of the face and neck, such as the forehead, nose bridge, cheeks, and chin, each layer leaving exposed the edges of the flesh tint preceding it. The features were then reinforced with additional painted detail. The eyebrows are sweeps of dark brown heavily outlined in black; the eyes have black outlines, the upper outline twice as thick as the lower one, and each eye has two short horizontal lines marking each corner. The pupil of the eye is solid black and the iris is light brown outlined in black. These details are placed high and centrally between the eyelids, but they do not touch the upper eyelids. To one side of the iris the eye is dark green and to the other it is light green. To the left of the iris, the eyes are highlighted with a white lime wash, overlaid with a further blob of thick lime highlight.

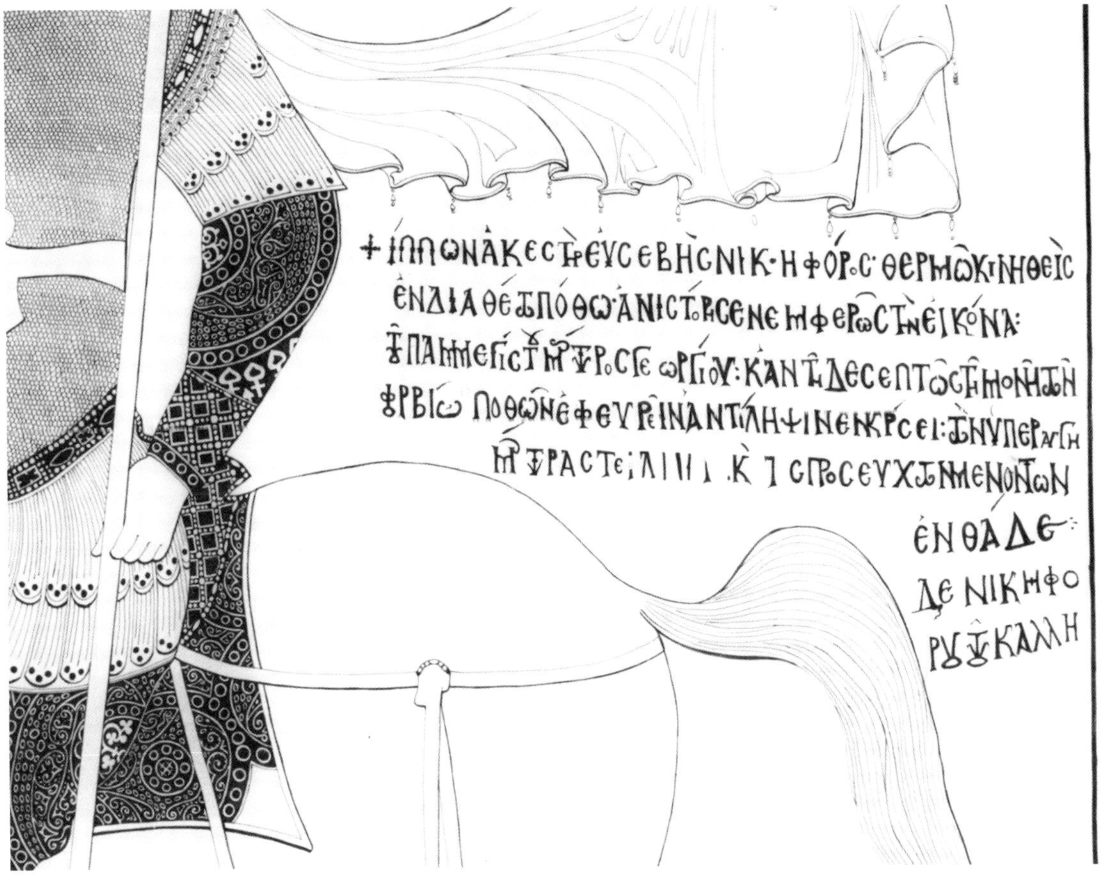

FIG. 4.8 Narthex, south conch. St. George. Drawing by June Winfield

Other highlights in the prominent areas of the face, neck, and earlobes are executed in creamy white lines and in blobs. Bright red is used to pick out the vertical of the nose bridge to the right of the cream highlight, and again for the upper and lower outlines of the lips, which themselves remain green with a central brown horizontal line parting them. Red is used as an added contour line for the pit of the throat and the scapular fossettes in the neck.

Altogether St. George's face is a sophisticated painterly exercise, and the definition of the features is so masterly and assured that it compels and holds the attention of the viewer.

Clothing

St. George wears a sumptuous outfit. His clothing must represent costumes that the painter had seen either at court or during high military occasions in Cyprus or Constantinople.[34]

Diadem: The diadem was originally of brilliant coloring with a ground of gold leaf. It has black outlines studded with white (in imitation of pearls) and with pear shapes in bright red and blue (in imitation of jewels). The structure between the outlines has rectangular sections similarly studded in imitation of pearls and jewels (Figs. 4.2, 4.7). The central crest is bright blue outlined in black and it is further picked out with pearls.

Chiton or Tunic: This can be seen at the elbow and at thigh level (Figs. 4.3, 4.8). It is decorated with circular and vermiculate patterns. The foreground color was bright blue applied over a black

34. For a scientific analysis of the complicated coloring of St. George's costume, see pp. 337–41 below.

base. The blue is overlaid with two distinct linear patterns: one includes vermiculation in bright red lines picked out with linear white circles; the other has black semicircular outline bands with solid red circles outlined in white. The cuff has a washer pattern at the wrist, and the body of the cuff is ornamented with a diaper pattern of pearl-lined corridors outlining square jewels—a pattern similar to the one that decorates the saddle.

Jacket or Jerkin: Over the tunic St. George wears a jacket or jerkin, which can be seen at the shoulder and below the belt. The fact that it was painted to imitate strips suggests that it was meant to indicate a gilded leather jerkin. Today, all that remains are the discolored mordant and the black outlines with a pattern of dots at the end of each strip.

Chain Mail: Chain mail covers St. George's body from the base of the torso upward (Figs. 4.3, 4.7). It was simulated with a field color of gold leaf but, except for a few fragments, all that remains is the discolored mordant. At one time, each chain mail link was meticulously outlined in black. In this figure of St. George, the chain mail is a substitute for the *thorakion*, or solid metal breastplate.

Sash: A sash painted to indicate a soft material winds round the chain mail at waist level. It is tied at the center with a decorative knot. It was originally a brilliant blue color with brown and black outlines. Its use or meaning is difficult to determine, but similar sashes can be seen on the costumes of archangels in other Byzantine churches.

Belt: The belt falling around St. George's groin is constructed of the same rectangular sections as the diadem (Figs. 4.3, 4.7). The areas of discolored mordant were originally gilded. The belt is damaged and most of the color has flaked off. Each segment once had black outlines and one of the segments was colored a brilliant blue. The black outlines were picked out in white dots to imitate pearls.[35]

Chlamys: The cloak has flowing folds that billow out behind the saint to give the impression of rapid movement. It was painted with a mixture of bright red and red ocher. The fold lines were rendered with a thin black wash. The highlights were bright red, but most of them have flaked away. The outlines were bright yellow with the indication of white pearls dangling from the hem. The cloak is fastened under the throat with a circular jeweled clasp or fibula. This accessory is painted in bright blue and red with a black outline and white dots to indicate pearls. To the right of the neck it can be seen that the cloak was extended so that it overlapped the finished bright blue of the background and the decorative border to the halo. The late adjustment was made presumably to improve the balance of the shoulders and to give greater substance to the neck.

Stocking: The close-fitted stocking is revealed at lower thigh and knee level. It has a dark red ground and small bright blue circles outlined in bright red. It is further decorated with bright red patches and yellow vermiculation.

Kampygra or Boot: The boot comes up to kneecap level and is painted plain black. Red and bright red cords along the side are painted to simulate braiding. Tassels at the ends of the cord have painted white ovals that probably represent stones or jewels to assist in pulling on the boots. The boot is neatly shaped to fit the calf.

Shield: The shield has a dark red ground and a wide border with a yellow ground that was finished with gilding (Figs. 4.2, 4.7). The border now has the dark greenish-yellow color that characterizes all the other areas where gilding has flaked away.

The gilding was enclosed by narrow black borders decorated to simulate white pearls and with elongated ovals of bright red to indicate jewels. The wide gilded border is punctuated at intervals

35. The rectangular sections of the diadem and the belt are quite accurately painted representations of the metal sections of ornate ceremonial belts. The linked sections gave necessary flexibility to the belt or the diadem. For the aristocracy these items could be made of gold or silver studded with precious jewels, while for the poor they were made of base metal studded with brightly colored glass or leather pieces. Fifty years ago such belts were commonly worn at weddings and other festivities in the Balkans and in Turkey.

by rectangular jewel shapes that are almost square. There are five of these, colored alternately in bright blue and bright red. All five are outlined in white. Between the rectangles the gilding is decorated with delicate vermiculate patterns painted in brown.

The dark red field color for the shield was painted before the final outlines of the horse were put in, and these outlines can be seen to overlap the red. The red field was decorated with four gilded circles and a gilded crescent moon and cross. These decorations have black borders, which are enriched by small bright blue ovals and larger, more elongated bright red ovals. Two of the other circles have crosses of equal arms at the center and the remaining two have floral patterning rendered in black lines. The red field is further studded with small jewel-like decorations. Two larger floral decorations are more irregularly painted than the rest of the work. They are of a light yellow very similar to the yellow used by the 1333 painter. This may indicate some repair work at that date, when the foreground below St. George was also repainted.

Lance: The shaft of the lance was originally gilded but this has now largely flaked off, leaving visible the discolored mordant. The gilding was probably relieved by decorative patterning, but the evidence for this is unclear.

The pointed head of the lance is of brilliant white. It is decorated with a bright red jewel and has some light blue highlights that help define its shape.

The Horse

Although the horse is portrayed in profile trotting eastward, his head is in three-quarter profile, revealing both eyes, both nostrils, and both ears (Figs. 4.4, 4.6). Three of the horse's legs are extended downward, though part of the left foreleg is missing due to damage. His raised right foreleg gives him a forward momentum. This movement is accentuated by the tail, which streams backward and downward, echoing the flowing movement of the saint's cloak. This is not a passive palfrey but a fiery warhorse, and the donor of the painting would surely have been proud of him.

The brilliant white body of the horse was made with raised lime as described above. The broadly brushed shadows are made with a thin wash of green and a darker olive green. These effectively outline the muscles and sinews. These shadows give a fine impression of realistic form to the body of the horse, even though they are not anatomically correct. The outlines of the horse are in black and the horse's hairs are drawn with black lines. A curved thin red line marks the tops of the fetlocks. The mane, the tail, and the fetlocks all have a green wash ground and are outlined in dark green and black.

The eye cavity is green with dark green shadow lines and black lines. The pupils of the eyes have been gouged out, but the remaining irises are bright blue. The tongue is bright red and the teeth are white.

Bridle: The bridle was originally all gilded but now shows only the discolored mordant. Over the horse's mane, there are three buckles or knots for adjusting the bridle. These were painted bright red with black outlines and some white blobs in imitation of pearls. A martingale, used to restrain the horse from raising its head, runs down from the bit around the horse's neck and chest, and disappears under the belly. It is rendered as a braided cord and is colored bright red. The bit and the noseband are decorated with jewels and pearls, and bejeweled phalerae (round metal ornaments) decorate the headband and the breast saddle tie.

The Girth of the Underbelly: The girth of the underbelly would have been made of leather. Here, it is brilliantly colored with a dark red ground and zigzag patterning in broad lines of white, gray-blue, bright red, yellow, black, and green.[36]

Saddle: The saddle, which juts slightly upward before and aft of the rider, is decorated with a diaper pattern of rows of pearls outlining rectangular jewels (Figs. 4.3, 4.6). The pattern is similar to that of the cuff of the saint's tunic.

36. The painting of the girth provides circumstantial evidence for the craft of coloring and embossing leather. It was later to become a popular craft in Spain and the Netherlands.

Lettering and Inscription

The Titular Lettering: The titular lettering, in brilliant white, is painted in ornate letters with a flourish of serifs and varied shaping. It is arranged symmetrically in cross patterns to either side of the saint's head.

The Donor's Metrical Inscription: The donor's inscription is a much less careful piece of lettering, painted in the same white as the titular inscription (Figs. 3.10, 4.8). The shaping of its letters suggests that it was written by the same painter who made the titular inscription. He has followed a fairly typical Byzantine wall-painter's habit of starting a line with grand, well-spaced lettering and ending it with smaller, crowded letters, to make room for the whole of his text.

The last two lines mar the general perfection of the whole painting by diverting from the horizontal and running uphill.[37] The white paint there is of a duller color than it is in the metrical inscription, and it appears discolored with a yellowish tinge, not unlike the discolorations of the face and hands. These last lines, therefore, may refer to a Nikephoros other than the donor featured in the metrical inscription. Or it could be the name of some Nikephoros unrelated to the painting, but who chose to commemorate himself on the image of a saint whom he admired (see also above, pp. 19 and 82–83).

Proportion

The figure of the rider appears to be disproportionately large in relation to the size of the horse. However, the painter has arranged the panel so that the disproportion is noticeable only when an analysis is made. The skillful simulation of natural size in both horse and rider is achieved by the dominant bulkiness of the white horse contrasting with the elaborately ornamented clothes and armor of the saint, which break up his form and distract the eye from his size.

It would be unsound to generalize about the proportion of a single mounted figure when this is the only painting by this painter in the church of Asinou. To determine with any certainty the proportional measures used by individual painters, one must have a sufficient number of their paintings available. Only by comparing and cross-checking between multiple figures is it possible to assess a painter's measuring system or canon of proportion.[38] However, with regard to the mural of St. George, some interesting observations may be made.

The saint's face is of unequal planes in relation to the center of his nose, the left side being wider than the right (from the figure's perspective; Figs. 4.2, 4.7). This is characteristic of post-Iconoclast frontal faces. The figure's left eye is larger than his right and his gaze is directed sideways to his left across the wider plane of his face. The pupils are centered within the eyes, but the deliberate placing of the strong white highlights within the irises reinforces the indirect sideways gaze. Both nostrils are shown, indicating that this is a three-quarter frontal face. The large head rests upon a comparatively thin neck, whose sides lie well in from the earlobes above. This is probably the reason why, at a final stage of the work, the painter extended the cloak to the right of the neck. This late addition gives the head a firmer base (see discussion under "Chlamys," above).

The center point of the halo lies to the right of the nose, within the wider plane of the face, on a level with the upper rim of the eyes. The vertical distance from the base of the nostril to the bridge of the nose, which is the nose length, is equal to the distance from the base of the nostril to the base of the chin. Byzantine faces, when measured from the base of the chin to the apex of the forehead, usually have three equal divisions based on nose

37. I am grateful to Nancy Ševčenko for pointing out the difference in the last two lines.

38. See Dionysius of Fourna, *Ἑρμηνεία*, appendix 1, pp. 237–39. For an analysis of Panselinos measures, and in particular of the mounted figure, see Winfield and Winfield, *Proportion and Structure*, 66–100, and for St. George specifically, pp. 81–82, fig. 14, and pl. 7. Further information on proportion is contained in Winfield, *La Maniera Greca*.

length. In the case of St. George, the apex of the forehead, which is one nose length above the bridge of the nose, would lie on the upper horizontal of the diadem. The upper area of the saint's head, from the top of the diadem to the crown of the head, is shorter than a nose length. The halo measures six nose lengths (or two faces) in diameter, a measure echoed in the width of the shoulders.

The only other certain reference points are within the sash marking the waistline, and the base of the belt marking the base of the torso and the divide of the legs. Measuring vertically, the waist could be said to lie six nose lengths (two face lengths) from the chin, and the base of the torso nine nose lengths (three face lengths) from the chin.

The figure of St. George is distorted so that his head and torso are portrayed in a stiff, frontal stance, while his left leg is firmly in profile. Both figure and horse are constructed around an implied central vertical. This runs down through the vertical diameter of the halo and through the inner corner of the saint's left eye, then continues through the sash knot and the center of the belt, runs tangent to the rear back leg of the horse, and finally meets the base line, where it marks the center of the dado pattern below.

Further proportional measures for the horse and rider would be speculative. This is because the painting is executed on a horizontally curved wall, while the horizontal measures that were taken, and the measures for the drawing in Figures 4.5–7, were taken along the flat of the wall. It is possible that the painter used preemptive devices for counteracting the curvature of the wall, since it is known that Byzantine painters used optical corrections. In this case, St. George, when seen at a distance, looms taller in the saddle than he appears when his figure is drawn on flat paper from measures taken along the flat of the wall.

The Dado

The dado is painted to imitate a rich marble revetment of opus sectile (Fig. 4.1). The squares of the dado pattern are about 30 cm wide. They are decorated with inscribed circles with a diameter of circa 20 cm for the solid colored circles, or 25 cm if one includes the black-and-white decorative border. The rectangular sections that separate the inscribed circles are circa 14 cm wide by 30 cm high. The upper red border dividing the dado from St. George is 8 cm high, including the two white borders.

A combination of damage and overpainting makes the dado colors very difficult to read. The upright rectangles may have been dark green and would have been picked out in light green spots, in imitation of verd antique. The circles within the squares were darkish red, probably in imitation of porphyry. The dentils, either rounded or pointed, which outline the porphyry were painted in black and the interstices in white.

Condition and Conservation

Condition: St. George was a very popular saint in Cyprus, and the fact that this painting is in the ground register means that it will have received a great deal of votive attention from worshippers. Candles, oil lamps, and the ritual kissing of St. George have all contributed to the buildup of grime on the surface. The monks would likely have periodically cleaned the painting, and this may be why so little gilding remains, and why most of the colors are thin in texture. Byzantine painters normally used thickly textured colors, as can be seen in the paintings from other periods at Asinou. Some of the damage marks suggest that a hard-bristled brush may have been used in past attempts at cleaning the painting.

Alternatively, the thin texture could be accounted for by the fact that the painter finished this painting in all its minute detail before he started gilding it with gold leaf. He may have wanted the smooth surface of the thin coloring so that his gold leaf had a better chance of adhering to the ground. This would be akin to the practice of Byzantine mosaic workers who painted a complete fresco of their subject before covering it with tesserae. The sad discoloration of the flesh colors could have come either by someone's cleaning it with some harmful liquid, or by someone's application of a surface preservative, which has now discolored it. Or a fault in the painter's technique could have allowed the green ground color of the flesh to permeate through the bright, lifelike finishing colors. At the top right-hand corner of the painting there has been some damage from water seepage, causing the blue of the background to turn green.

The lower area of the painting was already badly damaged by the early fourteenth century, and this must account for the rather crude repainting of the ground area when the narthex was further decorated in 1333.

Conservation: A diagonal crack, probably caused by earthquakes, runs across the painting from the top left-hand side down toward the bottom right-hand side. Earthquakes probably also loosened the plaster ground from the wall surface. It would not have been possible to draw the plaster edges together again across the crack without risking further cracks in the paint and plaster. In conserving this mural, we therefore reaffixed the plaster by injecting a lime slurry mixed with the addition of a small percentage of polyvinyl acetate (PVA) emulsion. The PVA was necessary because of the natural accumulation of dust, insect bodies, and other foreign matter in the hollow behind the painted plaster. We feared that lime slurry on its own would not have been able to coagulate efficiently in the presence of all the foreign matter.

The painting was first cleaned with soft india rubbers. The lower half of the painting from the horse's body downward was more thickly begrimed. It was cleaned with a general cleaning fluid consisting of a few drops of the nonfoaming detergent Lissapol N, a few drops of white spirit, and a few drops of ammonia dissolved in a large quantity of distilled water. No attempt was made at a definitive cleaning because of the fragile state of the few remaining fragments of gilding.

Conclusion

There is no certainty about the date of the painting of St. George. The addition of the well-built narthex of Asinou is unlikely to have been carried out after the conquest of Cyprus by Richard the Lionheart in 1191; how long before this date it was constructed is unclear, as indicated earlier in this chapter (pp. 93–95). St. George appears to represent the earliest layer of painting in the narthex, and stylistically a date in the second half of the twelfth century seems reasonable. The ornamental patterns, the high quality of the colors, the gilding, and the dado pattern all have parallels with the work at St. Neophytos, dating before and after 1183, and with work at Lagoudera, dating to 1192.

There are also some technical similarities with these two monuments, such as the use of an opalescent white to simulate pearls and the impressing of plaster and the fine incision lines to mark out the preliminary drawing. It therefore seems likely that St. George was painted by a master associated with the school of painting centered around St. Neophytos and Bishop Kinnamos.

There is no doubt that this fine equestrian portrait is one of the masterpieces of Byzantine wall painting and probably the finest of all equestrian paintings before the time of the Florentine painter Paolo Uccello (1397–1475). Even then, the comparison falls in favor of the Asinou St. George, since Uccello's horses appear frozen in a wooden stance, whereas St. George's horse ripples with lively movement and seems about to trot out of his painted panel. The horse and rider together form a majestic piece of artistry.

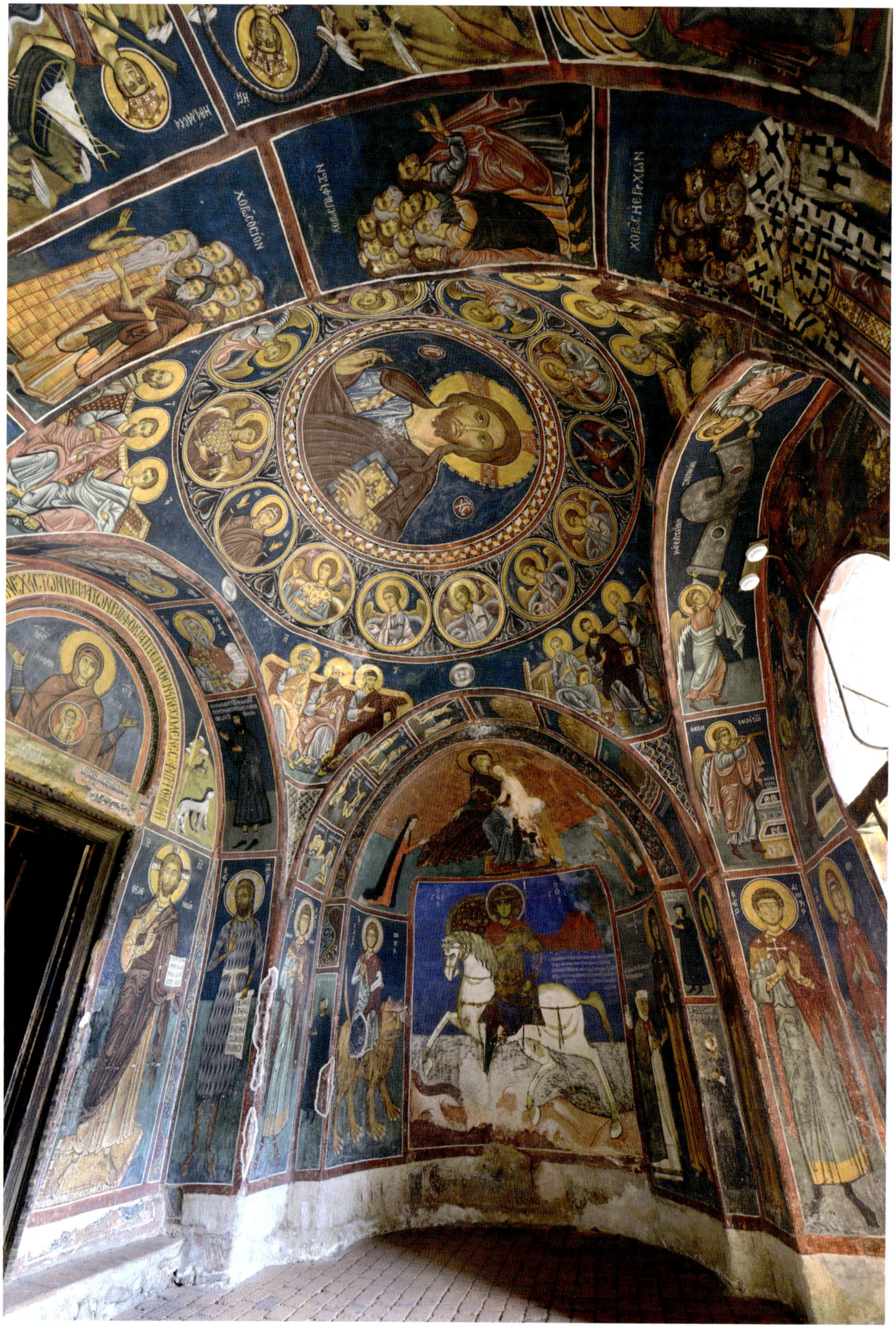

The church of Panagia Phorbiotissa: the narthex from the north apse
(photo courtesy of G. L. Carr)

CHAPTER FIVE

The Murals of the Narthex

The Paintings of the Late Thirteenth and Fourteenth Centuries

Sophia Kalopissi-Verti

This chapter turns to the paintings from Cyprus's Lusignan period (1192–1489) that adorn the narthex at Asinou, beginning with two private votive frescoes of the late thirteenth century that were integrated into the later cycle of 1332/33, which dominates the space. One of Orthodox and one of Latin dedication, the panels frame the twelfth-century ex voto of St. George in the south apse, harmonizing both with it and with each other.[1] The image of St. Anastasia Pharmakolytria (Poison-Curer) with her Orthodox devotee, Anastasia Saramalina, has been linked in style and technique with the paintings inside the church on the rebuilt apse conch and the naos responds. The Latin panel shows the Virgin of Mercy shielding three Frankish donors under her protective mantle (Fig. 5.1). Together the two panels cast light on the coexistence and correlation of local Cypriot and Latin patronage in an Orthodox monastery in Lusignan Cyprus.

The Late Thirteenth-Century Paintings in the Narthex

St. Anastasia Pharmakolytria and Donor Anastasia Saramalina

The panel of the Anastasias is on the wall of the south apse, to the right of the late twelfth-century image of St. George on horseback (Fig. 5.2). St. Anastasia Pharmakolytria is represented holding a white martyr's cross in her right hand and a white bottle with a long neck in her left. The accompanying inscription reads:

Research for this study was carried out while on a fellowship at Dumbarton Oaks in the autumn term of 2000.

1. On the program of the south apse, see Carr, "Correlative Spaces." On the frescoes of the narthex, see Buxton et al., "Church of Asinou," 335–40; Winfield, *Asinou,* 14–17, 19–20; Stylianou and Stylianou, *Painted Churches*, 134–40; Philotheou, "Μνημειακὴ ζωγραφική," 117; Hadjichristodoulou, *Our Lady of Asinou*, 29–41. On the fresco layers, see Winfield, *Asinou*, 26–27; Mango, "Summary of Work," 102–23.

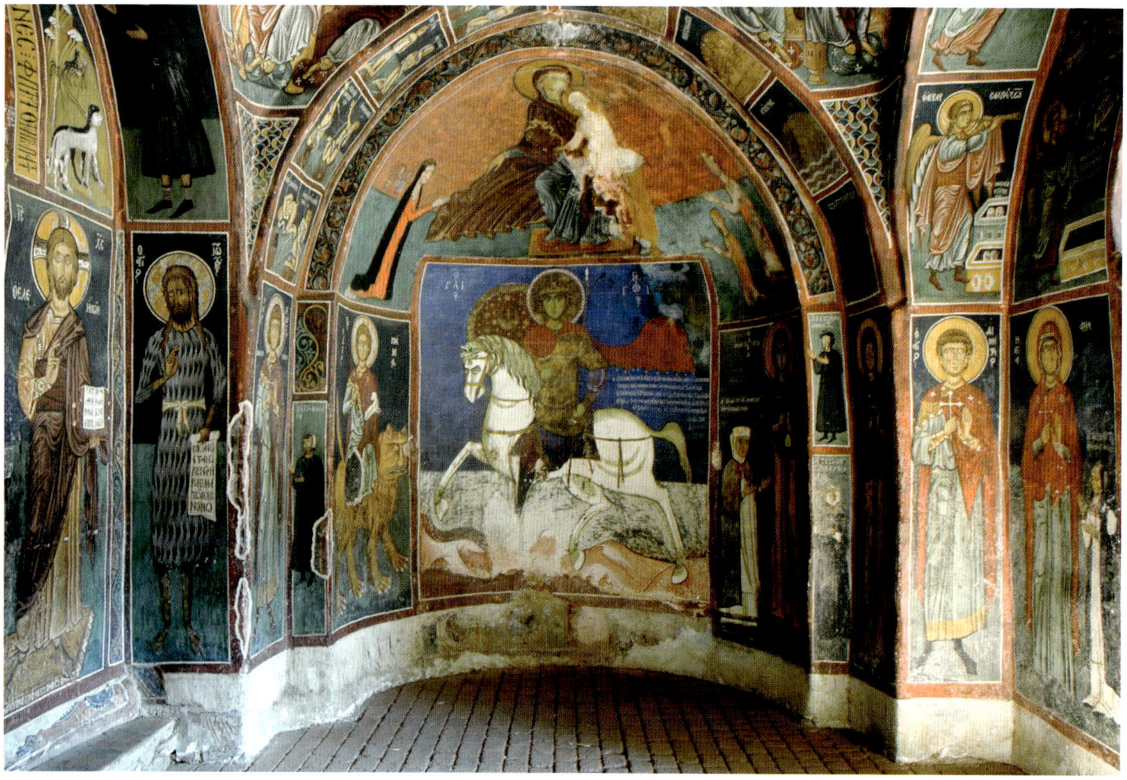

FIG. 5.1 Narthex, view toward south. Semidome: The Virgin of Mercy with three Latin donors. Arch: Torments of the Damned. Lower zone, left to right: Christ Eleemon, St. John the Baptist, St. George Machairomenos, lay supplicant Georgios, St. Mamas, St. George, St. Anastasia with donor, monk Kallinikos (above) and lay supplicant Basileios (below), St. Irene, St. Demetrios, St. Anna and donor (photo courtesy of G. L. Carr)

ἡ / ἁ/γί/α / Ἀναστασία, written in cruciform on the left, and ἡ / Φ/αρ/μα/κο/λυ/τρί/α, painted in a vertical line on the right.

A victim of the persecutions of Diocletian, St. Anastasia is commemorated by the Orthodox Church on 22 December.[2] After 458 her relics were transferred from Sirmium, where her cult originated, to the church of St. Anastasia (also called the Anastasis Church or the Anastaseion) in Constantinople, which was known as a place of healing and remained the center of her cult throughout the Middle Ages.[3] According to the synaxarion of the Constantinopolitan church, where Anastasia is characterized as φαρμακολύτρια, i.e., dissolver of poison, she used to cure those who suffered for their faith in Christ by cleaning their wounds and placing a remedy on them.[4] The verses in the Menaion of 22 December praise her: "Ἀναστασία, φάρμακον πιστοῖς μέγα, / πᾶν φάρμακον λύουσα. . . ." (Anastasia, great remedy to the faithful, dissolving

2. J. P. Kirsch, "Anastasie (sainte)," in *DACL* 1–2: 1919–24; *BS* 1:1041–49; *BHG* 1:24–26; idem, *Légendes grecques*, 86–157; *Life and Martyrdom*. St. Anastasia Pharmakolytria should not be confused with St. Anastasia Romana, commemorated on 29 October.

3. Janin, *Les églises et les monastères*, 23. For Anastasia's miraculous healings, especially in 10th-century texts, see Baun, *Tales from Another Byzantium*, 116–17. For a discussion of the cult of St. Anastasia in the 10th century, ibid., 117–20; Baun, "Apocalypse of Anastasia," 128–31; Rydén, "Church of St. Anastasia."

4. Delehaye, *Synaxarium*, 335.

every poison), playing upon the double meaning of φάρμακον as medicine and as poison.[5]

Anastasia's portrait, in which she usually holds the cross of martyrdom and a bottle of medicine as at Asinou, is found in several churches of the Lusignan period on Cyprus as, for example, in the earliest fresco layer of the church of the Virgin near Kophinou, dated to the late twelfth or thirteenth century;[6] in the church of St. Herakleidios in the monastery of St. John Lampadistes at Kalopanayiotis (ca. 1400); and in Palaia Enkleistra at Kouklia (after 1442).[7] She is also portrayed on a reliquary diptych made of steatite, now in the Cathedral Museum at Mdina in Malta, which has been attributed to a Cypriot workshop of the first half of the fourteenth century.[8]

Anastasia's appeal did not lie in her healing powers alone. On the basis of her name, a cognate of ἀνάστασις—that is, resurrection—she was linked iconographically and conceptually to the resurrection of Christ. In church programs, as Dragan Vojvodić points out, her image is often correlated with scenes of the Descent into Hell and the Last Judgment.[9] She is also depicted in funerary contexts, as in the cave church of the Palaia Enkleistra near Kouklia (after 1442), where she is painted along with the medical saints Cosmas, Damian, and Hermolaos.[10] As such, she evokes themes—of

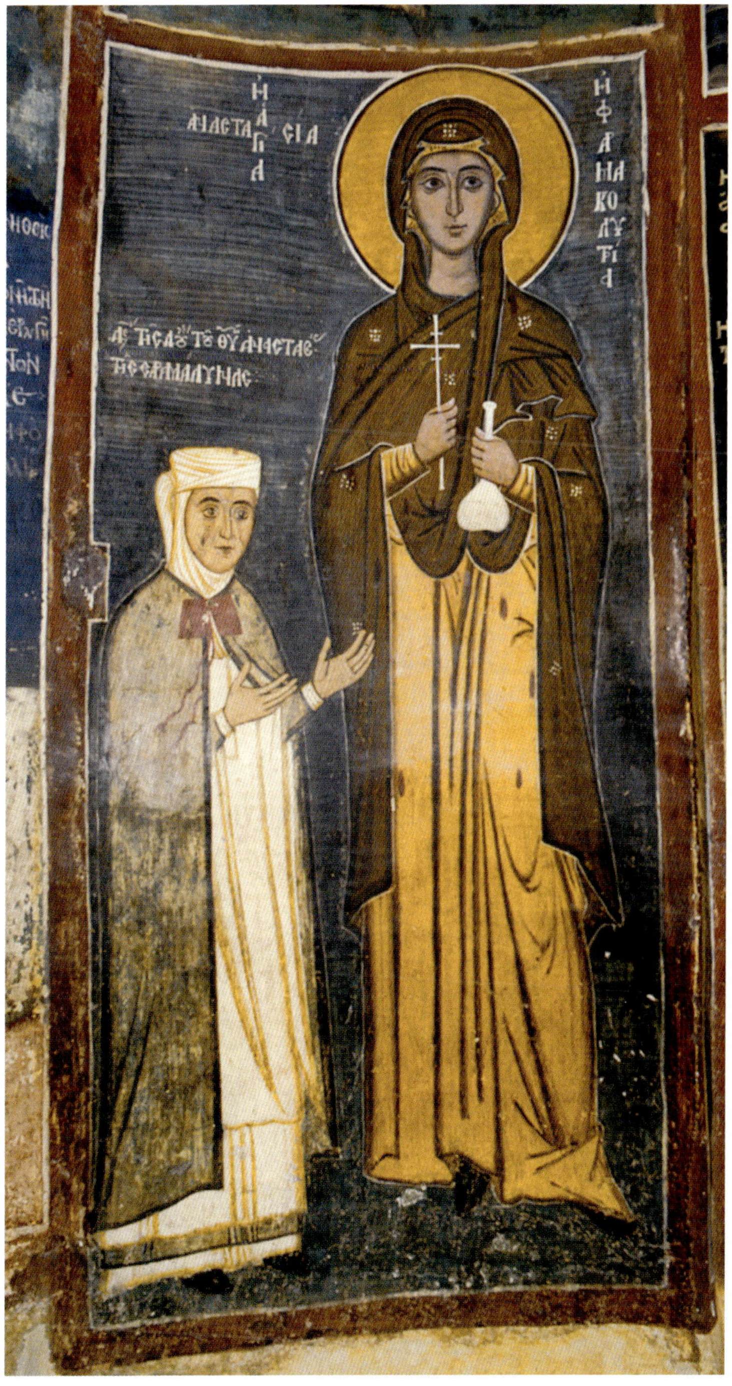

FIG. 5.2 Narthex, south conch. St. Anastasia with devotee Anastasia Saramalina (photo courtesy of the Leventis Foundation and the Archaeological Research Unit, University of Cyprus, No. 006326)

5. *Menaion*, 22 December, 588.
6. Gabelić, "Kophinou," 147, fig. 3 (late 12th c.). According to Mouriki, "Cypriot Saints," 252, this fresco layer should be dated to the 13th c. In the church of the Panagia at Moutoullas (1280) the portrait of St. Anastasia on the west wall, bearing no eponym, cannot be identified with either Anastasia Pharmakolytria or Romana; see Mouriki, "Church of the Panagia at Moutoullas," 197, fig. 25.
7. Stylianou and Stylianou, *Painted Churches*, 304, 398.
8. The reliquary belongs to the "Treasure of the Hospitaller Knights." Through the coats of arms represented on it, it has been linked to the Grand Master Hélion de Villeneuve (1319–46). See Hetherington, "Byzantine Steatites"; idem, "Byzantine Reliquary"; Kalavrezou-Maxeiner, *Byzantine Icons*, 180–84, no. 102.
9. Vojvodić, "Kult i ikonografija," 33.
10. Stylianou and Stylianou, *Painted Churches*, 398.

healing, resurrection, and salvation—that conform perfectly to the context of the narthex decoration as a whole at Asinou. Indeed, although her portrait belongs to an earlier phase, it was integrated seamlessly into the main phase of the narthex decoration, serving as a pendant to the fourteenth-century images of Cosmas and Damian on the wall of the north apse (see below, pp. 170–71).

The donor, Anastasia Saramalina, unknown from other sources but seemingly a respected elderly local woman, is depicted standing with raised arms, turned toward her patron saint. The accompanying inscription reads: δέ(ησις) τῆς δούλ(ης) τοῦ Θ(εο)ῦ Ἀναστασί(ας) / τῆς Σαραμάλυνας (prayer of the servant of God Anastasia Saramalina). Gilles Grivaud has now plausibly linked Anastasia's surname, Saramalina, to a village called Saramali in the nearby valley of Xyliatos; the name had been associated before with a village named Sarama in the district of Paphos.[11]

Anastasia the donor is dressed in the four garments customary for Byzantine lay women.[12] The first, the undergarment (ὑποκαμίσιον), is white and falls to the feet; besides its cuffs one can see its hem just above the black shoes. The second dress (καμίσιον), long and long-sleeved, is olive green. Its hem and the lower part of the sleeves are also visible. The third, a long, white T-shaped garment, is characterized by its very wide sleeves, which can be viewed as long, sharply pointed triangles with yellow ocher contours falling from the arms in front of the body. The T-shaped dress with wide sleeves has been identified with the *γρανάτζα,* which was originally a courtly gown.[13] A yellow line running horizontally under Anastasia's knees seems to indicate that she also wore the *porphyra*, a vertical band falling in front of the body, originally a distinctive element of the costume of court women.[14] The last garment is an olive-green mantle held together under the chin with a round brooch or button and strings sewn on red rectangular patches (ταβλία or ἐπιρράμματα). Rectangular or square patches on the mantle under the neck serve both to decorate and to reinforce the textile at those points where the strings are sewn, which are used to fasten the garment more or less tightly. Similar patches are seen in the portrait of Eirene, wife of the donor Ioannes in the village church of the Panagia at Moutoullas (1280; Fig. 5.3).[15] In certain cases, however, the patches are decorated and seem to represent the two parts of a brooch rather than cloth, as in the mantles of the wife of the donor Michael Katzouroumpos in St. Demetrianos, Dali (1317), of the πρεσβυτέρισσα Nenkomia in the church of the Holy Cross at Pelendri (ca. mid-fourteenth century; Fig. 5.48),[16] and of the donor Anna in the narthex of Asinou (see below, pp. 188–90; Fig. 5.47). Such patches also appear in several examples in churches on Crete.[17]

Anastasia's Byzantine attire was widely depicted in the eastern Mediterranean regions in the

11. See above, p. 27. For previous views, Goodwin, *Toponymy of Cyprus*, 611; Young, "Byzantine Painting," 341 and 377, n. 63.
12. On Byzantine dress, see Koukoules, *Βυζαντινῶν βίος καὶ πολιτισμός*, 2:5–59; Mylopotamitaki, "Βυζαντινή γυναικεία φορεσιά"; eadem, "Παρατηρήσεις στὶς τοιχογραφημένες παραστάσεις"; Bitha, "Ενδυματολογικές μαρτυρίες"; Kalamara, *Système vestimentaire*; Ball, *Byzantine Dress*. On female attire in medieval Cyprus, see Talbot Rice, "Costume of Cyprus," 105–6; Christoforaki, "Female Dress in Cyprus"; Frigerio-Zeniou, "Κυπριώτισσες Κυράδες"; cf. Rizopoulou-Hegoumenidou, *Αστική ενδυμασία*, 70, 74. For a discussion on the male and female dress and headcover and the fusion of Byzantine and Western elements in 14th–16th-century Cyprus, see Kalamara, "Vêtement byzantin ou syrien." I wish to thank my friend and colleague Ioanna Bitha for our discussions on Byzantine fashion.
13. Mylopotamitaki, "Βυζαντινή γυναικεία φορεσιά," 114. On the courtly γρανάτζα, see Cvetković, "Vizantijskog dvorskog kostima."
14. Mylopotamitaki, "Βυζαντινή γυναικεία φορεσιά," 117; Bitha, "Ενδυματολογικές," 2: 440–41.
15. Mouriki, "Moutoullas," 182, fig. 11; Stylianou and Stylianou, *Painted Churches*, 324–25, fig. 192.
16. Stylianou and Stylianou, *Painted Churches*, fig. 256; eidem, "Donors and Dedicatory Inscriptions," fig. 9. Cf. Christoforaki, "Female Dress in Cyprus," 15.
17. Gerola, *Monumenti Veneti*, 2: pls. 12.2, 13.1; Spatharakis, *Dated Byzantine Wall Paintings*, fig. 181.

fourteenth and fifteenth centuries, recurring especially in the female donor portraits of churches in Rhodes and Crete.[18] The figure of Kale in the monastery church of Panagia Kera in Pediada (Herakleion), Crete (fourteenth century) can be cited as a very close parallel.[19]

By contrast, Anastasia's white headdress seems to follow western style (Fig. 5.4). The barbette, a strap passing under the chin and pinned on top, as well as the *crespine*, which surrounds the hair at the back of the head, follows a fashion that Susan Young identified as having emerged in France.[20] Young dated its emergence in the mid-thirteenth century, but it seems to have appeared in France already in the twelfth century, as can be determined from a statue dated to the twelfth century in the Chapelle des Cordeliers at Nancy, representing the crusader Hugues de Vaudemont and his wife, who wears this type of headdress.[21] The barbette and the kerchief (*couvre-chef*) together formed the wimple (*la guimpe*), which was worn from the twelfth to the fifteenth centuries by elderly women and widows, and also by nuns, who continued to wear it in subsequent centuries. Occasionally, this headdress was supplemented by a band of rigid linen cloth, about ten centimeters high, which was pinned on the kerchief on the top of the head, as in the case of Anastasia.[22] This band is seen again on Cyprus in the portrait of Eirene at the church of the Panagia at Moutoullas dating to 1280 (Fig. 5.3).[23] Susan Young found yet another example of this headdress on the female donor of a bilingual Greek and Latin Psalter, circa 1300, known as the Hamilton Psalter. That manuscript is linked to Cyprus by an inscription indicating that it belonged to Carlotta Lusignan, Queen of Cyprus (1458–1475).[24] This type of headdress seems, in fact, to have been quite prevalent in the Mediterranean East in the second half of the thirteenth century, as attested by an Armenian Gospel book in Washington, D.C., Freer Gallery 32.18, sponsored by Prince Vasak and dated to about 1268. Painted by T'oros Roslin, the miniatures show this type of headdress worn not only by women of the aristocracy, such as Herodias

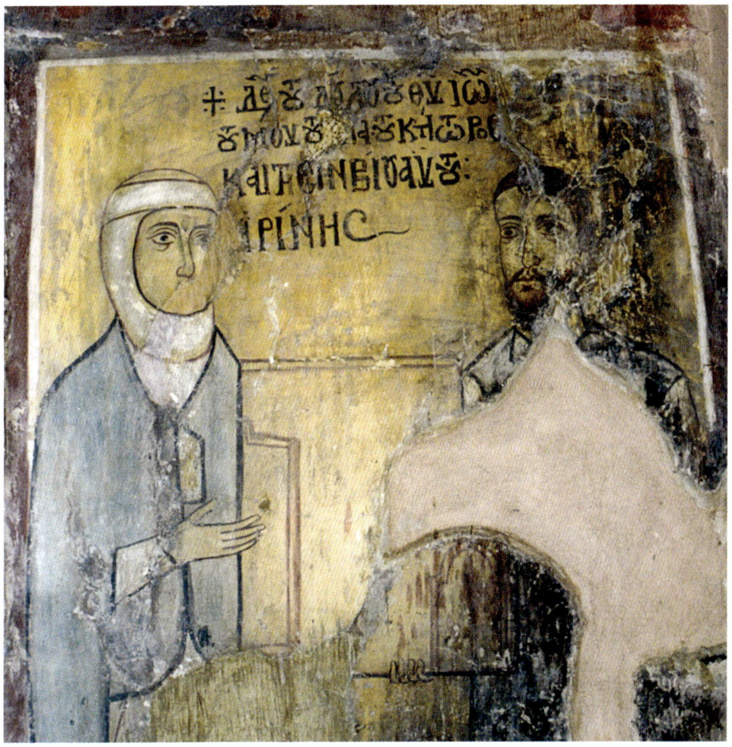

FIG. 5.3 Moutoullas, church of the Panagia, north wall of sanctuary. The donors Ioannes and Irene (photo courtesy of S. Kalopissi-Verti)

18. Bitha, "Ενδυματολογικές μαρτυρίες," pls. 170a, 175; Gerola, *Monumenti Veneti*, 2: pls. 8.2, 10.2–4, 12.2, 13.1, 15.1–2.

19. Mylopotamitaki, "Βυζαντινή γυναικεία φορεσιά," pl. 49.

20. Young, "Byzantine Painting," 341–42; Greenhill, *Incised Effigial Slabs*, 1:233–36, 2: pl. 133c; cf. Semoglou, "Portraits chypriotes de donateurs," 488–89. For a different opinion, see Emmanuel, "Hairstyles and Headdresses," 119.

21. Boucher, *Histoire du costume*, 175, fig. 302; Pinasa, *Costumes*, 72.

22. Viollet-le-Duc, *Encyclopédie médiévale*, 2:501; Boucher, *Histoire du costume*, 200, 441; Pinasa, *Costumes*, 99.

23. See above, note 15.

24. Fol. 39v, Havice, "Hamilton Psalter"; eadem, "Marginal Miniatures"; Spatharakis, *Portrait*, 45–48; N. P. Ševčenko in Vassilaki, *Mother of God*, 388–89, no. 54; A. W. Carr in Evans, *Byzantium: Faith and Power*, 153–54, no. 77; Carr, "Art," 309–10.

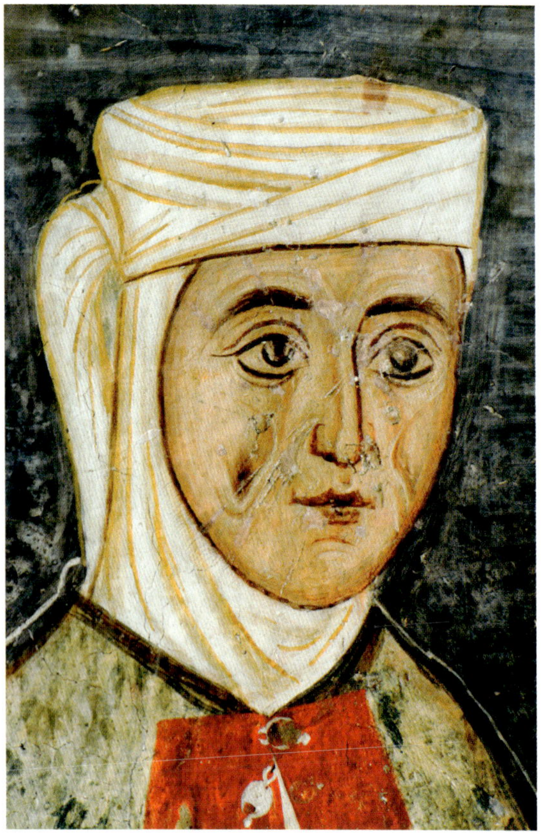

FIG. 5.4 Narthex, south conch. Face of Anastasia Saramalina (photo courtesy of G. L. Carr)

in Herod's banquet and Pilate's wife, but also by ordinary people, such as the woman in the scene of Peter's Denial.[25]

The plaster joins show that the panel of St. Anastasia overlies and therefore postdates the late twelfth-century image of St. George, but that it is earlier than the paintings of 1332/33. Chronologically and stylistically, the Anastasia layer has been associated with the late thirteenth-century murals of the bema at Asinou. David Winfield[26] and Ioanna Kakoulli have stressed the technical similarities between the Anastasia panel and the apse composition of the bema, which shows the Virgin orant, labeled ἡ Παντάνασσα, between archangels (see below, pp. 213–16, 341; Figs. 6.8, 6.9 and accompanying discussion). These similarities include the incised drawing on the still-damp plaster denoting the folds of the garments; the white lines on the contours of the figure of St. Anastasia and the figures of the angels in the apse (Figs. 5.5, 6.4); the horizontal brushstrokes with a splash of paint at the finishing point on the background (Fig. 7.28); the chemical consistency of the pigments; and the shape of certain letters in the inscriptions, such as C, N, and M (Figs. 5.2, 6.4). One should also note the bright green used to shade the face in both paintings; the shape of the eyes, with a curved upper eyelid, which exposes the full circle of the iris; the short horizontal line at the inner angle of the eye and the linear rendering of the shading under the eye; the nose, with its triangular green shading at the base and the short, vertical highlights at the top; the rectangular shape of the nostrils; and the endings of the upper lip (Figs. 6.8, 6.9). All these shared technical and stylistic traits lead to the conclusion that the compositions of the apse semidome and of the Anastasia panel belong to the same period and the same workshop or painter.

Close stylistic parallels for the figure of St. Anastasia are seen in wall paintings and icons of the late thirteenth century on Cyprus, including the murals of the church of St. George of Ancona at Ormedeia in the district of the metropolis of Kition; the icon of St. Marina from the homonymous church at Pedoulas; the icon of the Virgin and Child from the Monastery of St. John Lampadistes at Kalopanayiotis; the icons from the church of the Panagia at Moutoullas; and an icon at Sinai that has been associated with Cyprus.[27] Close affinities appear in the icon of the Virgin and Child in a variant of the Kykkotissa type that is currently exhibited

25. Der Nersessian, *Miniature Painting*, 1:55–57, 2: figs. 268, 272, 276; cf. eadem, *Armenian Manuscripts*, 26–54, figs. 77, 99, 160, 168, 171.
26. Winfield, *Asinou*, 26; Winfield, "Wall Painting Methods," fig. 11.

27. Spanou, "Τέχνη," 43, fig. 26; Papageorgiou, *Icons of Cyprus* [1992], 46, 55, figs. 28, 34; Hadzichristodoulou and Papaioakim, "Φορητὲς εἰκόνες," 131–32; Vocotopoulos, "Icons at Moutoullas"; Mouriki, "Thirteenth-Century Icon Painting," 63–64, fig. 26.

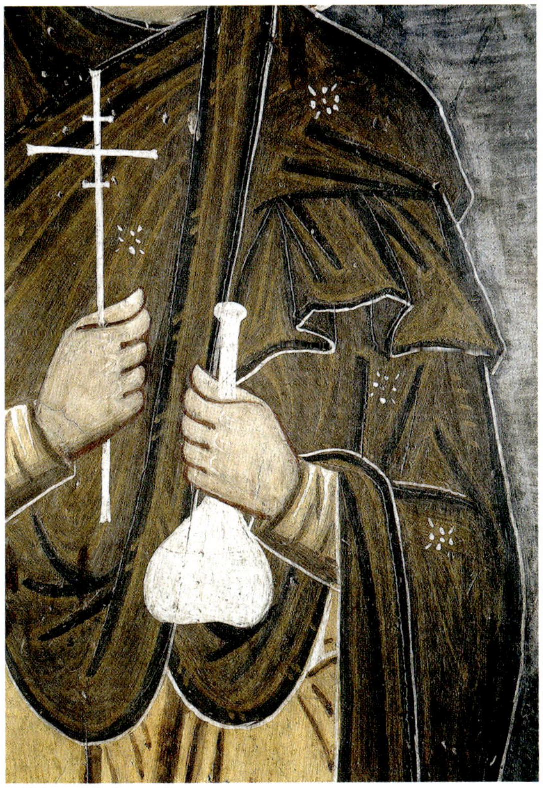

FIG. 5.5 Narthex, south conch. Detail of St. Anastasia showing incised drawing and white lines along the contours of the maphorion (photo courtesy of Dumbarton Oaks BF.T.As.L.4.2)

in the Museum of the Foundation of Archbishop Makarios III in Nicosia (Fig. 5.58).[28] This icon comes from the church at Asinou and has been assigned to the same late thirteenth-century restoration phase to which the Virgin in the apse and the Anastasia panel in the narthex belong.

The image of St. Anastasia exemplifies the linear style that dominated late thirteenth-century art production in Cyprus. This style was characterized by Doula Mouriki as the "maniera cypria" and was associated with a group of late thirteenth-century icons at Sinai, which she assigned to Cypriot painters.[29] Mouriki recognized in this stylistic idiom a fusion of Byzantine and Crusader/Latin features that took shape in Lusignan Cyprus during the thirteenth century, especially toward the end of that century.

Recent scholarship offers new insights in this subject matter. Jaroslav Folda called the style of this group of icons "Veneto-Byzantine Crusader style" and assigned the group to a workshop of Latin painters working at Acre or Sinai in the 1260s.[30] By contrast, Mat Immerzeel stressed the contribution of the east Christian communities in Syria and Lebanon in the formation of this refined linear style, and Annemarie Carr suggested that this style was probably formulated on the Levantine mainland and came to Cyprus as the refugees from the Mamluk invasions of 1264–68 settled on the island (see below, pp. 222–23).[31] In addition, her observations on the placement of the Sacrifice of Isaac on the triumphal arch at Asinou—which she associates with late twelfth- and thirteenth-century churches in Syria/Lebanon and Egypt—lends support to the hypothesis that the eastern Christian communities played a substantial role in shaping the maniera cypria (see below, pp. 221–23). It should be noted, however, that similar artistic developments—that is, the break with twelfth-century Constantinopolitan tradition and the development of simplified, schematic, and linear stylistic currents in the wake of Latin conquest—have also been observed in other Latin-held Byzantine provinces, such as the Peloponnese and Attica.[32] Nonetheless, the historical conditions that prevailed on Cyprus in the thirteenth century—including isolation from the Byzantine metropolitan tradition and the

28. Papageorgiou, *Icons of Cyprus* [1992], 55, fig. 35.
29. Mouriki, "Thirteenth-Century Icon Painting," 35, 67–77; eadem, "Moutoullas," 200–213. This group of icons was attributed by Kurt Weitzmann, "Icon Painting," 69–74, to the Master of the Knights Templar. For a recent discussion on the subject with bibliography, see Carr, "Art," 299–302, 311. For a different approach, see Kotoula, "Maniera Cypria."
30. Folda, "Figural Arts," 318; idem, *Crusader Art in the Holy Land*, 336–42.
31. Immerzeel, "Divine Cavalry"; idem, "Holy Horsemen"; Carr, "Art," 295, 300, 305; eadem, "Perspectives on Visual Culture," 106–10.
32. See Kalopissi-Verti, "Impact of the Fourth Crusade."

immigration of Latins, Syrians, and Armenians from the mainland[33]—seem to have favored the amalgamation of Byzantine, Latin, and east Christian stylistic features on the island, endorsing the process of simplification and linearization and encouraging its widespread application.

Unlike the painter, whose name and origin are unknown, Anastasia Saramalina's prominent placement in the narthex, her substantial role as a donor, and her well-appointed apparel indicate that Anastasia must have been a respectable member of the local community, perhaps an independently wealthy widow.[34] Whether she donated all of the late thirteenth-century decoration in the narthex, naos, and bema, or only the panel with her eponymous saint, however, remains an open question.

The Virgin of Mercy and Latin Donors

The panel depicting the Virgin of Mercy and Latin donors, in the semidome of the south apse, shows the enthroned Mother of God flanked by a kneeling woman to her right and two kneeling youths to her left (Figs. 5.1, 5.6). The Virgin leans slightly to the left while, with her outstretched right hand, she swings her maphorion toward the kneeling female supplicant. Her face and glance, in turn, are directed toward the kneeling supplicant youths. Her maphorion, highlighted with gold, is decorated with very fine rosettes, each one consisting of a red gem surrounded by pearls. The layers of paint on her face have peeled, revealing the underpainting and the drawing of the features (Fig. 5.7). The Christ child turns slightly to the left, bending his head and stretching out his right arm in a gesture of blessing toward the supplicant woman. His figure is quite damaged and little is visible, except for the drawing. The rims of the nimbi are ornamented with pearls. Traces of the abbreviations MP ΘY, painted in white, are visible on either side of the Virgin's head.

This particular image of the Mother of God represents an iconographic type that came from the West. It is called by scholars *Madonna della Misericordia*, or *Schutzmantelmadonna*, because Mary extends her mantle in protective mercy over supplicants.[35] The type is believed to have been created in Italy to serve the new religious orders that emerged in the early thirteenth century.[36] It spread through the missions of the Dominicans and the Franciscans to the Latin East, where it occurs in two well-known manuscripts of Armenian Cilicia: the Gospels of Prince Vasak in the Armenian Patriarchate of Jerusalem, dated shortly after 1272, and a miniature from the Gospel book of Marshal Oshin, formerly in the Feron-Stoclet Collection in Brussels and now in the Pierpont Morgan Library in New York, dated to 1274.[37] The Virgin of Mercy in the Asinou narthex is not an iconographic

33. Richard, "Peuplement latin et syrien." For the stylistic trends in Cyprus during the 12th century and their continuity in the early 13th, see Panayotidi, "Ζωγραφική του 12ου αιώνα"; Carr, "Art," 289–92 (with bibliography).

34. On the role of widows and their matronage in villages in the late Byzantine period, see Gerstel and Kalopissi-Verti, "Female Church Founders."

35. On the iconographic type, see Belting-Ihm, *Sub Matris tutela* (with bibliography); Bacci, "Madonna della Misericordia." On the panel of the south conch of the narthex of Asinou, see Young, "Byzantine Painting," 342–72; Carr, "Correlative Spaces"; Kalopissi-Verti, "Representations of the Virgin," 307–10; Bacci, "Madonna della Misericordia," 177–78.

36. Among the earliest examples of the Virgin of Mercy in the West are (a) an image on the enamel ornamentation of a chalice in the Cistercian abbey of Mehrerau in Bregenz, which dates back to the third quarter of the 13th century: Schmidt, "Madonna dei francescani," 36, fig. 11; and (b) the small panel of the Virgin of the Franciscans in the Pinacoteca Nazionale of Siena, painted by Duccio and variously dated around 1280 or in the 1290s, Deuchler, *Duccio*, 41, 208, figs. 42–43; V. M. Schmidt, in Bagnoli et al., eds., *Duccio: Alle origini*, 158–61, no. 24 (with bibliography).

37. Armenian Patriarchate of Jerusalem no. 2568, fol. 320; Pierpont Morgan Library MSS M740 and 1111. Der Nersessian, "Vierge de Miséricorde"; eadem, *Miniature Painting*, 1:158–59, 2: pls. 646–67; Young, "Byzantine Painting," 349–53; Evans, *Byzantium: Faith and Power*, 60–61, no. 30; Bacci, "Madonna della Misericordia," 179–83.

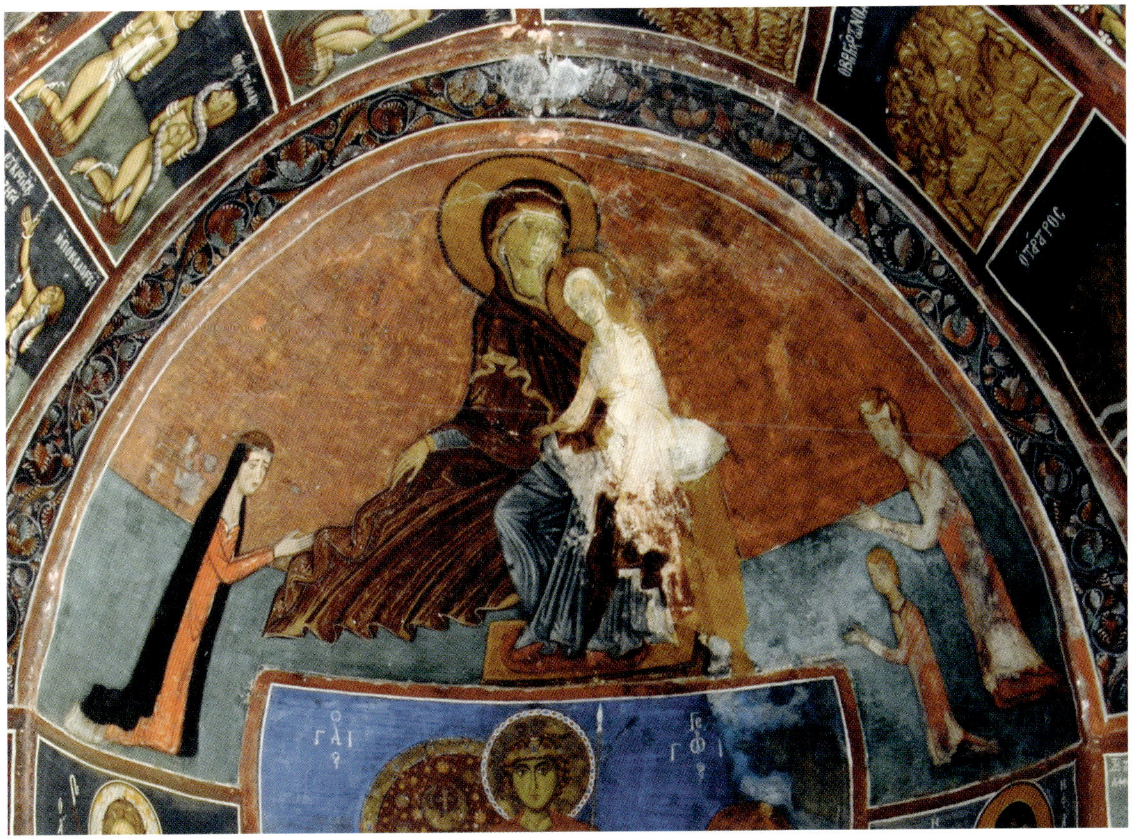

fig. 5.6

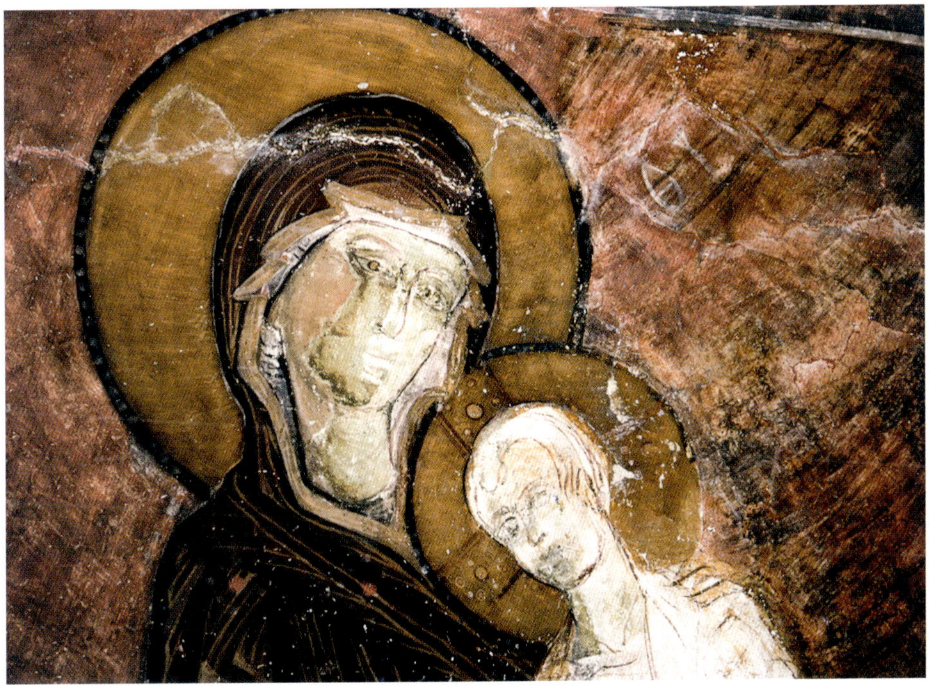

fig. 5.7

FIG. 5.6
Narthex, south conch. The Virgin of Mercy and Christ child with Latin donors (photo courtesy of G. L. Carr)

FIG. 5.7
Narthex, south conch. Face of Virgin of Mercy (photo courtesy of S. Kalopissi-Verti)

unicum in Cyprus. The same iconographic type appears on a Cypriot icon in the Museum of the Foundation of Archbishop Makarios III, where the Virgin protects a group of Carmelite monks under her mantle (ca. 1300).[38] In later centuries, the Virgin della Misericordia seems to have been well established in the Latin East, as illustrated by examples in Venetian-occupied Crete[39] and in Rhodes of the Hospitallers.[40]

While the iconographic type of the Virgin is Latin, certain details link her with local Orthodox artistic production in Cyprus. The ornamental motifs on her maphorion, for example, are distinctive to late thirteenth-century Cypriot icons, usually in the form of a lozenge-shaped central motif surrounded by pearls that are either painted or rendered in gesso relief.[41] Maphoria studded with a star-shaped decoration are also seen in the murals of the church at Moutoullas (1280).[42]

Other features, by contrast, were common throughout the eastern Mediterranean in the thirteenth and fourteenth centuries. Pearl-rimmed haloes, for instance, are encountered on the icons dating from the second half of the thirteenth century at Sinai, icons that have been connected either with the artistic activity of the Crusaders or with Cypriot painters.[43] Moreover, pearled haloes appear on a late-thirteenth-century icon of the Crucifixion from the church of St. Anna at Kalliana in Cyprus and in the figure of St. John of Damascus painted on the face of the apse arch in the church of Asinou itself (Fig. 6.7).[44] In addition, nimbi edged with pearls are often seen in thirteenth- and fourteenth-century miniatures from Sinai, Syria, and Cilician Armenia.[45]

The female Latin donor, who is not named, is depicted to the Virgin's right, kneeling and raising her arms in prayer (Fig. 5.8). Her placement on the dominant side of the image, and the fact that the men with whom she appears are youths, indicate that she must have been the head of the household, plausibly a widowed mother. Her upright posture, with hands clasped in prayer, mirrored in the suppliant boys, is typically western.[46] She appears young and attractive, although the raised eyebrows give

38. Papageorgiou, *Icons of Cyprus* [1992], 49, fig. 31; Folda, "Crusader Art in the Kingdom of Cyprus," 217–22, pl. 7 (with previous bibliography); Carr, "Art in the Court," 242; Bacci, "Tra Pisa e Cipro," 378–79; idem, "Madonna della Misericordia," 175–77.

39. For example, in the churches of the Virgin in Sklaverochori/Pediada Herakleiou (15th c.) and of St. Irene in Malatheros/Kisamos (first half of 15th c.), and on an icon in the National Gallery of Athens commissioned by a confraternity in Candia in the mid-15th c.: see Gallas, Wessel, and Borboudakis, *Byzantinisches Kreta*, 397; Borboudakis, "Παρατηρήσεις στή ζωγραφική," 2:362, pl. 134a; Vassilaki, "Καθημερινή ζωή και πραγματικότητα," 63, fig. 6; Chatzidaki, *Εικόνες Κρητικής Σχολής*, 48, no. 41; Constantoudaki-Kitromilides, "Pittura di icone," 467, pl. 16.

40. See the impressive examples in the church of St. George Chostos at Phileremos (ca. 1500), where, in the lower zone of the side walls, there is a procession of saints who stretch out their mantles to protect a good number of supplicants: kneeling knights, other lay persons, and whole families: Kollias, *City of Rhodes*, fig. 47; Christophoraki, "Χορηγικές μαρτυρίες," 2:455, pl. 176b. The Virgin of Mercy was probably depicted on the west façade of the church of the Panagia tou Kastrou, the Latin cathedral of Rhodes (after 1480). See Archontopoulos, "Παναγία η Φιλόστοργος," 1:322.

41. Papageorgiou, *Icons of Cyprus* [1992], figs. 29, 34, 35; cf. a Sinai icon of the Hodegetria, which has been linked to Cyprus: Mouriki, "Thirteenth-Century Icon Painting," 63–64, fig. 26; Evans, *Byzantium: Faith and Power*, 354, no. 213; *Pilgrimage to Sinai*, ed. Drandaki, no. 26.

42. Mouriki, "Moutoullas," figs. 2, 7, 13, 15.

43. Soteriou and Soteriou, *Εικόνες*, nos. 25, 28, 30–32, 81, 176; Weitzmann, "Thirteenth-Century Crusader Icons," figs. 1, 3–4, 9–12, 18–20, 22; idem, "Icon Painting," figs. 9, 11–12, 17–19, 21–25, etc.; idem, "Four Icons on Mount Sinai," figs. 1–7, 10–11; Mouriki, "Thirteenth-Century Icon Painting," 64–66, fig. 6; Weitzmann, *The Icon*, 211–16, 219–20, 223–24, 228–30, 235.

44. Kalliana: Papageorgiou, *Icons of Cyprus* [1992], 59, fig. 38.

45. Leroy, *Manuscrits syriaques*, 1:313–30, 2: pl. 101, 2, 4; Der Nersessian, *Miniature Painting*, 2: figs. 107–8, 580–87, 595–602, 608, 622, 653–54.

46. Young, "Byzantine Painting," 344 and 378, n. 69; Carr, "Correlative Spaces," 66 and n. 47. The Byzantine

her an expression of deep concern. She is clothed in a long scarlet dress with tightly fitted, wrist-length sleeves and a deep, V-shaped neckline. Beneath it she wears a long white undergown, which is visible around the ankles and feet as she kneels. The scarlet dress seems to be the so-called *cotte*, which appears in France in this form from the thirteenth century onward. The cotte is usually colored (green, blue, or red), has a tight bodice, and flares out from the hips downward. It is shorter for men but very long in the women's version, with a train at the back; the sleeves are long, often buttoned at the lower arm.[47] The deep, V-shaped neckline follows a western fashion of the late medieval period.[48] Scarlet-red dresses seem to have been in fashion among Latin women in Cyprus around 1300 for festive and formal occasions, as attested by the figure of the wife of the knight who commissioned the icon for the church of St. Nicholas of the Roof (τῆς Στέγης)[49] and by the woman depicted with her husband in the narthex of the same church (Fig. 5.9).[50] The painter renders the very long white undergown of the Latin donor at Asinou in a rather awkward manner as its folds cluster around her ankles and feet. More clearly depicted parallels can be seen in the garments of the two kneeling daughters of Queen Keran and King Levon III in the Gospels of Jerusalem (Armenian Patriarchate 2563), dated to 1272.[51]

The Latin lady wears a long black veil descending from her head to her feet. It is fastened on a transparent circlet around her head and is also held in place by means of narrow black ribbons visible on top of her brown hair. Long veils that are either monochrome or have multicolored designs and are sometimes cloaklike and heavy in appearance—falling from the top of the head down the back to the feet—were in vogue in the Levant. They were worn by both local and Latin women. One may assume that the western fashion of a short and very light veil attached to a circlet was mingled with the local fashion in the Latin east of a long, heavy cloak worn from the top of the head.[52] As a rule, veils are not fastened to the head in the manner seen on the Latin supplicant at Asinou. A headdress consisting of a band (*chapel* or *chapelet*) or diadem, and some kind of bonnet or net on top of which the veil is fastened, is seen being worn usually by Armenian women in late thirteenth- and fourteenth-century miniatures.[53] This manner of wearing the veil, falling from the top of the head, occurs in Cyprus on the figure of the wife of a nobleman, usually identified as John Lusignan (d. 1375), depicted in the north vessel of the church of the Holy Cross at Pelendri, as well as on a deceased woman named Maria, painted in the tympanum of the conch above the western entrance of the same church, and in certain fourteenth-century icons.[54] In other Cypriot examples, like the figure of Anna in the narthex at Asinou (see below, pp. 188–90; Fig. 5.47)

---

gesture of prayer has the hands separated, as depicted in all other donor portraits in the narthex.

47. On the history of costume at the time of the Crusades and the eastern–western reciprocal influences and exchanges, see Boucher, *Histoire du costume,* 173–89. On the cotte, see ibid., index; Viollet-le-Duc, *Encyclopédie médiévale,* 518–25, esp. 522–23; Pinasa, *Costumes,* 77.

48. See Kalamara, "Ενδυμα στο Μυστρά," 114.

49. Papageorgiou, *Icons of Cyprus* [1992], fig. 32a. In the case of the Hamilton psalter, however, the red color of the garments of all figures depicted on fol. 39v may be conditioned by the icon they are venerating, since the servants of the Hodegetria wore red. See Havice, "Hamilton Psalter"; eadem, "Marginal Miniatures"; N. P. Ševčenko, in Vassilaki, ed., *Mother of God,* 388–89.

50. Stylianou and Stylianou, "Ναὸς τοῦ Ἁγίου Νικολάου," 132–36, fig. 9; eidem, "Επανεξέτασις," 83–88; Kalopissi-Verti, "Church Inscriptions as Documents," 85, fig. 5; Carr, "Art," 288–89. The couple is dressed in western garments but the accompanying inscription is in Greek.

51. Fol. 380; Der Nersessian, *Miniature Painting,* 2: fig. 641.

52. Viollet-le-Duc, *Encyclopédie médiévale,* 462, fig. 9B; 499, fig. 22g.

53. Der Nersessian, *Miniature Painting,* 2: figs. 597, 599, 624, 627–28, 641.

54. Stylianou and Stylianou, *Painted Churches,* 231–32; Zarras, *Holy Cross,* 49, fig. 43 (see also note 70); Papageorgiou, *Icons of Cyprus* [1969], plates on pp. 38, 39. The external painting on the lunette above the western entrance door in Pelendri is not published.

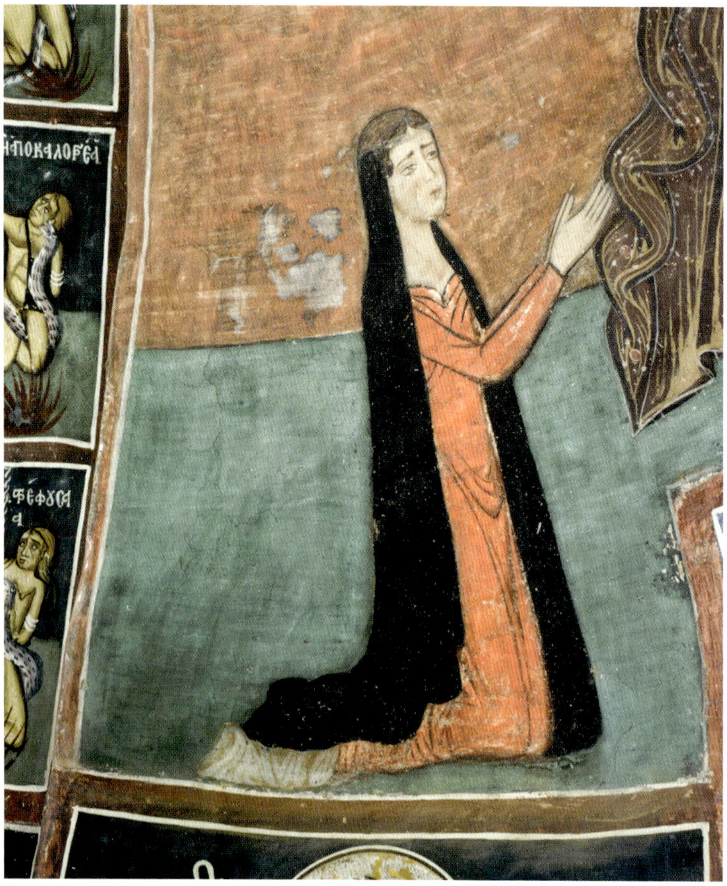

fig. 5.8

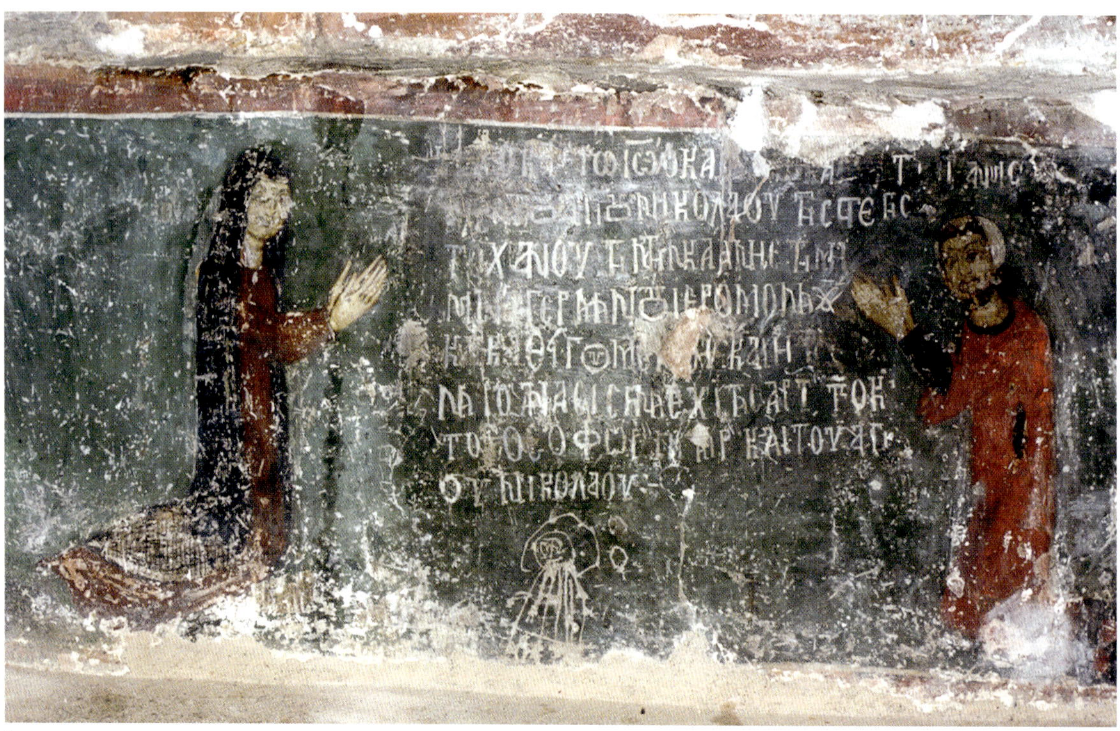

fig. 5.9

FIG. 5.8

Narthex, south conch. The Latin female donor (photo courtesy of the Leventis Foundation and the Archaeological Research Unit, University of Cyprus, No. 006429)

FIG. 5.9

Kakopetria, Church of St. Nicholas of the Roof (τῆς Στέγης), narthex. Donor couple (photo courtesy of S. Kalopissi-Verti)

or Nenkomia in the central vessel at Pelendri (Fig. 5.48),[55] the veil is worn over a peculiar local type of strapped garment that also covers the neck. Further images in Cyprus show the veil covering the entire head, beginning from the top of the forehead, as in the figure of the wife of Michael Katzouroumpos in the church of St. Demetrianos at Dali (1317). Sometimes it is tied around the head with a cord, the ends of which fall down along the back, as in the case of the female supplicants in the church of the Archangel Michael at Pedoulas (1474).[56]

The specific and very elegant manner in which the veil is worn by the Latin donor at Asinou—attached to a circlet and falling backward not from the top but from the back of the head—differs from the Cypriot examples given above, mostly local women. This manner of wearing the veil occurs in works from the Latin East such as the Arsenal Bible, produced in the scriptorium of Acre during St. Louis's sojourn in the Latin East (1250–54), and in the detached frescoes from a chapel in Beirut that have been associated with one of the Cistercian nunneries founded in Syria in the thirteenth century.[57] It is also worn in this way by the donor of the St. Sergios icon at Sinai, attributed to Latin Syria in the mid-thirteenth century.[58] Another Latin lady from the Crusader Levant, Simone Guers, wife of Renier de Gibelet, wore a similar veil, as shown on her funerary slab in the chapel of the Archangel Michael in Panagia Angeloktiste at Kiti (1304).[59] Moreover, the women with veils schematically represented on fourteenth-century Cypriot glazed bowls demonstrate the dissemination of this type of veil in medieval Cyprus.[60]

Closely parallel in attitude, gesture, and costume to the Latin lady at Asinou is the probably Latin donor couple depicted in the narthex of St. Nicholas of the Roof in Kakopetria (Fig. 5.9). The female donor kneels to the left with her hands raised together in the western gesture of prayer; she is clad in a red, long-sleeved dress and a black veil.[61]

The two supplicant youths in the narthex of Asinou are depicted kneeling to the right of the enthroned Virgin, raising their arms in prayer (Fig. 5.10). They both wear long tight pants: red for the older boy, red and black for the younger. The two figures are quite worn away but one can discern, especially in the image of the younger boy, that each wears a short white tunic reaching to the knees with tightly fitting sleeves and, over that, a light-red, knee-length mantle, open in front, with tight sleeves, shorter than those of the white tunic. The boys are beardless and have short, reddish-blond hair.

Two-colored costumes like the red and black pants of the younger boy follow a western fashion known as "Mi-Partie," which was also popular in Venetian-dominated Crete in the fourteenth and fifteenth centuries.[62] The boys' hair—cut rather short, combed backward, and falling behind the ears, with a large fringe forming a curve on the forehead—seems to follow a fashion for young boys that was widespread in the eastern Mediterranean,

55. Stylianou and Stylianou, "Dedicatory Inscriptions," 108, fig. 9; Zarras, *Holy Cross,* 19, fig. 13.
56. Stylianou and Stylianou, *Painted Churches,* 425–26, fig. 256 (Dali); 331, fig. 196 (Pedoulas).
57. Buchthal, *Miniature Painting,* pl. 73; Hunt, "Woman's Prayer," 2:84–85, fig. 9.
58. Hunt, "Woman's Prayer," 2:79–84, fig. 1.
59. Greenhill, *Incised Effigial Slabs,* 1:242–47, 2: pl. 138c; Foulias, *Our Lady Angeloktisti*, 20, fig. 13; Imhaus, *Lacrimae Cypriae*, 1:142–43, pl. 121 (F. 271); Piponnier, "Vêtement occidental à Chypre," 2:93–94, 100, pl. 285. For a discussion of female headcoverings and costume on 14th-century funerary slabs in Cyprus, see Piponnier, "Vêtement," 92–94. Young, "Byzantine Painting," 346, sees a chronological evolution in the way the veil is worn; the dated slab in Kiti (1302) is one of her arguments for dating the panel of the Virgin of Mercy at Asinou to about 1300.
60. Papanikola-Bakirtzis, *Medieval Cypriot Pottery*, nos. 12–18. Visual evidence challenges the claim of the traveler Jacopo da Verona, who visited Cyprus in the year 1335, that the black veil was adopted by Cypriot women as a sign of mourning after the loss of Acre in 1291. See Talbot Rice, *Icons of Cyprus*, 103; Young, "Byzantine Painting," 345–46 and 378, n. 73; Hunt, "Woman's Prayer," 82–84, 100–101.
61. See above, note 50.
62. Lymberopoulou, *Archangel Michael at Kavalariana*, 214–15.

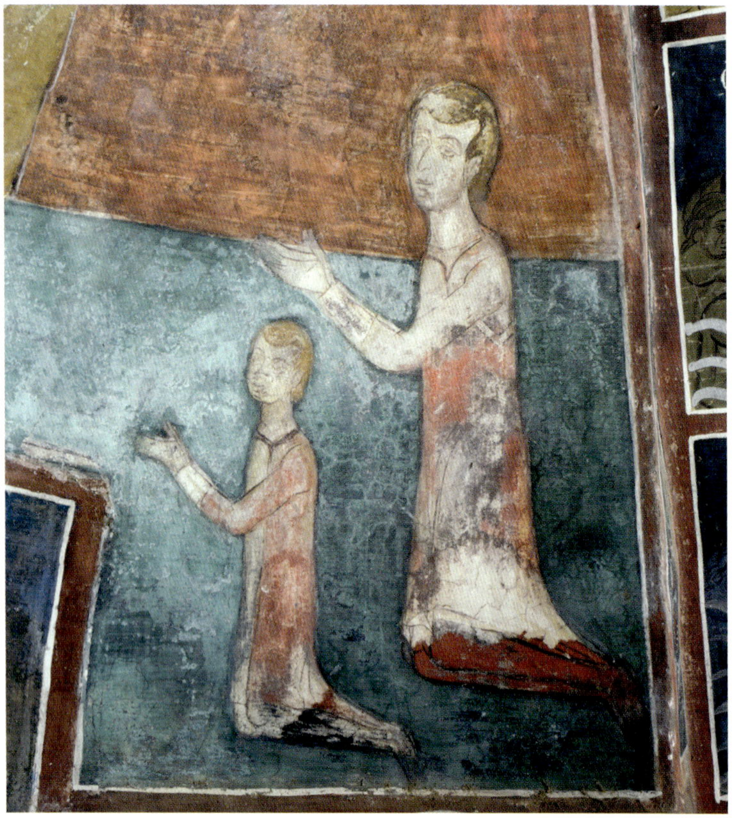

FIG. 5.10 Narthex, south conch. The two supplicant male youths (photo courtesy of the Leventis Foundation and the Archaeological Research Unit, University of Cyprus, No. 006428)

evident in miniatures of the second half of the thirteenth century in Armenian Cilicia and in early fourteenth-century frescoes in Crete.[63]

The red background seen in the panel with the Virgin of Mercy is typical of several artistic traditions that met in the East at the time of the Crusades. A common device in Byzantine painting during the Komnenian period, it recurs in Orthodox church decoration in regions under Latin rule, such as Attica and Cyprus.[64] It appears also in the West, especially in Romanesque painting. Moreover, it is encountered in the eastern Mediterranean, for example, in Syriac manuscripts and Sinai icons assigned to Christians of the Levant.[65] Thus it emerges as a device rooted in both eastern and western artistic traditions, and favored in the art of the areas affected by the Crusades.

Portions of the figures in the panel that are well worn allow certain observations of the painter's techniques. A light olive underlayer covers the whole of the Virgin's face (Fig. 5.7). The contour lines are drawn in black and the features in red-brown. Modeling of the flesh is based upon very gentle gradations of pink and a subtle green shade on the contour. In the figure of Christ, the initial drawing on the white plaster is visible. Moreover, the fresco preserves traces of the underlayer in a light olive green, and of the subsequent layer of paint in gold ocher on the *himation*. In the figures of the boys one can see the initial drawing in brown, the overall brown underlayer of the hair, and parts of the final red layer of the garments.

The figure of the female donor is in an excellent state of preservation (Fig. 5.8). Contour lines are black and relatively thick. Very fine brown brushstrokes outline the features of the face, sometimes reinforced in black. The modeling of the flesh on the face and neck is very subtly graduated in tones of pale pink ocher, with light brown shading and reddish touches on the cheeks. Her dress is covered with scarlet red unmodulated by highlights; a few fine black lines define the folds. The very delicate modeling and the pale coloring give the young woman an expression of exquisite elegance.

Of all the surviving works on Cyprus that are assigned to a Latin patron, the fresco at Asinou is the closest in style to the western artistic tradition. However, the multicultural character of Lusignan Cyprus raises questions as to the painter's likely

63. Der Nersessian, *Miniature Painting*, 2: figs. 646, 647; Lymberopoulou, *Archangel Michael at Kavalariana*, figs. 29, 50–53.

64. Mouriki, "Τοιχογραφίες τῶν παρεκκλησίων τῆς Σπηλιᾶς," 107A; eadem, *Τοιχογραφίες τοῦ Σωτῆρα*, 51; Papageorgiou, "Ἰδιάζουσαι βυζαντιναὶ τοιχογραφίαι," 2:209–10; Boyd, "Monagri," 321–22; Young, "Byzantine Painting," 211–13; Mouriki, "Moutoullas," 204–5.

65. Leroy, *Manuscrits syriaques*, 288, 298–99; Weitzmann, "Icon Painting," 70; Mouriki, "Thirteenth-Century Icon Painting," 25–26.

origin: Was he a Westerner from the Crusader states, an Orthodox refugee from the mainland, or a Byzantine Cypriot? It seems clear that local Byzantine painters worked quite often for Latin clientele in regions conquered by the Franks, the best documented example being the work of Cretan painters under Venetian rule.[66] These artists were capable of adopting iconographic and stylistic devices particular to the needs and tastes of their patrons and of blending these elements with the long-established Byzantine artistic tradition.

Despite the evidently western character of the composition, the gothic elegance of the figures, and the charm of a work of Crusader art, the image shares certain stylistic features with the painting in the main apse (Figs. 6.4, 6.8) and with the panel of St. Anastasia in the narthex (Figs. 5.2, 5.5, 6.9). Susan Young has, rightly I think, pointed to features in the modeling of the garments that appear in both the Virgin of Mercy and the archangels in the main apse, especially the sharp, agitated ends of the hems and the lines of the bent legs, which curve over thigh and calf to converge at the knee.[67] Moreover, the billowing ends of the archangels' himatia in the apse are similar in shape to the hem of the Virgin's maphorion, in front of her left knee, in the narthex; the large oval highlight with the small, dark V-shaped line in the middle of the shin is found in both the Gabriel of the apse and the Virgin in the narthex; the tunics of the Virgin Pantanassa in the main apse and the Latin lady in the narthex have black linear V-shaped folds in front of the body. Additionally, the white contour line, next to the black line, is a common feature of the images of the Virgin of Mercy, of St. Anastasia in the narthex, and of the archangels in the main apse. Moreover, the Virgin of Mercy and St. Anastasia each wear a maphorion studded with rosettes. These kinships suggest that the painter(s) of the main apse and of the Latin lady had similar training and background. Thus, as Susan Young has noted, the fresco of the Virgin of Mercy with Latin donors may be assigned to the same workshop that executed the composition of the main apse and the fresco of St. Anastasia in the narthex, toward the end of the thirteenth century, either during the same campaign (ca. 1290–1300) or slightly later (ca. 1300).[68]

This workshop has so far been considered a local Greek Orthodox painters' shop. However, Annemarie Carr's suggestion that the late thirteenth-century apse program of Asinou should be associated with the art of the Christian communities on the Levantine mainland may introduce a new factor into the question of the painter's (or painters') identity, for artistic interchange among local and Latin Christian groups was already extensive in the mainland Crusader states (see below, pp. 221–23). What stands out most strongly in the case of this painting, though, is the close interaction of Greek and Latin cultures. This fresco is a clear example of Crusader art because its patrons, iconography, and style are Latin; at the same time, it bears a Greek inscription because it is addressed to Greek-speaking viewers, and it is offered—probably with a donation—by a Latin lady to an Orthodox church dedicated to her patron saint—the Virgin—presumably in thanksgiving for her own and her sons' survival after the fall of Acre (1291) and very likely in memory of her late husband.[69]

66. M. Chatzidakis, *Ἕλληνες Ζωγράφοι*, 79–82; N. Chatzidakis, "Icon Painting in Crete"; Constantoudaki-Kitromilides, "Taste and Market"; eadem, "Pittura di icone a Creta Veneziana," 461–62; Kazanaki-Lappa, "Βυζαντινή παράδοση." For a possibly similar situation in the Holy Land in the 12th c., see Folda, *Art of the Crusaders*, 318.

67. Young, "Byzantine Painting," 328–29, 362, 368–72.

68. Ibid. Technically, the overlapping plaster joins (*pontate*) indicate that the image of the Latin donors postdates the late 13th-c. fresco of St. Anastasia but precedes the narthex decoration of 1332/33. See Fig. 7.29. However, it does not tell us how long a time intervened. It could be a different phase between the late 13th c. and 1332/33, as David Winfield believes (*Asinou*, 26), or it could be a *giornata*, i.e., the painter's work in a day during the same campaign as the fresco of St. Anastasia.

69. On the migratory waves of settlers, refugees, merchants, and others from the Eastern Mediterranean to Cyprus in the Lusignan period, see Coureas, "Place to Be," 125–26; cf. Edbury, *Cyprus and the Crusades*, 19, 22.

The paintings closest in context to the Asinou fresco are the two large and much-discussed icons now in the Museum of the Foundation of Archbishop Makarios III: the icon of St. Nicholas of the Roof, dedicated by a knight of the Ravendel/ Ravandel family, most probably Mellours de Ravendel, one of the last lords of Maraclea on the coast of Syria; and the icon of the Virgin of Mercy, offered by Carmelite monks. Commissioned by Latins and painted in a hybrid style mingling Byzantine and Latin traditions around 1300, these two icons have been assigned to Cypriot workshops. It is a point of controversy, however, whether these were Cypriot Greek (Mouriki, Carr) or Cypriot Crusader (Folda) workshops.[70] In any case, they reflect the multicultural milieu that developed in Cyprus in the late thirteenth century, at the time of the displacement of the last Crusaders from the Syro-Palestinian coast to the islands of the southeastern Mediterranean, especially Cyprus and Rhodes. Thus, Latin donors, who evidently took refuge in Cyprus after the fall of the last strongholds of the Crusaders on the Syro-Palestinian coast, seem to have commissioned votive paintings from Cypriot workshops and offered them to Orthodox shrines in thanksgiving.[71] This evidence is confirmed, moreover, by written sources referring to donations made by Latins to Orthodox religious foundations during the fourteenth century.[72]

In the south apse of the narthex at Asinou, three votive images—painted in different periods and representing separate identities—interact in a shared space (Fig. 5.1), as Annemarie Carr has shown.[73] Though reflecting different backgrounds, these three images—the impressive late twelfth-century mural icon of St. George on horseback, an ex-voto of a healer of horses, Nikephoros [Kallias];[74] the late thirteenth-century image of St. Anastasia Pharmakolytria with her namesake devotee, Anastasia Saramalina, a respected elderly local woman; and the exquisite panel of the Virgin of Mercy protecting a young elegant Latin lady with her two boys beneath her maphorion—all correlate harmoniously in the same space. The Latin supplicants, presumably refugees from the Crusader Levant after the fall of Acre in 1291, offer a panel of private devotion to an Orthodox church. Accepted by the Orthodox community, they place themselves under the protection not only of the Virgin of Mercy but also of St. George, a saint highly venerated both East and West whose cult center was at Lydda (Diospolis) in Palestine. In the late thirteenth century, the space of the south apse seems to have served as a quasi-private chapel for individual devotion, with the Orthodox and Latin votive panels framing the twelfth-century image of St. George in a harmonious interplay. For the late thirteenth-century viewer, this apse reflected strong bonds with the Syrian mainland and the interaction of Orthodox and Latin traditions in the multicultural milieu of Cyprus.[75]

70. Papageorgiou, *Icons of Cyprus* [1992], 46, 49, figs. 31–32; N. P. Ševčenko, *Life of Saint Nicholas*, 38, no. 14; Mouriki, "Thirteenth-Century Icon Painting," 38–47, figs. 48–53; Folda, "Crusader Art in the Kingdom of Cyprus," 216–22; Carr, "Art in the Court," 242.

71. For later, fourteenth-century examples, see the frescoes of the north vessel of the church of the Holy Cross at Pelendri, which have been associated with John de Lusignan, brother of King Peter I (1359–69) and lord of the casale of Pelendri from 1353 to his death in 1375: Stylianou and Stylianou, *Painted Churches,* 223–32; Carr, "Byzantines and Italians," 347–48; Christoforaki, "Unusual Representation." For the identification of the donor with John de Lusignan, see Enlart, *Gothic Art*, 352–53, figs. 313–14; for another possible identification with Thomas, John's younger brother, see Carr, "Art in the Court," 245–46; see also the Latin couple depicted in the narthex of St. Nicholas of the Roof at Kakopetria, above, note 50.

72. See below, p. 367, nn. 10 and 11. On the relations between the Latin and the Orthodox churches in Cyprus, see Coureas, *Latin Church in Cyprus*, 251–317.

73. Carr, "Correlative Spaces," 59–80.

74. According to N. Ševčenko, the part of the inscription mentioning Kallias is a later addition. See above, p. 83.

75. Kalopissi-Verti, "Representations of the Virgin," 305–10.

In the campaign of 1332/33, the figure of St. Mamas, a healer of flocks and of people venerated in both Byzantium and the West, was depicted riding a lion (Fig. 5.33; see below, pp. 161–64) on the wall of the south apse opposite the image of St. Anastasia, thus complementing the therapeutic and protective connotations of the program of this space and serving as a pendant to St. George mounted on a horse. In this same campaign, as will be shown in the following, scenes of individual punishment as part of the Last Judgment were painted on the soffit of the south arch, thus limiting the space of the south apse.

The Wall Paintings of 1332/33

The fourteenth-century program is dominated by the Last Judgment and contextually focuses on salvation through repentance. At the same time, the sanctoral cycle, mingling Cypriot saints with universally venerated ones, acquires a strong local character. Lay and monastic supplicants, depicted among the saints' figures in the lower zone, join their prayers to those of the saints; together, they address their invocations to the holy persons of the Deesis on the east wall, who act as responding recipients. Individual devotion thereby becomes corporate and collectively embraces not only the monastic and lay donors but also the members of the congregation.

Last Judgment

The composition of the Last Judgment dominates the narthex at Asinou (Fig. 5.11).[76] The scene's various elements are distributed across the vault, the west lunette, the northern semidome, and the soffits of the north, south, and west arches. They could not expand symmetrically into the southern semidome, because that was already occupied by the votive with the Latin donors, which had to be respected and integrated into the iconographic program of the narthex.

The Last Judgment is based on a synthesis of scripture, homilies, and poetic works.[77] Thus it embraces several constituent scenes. Eschatological visions, written mostly in the tenth century,[78] and apocalypses dating to the middle Byzantine period[79] reflect the literary background of the artistic depictions of the Second Coming, which took shape almost simultaneously. The Byzantine rite also had an important impact on its iconography. The services on Meatfare Sunday (Κυριακὴ τῆς Ἀπόκρεω), dedicated to the Second Coming, and the vespers on the preceding Saturday (one of the Saturdays of Souls [Ψυχοσάββατα], which commemorate all the deceased) not only include the canon of the Second Coming by Theodore Stoudites and the beginning (prooimion and first oikos) of the relevant kontakion of Romanos Melodos but also incorporate in the troparia nearly all the elements of the Second Coming in the Old and New

76. On the iconography of the Last Judgment, see Millet, *Dalmatique du Vatican*; Milošević, *Das Jüngste Gericht*; Brenk, "Anfänge der byzantinischen Weltgerichtsdarstellung"; idem, *Tradition*; Christe, *Jugements derniers*; Angheben, "Jugements derniers byzantins"; Pace, ed., *Le Jugement dernier*. For the post-Byzantine period, see Garides, *Jugement dernier post-byzantin*.

77. Ezek. 18:4–20, 24:14, 34:17, Dan. 7:1–28, 12:2–3, Amos 5:18–20, Psalms 7, 9, 97, 102, Mark 13:24–37, Matt. 24, 25, John 5:25–30, Paul's epistles to the Thessalonians (I, 4:13–17; II, 1:8–10) and the Corinthians (II, 5:10), Apocalypse (5, 20:11–15, 22:12); Hemmerdinger-Iliadou, "Données archéologiques"; eadem, "Éphrem le Syrien"; Gavrilović, "St. Ephraim the Syrian"; Brock, "Ephrem's Letter to Publius"; idem, *Hymns on Paradise*; Grosdidier de Matons, *Romanos Le Mélode*, 5:209–67.

78. Angelidi, "Version longue"; eadem, "Βίος τοῦ Ὁσίου Βασιλείου"; Veselovskij "Razyskanija," and Vilinskij, "Žitie sv. Vasilija novago"; Rydén, *Life of St. Andrew the Fool*, 2:164–69. On the life of Andreas Salos and its date, idem, "Date of the Life"; idem, "St. Basil the Younger."

79. James, *Apocrypha Anecdota*, 109–26; Pernot, "Descente de la Vierge"; Bauckham, "Four Apocalypses." On the impact of Marian apocalyptic texts on the composition of the Last Judgment, see Semoglou, *Voyage outre-tombe*, 69–72. On the apocalyptic tours of hell, Himmelfarb, *Tours of Hell*. On the apocalypse of St. Anastasia, see Baun, "Apocalypse of Anastasia"; eadem, "Middle Byzantine 'Tours of Hell'"; eadem, *Tales from Another Byzantium*.

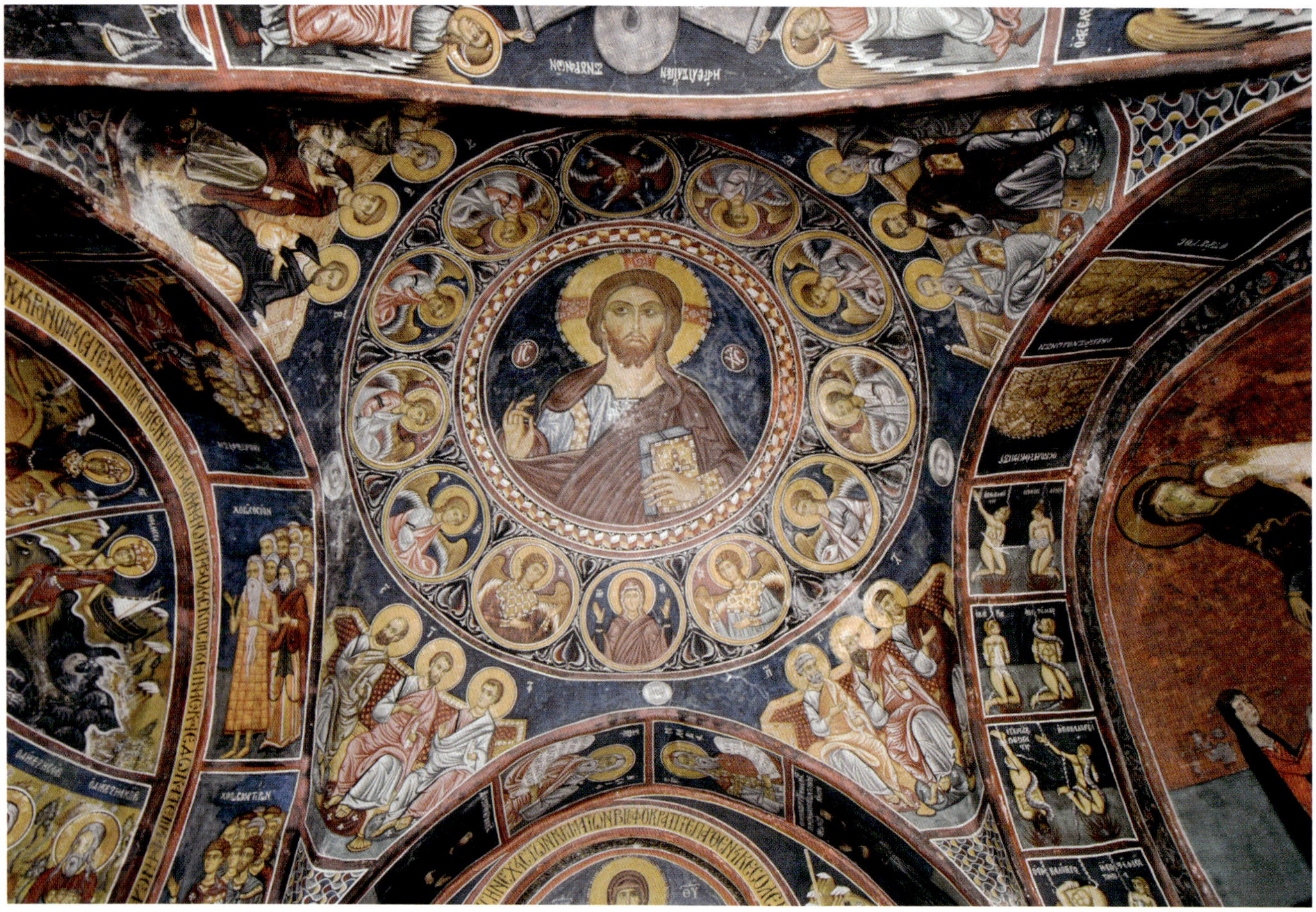

FIG. 5.11 Narthex. Vault: The Pantokrator surrounded by medallions depicting the Mother of God, angels, and a seraph. Pendentives: The Apostles. South arch: Torments of the Damned. North arch: Choirs of the Elect (photo courtesy of G. L. Carr)

Testaments that are depicted in art.[80] The throne of glory, the fiery stream, the open books, the sounding trumpets, the outer darkness, Tartarus, the gnashing of teeth, and the terrible worm are some of the subjects included in the hymnography sung during these services. Moreover, the synaxarion of Meatfare Sunday repeats almost verbatim Matthew 25:35–46, which expresses the principal ideological basis of the Last Judgment and is often inscribed in compositions of the Second Coming, as it is at Asinou itself.[81]

The earliest surviving middle Byzantine compositions of the Second Coming in monumental painting are found in regions of the Byzantine periphery such as Cappadocia and Kastoria and belong to the late ninth and tenth centuries.[82] By the beginning of

80. *Τριώδιον*, 27ff. (Canon of Stoudites), 31 (Kontakion of Romanos). Similar content is found in the hymns included in the service of Saturday before Pentecost, a ψυχοσάββατον on which the dead are honored: *Πεντηκοστάριον*, 198.

81. *Τριώδιον*, 32.

82. Cappadocia: Yılanlı kilise in the valley of Ihlara, St. John at Güllü dere (913–20), funerary church no. 2b in Göreme: see Thierry and Thierry, *Nouvelles églises rupestres*, 93–102, fig. 22, pls. 49–50; eidem, "Ayvalı Kilise," 131–41, figs. 28–29, 31; N. Thierry, *Haut Moyen Age*, 1:153–73; eadem, "Apocalypse de Jean," 325–30, figs. 5–8; eadem, "Église au Jugement dernier"; Jolivet-Lévy,

the eleventh century the scene was fully developed, as seen in Panagia ton Chalkeon in Thessalonike (1028), and at that point it appears not only in monumental painting but also on icons (Sinai, second half of eleventh and early twelfth century) and in manuscripts (Paris. gr. 74, eleventh century).[83]

The Last Judgment is a popular subject in Cyprus. The twelfth-century composition in the narthex of St. Nicholas of the Roof at Kakopetria is the earliest extant example.[84] The representations in the church of the Transfiguration at Sotera near Famagusta (ca. 1280–1300), in the narthex of Asinou (1332/33), in Panagia Kanakaria at Lythrankomi (fourteenth-century fresco layer), and in the narthex of St. John Lampadistes at Kalopanayiotis (after 1453) reveal the popularity of the subject in the Lusignan period.[85] The composition is widespread in the Venetian period as well, especially in church ambulatories, as in the Panagia at Moutoullas, the Holy Cross of Agiasmati at Platanistassa (1494), and St. Sozomenos at Galata (1513), and on icons.[86]

A notable peculiarity in the composition on the Last Judgment at Asinou is the unusual representation of its central subject, the HEAVENLY COURT, traditionally depicted as an entity consisting of Christ enthroned as supreme judge with the Virgin, John the Baptist, the apostles, and the escorting angels. Instead of this well established unified configuration, in Asinou the particular elements of the scene are dispersed spatially on the vault, the pendentives and the east wall. Thus, Christ (with accompanying inscription Ι(ησοῦ)ς Χ(ριστό)ς) is represented half-length at the center of the vault in the iconographic type of the Pantokrator (All-Ruler); he is surrounded by twelve medallions that contain, at the east, the Mother of God (Μ(ήτ)ηρ Θ(εο)υ) depicted frontally with raised hands in supplication; the archangels Michael (ο αρχ(άγγελος) Μιχ(αήλ) and Gabriel (ο αρχ(άγγελος) Γαβρι/ήλ) to either side of her; a seraph in the west; and eight more angels (Fig. 5.11). The apostles are depicted in the pendentives, and the Deesis, which may be considered also as part of the Second Coming, is placed on the east wall of the narthex (see below, pp. 154–58 and Fig. 5.30).

Abbreviations written beside each of the ten angels allow their identification.[87] Angels with these names occur very rarely in art.[88] Following Gabriel,

Cappadoce médiévale, 270–74; eadem, "Premières images." Kastoria: St. Stephen, Taxiarches Metropoleos: see Panayotidi, "Peinture monumentale," 79–82, figs. 6, 8, 9; Siomkos, *Église Saint-Etienne*, 91–99, schémas 18–22, figs. 33–49.

83. Papadopoulos, *Wandmalereien*, 57–76; Brenk, *Tradition*, 82–84, fig. 5; Soteriou and Soteriou, *Εἰκόνες*, nos. 150 and 151; Weitzmann, *Manuscript Illumination*, 301, 304, 306, figs. 303–4; Vocotopoulos, *Βυζαντινές Εικόνες*, pl. 20; Galavaris, *Eleventh Century Hexaptych*, 133–35, pls. 15–16. For Paris. gr. 74, ff. 51v and 93v, see Omont, *Évangiles avec peintures byzantines*, 1: pls. 41, 81; Brenk, "Anfänge," 106–8, Abb. 1; idem, *Tradition*, 84–85, fig. 24; Tsuji, "Byzantine Gospel Illustrations," 53, 54, n. 42; for a color plate of fol. 93v, see *Trésors de Byzance*, no. 23. Tsuji, in "Headpiece Miniatures," dates the manuscript between 1060 and 1080.

84. Stylianou and Stylianou, *Painted Churches*, 59–62, figs. 23–24.

85. Megaw and Hawkins, *Lythrankomi*, 153–55; Stylianou and Stylianou, *Painted Churches*, 306–11; Cholet, "Fresques du Jugement dernier." For the church at Sotera, see A. Papageorgiou in *ARDAC* 1989, 29–30. On the theological controversies between Latins and Greeks in Cyprus concerning beliefs about the afterlife, see Duba, "Afterlife."

86. For Moutoullas, see Nicolaïdès, "Jugement dernier" (14th century); Emmanuel, "Ναός της Παναγίας στο Μουτουλλά" (second quarter of 16th century); for the other churches, see Stylianou and Stylianou, *Painted Churches,* 88, 218. For the icon from Phoini, in the district of Paphos, now in the Byzantine Museum of the Foundation of Archbishop Makarios III (first half of 16th c.), see Papageorgiou, *Ιερά Μητρόπολις Πάφου*, fig. 112.

87. For the identification of the angels depicted in the vault, see J. Michl, "Engel V (Katalog der Engelnamen)" in *RAC* 5:200–239. I am indebted to Professor Franz Tinnefeld for his suggestions.

88. Cf. the 13th-century icon of Archangel Michael on the screen of St. Herakleidios at Kalopanayiotis, which has six other archangels in its two vertical frames. They are labeled, according to Papageorgiou, *Αγίου Ιωάννου*

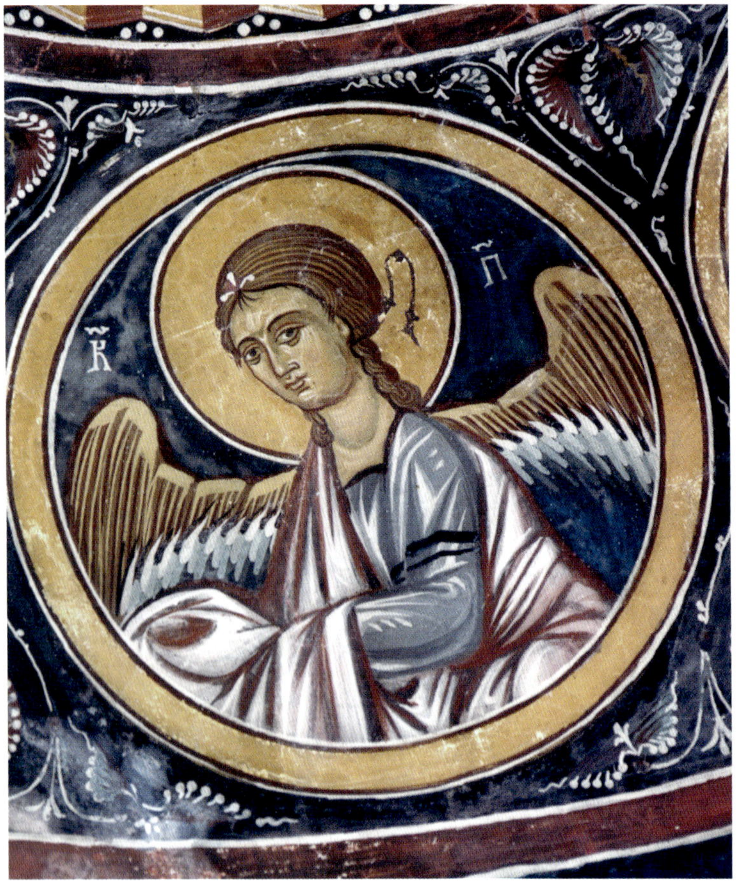

FIG. 5.12 Narthex, vault. The archangel Kopiel (photo courtesy of S. Kalopissi-Verti)

who in magical texts is considered to be an angel of the moon,[89] those on the southern part of the vault may be identified as follows: Κ Π = Κ(ο)π(ιήλ), Kopiel, mentioned in magical texts as an angel of the moon (Fig. 5.12); Κ Ν = Κ(άι)ν or Κ(αινά)ν, Kain or Kainan, a gnostic ἐξουσία ("authority") identified with the sun; C Τ = C(αλ)τ(αήλ), Saltael (or Salathiel), thought to be one of the seven archangels and characterized as a supplicant whose name is interpreted as "request of God"; in magic he is regarded as an angel of Hermes; C ΑΥ = Cαυ(σιοῦ), Sausiou, a Christian angel related to the wind of sweet scent.[90] In the northern part of the vault, after the archangel Michael, who in magical texts is believed to be the first of the five angels of the sun,[91] we can identify the following: Θ ΟΥ = Θου(ριήλ), Thouriel, considered in superstition to be an archangel; ΓΓ Λ = Γ(αλ)γ(αλιή)λ, Galgaliel, a Jewish angel who, together with ninety-six other angels, moves the sun; Τ Α = Τα(ρταροῦχος) or Τα(ρταριήλ),Tartarouchos or Tartariel, an angel who watches over the torments of sinners in hell, in magic one of the masters of the underworld and a demon of the moon and of the sun;[92] Τ Π = Τ(ε)π(ταδαήλ), Teptadael, an angel serving the Just (or Elect) and in astrology an angel of winter.

In sum, the angels escorting the Pantokrator in the vault include two angels of the sun, Kain and Galgaliel; an angel-demon who is master of the torments in hell, Tartarouchos; an angel serving the Just, Teptadael; and an angel who is considered to be a supplicant par excellence, Saltael. Consequently, the Pantokrator in the vault of the narthex at Asinou is encircled by angels serving as escorts and extollers of God, by angels related to cosmological symbols, and by angels directly connected to the Second Coming, who watch over the Just and the Unjust and beseech God for mercy. All escorting angels, together with the Virgin, direct

του Λαμπαδιστού, 53, fig. 57: on the viewer's left, Gabriel, Sychael, Ioel; and on the viewer's right Ouriel, Raphael, and Phlogael. I thank Annemarie Carr for pointing out this icon to me. Moreover, two angels rarely depicted in art—Γιήλ and Γιδαήλ—occur in the dome of St. Hierotheos close to Megara in Attica (ca. 1180): see Mouriki, "Ὁ ζωγραφικὸς διάκοσμος τοῦ Ἁγίου Ἱεροθέου." On the representation of angels in Byzantine art, see Peers, *Subtle Bodies*.

89. Delatte, "Traité de Magie," 404, l. 8; 435, l. 10; 438, l. 31.

90. For Kopiel, see Delatte, "Traité de Magie," 435, ll. 13–14. For Saltael, ibid., 437, l. 1. Saltael appears in a 14th/15th-century fresco in Palermo: see Perdrizet, "L'archange Ouriel," with the inscription "orator" (he who prays). Under this abbreviation C T we could also understand Satanael, an angel who, after his fall, became Satan. For Sausiou, see Cumont, "Les vents."

91. Delatte, "Traité de Magie," 403, l. 25; 434, l. 15.

92. Ibid., 404, l. 10; 435, l. 6. On the basis of his abbreviated name T A, he could also be identified with Tahariel or Tathiel.

their entreaty toward Christ for the salvation of humankind.

The apostles, as members of the heavenly court on the Day of Judgment (Matt. 19:28), usually flank the central trio of Christ the Judge, the Virgin, and John the Baptist. Here they have been transferred to the pendentives (Fig. 5.11). They are depicted in groups of three, seated on wooden thrones. Each holds a scroll in his left hand, with the exception of the four evangelists, who hold gospel books. Reading counterclockwise from the southeast pendentive (Fig. 5.13), we begin with Peter (Π = Π(έτρος)), Paul (Π = Π(αῦλος)), and Luke (Λ = Λ(ουκᾶς)). The next group, in the southwest pendentive (Fig. 5.14), includes the other three evangelists: Matthew (M = M(ατθαῖος)), Mark (M = M(άρκος)), and John (IΩ = Ἰω(άννης); Fig. 5.15).[93] The third group, in the northwest pendentive (Fig. 5.16), consists of Andrew (A = A(νδρέας); Fig. 5.17), Thomas (Θ = Θ(ωμᾶς)), and Bartholomew (B = B(αρθολομαῖος)). Finally, the northeast pendentive (Fig. 5.18) contains Simon (C = C(ίμων)), James (I = I(άκωβος)), and Philip (Φ = Φ(ίλιππος)).

Rhythmic alterations in the figures' postures and gestures, as well as in color and design, give the composition internal coherence. For example, the heads of the apostles are slightly turned so as to compose pairs. In each group the pair closest to the east-west axis face each other, while the third, closest to the north-south axis, forms the corner of an interactive rectangle. Each "third" apostle turns to the one across from him on the north-south axis, yet looks and gestures to the group in the next pendentive counterclockwise. Thus the apostles, although depicted in four separate compartments, are conceived not only as a continuous but also as a symmetrical and complex entity which bridges the space under the image of the Pantokrator. Moreover, the groups of apostles depicted in the south and in the north pendentives seem to form through their posture and gesture two coherent unities that correspond to the two choirs of apostles who usually flank Christ, the supreme judge, in the scenes of the Last Judgment.

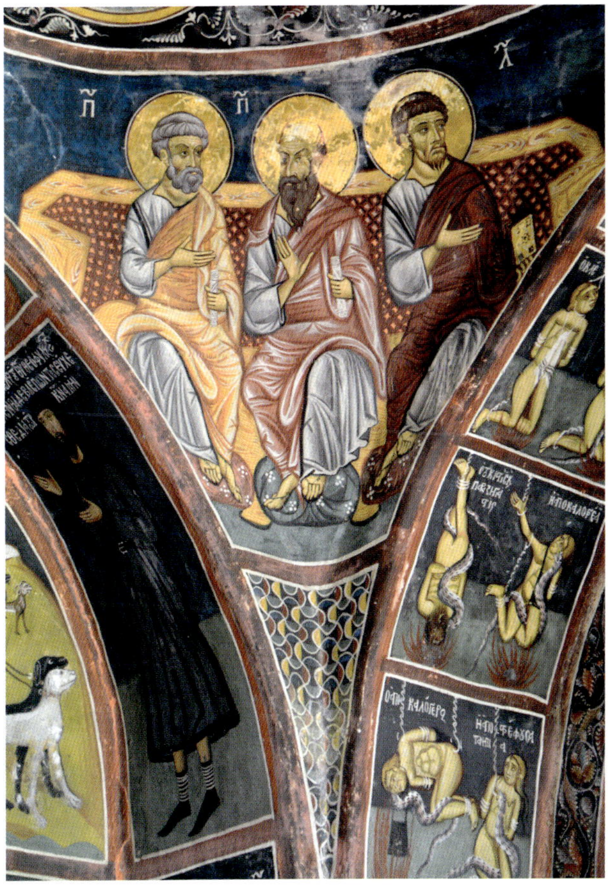

FIG. 5.13 Narthex, southeast pendentive. SS. Peter, Paul, and Luke (photo courtesy of G. L. Carr)

In sum, all the figures of the heavenly court—the traditional central theme in a Last Judgment scene—are present in the vault of the narthex at Asinou: Christ as the supreme judge, the angels, the Virgin, and the apostles; only John the Baptist is missing. However, they are rendered in an iconographic scheme that recalls a typical dome composition.[94]

93. On the inclusion of the four evangelists in the group of the apostles and the prominence given to them, see Mouriki, "Unusual Representation," 154.

94. To recall a dome composition, the vault is separated from the pendentives by a painted border; see Underwood, "Third Preliminary Report," 241, n. 4. For dome compositions in Cypriot churches, see

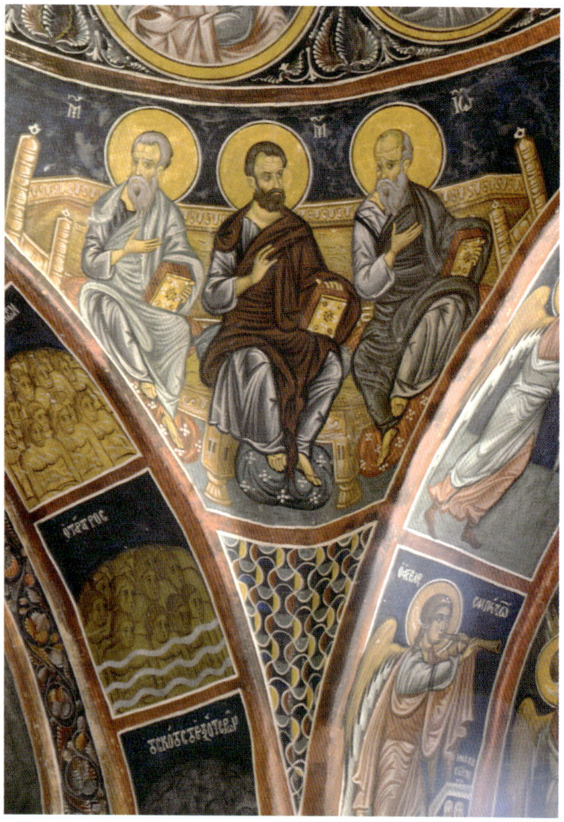

fig. 5.14

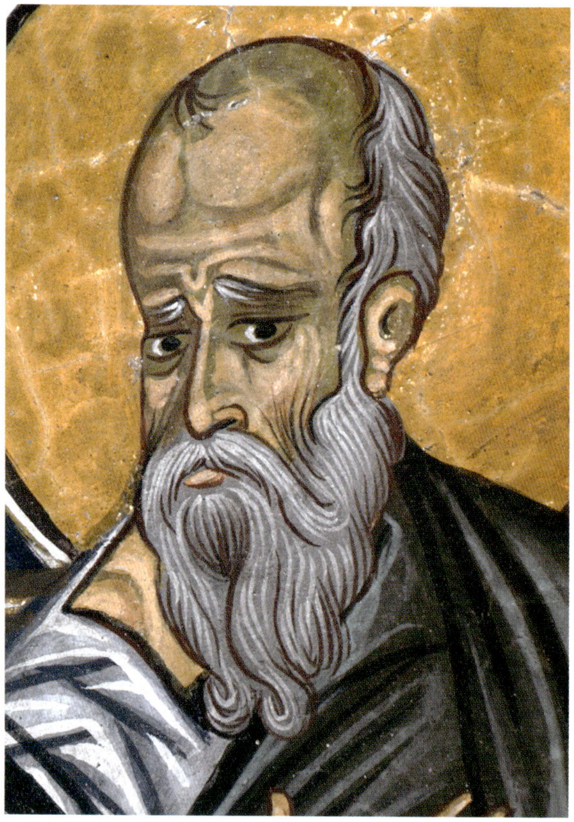

fig. 5.15

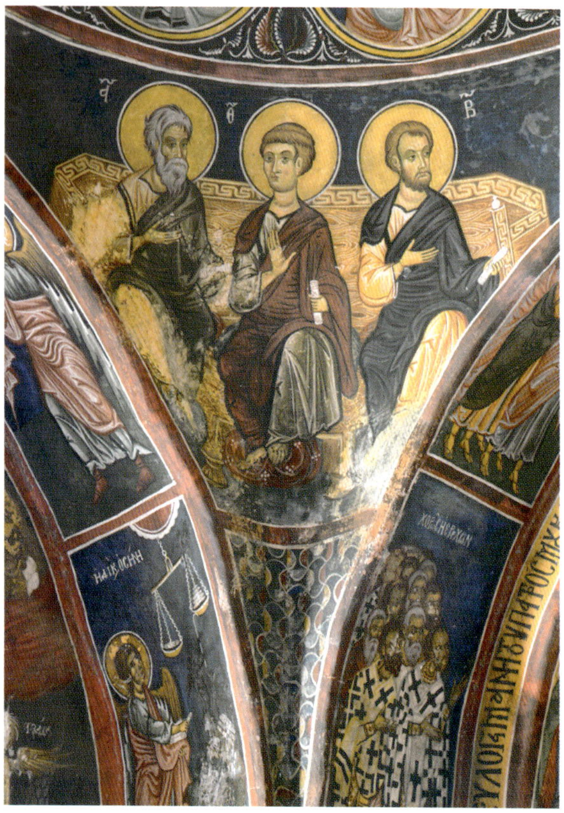

fig. 5.16

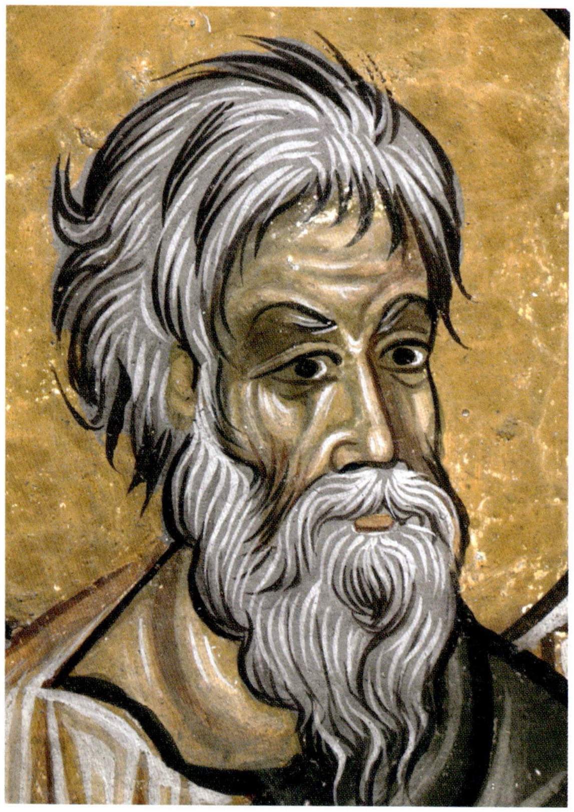

fig. 5.17

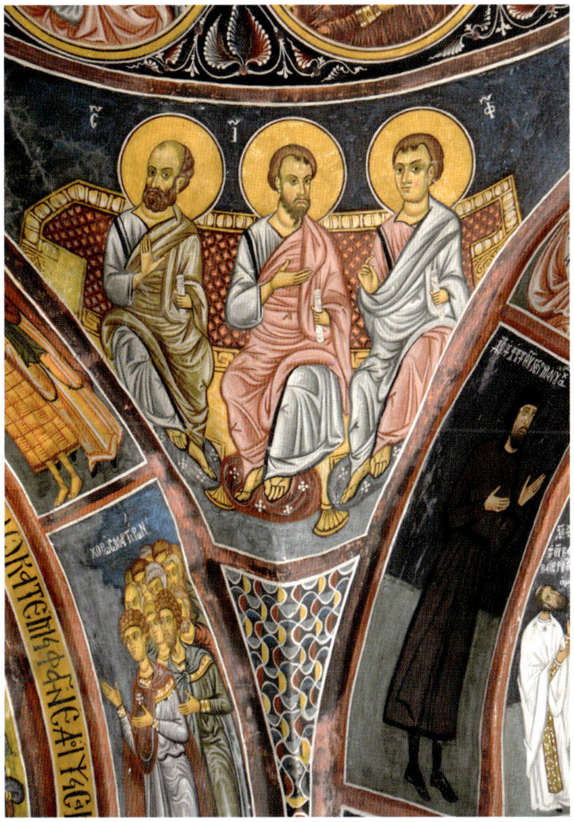

fig. 5.18

FIG. 5.14
Narthex, southwest pendentive. SS. Matthew, Mark, and John (photo courtesy of G. L. Carr)

FIG. 5.15
Narthex, southwest pendentive. St. John the Evangelist (photo courtesy of G. L. Carr)

FIG. 5.16
Narthex, northwest pendentive. SS. Andrew, Thomas, and Bartholomew (photo courtesy of G. L. Carr)

FIG. 5.17
Narthex, northwest pendentive. The Apostle St. Andrew (photo courtesy of G. L. Carr)

FIG. 5.18
Narthex, northeast pendentive. SS. Simon, James, and Philip (photo courtesy of G. L Carr)

A distinctive element in the scene of the Last Judgment at Asinou is the depiction of four discs at the cardinal points between the pendentives (Figs. 5.11, 5.19, 5.37). Each disc consists of three concentric circles, painted in a shiny gray that gives the impression of polished metal. Such discs occur in certain late medieval monuments, especially in Serbia.[95] More rarely, metallic discs consisting of concentric circles are held by angels, as in the scene of the Last Judgment in the narthex of St. Demetrios in Mistra (ca. 1310–20).[96] In Cyprus, metallic discs are painted in the church of the Holy Cross at Pelendri, under the vault of the central vessel (ca. mid-fourteenth century). Pictorial evidence thus suggests that this iconographic feature developed in Palaiologan times and that it was employed in the upper zones of churches in places that either symbolize or are close to the heavenly sphere; they may also occur in connection with angels.

It has been argued that discs, often diaphanous, more rarely enclosing figures, and mostly held by angels, symbolize mirrors through which angels apprehend God's will.[97] Zaga Gavrilović has probed the theological background of the image of the disc as mirror, by drawing on biblical references, Neoplatonic concepts, and church hymns.[98] The shiny metallic discs depicted in zones of a church

Velmans, "Quelques programmes iconographiques"; Papamastorakes, *Ὁ διάκοσμος τοῦ τρούλου*, 21–25; for the composition in the vault of the narthex of Asinou, Velmans, "Programmes," 148.

95. Schwartz, "Whirling Disc." The author records six examples in Serbia, Kastoria, and Bosnia dating from the 13th to the 16th centuries.

96. *Πολιτεία του Μυστρά*, fig. 144.

97. Grabar, "Sphaira, Globus und Reichsapfel," 111; cf. Prolović, *Heiliger Andreas an der Treska*, 196, n. 314; figs. 109, 110, 112; and the following note.

98. Gavrilović, "Discs Held by Angels."

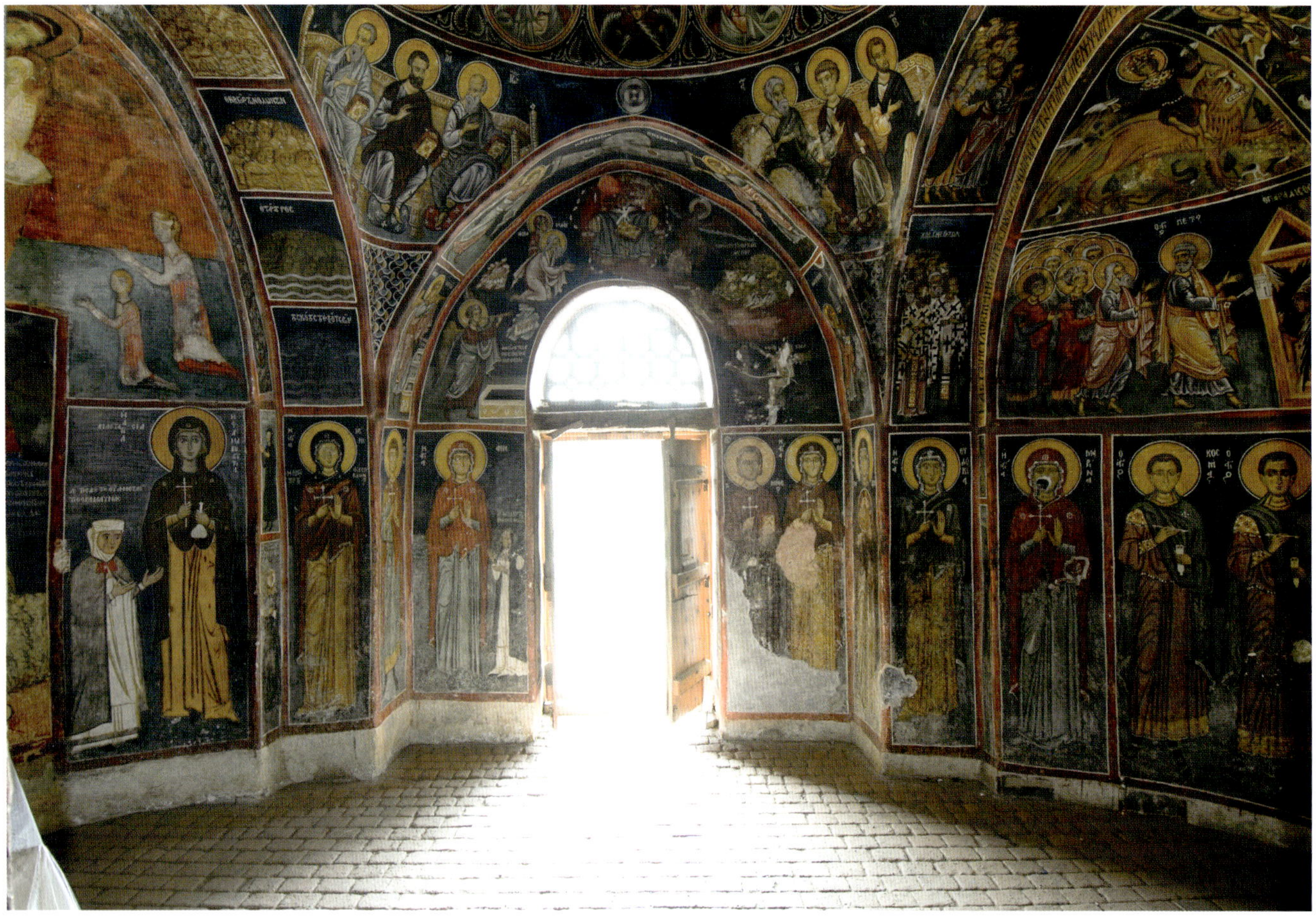

FIG. 5.19 Narthex, view toward west. Pendentives: Apostles. Lunette and arches: scenes of the Last Judgment. Lower zone, left to right: St. Anastasia and donor, monk Kallinikos (above) and lay supplicant Basileios (below), St. Irene, St. Demetrios, St. Anna and donor, SS. Timotheos and Mavra, St. Paraskeve, St. Eudokia, monk Babylas, St. Marina, SS. Cosmas and Damian (photo courtesy of G. L. Carr)

that symbolize heaven, then, near the angels and Christ, may be interpreted as mirrors that reflect the image of God according to medieval theological symbolism; they may thus be considered as cosmological symbols related to angels and mirroring the incarnate Logos.[99] Consequently, the composition in the vault of the narthex at Asinou combines a cosmological image of God, praised by angels in heaven, with a reflection of the incarnate Word on earth, through whom the salvation of humankind in the hour of Judgment becomes possible.

Scenes belonging to the Last Judgment continue on the lunette and arch over the western doorway of the narthex (Figs. 5.19, 5.20). The PREPARATION OF THE THRONE (Ps. 9:4, 88 and 102:19, Matt. 25:31 and 19:28), labeled η ετιμα/σία του θρό/νου = ἡ ἑτοιμασία τοῦ θρόνου, is depicted on the upper part of the west wall. A double-armed cross with the crown of thorns stands before the throne; in front of it are the gospel book and the Holy Spirit in the form of a white dove. Flanking the cross are symbols of the Passion—spear and sponge—and the sigla Ι(ησοῦ)ς Χ(ριστὸ)ς ν(ι)κ(ᾷ). The throne is

99. Cf. Radojičić, *Mileševa*, 16; Schwartz, "Whirling Disc," 26–29, associates these discs with the burnished discs on late Komnenian and 13th-century icons.

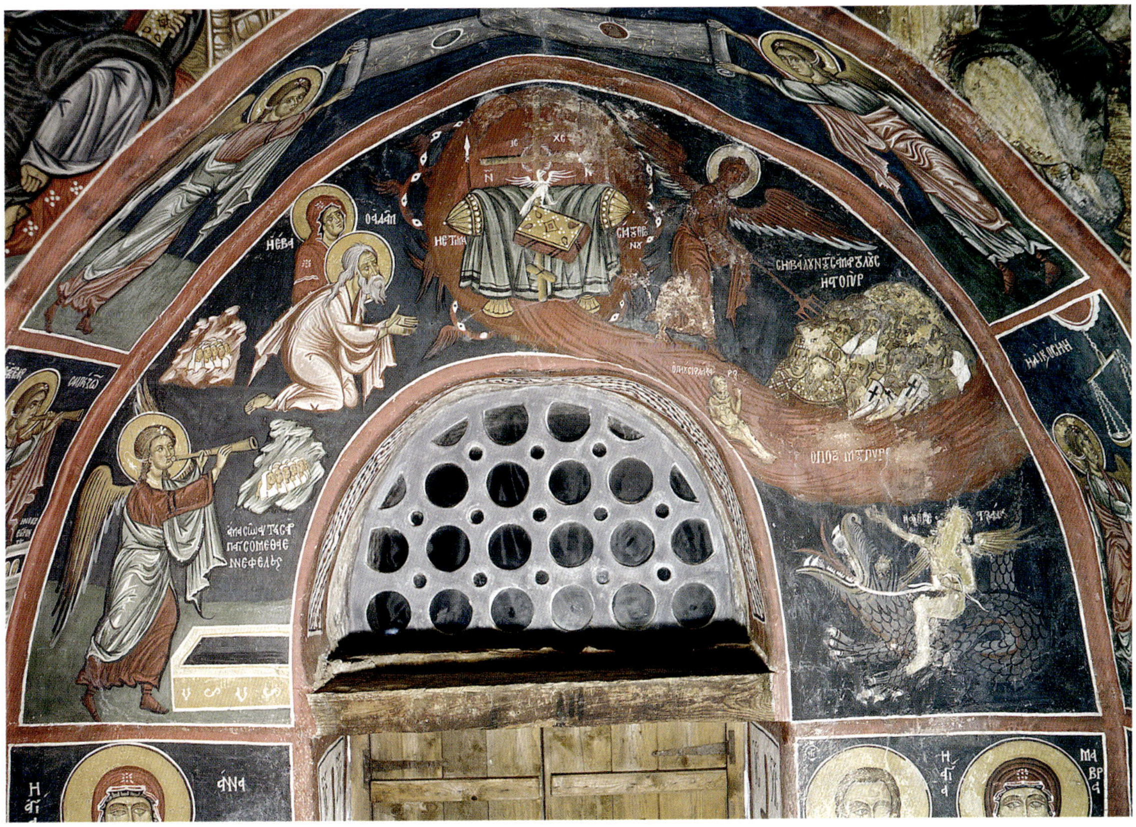

FIG. 5.20 Narthex, west lunette. Clockwise from top: The Preparation of the Throne, The Fiery Stream, Hades, Trumpeting angel, Adam and Eve. Soffit of west arch: Two angels rolling up the scroll of heaven (photo courtesy of Dumbarton Oaks BF.T.As.K.8.2)

enclosed in a round red mandorla surrounded by wheels bearing eyes and wings (Ezek. 10:12–13). At the right hand of the throne Adam (ο Ἀδᾶμ) kneels in prayer with raised arms, while Eve (ἡ Ἔβα) stands behind him.

The Preparation of the Throne is a symbolic image par excellence, with semantically multivalent meanings.[100] Its principal, eschatological content is amplified by the instruments of the Passion—spear, sponge, and crown of thorns—that symbolize Christ's sacrifice. Moreover, throne, cross and Gospel book, and dove allude to the Holy Trinity. The gospel book symbolizing Christ conforms to tradition; its omission in certain churches found in Frankish- or Venetian-held regions, as in the church of St. Herakleidios at Kalopanayiotis (ca. 1265–80), has been interpreted as an anti-Latin response to the disputed issue of the *filioque*.[101]

Issuing from the lower part of the throne and flowing to its left is the FIERY STREAM (Fig. 5.20). An angel painted entirely in red pushes the crowd of sinners into the flames with a trident. A king and a queen wearing crowns and *loroi* as well as three hierarchs occupy the first row; two of the latter wear Latin tiaras. The inscriptions read: σημβάλουν τοῦς ἁμαρτολοὺς / ἡς το πὺρ = συμβάλλουν τοὺς ἁμαρτωλοὺς εἰς τὸ πῦρ (they place the sinners into the fire) and ο ποταμ(ός) του πυρ[ός] = ὁ ποταμὸς τοῦ

100. Brenk, *Tradition*, 71–73, 98–100; Bogyay, "Geschichte der Hetoimasie"; idem, "Hetoimasia," *RbK* 2:1189.

101. Gkioles, "Λειτουργικὲς πηγὲς τῆς Ἀνάληψης," 521, n. 41; Papamastorakes, "Ένταξη των προεικονίσεων," 323, 326; Kepetzi, "Représentation du Jugement dernier," 401.

πυρός (the fiery stream). Based on passages of the Old and New Testaments (Dan. 7:10, Ps. 49:3–4, Matt. 25:34, 41, Apoc. 11:10, 14), the Fiery Stream frequently occurs in texts referring to the Second Coming, as in a homily attributed to Hippolytos, in a homily addressed to Emperor Constantine V, and in the *Apocalypse of Anastasia*.[102]

Imperial figures are often depicted in hell, frequently within the fiery stream.[103] Church officials are also commonly included among sinners damned to eternal fire in scenes of the Last Judgment.[104] Two hierarchs and an emperor are painted among the damned in the fiery stream in St. Nicholas of the Roof at Kakopetria (twelfth century); bishops are included among sinners in the narthex of St. John Lampadistes at Kalopanayiotis (after 1453).[105] The depiction of bishops wearing the mitre alludes either to sinful Latin hierarchs or to Orthodox bishops who promised obedience to the pope, thus registering the critical response of the Orthodox population in Latin-occupied regions. Hierarchs with a mitre appear among the sinners engulfed in flames, not only in Cypriot churches like the Panagia at Moutoullas and the Panagia Katholike at Pelendri (1502),[106] but also in monuments of Venetian-occupied Crete, as, for example, in St. Paraskeve at Episkope of Pediada (fourteenth/fifteenth century).[107]

Across from the group of sinners and surrounded by the flames of the lake of fire is the naked figure of the Rich Man, who raises his hand to his mouth as he entreats Abraham to send Lazaros to cool his tongue (Lk. 16:19–31; Fig. 5.20). He is labeled ὁ πλούσιος Λάζα/ρος (the rich Lazaros). Already represented in the church of St. Stephen at Kastoria in the tenth century,[108] the parable of the rich man suffering the torments of hell and poor Lazaros enjoying the blessings of paradise in Abraham's bosom occurs in Cyprus in the church of St. Nicholas of the Roof at Kakopetria.[109] The parable is commonly depicted in monumental ensembles of the thirteenth and fourteenth centuries and is very widespread in the late medieval churches of Crete.[110] In many cases, as at Asinou, the labeling is confused, with the rich man instead of the poor one being called Lazaros. Hades, at the right corner in front of the fiery stream, is personified as a naked winged figure riding on a monster and is labeled ο ἀκόρε/στος Ἅδης (the insatiable Hades; Fig. 5.20).

Scenes of the TRUMPETING ANGELS (Matt. 24:31) occupy the south part of the west wall and

102. PG 10:904–52; PG 95:324–25; Baun, *Tales from Another Byzantium*, 407, §29, 407–8, §32.
103. For example in Paris. gr. 74, fol. 51v, Omont, *Évangiles*, 1: pl. 41; in Torcello, see Andreescu, "Torcello" (1972), 195–207, pls. 15ff.; (1976), 245–76; in the churches of Episkope and Agetria in Mani, see Drandakes, *Τοιχογραφίες τῆς Μέσα Μάνης*, 207, fig. 56; 251, fig. 29; Tomeković, "Jugement dernier inédit"; in Mileševa, see Radojičić, *Mileševa*, pl. 44; and in the Metropolis of Mistra, see Millet, *Mistra*, pl. 81/2. In St. George at Kalyvia Kouvara, the imperial couple is labeled Herodes and Herodias: see Mouriki, "Unusual Representation," 157–58, pl. 87. On representations of emperors in Last Judgment scenes, see Kepetzi, "Empereur, piété et rémission," 235–44.
104. For examples, see Mouriki, "Unusual Representation," 158–59, pl. 88. For examples in Cappadocia, see Jolivet-Lévy, "Images et espace cultuel," 179–80, fig. 23; eadem, *Cappadoce Médiévale,* 274–76. For textual parallels, see Baun, *Tales from Another Byzantium,* 410, §41–42.
105. On the fresco at Kakopetria before cleaning, see Stylianou and Stylianou, "Ὁ ναὸς τοῦ Ἁγίου Νικολάου," 118–22 (this detail is not published). On Kalopanayiotis, see Cholet, "Fresques du Jugement dernier," 110.
106. Nicolaïdès, "Jugement dernier"; Emmanuel, "Ναός της Παναγίας στο Μουτουλλά"; Stylianou and Stylianou, *Painted Churches*, 233.
107. Drakopoulou, "Φόβοι της τιμωρίας," 101. In another church of Crete, St. Prokopios at Leibada in Kandanos Chanion (14th century), Franciscan monks are depicted in the fiery river: see Bougrat, "Trois Jugements derniers," 19.
108. Siomkos, *Saint-Etienne à Kastoria*, 96–98, schéma 19, figs. 46–47. The first fresco layer of the church has been dated by Siomkos, *Saint-Etienne*, 132, to about 900. On the iconography of the parable, see Mantas, *Die Ikonographie der Gleichnisse,* 301–9.
109. Stylianou and Stylianou, *Painted Churches*, 62.
110. Mouriki, "Unusual Representation," 156–57, pl. 85; Underwood, *Kariye Djami,* 3:390, 397; Živković, *Gračanica*, 10:1. Vassilaki, "Οἱ πλούσιοι," 473–76, figs. 1–7.

the south side of the soffit of the west arch. On the west wall an angel stands trumpeting before an empty sarcophagus.[111] Two groups of souls, depicted as children wearing white garments and with covered heads, are carried on clouds. The accompanying inscription quotes 1 Thessalonians 4:17: ἅμα σῦν αυτεις ἁρ/παγισόμεθα ε/ν νεφέλαις = ἅμα σὺν αὐτοῖς ἁρπαγησόμεθα ἐν νεφέλαις (we will be caught up together with them in the clouds). Another trumpeting angel is represented on the soffit of the western arch (Fig. 5.21). A pair of souls rises from each of two uncovered sarcophagi painted in front of him. The inscriptions read: ὁ ἀγκελος / σαλπείζω(ν) = ὁ ἄγγελος σαλπίζων (the trumpeting angel) and η νεκρὶ / εγίρον/ται = οἱ νεκροὶ ἐγείρονται (the dead rise).

On the soffit of the western arch two angels with upraised arms roll up the Scroll of Heaven, which forms a loop in the center; golden stars are scattered on the blue-gray scroll, and two heads in profile, enclosed in radiating medallions, personify the moon and the sun (Fig. 5.22). The inscription reads: η ἀγγελει τηλῖγοῦν / των οὐρανῶν = οἱ ἄγγελοι τυλίγουν τὸν οὐρανόν (the angels are rolling up the [scroll of] heaven).

Apocalypse 6:13–14 is the main source of inspiration for the scroll of heaven and its stars: καὶ ὁ οὐρανὸς ἀπεχωρίσθη ὡς βιβλίον ἑλισσόμενον (and the heaven departed as a scroll when it is rolled together). The comparison of heaven to a book-scroll is also inspired by Isaiah 34:4: ἑλιγήσεται ὁ οὐρανὸς ὡς βιβλίον (and the skies [shall] roll up like a scroll), as Herbert Hunger has pointed out.[112] Moreover, an extract of a homily on the Second Coming attributed to Hippolytos illustrates not only the scroll of heaven but also the stars, the sun, and the moon depicted on it: ὁ οὐρανὸς ὡς βιβλίον εἱλίσσεται. . . . τὰ ἄστρα τοῦ οὐρανοῦ πεσοῦνται, ὁ ἥλιος καταστραφήσεται εἰς σκότος, καὶ σελήνη εἰς αἷμα (the heaven will be rolled up as a book, the stars of heaven will fall, the sun will be destroyed into darkness, and the moon into blood).[113] The scroll of heaven, looped in the center, studded with stars, and held by two angels, is seen

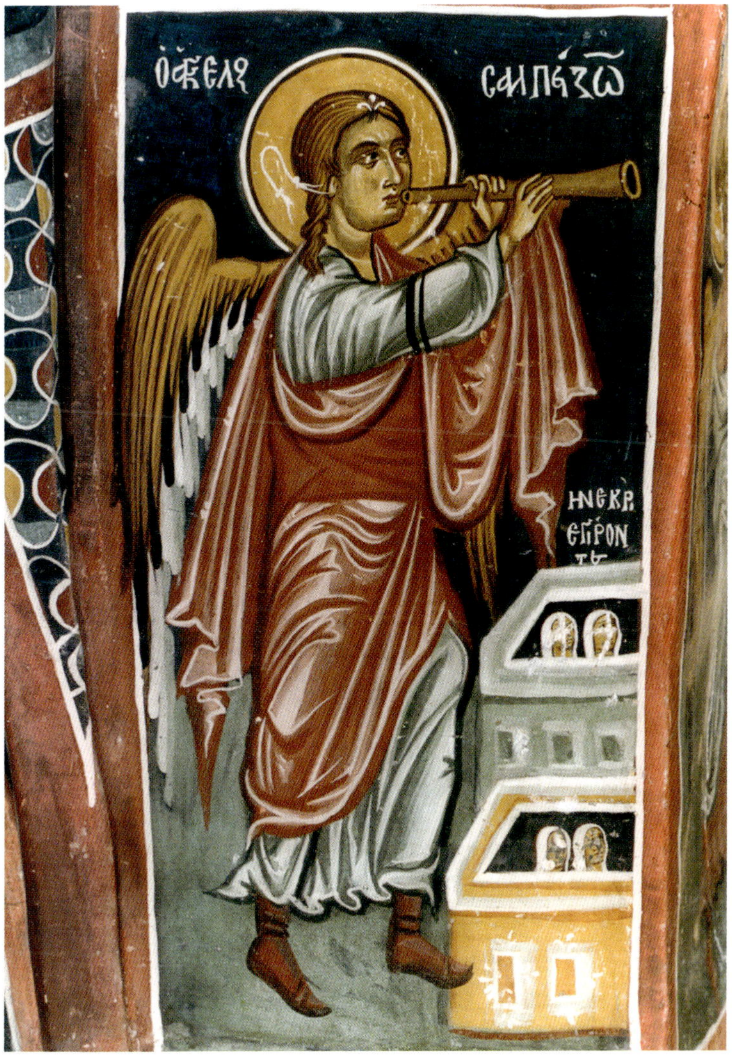

FIG. 5.21 Narthex, soffit of west arch, south side. Trumpeting angel (photo courtesy of S. Kalopissi-Verti)

111. Maliaras, *Βυζαντινά Μουσικά Όργανα*, 234, fig. 150.
112. Hunger, "Ἑλιγήσεται ὁ οὐρανὸς ὡς βιβλίον." The author has collected all literary evidence—apocalyptic texts, hymnography, homilies, etc.—where heaven is compared to a book-scroll.
113. PG 10:940. On the development, variants, and examples of this iconographic motif, see Kepetzi, "Quelques remarques." In addition, see Gospel book 212 of the Matenadaran in Erevan, fol. 80r (1337): Velmans, in *Βυζάντιο ως Οικουμένη*, 214, fig. 53. One of the earliest examples of the two angels holding the scroll of heaven between them is found in the 10th-century fresco layer of St. Stephen at Kastoria: Siomkos, *Saint-Etienne à Kastoria*, 93, fig. 38.

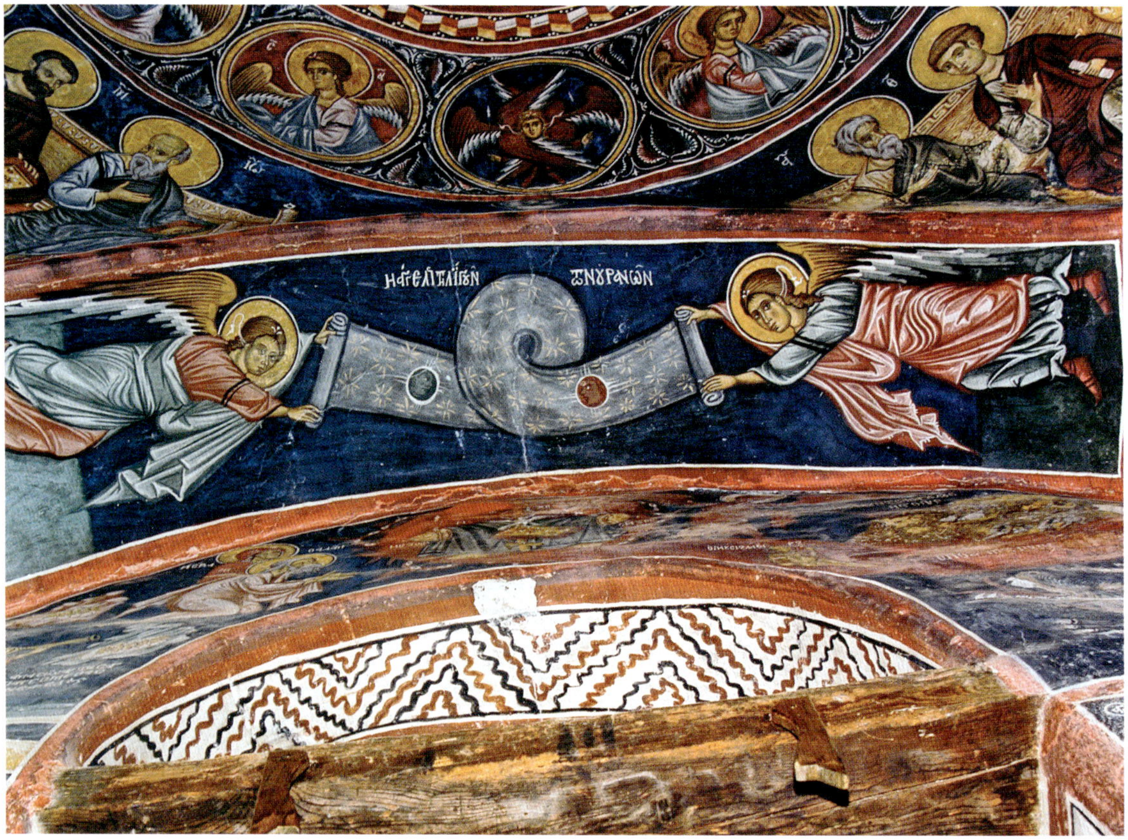

FIG. 5.22 Narthex, soffit of western arch. Angels rolling up the scroll of heaven (photo courtesy of S. Kalopissi-Verti)

again in Cyprus in the narthex of St. Nicholas of the Roof at Kakopetria (twelfth century), where, as at Asinou, it is placed in the soffit of an arch.[114] In St. John Lampadistes at Kalopanayiotis (after 1453), only one angel is depicted holding the scroll of heaven. Semantically, the scroll forming a loop in the middle has been interpreted as a sign that heaven is in the process of disconnecting, and the end of the world has begun.[115]

On the north side of the soffit is the scene of the WEIGHING OF SOULS (Ψυχοστασία; Dan. 5:27, Job 31:6), labeled ἡ δικ(αι)όσήνη = ἡ δικαιοσύνη (Justice, Fig. 5.23). The scales hang by a chain from a red semicircle symbolizing heaven. An angel holds scrolls with records of the souls about to be judged. On the other side of the scales, devils carry scrolls on their back or in their hands with the records of sins to be put on the balance; little winged black demons climb on top of each other and attempt to cheat by pulling the scale to their side with a hooked stick, while another black creature has climbed on top of the scale trying to push it down. In the monuments of Cyprus the Weighing of Souls already occurs in the narthex of St. Nicholas of the Roof at Kakopetria (twelfth century), where a sole winged black demon is depicted holding a heap of scrolls. In the narthex of St. Herakleidios at Kalopanayiotis (after 1453), the scales hang by a chain from the prepared throne.[116]

The belief that the dead will be judged according to their deeds, which are inscribed in books, is based

114. Stylianou and Stylianou, "Ὁ ναὸς τοῦ Ἁγίου Νικολάου," 121, fig. 2.
115. Kepetzi, "Quelques remarques," 108.
116. Stylianou and Stylianou, *Painted Churches*, 59–62; Cholet, "Jugement dernier," 110.

on Apocalypse 20:12. The black demons,[117] often called Ethiopians in medieval texts, place the scrolls in which the crimes of sinners are recorded on one side of the scales, while angels place their documents, with the good deeds of the deceased, on the other side. This is standard in Byzantine literary texts, as, for example, in the homily on the sixth Psalm by Anastasios Sinaites (early eighth century) and in the *Life of St. Basil the Younger* (tenth century).[118]

Scenes of Hell continue in the soffit of the south arch, where eight rectangular compartments display the Torments of the Damned (Figs. 5.1, 5.19). On the western side are four scenes of collective punishment, labeled (top down) as: ο σκόληξ ὁ ἀκήμιτος = ὁ σκώληξ ὁ ἀκοίμητος (the worm that sleepeth not, Mark 9:48); ὁ βριγμõς τῶν ὀδώντων = ὁ βρυγμὸς τῶν ὀδόντων (the gnashing of teeth, Matt. 8:12, Fig. 5.24); ὁ Τάρατρος = ὁ Τάρταρος (Tartarus); and το σκότος το ἐξότερῶν = τὸ σκότος τὸ ἐξώτερον (the outer darkness, Matt. 8:12, Fig. 5.25). The sinners are depicted in groups against a dark blue background. The dozen or so figures in the front row of each group are represented half-length; in the back rows only heads or parts of heads are visible. Virtually identical, they turn together toward the center of the narthex: that is, toward Christ, the supreme judge. The four groups are differentiated only through inscriptions and symbols: a multitude of white worms devouring bodies, limbs, and faces in the panel of the Worm that Sleepeth Not; visible teeth in the scene of the Gnashing of Teeth; dim light for Tartarus; and deep darkness for the Outer Darkness. Raised eyebrows and brown brushstrokes running obliquely across their cheeks express sorrow and agony in the faces of the damned.

Collective torments occur in apocalyptic texts, such as the mid-third-century *Apocalypse of Paul* and the middle Byzantine apocalyptic texts of the Virgin and of Anastasia, as well as in church hymnography. For example, three of the torments at Asinou (the Worm, the Gnashing, and the Darkness), inspired by the Gospels of Mark and Matthew, are repeatedly mentioned in the troparia sung during vespers on the Saturday of Souls before Meatfare Sunday, in odes 1, 5, and 7 of Theodore Stoudites' poem included in the matins of Meatfare Sunday, and in a troparion sung during the matins of the Saturday of Souls before Pentecost.[119] By contrast, Tartarus, which goes back to an ancient Greek tradition, occurs more rarely in iconography and in hymnography.[120]

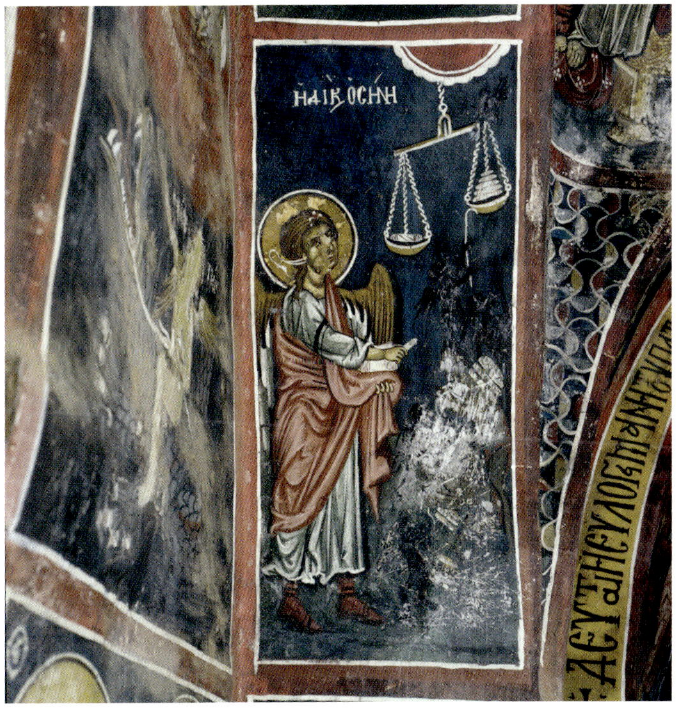

FIG. 5.23 Narthex, soffit of west arch, north side. The Weighing of Souls (photo courtesy of the Leventis Foundation and the Archaeological Research Unit, University of Cyprus, No. 006444)

117. On the demons, especially in the post-Byzantine period, see Garides, *Études sur le Jugement dernier,* 31–62; Probatakes, *Διάβολος*, 63, 80.

118. PG 89:1112–16; Veselovskij, "Razyskanija," 25.31, 28.19ff.

119. Tischendorf, *Apocalypses apocryphae*, 62 (Gnashing of Teeth); Pernot, "Descente de la Vierge," 253 (Gnashing of Teeth); Baun, *Tales from Another Byzantium*, 407, §30 (Sleepless Worm). *Τριώδιον*, 27–28, 30, 32; *Πεντηκοστάριον*, 198.

120. See, for example, the Sinai icons, n. 83 above, and the church of Boubas at Sphakia, Crete, in Gerola,

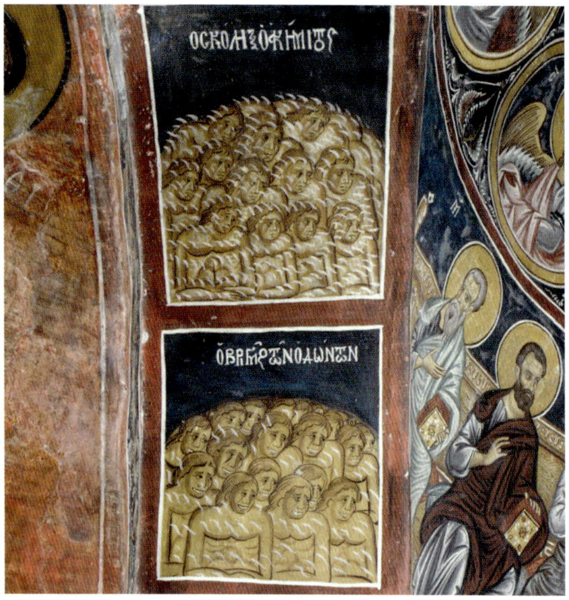

FIG. 5.24 Narthex, soffit of south arch, west side. Collective torments: the Worm that Sleepeth Not, the Gnashing of Teeth (photo courtesy of the Leventis Foundation and the Archaeological Research Unit, University of Cyprus, No. 006425)

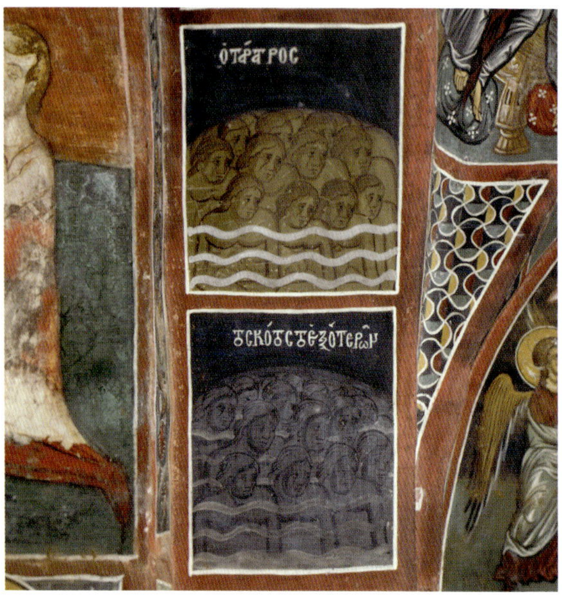

FIG. 5.25 Narthex, soffit of south arch, west side. Collective torments: Tartarus, the Outer Darkness (photo courtesy of the Leventis Foundation and the Archaeological Research Unit, University of Cyprus, No. 006426)

Collective punishments arrayed in rectangular or round-headed compartments are depicted in scenes of the Second Coming from the eleventh century onward.[121] From an iconographical perspective, the composition at Asinou follows a long-established tradition according to which the damned are depicted in the form of unvarying heads, skulls, or busts.[122] By contrast, in the Palaiologan period, the damned are most often represented full length and differentiated, as in Bogorodica Ljeviška in Prizren (1307–13), in the Chora Monastery (1315–21), and in the church of the Pantokrator at Dečani (1340–50).[123] Collective punishments depicted in churches of Cyprus are encountered in the narthex of the Panagia at Moutoullas and in the church of the Archangel Michael at Choli in the district of Paphos (fifteenth/sixteenth century); Tartaros is included in both.[124] They are also recurrent in churches of Venetian Crete.[125]

The individual torments (Fig. 5.1) are prominently displayed on the eastern part of the south arch, where they are readily visible to anyone entering the narthex. They are depicted in pairs in four square compartments and are identified by

---

Monumenti Veneti, 2:343. Cf. a hymn sung in the vespers of Saturday before Meatfare Sunday, *Τριώδιον*, 27.

121. Garides, *Études sur le Jugement dernier*, 82–117.

122. For example, in Paris. gr. 74, fols. 51v and 93v, on the Sinai icons, and in Torcello, see above, notes 83 and 103; in the now-destroyed church of the Pantokrator in Nereditsa close to Novgorod (1198/99), see Pivovarova, *Freski crkvi Spasa*, 80f, fig. 6, 180; in the churches of Episkope, Agetria, and Ἀϊ-Στράτηγος in Mani, see Drandakes, *Βυζαντινὲς τοιχογραφίες*, 204–7, figs. 53, 57–58; 251–52, figs. 28–29; 462, fig. 75.

123. Živković, *Bogorodica Ljeviška*, 76; Underwood, *Kariye Djami*, 3:398–403; Davidov-Temeriskij, "Ciklus strašnog suda," fig. 17.

124. Nicolaïdès, "Le Jugement dernier," 76; The fresco in Choli has not been published. See also a 16th-century Cypriot icon from Phoini, close to Paphos, representing the Second Coming, today in the Museum of the Foundation of Archbishop Makarios III. Papageorgiou, *Icons of Cyprus* [1969], pl. on 93.

125. Gerola, *Monumenti Veneti*, 2: 343–44; Karapidakis, "Jugement dernier," 81.

FIG. 5.26

Narthex, soffit of south arch, east side. Individual punishments (from top left): He who ploughs over the boundaries and the dishonest miller; the thief and the slanderer (photo courtesy of the Leventis Foundation and the Archaeological Research Unit, University of Cyprus, No. 006449)

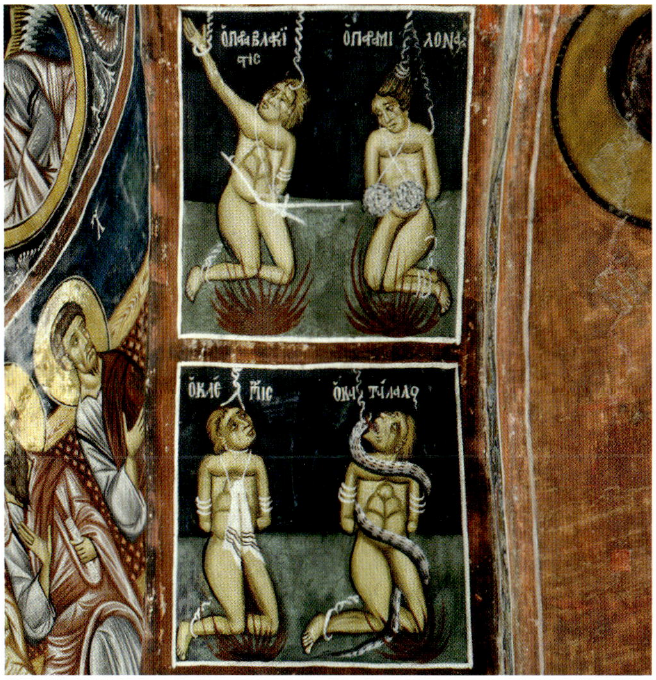

inscriptions: he who ploughs over the boundaries (ὁ παραβλακϊ/στις = ὁ παραυλακιστής) and the dishonest miller (ὁ παραμι/λονὰς – ὁ παραμυλωνᾶς); the thief (ὁ κλέ/πτις = ὁ κλέπτης) and the slanderer (ὁ κα/τάλαλος, Fig. 5.26); the usurer and falsifier of weights (ὁ τοκιστὶς κ(αὶ) / παραζηγγιά/στὶς = ὁ τοκιστὴς καὶ παραζυγιαστής); and the faithless nun (ἡ ἀποκαλογρέὰ = ἡ ἀποκαλογραία), the faithless monk (ο ἀπο/καλόγερος), and the woman who refuses to nurse her children (ἡ ἀπο/στρέφουσα / τα νήπι/α; Fig. 5.27).

All figures are naked, bound with shackles, and suspended by hooks over flames. Not only the accompanying inscriptions but also the implements and symbols of their torments make the sinners' identities clearly identifiable. Thus, he who ploughs over the boundary in his neighbor's plot has a plough hanging from his neck. Two millstones hang from the neck of the dishonest miller. A cloth, probably a purse, is hanging from the neck of the thief. A hooked chain suspends the slanderer by the tongue, and a serpent surrounding him bites his tongue. A black rectangular cloth, evidently the scapular (ἀνάλαβος), is suspended from the neck of each monastic—the faithless nun and the faithless monk. The woman who refuses to nurse her children is bitten on the breast by a serpent.

The individual sins depicted at Asinou can be classified into the following groups: (a) sins concerning agricultural economy specifically (he who ploughs over the boundaries, the dishonest miller); (b) sins related to financial life and social interaction in general, but also affecting rural communities (the usurer and falsifier of weights, the thief, the slanderer); (c) sins of women affecting the life of children and, in a wider sense, the survival of the community (the woman who refuses to nurse

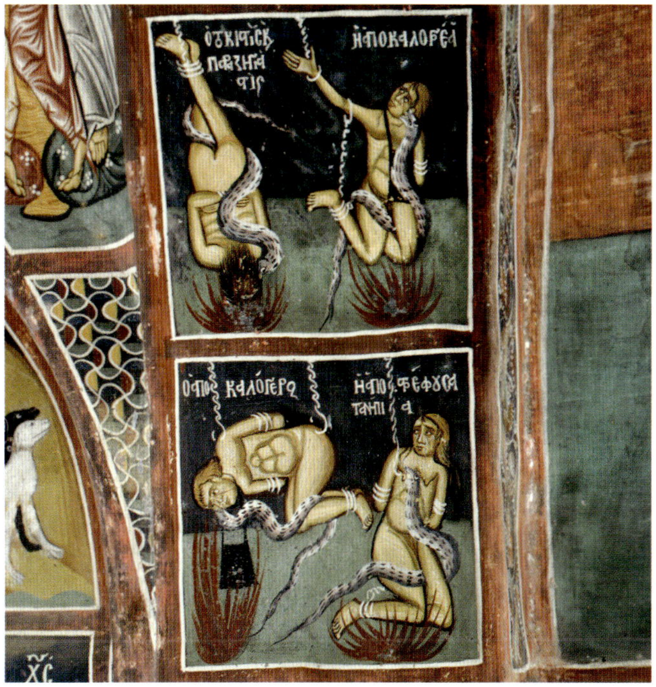

FIG. 5.27

Narthex, soffit of south arch, east side. Individual punishments (from top left): the usurer and falsifier of weights, the faithless nun; the faithless monk, and the woman who refuses to nurse her children (photo courtesy of the Leventis Foundation and the Archaeological Research Unit, University of Cyprus, No. 006448)

her children or wetnurse other women's babies);[126] and (d) monastic sins (the faithless monk, the faithless nun). Consequently, the individual sinners depicted in the narthex of Asinou reflect the rural and monastic milieu of the Phorbiotissa monastery. As has been noted of images elsewhere, the individual punishments are calibrated to local historical and social conditions.[127]

Certain of the sins depicted in the narthex of Asinou find their literary parallels in apocalyptic texts. Thieves and slanderers are punished in hell in the early Christian *Apocalypse of Paul*.[128] The ninth-century *Apocalypse of the Virgin* includes slanderers, usurers, and thieves among the damned in hell.[129] Closer literary parallels to the sinners of Asinou are evident in the *Apocalypse of Anastasia*, a text compiled in the late tenth or eleventh century that reflects the realities and social perceptions of a provincial community in the Macedonian period. Those who plough over their neighbor's boundaries (παραυλακισταί) and monks who cast off the great and angelic schema are mentioned next to thieves, suffering the horrible torments of hell.[130] The tenth-century hagiographic text of the *Life* of St. Basil the Younger includes a chapter on the death of Theodora, his faithful servant. On her way to the other world she has to pass through tollhouses (τελωνεῖα) guarded by demons that keep records of crimes and sins committed in life. Among the twenty-one sins enumerated in the narration—such as envy, lying, arrogance, drunkenness, idolatry, gluttony, adultery, fornication, and so on—those of slander, usury, and theft are depicted at Asinou.[131]

The measure-for-measure character of the punishments in hell, based on very ancient Hebrew and Roman traditions, is evident especially in the cases of the slanderer and the woman who refuses to nurse children, who are tormented on their tongue and their breast, respectively. Scholars have emphasized the correspondence of certain torments to punishments in Byzantine penal codes, especially the *Ecloga*.[132]

Groups of naked sinners, mainly women, surrounded and bitten by snakes appear in Yılanlı kilise in Cappadocia (end of ninth/beginning of tenth century) and in the tenth-century *Life* of St. Andrew the Fool,[133] which probably reflects an existing image of the Second Coming in Constantinople. Nonetheless, depictions of punishments of individual sins become common only in the late Byzantine period.[134] Individual punishments are represented in

126. It is probable that this sin refers to a mother's refusal not only to feed her own children but also to suckle the children of other women. The practice of wetnursing continued in Greek villages and towns through the mid-20th century.

127. According to Garides, *Études sur le Jugement dernier*, 90, the individual punishments are linked to agricultural and monastic societies and are not depicted in churches of urban centers; cf. Drakopoulou, *Φόβοι της τιμωρίας*, 93–110, esp. 101.

128. Tischendorf, *Apocalypses apocryphae*, 58, 60. For a comparative study of sin and punishment among apocalyptic texts (Jewish, early Christian, and Byzantine), see Himmelfarb, *Tours of Hell*, 69–75.

129. Pernot, "Descente de la Vierge," 245 (καταλαλοῦντες), 249 (κατάλαλοι), 252 (κατάλαλοι, κλέπται), 246 (οἱ λαμβάνοντες τὸν τόκον ἐκ τοῦ χρυσίου αὐτῶν); James, *Apocrypha Anecdota*, 109–26, esp. 118 (ὁ τόκον λαμβάνων ἐκ τοῦ χρυσίου αὐτοῦ), 119 (καταλαληταί).

130. Baun, *Tales from Another Byzantium*, 407, §29 (thieves), §30 (παραυλακισταί), 408, §36 (monks who cast off the great and angelic schema).

131. Veselovskij, "Razyskanija," 19, 22, 33.

132. Himmelfarb, *Tours of Hell*, 75–82; Baun, "Middle Byzantine 'Tours of Hell'," 56–57; Gerstel, "Sins of the Farmer," 215–16. On punishments in Byzantine law, see Troianos, "Ποινές στο βυζαντινό δίκαιο."

133. Thierry and Thierry, *Nouvelles églises rupestres*, 101, pls. 49b, 50; Rydén, *Life of St. Andrew*, 2:36–67, 370–73.

134. Garides, "Punitions collectives et individuelles"; Gerstel, "Sins of the Farmer," 211ff. In the late Byzantine period they are encountered, for example, in Panagia Mavriotissa near Kastoria (beginning of the 13th c.); see Moutsopoulos, *Καστοριά*, figs. 52, 53; in the church of St. George at Kalyvia Kouvara (mid-13th c.), see Mouriki, "Unusual Representation," 145–71; in Episkope (ca. 1200) and Ἅϊ Στράτηγος at Boularioi in Mani (2nd half of the 13th c.), see Drandakes, *Βυζαντινὲς τοιχογραφίες*, 206, figs. 27, 57; pl. 53, 462–63, fig. 75; in Sopoćani (1272–74) and Bogorodica Ljeviška in Prizren (1307–13), see Djurić, *Sopoćani,* 253; Živković, *Bogorodica Ljeviška*, 76–77.

the scene of the Last Judgment in Cypriot churches, such as the Transfiguration at Sotera near Famagusta (ca. 1280–1300), the narthex of St. Herakleidios at Kalopanayiotis (after 1453), where—among others—the inscription [ἡ ἀποστρέφου]σα τὰ νήπια can be read, and the narthex of the Panagia at Moutoullas.[135]

The great number of parochial and private village churches scattered in the countryside of Venetian Crete offer many examples of individual punishments mirroring the crimes of a typical agricultural society of late medieval times.[136] A number of the sinners present in the village churches of Crete in the late thirteenth and particularly in the fourteenth and fifteenth centuries are identical to those found at Asinou, such as:

- ὁ παραυλακιστής, in the churches of Panagia Kera at Kritsa (end of thirteenth century), St. Paraskeve at Kantanos Selinou (1362), St. Paraskeve at Kitiros Selinou (1373), St. John Chrysostom near Kritsa Merambellou (1370), St. John at Axos Mylopotamou (ca. 1400), and St. John at Seli Rethymnou (1412);[137]
- ὁ μυλωνᾶς, in the churches of St. Paraskeve at Kitiros Selinou, Panagia at Anisaraki in Kantanos Selinou (last decades of fourteenth century), St. John at Axos Mylopotamou, and St. John at Seli Rethymnou;[138]
- ὁ κλέπτης, in the churches of Panagia Kera at Kritsa, St. John near Kritsa (1370), St. Paraskeve at Kitiros Selinou, St. John Chrysostom at Kadros Selinou (second half of fourteenth century), Panagia at Anisaraki in Kantanos Selinou, St. John at Axos Mylopotamou, and St. John at Seli Rethymnou;[139]
- ἡ αποστρέφουσα or ἡ μὴ βυζάνουσα τὰ νήπια, in the churches of St. Paul at St. John Priotissas (1304), St. Pelagia at Apano Viannos (1361), St. Paraskeve at Kitiros Selinou, St. John Chrysostom at Kadros Selinou, Panagia at Anisaraki in Kantanos Selinou, and St. John at Axos Mylopotamou; and so forth.[140]

Cretan churches sometimes label the usurer as ζουράρης, from the Italian *usuraio*, whereas at Asinou he is named ὁ τοκιστής. They also have examples of the καταλαλοῦσα;[141] at Asinou there is the male κατάλαλος.

The similarities in the iconography of the Torments of the Damned in churches of Lusignan/Venetian Cyprus and Venetian Crete reflect the rural social milieu shared by these regions, both under Latin rule. Affinities may also be interpreted in terms of shared schemes of patronage in both regions. The dedicatory inscription at Asinou, for example, testifies that the common people (ὁ κοινὸς λαός) were among the main contributors to the painting campaign of 1332/33 (Fig. 5.37 and discussion, pp. 176–79). Hence, it is evident that ordinary peasants played a decisive role, both as patrons and as viewers of the paintings in the narthex. In village

135. On the subject, see Chatzioannou, "Παραστάσεις τῶν κολαζομένων." See also A. Papageorgiou in *ARDAC* 1989, 29–30; Cholet, "Jugement dernier"; Nicolaïdès, "Jugement dernier," 73–74; Carr, "Art," 296–97.

136. Gerola, *Monumenti Veneti*, 2:340–46; Gerola and Lassithiotakes, *Τοπογραφικὸς κατάλογος*, 123–27; Maderakes, "Κόλαση"; idem, "Αναζητήσεις," 80–91; Bougrat, "Trois Jugements derniers," 13–40; Karapidakis, "Jugement dernier," 67–92; Vassilaki, "Οἱ πλούσιοι."

137. Gerola, *Monumenti Veneti*, 2:342–43; Gerstel, "Sins of the Farmer," 21, fig. 6; Borboudakis, *Panaghia Kera*, fig. 64; Albani, "Τοιχογραφίες," 184; Karapidakis, "Jugement dernier," 74–75.

138. Gerola, *Monumenti Veneti*, 2:342, 344; Bougrat, "Trois jugements derniers," 26; Albani, "Τοιχογραφίες," 183; Karapidakis, "Jugement dernier," 75 .

139. Gerola, *Monumenti Veneti*, 2:342–44; Borboudakis, *Panaghia Kera*, fig. 64; Bougrat, "Trois Jugements derniers," 26; Albani, "Τοιχογραφίες," 184; Karapidakis, "Jugement dernier," 75.

140. Gerola, *Monumenti Veneti,* 2:342, 344, 346; Gerstel, "Sins of the Farmer," fig. 6; Bougrat, "Trois Jugements derniers," 26; Albani, "Τοιχογραφίες," 182.

141. For the ζουράρης, see Gerola, *Monumenti Veneti,* 2:344; Borboudakis, *Panagia Kera,* fig. 64; Vassilaki, "Οἱ πλούσιοι," 476–81, figs. 9–10, 12. For the καταλαλούσα, St. Pelagia in Apano Viannos at Belvedere (1361), see Gerola, *Monumenti Veneti*, 2:346.

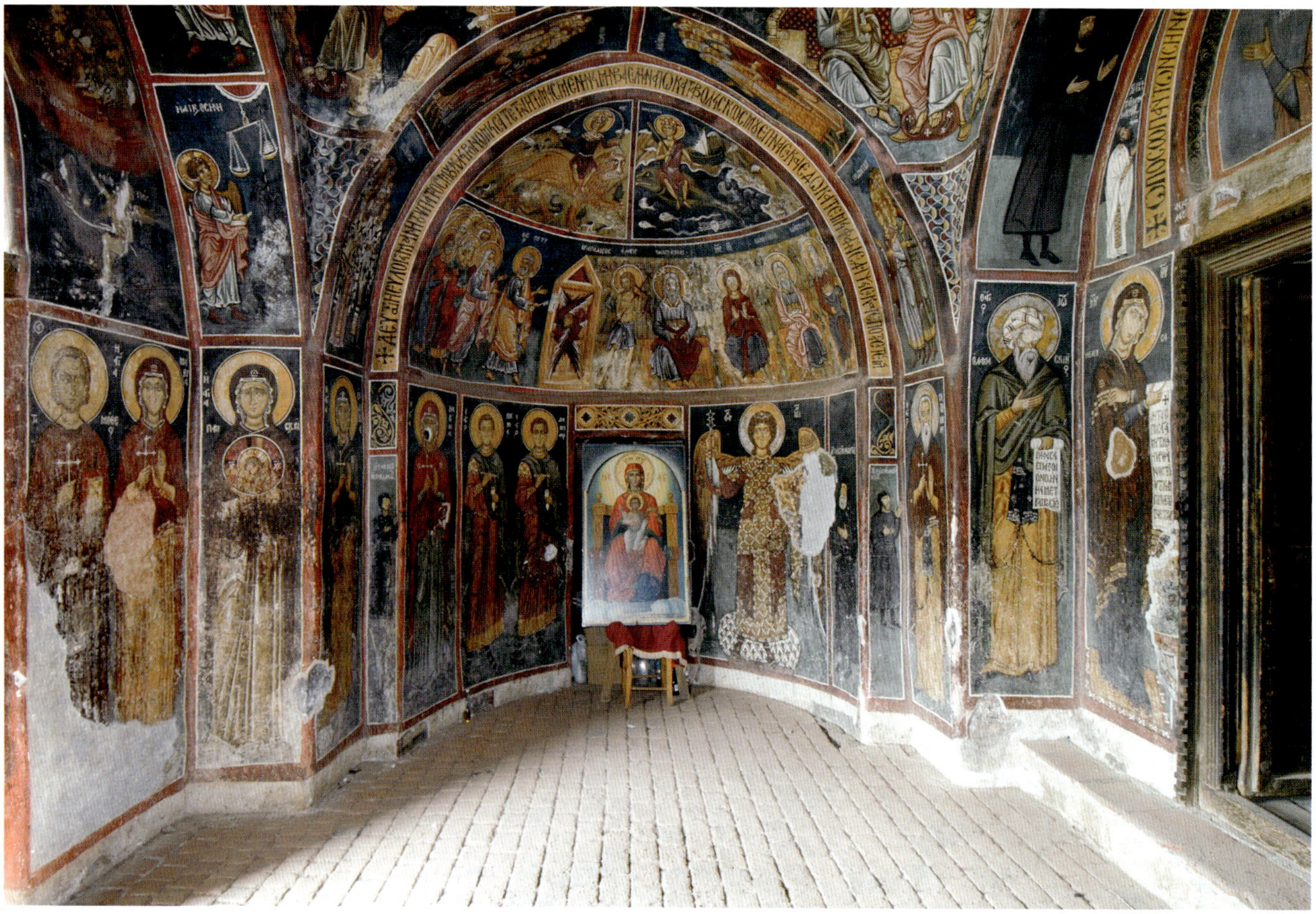

FIG. 5.28 Narthex, view toward north. Soffit of arch: The Choirs of the Elect. Semidome: Personifications of Earth and Sea and the Garden of Paradise. Lower zone, left to right: SS. Timotheos and Mavra, St. Paraskeve, St. Eudokia, the monk Babylas, St. Marina, SS. Cosmas and Damian, Archangel Michael, the monk Leontios, the monk Laurentios, St. Sozomenos, St. John of Damascus, Virgin Paraklesis (photo courtesy of G. L. Carr)

churches of the fourteenth and fifteenth centuries on Crete, too, collective contribution by large numbers of lay and monastic or ecclesiastic donors is among the most common patterns of patronage.[142]

The representation of very specific sins corresponding to crimes familiar to the viewers, the realistic and grisly rendition of tortures, and the unmistakable identification of sins through the implements hanging from the sinners' necks make it clear that these images were to be understood by every single peasant who belonged to the church congregation. Both the didactic aim of these narrative scenes, addressed to a mostly illiterate public, and their apotropaic function are clear.[143]

As a pendant to the Torments of the Damned in the southern arch, four CHOIRS OF THE ELECT are represented in the soffit of the northern arch (Figs. 5.28, 5.29). They are labeled, from west to east: χόρῶς ἡεραρχῶν = χορὸς ἱεραρχῶν (choir of

142. Kalopissi-Verti, "Collective Patterns of Patronage."

143. Cf. Gerstel, "Sins of the Farmer," 212. It is characteristic that in the marginal notes of scribes, potential thieves of codices are threatened with the fear of the Second Coming and are classified among the ranks of the damned to eternal punishment. See Evangelatou-Notara, *Χορηγοί–Κτήτορες–Δωρητές*, 152.

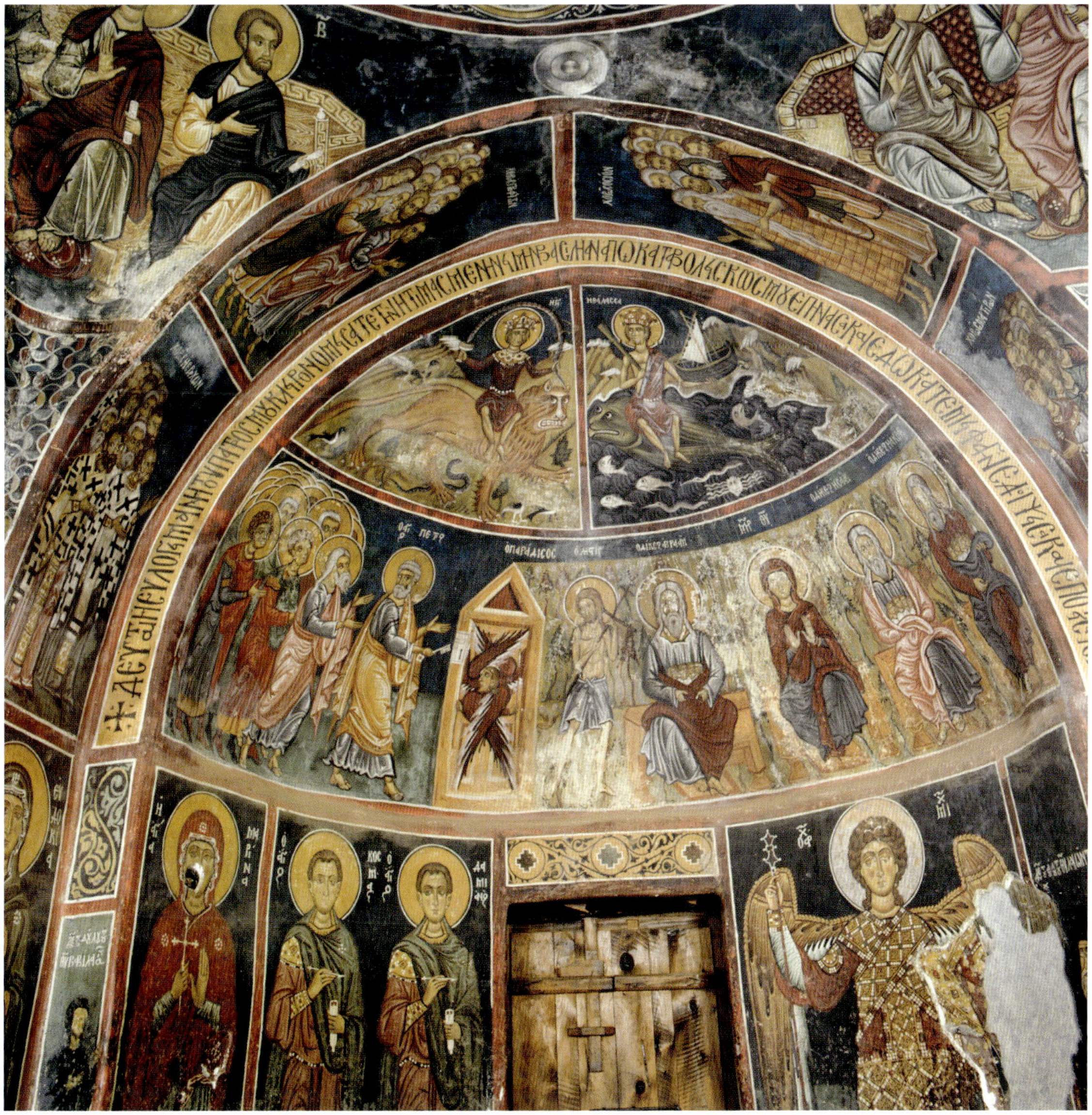

FIG. 5.29 Narthex, north conch. Personifications of Earth and Sea, Garden of Paradise. Soffit: Choirs of the Elect. Face of arch: inscription (photo courtesy of the Leventis Foundation and the Archaeological Research Unit, University of Cyprus, No. 006434)

bishops); χορῶς προφειτῶν = χορὸς προφητῶν (choir of prophets); χορῶς ὁσίον = χορὸς ὁσίων (choir of the blessed); and χορῶς μαρτίρων = χορὸς μαρτύρων (choir of martyrs). The Elect are arranged in groups of twelve or thirteen people, standing full-length in successive rows. Raising their arms in supplication, they turn toward Paradise, depicted in the northern semidome. At the head of the choir of bishops are John Chrysostom and Basil in the first row, while Gregory the Theologian may be identified between them in the second row. The prominent place given to John Chrysostom and to Basil at the head of the choir of church fathers may be associated with their significance as authors of the liturgies.[144] The choir

144. Moreover, John Chrysostom's distinguished position could possibly be linked to the *Spiritual Meadow* of John Moschos (7th c.), a text popular throughout

of the prophets is preceded by a brown-haired and bearded prophet (Moses?) followed by an elderly figure (Elijah?) with long white hair and beard. An old anchorite who wears a straw garment and an elderly monk clad in the *koukoullion* (κουκούλιον; hood), cloak (μανδύας), and *analabos* (ἀνάλαβος; scapular) of the monastic schema lead the choir of the blessed. SS. George and Theodore are discernible in the first rank of the choir of martyrs.

The iconography of the groups of Elect at Asinou, standing in rows, follows the middle Byzantine tradition,[145] which in general continues in the late Byzantine period. However, in Palaiologan times the Just are occasionally depicted in *proskynesis* and carried by clouds—as, for example, in the Chora monastery in Constantinople.[146] A peculiar feature in the composition at Asinou is the fact that, contrary to the norm, the scenes of the Elect and of Paradise are not depicted on the right hand of the prepared throne but on its left. Nonetheless, they are on the right hand both of the Pantokrator, painted in the vault, and of Christ Eleemon in the Deesis composition on the east wall.[147]

The Personifications of Earth and Sea are depicted in the upper zone of the northern semidome in two separate compartments (Figs. 5.29, 5.30). They are both represented as crowned youths of ambiguous gender, although they are usually depicted as women in accord with the gender of their names (ἡ γῆ, ἡ θάλασσα). In the western part, seated frontally on the back of a lion that strides across a mountainous background, the Personification of the Earth (ἡ γῆ) holds in the left hand the tail of a serpent, its body forming an arch and its head ending in a goblet. Trees, birds, a serpent, and a feline are painted in the background. In the eastern compartment the sea (ἡ θάλασσα) is seated on a sea monster and holds a sailing boat in the left hand and an oar in the right. Two different kinds of fish and a stylized octopus inhabit the waves of the sea, while trees grow on the mountainous shore. The Personifications of Earth and Sea,[148] which are usually shown giving up their dead (Apoc. 20:13), have been separated from the trumpet-blowing angels painted on the western wall and arch, and are depicted above the Garden of Paradise, rather like cosmological symbols.

The Personification of the Sea appears already in the early Cypriot examples of the Second Coming. In St. Nicholas of the Roof at Kakopetria (twelfth century) the Sea is depicted with a halo, riding a monster and holding an oar. She is painted seated on a fish and bearing a double-masted boat in the church of the Transfiguration at Sotera, close to Famagusta (ca. 1280–1300). The preserved fragments of Paradise in Panagia Kanakaria at Lythrankomi (first half of the fourteenth century) show the personified sea seated upon a black monster, raising a ship with mast and lateen sail in the left hand and holding a rudder in the right. In the later example of the Panagia at Moutoullas, the sea supports the boat with raised hands over her head.[149]

The boat held by the Sea at Asinou has a slightly raised stern, two oars serving as rudders on both sides of the stern, a vertical mast, and a triangular sail fastened to the diagonal yard by rope loops. It has no deck. This kind of merchant boat with a triangular sail, called lateen, was typical of the vessels in the Mediterranean Sea from the sixth century until the thirteenth, when the Italian ships with

---

the medieval period. A pious woman who lamented Chrysostom's death was led in her dream to a "bright and glorious place" where it was explained to her that John Chrysostom "stands in the presence of the Lord's throne." See Moschos, *Spiritual Meadow*, 106. I wish to thank Karin Krause for drawing my attention to this passage.

145. For Sinai icons, Torcello, etc., see above, notes 83 and 103.

146. Underwood, *Kariye Djami*, 3:384–85.

147. Cf. Jolivet-Lévy, "Images et espace cultuel," 178.

148. On the Personification of the Sea, see Mijović, "Personnification de la Mer"; cf. Kono, "Personifications." On the Personification of the Earth at Asinou, see Frigerio, "Una raffigurazione."

149. Stylianou and Stylianou, *Painted Churches*, 62, fig. 24 (Kakopetria); Megaw and Hawkins, *Lythrankomi*, 154, fig. 105 (Kanakaria); Nicolaïdès, "Jugement dernier," 75 (Moutoullas).

"castles" and bows became prevalent.[150] However, this type of rigging remained long in use in smaller boats, and several fourteenth-century paintings still depict ships with lateen rigs.[151]

The lower zone of the northern semidome is occupied by the Garden of Paradise (ὁ παράδισος = ὁ παράδεισος), well confined behind its gate in a rectangular enclosure full of trees (Figs. 5.29, 5.30). In front of the locked gate, guarded by a cherub (Gen. 3:24), a group of the Elect approaches, led by Peter (ο ἅγι/ος Πετρος) who holds the key of the kingdom of heaven (Matt. 16:19). The Elect are preceded by an elderly figure, probably a prophet (Elijah?), and two martyrs (Demetrios and George?). Within the garden of paradise, distributed evenly on both sides of the Virgin and among stylized trees, the good thief and the three patriarchs Abraham, Isaac, and Jacob are depicted. The inscriptions, written with white capital letters on a dark blue ground, read: ὁ ληστὶς = ὁ ληστής (the thief); ο δίκεος Ἀβραὰμ = ὁ δίκαιος Ἀβραάμ (the just Abraham); Μ(ήτ)ηρ Θ(εο)υ (Mother of God); ο δήκεος Ἡσαὰκ = ὁ δίκαιος Ἰσαάκ (the just Isaac); and ὁ δήκεος Ἡὰκōβ = ὁ δίκαιος Ἰακώβ (the just Jacob).[152]

The figure of the good thief (Luke 23:39–43), depicted stepping into paradise and bearing a wooden double-armed cross, is contextually significant because, due to his repentance, he is regarded as the model of salvation. He is cited in apocalyptic texts, such as the late tenth- or eleventh-century *Apocalypse of Anastasia*,[153] and is a constant component of Last Judgment scenes, at least from the beginning of the eleventh century.[154]

The Virgin and the Patriarchs sit frontally on backless wooden thrones and rest their feet on rectangular wooden footstools. Each patriarch, painted in a very similar posture and displaying very similar physiognomic traits, folds a group of souls to his bosom within his himation. The souls are represented as youths turning their heads to the east. Based on Matthew 8:11 and Luke 13:28, the three patriarchs—Abraham, Isaac, and Jacob—are a typical component of paradise in Last Judgment scenes. Besides their eschatological content, they probably also allude to the Holy Trinity.[155] The peaceful repose in Abraham's bosom figures in the "tours of hell," apocryphal narratives of visits to or visions of the other world by biblical, monastic, or other persons. It is also commonplace in Orthodox hymnography, especially in the service of the two great feasts dedicated to the dead, namely in the Saturday of Souls before Meatfare Sunday and the Saturday of Souls before Pentecost. In addition, prayers in the funerary service (ἀκολουθία τοῦ ἐξοδιαστικοῦ) for both laymen and monks include pleas to God for the repose of the soul of the deceased in the bosoms of Abraham, Isaac, and Jacob.[156]

Already represented in the early depictions of the Last Judgment in the tenth century,[157] the

150. Landström, *Das Schiff*, 70, 80–83, 86–89; for middle Byzantine examples, see Aidoni et al., *Journeys*, 37; 21, fig. 7 (12th c.); 70, fig. 1 (11th c.), etc.

151. For examples, see N. P. Ševčenko, *Life of St. Nicholas*, figs. on 250 (Staro Nagoričino, 1318), 253 (Gračanica, 1321), 260 (St. Nicholas Orphanos, 1320–30), 281 (Platsa, 1348/49), 288 (Drapeti, Crete, mid-14th c.), 297, 305 (Dečani, 1340–50), etc. The lateen sail is still in use today in small fishing boats in Greece.

152. On the Garden of Paradise in the Last Judgment scenes, see Angheben, "Jugements derniers," 108–21.

153. Baun, *Tales from Another Byzantium*, 408, §37. It also occurs in the early 8th-century *Homily on the Sixth Psalm* by Anastasios Sinaites, PG 89:1112–16.

154. For example, in Panagia ton Chalkeon, see Papadopoulos, *Wandmalereien*, 64–65.

155. Brenk, *Tradition*, 33. On the origins of the motif of the cloth enclosing the souls of the Just held by the frontal figure of Abraham, and on the process of the *interpretatio christiana* of an ancient iconographic topos, see Schmidt-Colinet, "Velum und Kolpos," 31.

156. Tischendorf, *Apocalypses apocryphae*, 54; Angelidi, "Version longue," 84; *Τριώδιον*, 18, vespers on Friday; *Πεντηκοστάριον*, 191; 194, vespers on Friday; 199, matins on Saturday; Goar, *Euchologion*, 434, 450.

157. Yılanlı kilise, see Thierry and Thierry, *Nouvelles églises rupestres*, 100, pl. 45b; Taxiarches Metropoleos, see Panayotidi, "Peinture monumentale," 82, figs. 8–9. For the medieval West, see Baschet, *Sein du Père*. Cf. the aniconic illustration in the chapel of St. Basil near Ortahisar in Cappadocia (ca. 900), where three crosses, depicted in the central apse and labeled as Abraham,

three patriarchs became a popular motif in eastern Mediterranean art in the Crusader era, probably in conjunction with the escalation of pilgrimage to their tombs in Hebron. Thus they are encountered in two twelfth-century churches in Palestine and Syria: in the Hospitaller church of Abu Ghosh at Emmaus (third quarter of twelfth century), and in the monastery church of Mar Musa al-Habashi near Nebek in Syria (layer of 1192/93).[158] In the latter church, the Virgin is seated frontally next to the three patriarchs; all four figures fold souls to their bosom within their mantles. The now-lost eleventh-century mosaic of the Last Judgment in the church of the Holy Sepulchre is considered a source for the two Syro-Palestinian examples of the twelfth century.[159]

The patriarchs hold the souls in varying ways, especially in monuments of the periphery. In Karşı kilise at Gülşehir in Cappadocia (1212) all three patriarchs hold the souls in their laps.[160] Similarly, the three patriarchs with the souls of the dead in their bosoms are depicted frontally and half-length in the margin of an Armenian miniature representing an abbreviated form of the Last Judgment (Erevan, Matenadaran 7651, thirteenth century and 1320).[161] In the church of St. Prokopios in Leibada at Kantanos Selinou, Chania, Crete (fourteenth century), by contrast, Isaac and Jacob hold souls jointly, while Abraham holds them alone.[162]

On an icon assigned to the thirteenth century at Sinai, Abraham, Isaac, and Jacob stand full-length, in frontal position, blessing with the right hand and holding a scroll in the left.[163] They are strikingly similar to the patriarchs in Paradise in the narthex of Asinou in their strict frontality; in the linearity of their drapery, faces, and hair; and above all in the identity of the three figures' forms.

The Three Patriarchs seem to have been a popular subject in representations of the Second Coming in Cypriot monuments of the twelfth and thirteenth centuries, appearing in the church of the Transfiguration at Sotera Famagusta and in Panagia Kanakaria at Lythrankomi. In addition, Abraham with Lazaros resting in his bosom occurs among the pen drawings in the margins of a model book—originally a volume of John Chrysostom—that has been attributed by Irmgard Hutter to painters working in Cyprus in the late twelfth or early thirteenth century.[164]

On the vault-head arch above the northern semidome, an INSCRIPTION in black capital letters on a yellow-ocher ground (Figs. 5.28, 5.29) proclaims the passage of Matthew 25:34–35. + δεῦται ἡ εὐλογειμαινη του πατρός μου κλειρονομείσατε τὴν ἡτιμασμένηην ειμῆν βασιλήαν ἀπὼ καταβολεὶς κώσμου. ἐπήνασα κὰι ἐδώκατέ μει φαγῆν ἐδοίψεισα καὶ ἐποτείσατέ μει = + δεῦτε οἱ εὐλογημένοι τοῦ πατρός μου, κληρονομήσατε τὴν ἡτοιμασμένην ὑμῖν

Isaac, and Jacob, symbolically represent paradise or heavenly Jerusalem. Teteriatnikov, "Chapel of St. Basil," 109–12, has stressed the funerary context of this representation.

158. On Abu Ghosh, attributed to a Byzantine painter, see Carr, "Paintings of Abu Ghosh"; Kühnel, *Wall Painting*, 155–57, 173–80, pls. 42–47; Folda, *Art of the Crusaders*, 388. On Mar Musa, signed in Arabic by a painter-monk named Sarkis, see Westphalen, "Byzantinisierende Wandmalereien," 388–95, fig. 3; Dodd, *Frescoes of Mar Musa*, 84–90, 141, color pls. 2, 16; pls. 64, 69, 70.

159. Dodd, *Frescoes of Mar Musa*, 85. The three patriarchs as a symbol of paradise are also a popular subject in the Italo-Byzantine art of the late 12th/13th century, as for example in San Marco in Venice. See Demus, "Paradies von San Marco," 55ff; idem, *Mosaics of San Marco*, 2/1:21–22.

160. Jolivet-Lévy, "Images et espace cultuel," 178, figs. 5, 22. In a 9th-century manuscript of the Homilies of Gregory Nazianzen, when the iconography was not yet established, the three patriarchs were depicted not frontally, with the souls in their laps, but turning and raising their arms to receive the approaching souls: see Grabar, *Miniatures du Grégoire de Nazianze*, pl. 35/2.

161. Fol. 70v, Der Nersessian, *Miniature Painting*, 116, fig. 475.

162. Bougrat, "Trois Jugements derniers," 16–17, fig. 3.

163. Soteriou and Soteriou, *Εἰκόνες*, no. 181.

164. A. Papageorgiou in *ARDAC* 1989, 29–30; Megaw and Hawkins, *Lythrankomi*, 154, fig. 104; Hutter, "Magdalen College 'Musterbuch'," 117–29, fig. 4. For a complete publication of the manuscript, see eadem, *Corpus*, nos. 28, 71–83, figs. 237–357.

βασιλείαν ἀπὸ καταβολῆς κόσμου. ἐπείνασα γάρ, καὶ ἐδώκατέ μοι φαγεῖν, ἐδίψησα, καὶ ἐποτίσατέ με (Come, you that are blessed by my Father, inherit the kingdom prepared for you from the foundation of the world; for I was hungry and you gave me food, I was thirsty and you gave me something to drink).[165]

This passage is incorporated in the synaxarion read on Meatfare Sunday, which is dedicated to the Second Coming. Moreover, a great part of the homily on the Last Judgment attributed to Hippolytos is dedicated to the interpretation of this excerpt from Matthew (25:31–46).[166] In addition, it is interesting to note that in the tenth-century *Life of St. Basil the Younger,* Theodora's narrative about the other world singles out charity (ἐλεημοσύνη) as the virtue most able to benefit the souls who are on their way to the other world, passing through the tollbooths, which are guarded by demons keeping records of their sins: ἵνα τὰς ἀρετὰς κατεργαζόμενοι, καὶ μᾶλλον τὴν ἐλεημοσύνην ἥτις πλείονα τῶν ἄλλων τὴν ἰσχὺν ἐνταῦθα κέκτηται καὶ ὠφελεῖν δύναται τοὺς ἐνταῦθα διοδεύοντας τὴν ὁδὸν ταύτην, . . . (so that those who cultivate virtues, and most of all charity, which has here more power than the other [virtues] and can benefit those who pass here along this way).[167]

Matthew 25:34–35 conveys the principal idea behind the composition of the Second Coming—salvation through good deeds and mercy to one's neighbor—and it is often written in scenes of the Last Judgment together with its pendant, Matthew 25:41, implying eternal punishment for unjust deeds: "You that are accursed, depart from me into the eternal fire prepared for the devil and his angels." At Asinou only the first passage has been written (Matt. 25:34–35), on the front of the northern arch, referring to salvation and the attainment of eternal life. Matthew's second passage (Matt. 25:41), alluding to eternal punishments, has been replaced by the horrible punishment scenes represented in the soffit of the southern arch, which serve as a pictorial pendant to the facing inscription of Matthew's first passage, referring to salvation. This interplay of inscribed text and image shows that the inscription on the head of the northern arch forms an integral part of the painted decoration, supplementing contextually the iconographic program.[168]

In conclusion, the theme of the Second Coming adopted at Asinou was deeply rooted in the middle Byzantine iconographic tradition and widely used in eastern Mediterranean art in the Crusader period.[169] Asinou is distinctive, however, in its adaptation of the scene to fit into the available surfaces of the narthex. The vault offers a unique combination of the central, narrative subject of the Last

165. Uncial characters on yellow-ocher ground. Minuscules: α in δεῦται, ἐπήνασα, ἐδοίψεισα, ἐποτείσατέ, and καὶ. Accents and breathings indicated. Ligatures: ει, αι, νη, τρ, ου, την, νην, μηνβ, λη, αν, απ, αβ, πην, αγην. Spelling mistakes in 22 out of 62 syllables.
166. *Τριώδιον*, 32; PG 10:944–49.
167. "Περὶ τῆς τελευτῆς τῆς ἀμμᾶς Θεοδώρας," in Veselovskij, "Razyskanija," 46 (1889–90) 10–52, esp. 24–25. Cf. Angelidi, "Βίος τοῦ ὁσίου Βασιλείου," 178–87. Although crucial for the concept of the Last Judgment, Matt. 25:35–36 was not illustrated in Byzantine art before the post-Byzantine era. The Six Deeds of Charity first appear as an iconographic subject in western medieval art in the 12th century; they are illustrated in one of the most conspicuous works of the Crusader East, namely on the back leaf of the ivory cover of Queen Melisende's psalter (ca. 1135); see Kühnel, *Crusader Art*, 70–71, 75–79, 88–90, figs. 72, 76–78, 89; Buckton, *Byzantium*, 165–66, no. 181 (J. Lowden); Folda, *Art of the Crusaders*, 158, pl. 6. 10b.
168. Inscriptions, when placed high up so that they are illegible or when addressed to an illiterate audience, may have had an ornamental function. James, "And Shall These Mute Stones Speak?"; cf. Rhoby, *Byzantinische Epigramme*, 70, discussing the cryptogram on the eastern arch of the narthex at Asinou.
169. Characteristic examples are attested in the Syrian wall painting in the monastery church of Mar Musa (1192/93); in the Armenian gospel book in the Walters Art Museum, Baltimore (W539, fol. 109r), painted in 1262 by T'oros Roslin in Armenian Cilicia; and in a 13th-century icon in St. Catherine's monastery in Sinai, assigned by Weitzmann to a French artist of a Crusader atelier; see Der Nersessian, *Miniature Painting*, fig. 222; Westphalen, "Byzantinisierende Wandmalereien," 390–93, fig. 3; Weitzmann, "Icon Painting," 58–59, figs. 14a–b.

Judgment—Christ as supreme judge assisted by angels and apostles—with a typical dome composition. Most of the iconographic features of the composition at Asinou are already well attested in the twelfth-century Last Judgment in St. Nicholas of the Roof at Kakopetria and continued to be used in the monuments of the Lusignan era. Like Asinou, some earlier examples, including St. Nicholas of the Roof and Sotera, distribute constituent scenes in different areas of the narthex; in other cases, as at St. Herakleidios, the whole composition is confined to one panel. In accord with the art of other rural communities under Latin rule, like Venetian-occupied Crete, special emphasis is given to the didactic details of the collective and individual punishments, which are addressed to monastic and lay, male and female viewers alike. Even in our own era, the impact of these scenes in the same monastic and agrarian milieu is reflected in a poem of 1953 by the Greek poet and Nobel laureate George Seferis:

> Then the monk appeared: skullcap, frock, leather belt,
> and went to work decorating the gourd.
> He began at the neck: palm trees, fish-scales, rings.
> Then, cupping its round belly with a broad palm,
> he added the cheating farmer, the cheating merchant, the cheating miller, and the slanderer;
> Then the infant-hater and the defrocked nun;
> and at the bottom, almost hidden, the sleepless worm.[170]

Deesis

The figures of Christ and the Virgin are portrayed full-length on either side of the entrance to the naos (Fig. 5.30). They are joined at Christ's left by the figure of John the Forerunner (Fig. 5.1), thus constituting a Deesis.[171] As an intercessional composition, the Deesis in the narthex of Asinou belongs to the scene of the Last Judgment as one of its most central and essential parts.[172] At the same time, through its placement in the lower zone of the wall, within the sanctoral cycle, it plays a leading role in the saints' prayers for the redemption of humankind.

Christ, painted frontally to the south of the doorway, blesses with his right hand and holds an open book in his left. His nimbus is raised and bears traces of a stamped decoration. The inscriptions next to the nimbus read: Ι(ησοῦ)ς / Χ(ριστό)ς / ὁ ἐλε/ή̔μῶν (Jesus Christ the Merciful). His book displays John 13:34: ἐντο/λῆν κὰι/νῆν δί/δομε / ἡμῆν / ἥνα ἁ/γαπάτε / ἀλλΐλ(ους) = ἐντολὴν καινὴν δίδωμι ὑμῖν, ἵνα ἀγαπᾶτε ἀλλήλους (I give you a new commandment, that you love one another).

Although the text on Christ's book varies in Cypriot monuments, it is generally redemptive in content. In Lagoudera the passage is taken from John 8:12: ἐγώ εἰμι τὸ φῶς τοῦ κόσμου. ὁ ἀκολουθῶν ἐμοὶ οὐ μὴ περιπατήσῃ ἐν τῇ σκοτίᾳ ἀλλ᾽ ἕξει τὸ φῶς τῆς ζωῆς (I am the light of the world. Whoever follows me will never walk in darkness but will have the light of life). In Moutoullas it reproduces John 10:9: ἐγώ εἰμι ἡ θύρα. δι᾽ ἐμοῦ ἐάν τις εἰσέλθῃ σωθήσεται (I am the gate. Whoever enters by me will be saved).[173] The text used in the narthex at Asinou, and repeated in the naos (see below, p. 238), is particularly interesting for its relation to Matthew 25:34–35, the text of the dominant inscription surrounding the scenes of paradise in the northern apse (see above, pp. 152–53). Together, they say that Paradise will be gained by showing love for one another and charity to those

170. Seferis, *Collected Poems*, 340–41 ("Details on Cyprus").

171. On the subject, see Bogyay, "Deesis und Eschatologie"; Walter, "Two Notes"; idem, "Further Notes"; idem, "Bulletin"; Mouriki, "Deesis Icon"; Andaloro, "Note sui temi iconografici"; Cutler, "Under the Sign"; Zervou Tognazzi, "Δέησις"; Mantas, "Überlegungen zur Deesis"; Kazamia-Tsernou, *Ιστορώντας τη Δέηση*. On the Deesis in the apse of churches in Georgia and Cappadocia, see Thierry, "Peintures d'Ayvalı köy," 16–20; Velmans, "Image de la Déisis"; Jolivet-Lévy, *Cappadoce médiévale*, 125–28; Warland, "Deesis–Emmanuel–Maria."

172. On the Deesis icorporated into the Last Judgment, see Walter, *Art and Ritual*, 183–84.

173. Nicolaïdès, "Étude iconographique," 106; Mouriki, "Moutoullas," 191.

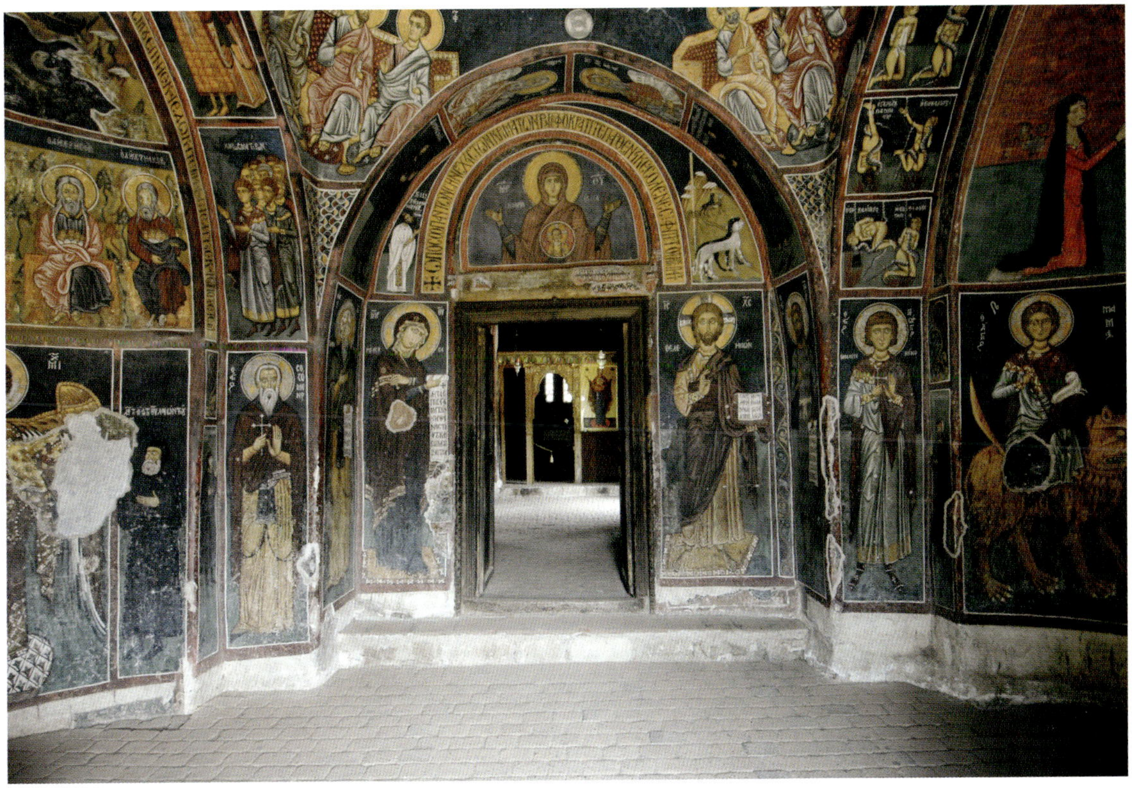

FIG. 5.30 Narthex, view toward east. Lunette: Virgin Phorbiotissa. Soffit of arch, left to right: monk Germanos, prophet Isaiah, prophet Zacharias, monk Theophilos. East wall, upper zone: priest-monk Barnabas on the left, mouflons and hounds on the right. Lower zone, left to right: monk Leontios, monk Laurentios, St. Sozomenos, St. John of Damascus, the Virgin Eleousa (Paraklesis), Christ Eleemon, St. John the Baptist, St. George Machairomenos, lay supplicant Georgios, St. Mamas (photo courtesy of G. L. Carr)

who are in need. This central message of the narthex at Asinou can be linked to the epithets given to Christ and the Virgin: ἐλεήμων and ἐλεοῦσα, meaning merciful, benevolent.[174]

The Virgin (Figs. 5.30, 3.12) occupies the north jamb of the door, turning toward her Son and holding an open scroll. Its inscription is discussed by Nancy Patterson Ševčenko in Chapter 3 (pp. 85–88). Mary is labeled Μ(ήτ)ηρ / Θ(εο)υ / ἡ ἐλεού/σα (Mother of God, the merciful). Traces of an earlier layer of painting are visible in the lower right corner of her panel, where the segment of a dado and some green ground with a small plant are exposed (evident especially in Fig. 3.12).

The Virgin assumes the type known as the Paraklesis (Intercession).[175] A variant of the Hagiosoritissa, the Paraklesis emphasizes Mary's role as the chief intercessor for humankind, based on her maternal relationship with Christ. Her

174. For a discussion of the epithets Eleousa and Eleemon and their funerary and soteriological connotations, see Pentcheva, *Icons and Power*, 177–83. It is interesting to note that in Cypriot examples, such as those at Lagoudera and Moutoullas, the Virgin Paraklesis is usually labeled Eleousa.

175. For a thorough study of the iconography and dissemination of the Virgin Paraklesis and of the dialogue written on her scroll, see Djordjević and Marković, "Dialogue Relationship" (with previous bibliography). For a discussion on the Paraklesis in the narthex of Asinou, see Kalopissi-Verti, "Representations of the Virgin," 305–7.

open scroll bears intercessory prayers to Christ, especially a poetic dialogue in which the Virgin prays for the salvation of humankind, and Christ responds to her supplication. The idea of the dialogue between the Virgin and Christ as found on the scroll of the Virgin Paraklesis seems to have originated in a canon of Theodore Stoudites (759–826).[176] The iconographic type may have emerged quite soon thereafter, as suggested by two epigrams preserved in a manuscript made most probably for a south Italian monastery around 900.[177] If the epigrams in fact accompanied images, it would imply that the iconographic type of the Paraklesis was crystallized by the end of the ninth century. Examples of the Paraklesis multiplied during the Komnenian and especially the Palaiologan period. In monumental painting the Paraklesis most often appears as a pendant figure to the image of Christ on the west face of the eastern piers or responds of the church flanking the templon. It also occurs in the narthex, on the west face of the piers or on the east wall flanking the entrance to the naos.[178] In certain churches, as at Asinou, the Virgin Paraklesis and Christ are painted in both naos and narthex, as discussed below. Finally, the Virgin Paraklesis may also be incorporated into the Deesis,[179] as in most of the Cypriot examples that follow.

The type of the Panagia Paraklesis is interesting in its dual appeal. In beseeching Christ for mercy on behalf of all humanity, it has a global character. Yet it has also been used for images of private devotion.[180] In Cyprus its use in individual contexts is rare. A niche over the tomb of St. Neophytos in the Enkleistra (ca. 1183) shows the Virgin enthroned with the Child, holding a scroll with a prayer addressed to Christ for the salvation of Neophytos himself. The prayer on the scroll is an individualization of the usual universal prayer of the Paraklesis.[181] The Paraklesis again assumes an aura of private devotion in the church of the Archangel Michael (or of the Virgin) at Galata (1514), where portraits of the patrons' family are included in the composition of the Deesis.[182] By contrast, in the narthex

176. Eustratiades, *Θεοτοκάριον*, 84–87, no. 26; Salaville, "Marie dans la liturgie," 315–16. On the impact of the canon of Theodore Stoudites on the iconography of the Paraklesis, see Tatić-Djurić, "Steatitska ikonica," 77, n. 65; Butyrskij, "Bogomater' Paraklesis." On the relationship of the Paraklesis type with *parakletikoi kanones* addressed to the Virgin, see N. P. Ševčenko, "Icons in the Liturgy," 55; with apocalyptic texts of the Virgin, see Semoglou, *Voyage outre-tombe*, 56; with civil and ecclesiastical administration, see Belting, *Illuminierte Buch*, 35–36, n. 115, figs. 23–24; Walter, "Two Notes," 317; Cutler, "Under the Sign," 146, n. 7; Cotsonis, "Virgin and Justinian," 52–53. For an overall discussion of possible connections with literary and ecclesiastical texts, see Djordjević and Marković, "Dialogue Relationship," 36–40.

177. Cod. Bodl. Barocci 50: see Lauxtermann, "Byzantine Epigram," 33–35.

178. For examples, see Djordjević and Marković, "Dialogue Relationship."

179. For a comprehensive study of this iconographic variant, see Papadaki-Oekland, "Τοιχογραφίες τῆς Ἁγίας Ἄννας"; cf. Hadermann-Misguich, *Kurbinovo*, 224–34, figs. 165, 117, 118.

180. In the above-mentioned south Italian epigrams dated around 900 (n. 177 above) the Virgin addresses her interceding prayers on behalf of mankind. By contrast, in other south Italian epigrams written by the poet Patrician in the years 940–70 the Virgin explicitly intercedes on behalf of an individual, namely Constantine VII: see Lauxtermann, "Byzantine Epigram," 35–36. For the use of the Paraklesis type in images of private devotion, see Papadaki-Oekland, "Τοιχογραφίες τῆς Ἁγίας Ἄννας," 41–47. In the 12th century this iconographic type was applied for individual prayer by renowned individuals such as George of Antioch (1143), see Kitzinger, *St. Mary's of the Admiral*, 197–206, 316–18, figs. XXII, XXIV, XXVI, 119, 123–25, 170, and the Grand Duke Andrej Bogoljubski (1158). In later copies, the Virgin Bogoljubskaja is represented before groups of monks or other pious persons: see Vloberg, "Types iconographiques," 439–42; Bentchev and Haustein-Bartsch, *Gottesmutterikonen*, 146–47; Smirnova, *Ikony*, 66. For the different variants and contexts of the image of the Virgin in an intermediary role between private individuals and Christ, see N. P. Ševčenko, "Close Encounters," 264–77.

181. Mango and Hawkins, "Hermitage," 184, fig. 107.

182. Stylianou and Stylianou, *Painted Churches*, 90, fig. 40; Constantoudaki-Kitromelides, *Ναοί*, 51–55.

at Asinou the individual prayers of the supplicants depicted on the walls are merged together in the global context of Mary's intercession with her Son for the salvation of humankind (πρὸς βροτῶν σωτηρίαν), as written on her scroll. Here, humans as a whole will be saved through love and good deeds toward one another, through the supplicatory prayers of the Virgin ἐλεοῦσα, and the mercy of the supreme judge, Christ ἐλεήμων.

The Virgin Paraklesis was popular in the monumental art of Cyprus from the second half of the twelfth century onward, as shown by Nancy Ševčenko (above, pp. 86–88), and a yet earlier example in Panagia Apsinthiotissa near Sychari (early twelfth century) is discussed by Annemarie Carr (see p. 238). Usually depicted on the north pier of the templon as the counterpart to the image of Christ on the south pier, in most cases it is accompanied by John the Forerunner, thus together constituting the three main figures of the Deesis. A very well-preserved example is found on the north respond in the church of the Panagia tou Arakos at Lagoudera (1192).[183] The images at Asinou belong to this category, as well.

John the Forerunner (ο / ἁγι/ος / Ιω(άννης) / πρ(ό)δρ(ο)μος) in the narthex at Asinou is clad in a gray, sleeved goatskin with a sash knotted in front (Fig. 5.1). Shown in a frontal stance with his head inclined toward Christ, he blesses with the right hand and holds in his left an open scroll inscribed μετανο/είται ἤγγι/κεν γὰρ ἡ / βασιλεία / τῶν οὐρα/νōν {ῶ} / = μετανοεῖτε ἤγγικε γὰρ ἡ βασιλεία τῶν οὐρανῶν (Repent, for the kingdom of heaven has come near, Matt. 3:2 and 4:17). Because John figures in most of the Cypriot examples of the Virgin Paraklesis with Christ, the evocation of the Deesis is familiar. In most cases, however, John stands behind Mary on the north wall, forming an asymmetrical Deesis, as at Lagoudera and Moutoullas.[184] In the narthex of Asinou, by contrast, he is depicted next to Christ, as a figure parallel and equal to the Mother of God. The quotation on his scroll is customary for the Baptist and is reproduced in the late twelfth-century church of the Archangel Michael at Kato Lefkara and in the church of the Panagia at Moutoullas (1280; see below, p. 239). The explicit eschatological allusion of the passage links the image of the Deesis specifically to that of the Second Coming. As such, it underlines the power of repentance (μετάνοια) during life, which is one of the preconditions for the salvation of the soul, as is often stressed in eschatological texts.[185]

The Deesis on the east wall of the narthex at Asinou repeats the iconography of the templon in the naos.[186] This duplication—of Christ and Mary alone, or of the Deesis—on the east wall of the narthex and on the sanctuary screen occurs primarily in late Byzantine monastic foundations.[187] Examples on Cyprus include the Panagia at Moutoullas and St. Nicholas of the Roof at Kakopetria.[188] It seems that these images, by their duplication, marked liminal zones defining spaces of graduated holiness in

183. Nicolaïdès, "Étude iconographique," 107–9, figs. 18, 77, 78 (with previous bibliography). There is a probably earlier example of the Paraklesis type in the church of the Holy Apostles in Perachorio (1160–80), where only part of the Virgin on the northern pier has been preserved: see Megaw and Hawkins, "Holy Apostles at Perachorio," 333, fig. 48.

184. Nicolaïdès, "Étude iconographique," [1996], 109; Mouriki, "Moutoullas," 191.

185. Apocalypse of Paul (mid-3rd c.): Tischendorf, *Apocalypses apocryphae*, 58, §33; homily on the Sixth Psalm of Anastasios Sinaites (early 8th c.), PG 89:1112–16; cf. Ivanov, "Dushepoleznaya istoriya"; Apocalypse of Anastasia (late 10th/early 11th c.), Baun, *Tales from Another Byzantium,* 409, §40.

186. The 14th-century program of the templon copies the early 12th-century iconography; see below, pp. 236–40.

187. For a discussion of the duplication of imagery on the east wall of the narthex and on the proskynetaria of the templon and sometimes also on the west façade of the church, particularly in monastic foundations of the late Byzantine period, see Kalopissi-Verti, "Proskynetaria of the Templon and Narthex."

188. In Moutoullas, the figure of Christ is repeated on the south part of the templon (1280) and on the east wall of the narthex (14th c.); in Kakopetria, Christ and the Virgin are painted in the narthex on both sides of the naos entrance (3rd quarter of 14th century), Kalopissi-Verti, "Proskynetaria," figs. 27–30.

the church: from narthex to naos, and from naos to sanctuary. As the imagery indicates, these thresholds also mark specific areas for prayer for the salvation of humankind. The representation of the Deesis is, moreover, closely related to the symbolism of the narthex, to the rituals performed there, and to its iconography, which often includes the Last Judgment, as at Asinou. As stated by Symeon, archbishop of Thessalonike (fl. 1416/17–1429), the priest entering the narthex symbolizes the descent of Christ into Hades in order to save the souls held there.[189] Accordingly, funerary and commemorative ceremonies were performed in the narthex, as attested in monastic typika and in euchologia.[190] Moreover, the office of the *lite*, celebrated in the narthex as part of the vespers preceding vigils, in accordance with the monastic rite, included prayers for the salvation of the living and for the deceased. The final prayer in particular, as Symeon explains it, invoked the benevolent Lord to show mercy through the intercession of Mary, the angels, the apostles, the martyrs, the church fathers, the beatified, and all the saints.[191] Accordingly, the epithets accompanying Christ and Mary in the image—ἐλεήμων and ἐλεοῦσα—indicate that they are the benevolent recipients of the prayers not only of all the saints and supplicants depicted on the wall of the narthex, but also of all those attending the church ceremonies, whether monastic or lay.

In sum, the Deesis depicted at Asinou can be considered a key image in the iconography of the narthex. It fulfills multiple roles. It constitutes part of the Last Judgment; it duplicates the imagery of the templon, marking liminal zones of prayer in the church; in addition, it functions as the recipient of the intercessions of the saints painted in the narthex, as well as of individual and corporate prayers for the salvation of the donors depicted on the walls of the narthex, of all the brethren of the monastic community, and of the congregation of the laity attending the services. Gestures of the figures and inscriptions on the scrolls of the holy persons of the Deesis illustrate the cyclical process of response. John foretells the imminence of the heavenly kingdom and urges repentance as a means of salvation; Mary, as a clement intercessor—a true Eleousa—addresses her mediatory prayers to Christ for the salvation of humankind; and Christ responds by giving a new commandment, "that you love one another." Consequently, prayer, repentance, intercession, and love for one another are bound together as the means that will lead to salvation. Provided that these conditions are fulfilled, Christ Eleemon responds benevolently by blessing the faithful and granting mercy.

Prophets

Two half-length figures of prophets are painted in the soffit of the eastern arch above the lunette with the Virgin Phorbiotissa. The prophet on the north side, labeled Isaiah (ο / πρ(ο)φ(ή)τ(η)ς / Ἡ/σα/ΐ/ας), holds a scroll with Isaiah 1:19: Ἐὰν θ/έλετε / καὶ ἠσα/κούσατε / μοῦ τα ἀγα/θα της γης / [φά]γεσ[θε] = καὶ ἐὰν θέλητε καὶ εἰσακούσητέ μου, τὰ ἀγαθὰ τῆς γῆς φάγεσθε (If you are willing and obedient, you shall eat the good of the land, Fig. 5.31). The pendant figure on the south side of the soffit, the prophet Zechariah/Zacharias (ο / πρ(ο)φ(ή)τ(η)ς / Ζα/χα/ρί/ας), is depicted as an old man, with gray hair falling to his shoulders and a long, sharply pointed beard (Fig. 5.32). His gray tunic has ornamented cuffs and a richly decorated collar extending to the chest. Over the tunic he wears a *paludamentum* bordered with pearls and gems and held together with a brooch. On his head he wears the priestly hat (κίδαρις). The inscription on the scroll, from Luke 1:68, reads: εὐλο/γιτος κ(ύριο)ς / ὁ θ(εὸ)ς τοῦ / Ἴσραὴλ / ὅτη ἐπε/[σκέ]ψατο = εὐλογητὸς κύριος ὁ θεὸς τοῦ Ἰσραήλ, ὅτι ἐπεσκέψατο (Blessed be the Lord God of Israel, for he has looked favorably. . . .).

The identification of the figure of Ζαχαρίας is problematic. Its placement as counterpart to the

189. "τὰς κατεχομένας ἐκεῖσε τῶν ἀπ' αἰῶνος ψυχὰς ῥύσασθαι," PG 155:292B.

190. On the funerary functions of the narthex, see Bache, "Fonction funéraire du narthex"; Nicholl, "Archaeological Interpretation"; cf. below, n. 398.

191. PG 155:616, κεφ. τμ'. Περὶ τῆς τελευταίας εὐχῆς τῆς ἐν τῇ λιτῇ.

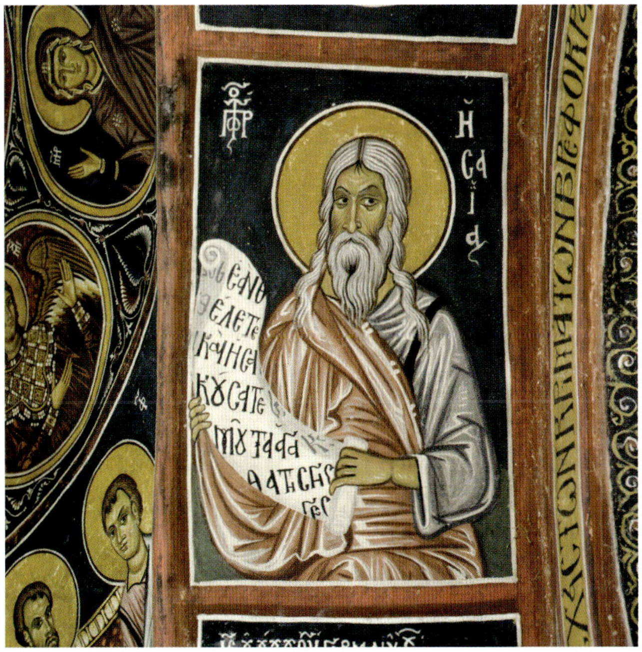

FIG. 5.31 Narthex, soffit of east arch, north side. The prophet Isaiah (photo courtesy of the Leventis Foundation and the Archaeological Research Unit, University of Cyprus, No. 006295)

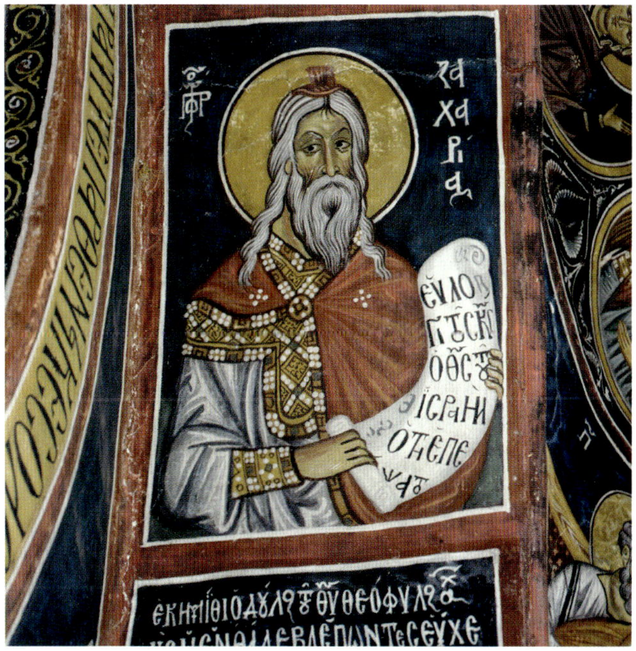

FIG. 5.32 Narthex, soffit of east arch, south side. The prophet Zacharias (photo courtesy of the Leventis Foundation and the archaeological Research Unit, University of Cyprus, No. 006298)

prophet Isaiah, as well as the label ο προφήτης, points to the prophet Zechariah, one of the twelve minor prophets of the Old Testament. However, Zechariah is usually depicted as a beardless, bareheaded youth with short brown hair, wearing a tunic and himation, and sometimes holding a sickle.[192] The advanced age of the figure at Asinou, the priestly hat and vestments, and the text on the scroll indicate an identification instead with the high priest Zacharias, the father of St. John the Baptist.[193] In Greek, the two figures share precisely the same name (Ζαχαρίας).

In painted dome compositions in Cypriot churches of the Lusignan period, the priest Zacharias outnumbers the prophet, appearing three times, while Zechariah appears just once. Thus the priest is depicted in the dome of St. Herakleidios in the monastery complex of St. John Lampadistes at Kalopanayiotis (third quarter of the thirteenth century) and in the dome of St. Nicholas of the Roof in Kakopetria (second half of the fourteenth century);[194] then both figures—priest and prophet—are portrayed in the dome of the Holy

192. Cf. Chatzidakis, "Εκ τῶν Ἐλπίου τοῦ Ρωμαίου," 410, ll. 20–21. On the iconography of the prophet Zechariah, see Stylianou and Stylianou, "Prophet Zechariah"; Van Rompay, "Une faucille volante."

193. Dionysios of Fourna, *Ἑρμηνεία τῆς ζωγραφικῆς τέχνης*, 79: "Ὁ προφήτης Ζαχαρίας, ὁ πατὴρ τοῦ Προδρόμου, γέρων μακρυγένης, φορῶν ἱερατικὴν στολὴν λέγει 'Εὐλογητὸς Κύριος ὁ Θεὸς τοῦ Ἰσραήλ,' ὅτι ἐπεσκέψατο καί."

194. Papamastorakes, *Διάκοσμος τοῦ τρούλου*, 21–22, no. 50, pl. 58; 24, no. 54, pl. 63a. According to Papamastorakes' study, the prophet Zechariah is represented in the cupola of 19 late Byzantine churches; the priest Zacharias is included among the prophets of the dome and labeled as prophet in 10 examples; in 5 cases both Zechariah and Zacharias are depicted: ibid., 238–41 (prophet), 195–97 (priest).

Cross at Pelendri (third quarter of the fourteenth century).[195] The prophet is represented as a young, beardless man dressed in tunic and himation, holding a sickle, with a passage from the book of Zechariah (9:9) written on his scroll; the priest is depicted as an old man, wearing the traditional priestly mantle and hat and holding a scroll with a passage from Zacharias's ode (Luke 1:68).

From the late twelfth century onward, the two figures are often fused in iconography. Thus John Lowden has pointed to the representation of the prophet as an old man, with shoulder-length gray hair and beard, wearing the priestly hat, in the Prophet Book Oxford, New College 44, fol. 28v (late twelfth–early thirteenth century); and again in the Prophet Book Vat. gr. 1153, fol. 59v (1260–70) he is depicted as an old man but bareheaded.[196] In turn, Luke's passage (1:67) recounting that Zacharias was filled with the Holy Spirit and spoke a prophecy, the frequent mentions of the high priest as a prophet in the Menaion on his feastday (5 September), and the illustration of the Psalter which often included his Ode (Luke 1:68–79), thus associating him with the prophetic Odes of the Old Testament, contributed to the association of the high priest with the prophet Zechariah.[197] The relation between the two figures is also evident in the Cypriot examples mentioned above, for passages from the prophecy of Zechariah (Zech. 8:19 and 1:4) are written on the scroll of the priest Zacharias in the domes of St. Herakleidios and St. Nicholas of the Roof.[198]

In sum, the figure labeled ὁ προφήτης Ζαχαρίας in the narthex of Asinou may be identified with the father of John the Forerunner, the priest Zacharias, who was considered a prophet and was a popular figure in Cypriot iconography.[199]

With regard to the content of the passages on the scrolls of the two prophets, the following observations can be made. Isaiah's text, with its Old Testament promise of obtaining the goods of the earth by being obedient to God's commands, may be related to the new commandment (John 13:34) proclaimed on the book of Christ just below (see above, p. 154). This new commandment, to love one another, has to be followed from now on in order to secure eternal salvation for the soul in the other world, rather than the goods of this world. On the other hand, Zacharias's passage refers to the realization of the promise of salvation according to the New Testament, since the full text of the opening verse of the Ode of Zacharias, found in Luke 1:68, is "Blessed be the Lord God of Israel, for he has looked favorably on his people and redeemed them." This passage may be associated with the inscription "Repent, for the kingdom of heaven has come near" (Matt. 3:2 and 4:17), depicted on the scroll of John the Forerunner in the socle zone (see above, p. 157), a passage that alludes to salvation through repentance and, consequently, to the salvific content of the entire iconographic program of the narthex.

Sanctoral Cycle

The lower zone of the narthex contains images of standing saints. Red borders segment the register into successive panels that the saints occupy individually, in pairs, or with a donor figure. With the exception of St. Mamas, who rides a lion, the saints stand in a frontal position. The background throughout is divided into two parallel zones: the lower, symbolizing earth, is green; the upper, corresponding

195. Stylianou and Stylianou, *Painted Churches,* 224, fig. 128a; eidem, "Prophet Zechariah"; Papamastorakes, *Διάκοσμος τοῦ τρούλου,* 23–24, no. 53, pl. 60a (prophet), 61a (priest).

196. For the fusion of the two figures and the relevant examples in the Prophet Books, see Lowden, *Illuminated Prophet Books*, 71, 73, figs. 66, 84, pl. 8.

197. *Menaion*, 5 September, 57–59, 61, 63; Lowden, *Prophet Books*, 71.

198. Papamastorakes, *Διάκοσμος τοῦ τρούλου,* 22, 24.

199. One of the earliest representations of the priest Zacharias in the monumental painting of Cyprus is preserved in the niche of the diakonikon of the church of St. Nicholas of the Roof at Kakopetria (11th c.). He is depicted as an old man, wearing the *kidaris* and the priestly cloak, and is accompanied by the inscription Ο ΑΓΙΟϹ ΖΑΧΑΡΙΑϹ: see Stylianou and Stylianou, *Painted Churches,* 55. For an illustration, see Mouriki, *Nea Moni,* pl. 333c.

to the sky, is blue. The inscriptions are painted in white capital letters on the blue ground. Traces of raised and decorated haloes are visible in most cases. As Ioanna Kakoulli shows below (p. 330–34), a layer of lime-plaster applied over the already painted halo was modeled, probably with a wooden mold; then tin leaf was applied with linseed oil and glazed with yellowish resin to imitate gilding.

On the southern side of the narthex, images of five saints belonging to the campaign of 1332/33—three male and two female—harmoniously incorporate the two earlier ex-votos: the impressive late twelfth-century figure of St. George on horseback and the late thirteenth-century panel of St. Anastasia Pharmakolytria with her homonymous devotee, discussed above (pp. 93–101, 115–22). Moving clockwise from St. John the Baptist, one meets on the west face of the southeast respond a rarely represented local saint, St. George Machairomenos (the Knifed), labeled ὁ / ἁγί/ος / Γε/ώρ/γι/ος / ὁ μαχερε/μένος, a local dialectical form of μαχαιρωμένος (Figs. 5.1, 5.33).[200] He is depicted as a handsome, beardless youth, clad in a tunic with a broad embroidered collar and holding a cross; his halo is raised. Unknown in the synaxarion of the church of Constantinople, he is mentioned by the fifteenth-century Cypriot chronicler Machairas, who characterizes him as a τοπικὸς θαυματουργός, i.e., a local worker of miracles, and locates his cult center in the village Ἀχλίοντας, today Ἀναλιόντας, south of Nicosia.[201] The eighteenth-century Cypriot historian, the archimandrite Kyprianos, considers this figure as one of the three hundred "Alaman" saints, who are thought to be either Orthodox Syro-Palestinians who found refuge in Cyprus after the Arab conquest of Jerusalem in 638 or Crusader Christians who came to the island when the Arabs reconquered Palestine at the end of the twelfth (1187) and the end of the thirteenth century (1291). It seems that this ambiguous legend reflects the repeated population displacement from the mainland to Cyprus during the long period of the Arab occupation.[202] Eustratiades' *Hagiologion* commemorates St. George Machairomenos on 31 December, but the recently edited Cypriot Menaion of December does not include him.[203] He should not be confused with St. George the Chozibite, commemorated on 8 January, a native of Cyprus who took the monastic habit and became abbot of the Choziba Monastery near Jerusalem (d. ca. 625), since the Chozibite died in peace,[204] whereas the St. George depicted in the narthex of Asinou was slain by a sword or stabbed with a knife, as his name indicates. A more or less contemporaneous portrait of St. George, accompanied by the same epithet, μαχερεμένος, appears in the central vessel of the church of the Holy Cross at Pelendri (third quarter of the fourteenth century).[205]

The next figure is one of the earliest Cypriot images of St. Mamas (ὁ / ἅ/γι/ος / Μά/μ/ας, Figs. 5.1, 5.33). He is shown frontally, riding a lion and holding a white lamb in his left hand and the shepherd's crook in his right. Mamas is youthful and beardless, with full, medium-length hair that partly covers the ears. A large area over his right leg is damaged. Traces of the raised halo are discernible. St. Mamas, who is considered to have incorporated the cults of ancient deities of Asia Minor, was born in Paphlagonia and suffered martyrdom in Caesarea of Cappadocia in the year 275 during the reign of the Roman emperor Aurelian.[206]

200. For the change of ο (ω) into ε in the Cypriot dialect in medieval and modern times, see Beaudouin, *Étude du dialecte chypriote*, 32; Sakellarios, *Τὰ Κυπριακά*, 2:38. I wish to thank my Cypriot colleague Dr. Stella Zeniou-Frigerio for this information.
201. Machairas, *Recital*, 1:34–35, §36, 2:65; Delehaye, "Saints de Chypre," 256.
202. Kyprianos, *Ἱστορία*, 526; Hackett, *History*, 418–30; Delehaye, "Saints de Chypre," 249–51; Kyrris, "Three Hundred Alaman Saints."
203. Eustratiades, *Ἁγιολόγιον*, 95.
204. Olster, "Construction of a Byzantine Saint"; Eustratiades, *Ἁγιολόγιον*, 91: "ἐν εἰρήνῃ τὸν βίον ἀπέλιπε."
205. Stylianou and Stylianou, *Painted Churches*, 231; Zarras, *Holy Cross*, fig. 32.
206. On the textual tradition, cult, and iconography of St. Mamas, see Marava-Chatzinikolaou, *Ἅγιος Μάμας*; see also Kyrris, "Δύο Κυπριακά," 90–119.

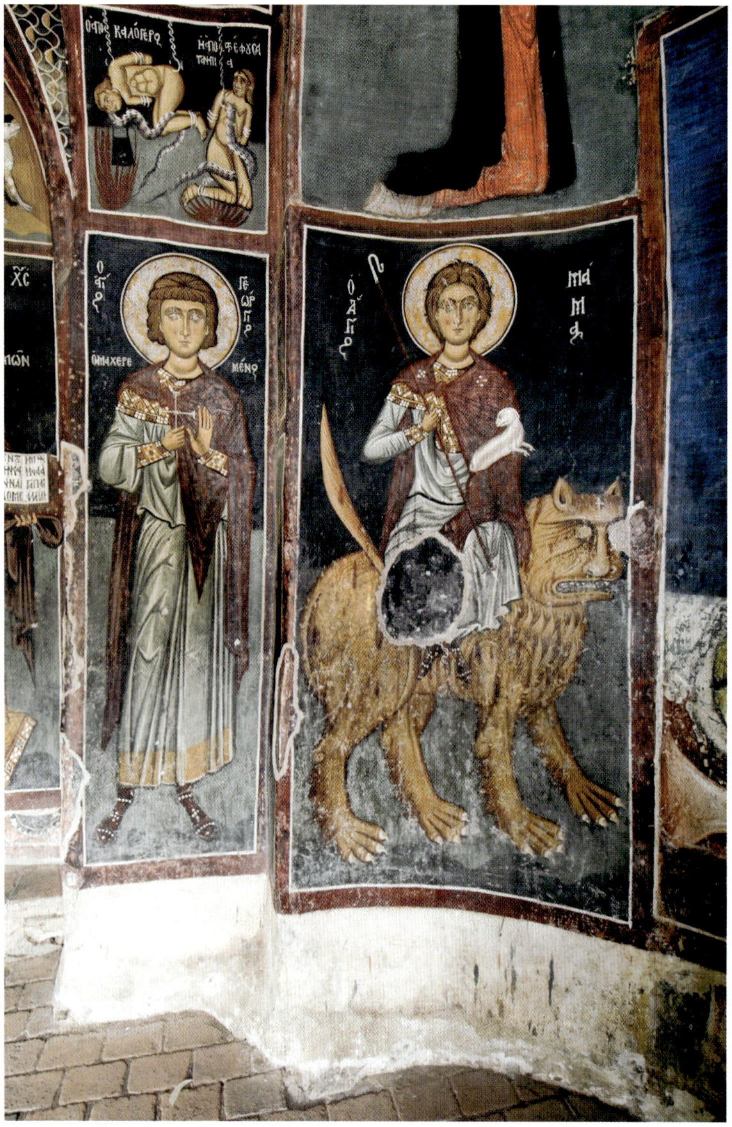

FIG. 5.33 Narthex, south-east respond and south conch. St. George Machairomenos and St. Mamas (photo courtesy of G. L. Carr)

St. Mamas's *Life* was included in the Synaxarium Constantinopolitanum and in the Metaphrastian Menologion, while prayers attributed to him for the curing of flocks are incorporated in the Euchologion.[207] His feast day is 2 September.

207. Delehaye, *Synaxarium,* cols. 5–7; *BHG* 2:72–74; *BS* 8:592–612; PG 115:565–74; N. P. Ševčenko, *Illustrated Manuscripts*, 17, 175; Dmitrievskij, *Opisanie*, 2:473; Meester, *Liturgia Bizantina*, 379–81.

St. Mamas was known in Cyprus from early Christian times.[208] Toward the end of the twelfth century, Neophytos the Recluse dedicated a panegyric (no. 2) to him that repeats the official *Life* by Metaphrastes but ignores local tradition, which was recorded by Leontios Machairas at the beginning of the fifteenth century.[209] According to Machairas, St. Mamas was born in Pamphylia and martyred by the Seljuk Turks. After his martyrdom, the coffin with his relics floated miraculously across the sea from Asia Minor and landed on the northern shore of Cyprus near Morphou, where a monastery was erected in his honor; from that time onward the saint worked miracles, especially healing incurable wounds. There is a Cypriot service in his honor, and the Cypriot Menaion at 2 September, the date of his commemoration, contains the Cypriot version of his life, mingling the Metaphrastian tradition with the legend recounted in Machairas, as well as many hymns in his honor.[210] St. Mamas's relics were housed not only in Morphou but also in the Troodos Mountains in the monastery of Kykkos.[211]

In Byzantine iconography St. Mamas is depicted holding the shepherd's crook in one hand and a lamb in the other; he is represented either as a standing figure—as in the church of the Virgin near Kophinou—or riding a lion.[212] The type with

208. For the cult and pictorial tradition of St. Mamas in Cyprus, see Marava-Chatzinikolaou, *Ἅγιος Μάμας*, 76–84; Gabelić, "Predstava Sv. Mamasa"; Mouriki, "Cypriot Saints," 249–51.

209. Hackett, *History,* 415–18; Delehaye, "Saints de Chypre," 272, 280; Machairas, *Recital*, 1:32, §33; Tsiknopoullos, "Ἅγιοι τῆς Κύπρου," 133–37; *Ἁγίου Νεοφύτου συγγράμματα*, 116–24. Another version, according to which the relics of St. Mamas were brought to Cyprus by the Mardaïtes Akrites sent to the island by Tiberios III (698–705), is recorded by Kourres, "Ἅγιος Μάμας," 233, 235. For other, more recent Cypriot traditions, see Marava-Chatzinikolaou, *Ἅγιος Μάμας*, 71–72.

210. Klerides, "Προλεγόμενα καὶ κείμενον"; *Κύπρια Μηναῖα*, 2 September, 9–30.

211. Meinardus, "Relics," 34.

212. Gabelić, "Kophinou," 147–48, fig. 3. The author dates the layer of frescoes, including that of Mamas, to

Mamas riding a lion goes back to the iconography of early Christian *eulogiai* given to the pilgrims who visited Mamas's martyrion in Caesarea of Cappadocia.[213] His image in Cypriot murals and icons from the fourteenth century onward may also have been affected, however, by the painted decoration of his funerary monument at Morphou. His tomb presently consists of a sixth-century marble sarcophagus under an arched niche richly decorated with Gothic relief foliage of the fourteenth century, a panel fitted into the lunette of the arch with thirty-eight miniature scenes of the saint's miracles, and a triptych of three large painted panels representing St. Mamas mounted on a lion between SS. George and Demetrios on horseback.[214] The present panels are from the nineteenth century, but it is probable that the tomb was already adorned with paintings in the fourteenth century, given the Gothic date of the sculpture on the one hand and, on the other, the particular popularity of the mounted Mamas in Cypriot imagery from the fifteenth century onward. St. Mamas riding a lion is not unknown in other regions; what is specifically Cypriot, however, as Smiljka Gabelić has pointed out, is the iconographic variant of St. Mamas riding a lion *and* holding his attributes, the lamb and the shepherd's crook.[215] The image of St. Mamas in the narthex of Asinou is among the earliest examples of this variant.[216]

Mamas, who was venerated as a protector of shepherds and curer of their flocks, was popular not only in Cyprus but also in other sheep-breeding areas, such as Cappadocia, Crete, Macedonia, and Serbia.[217] His cult was known in the Latin West as well, for the twelfth-century cathedral of Langres in Champagne possessed important relics, including his head, which was brought from Constantinople after 1204.[218] It seems that this Latin familiarity with St. Mamas favored the development of his cult in both ethnic groups of Cyprus, Latin as well as Greek. The Lusignan court promoted his cult;[219] at the same time, the veneration of St. Mamas by the Orthodox population is seen in the mounting frequency with which he is represented in Cypriot Orthodox churches and icons dating to the late Lusignan and Venetian periods.

St. Mamas, in sum, a very popular saint in Cyprus, was depicted in the narthex of Asinou as protector of shepherds and curer of flocks, in accordance with the monastery's agrarian setting. His portrait at Asinou may also be linked, however, to

---

the 12th c.; Mouriki, "Cypriot Saints," 251, dates it to the 13th c., which seems to be more probable; cf. Marava-Chatzinikolaou, *Ἅγιος Μάμας*, 93–97.

213. Marava-Chatzinikolaou, *Ἅγιος Μάμας*, 70–84; eadem, "Εὐλογία τοῦ Ἁγίου Μάμα," pl. 51.

214. Enlart, *Gothic Art*, 367–70, fig. 333; Marava-Chatzinikolaou, *Ἅγιος Μάμας*, pl. 11. Kourres, "Ἅγιος Μάμας," 234–38, figs. 1, 4.

215. Gabelić, "Iconography of Saint Mamas."

216. An icon with a painted image of Mamas in this iconographic type, now in the church of Panagia Katholike at Pelendri, has been dated to the late 13th century but is probably of later date (14th/15th c.). See Sophocleous, *Icons of Cyprus*, 89–90, fig. 27; idem, *Cyprus the Holy Island*, 156–59, no. 23; idem, *Icônes de Chypre*, 131–32, 218, fig. 15. Cf. a 14th-century vita icon of Mamas from Moutoullas, now in the Kykkos Monastery, *Ἱερὰ Μητρόπολις Μόρφου*, 274, no. 15.

217. Gabelić, "Predstava Sv. Mamasa," 73–75. For examples in Cappadocia, see Jolivet-Lévy, *La Cappadoce médiévale,* 340. For St. Mamas's cult in Crete, see Detorakes, "Λαϊκὴ λατρεία"; Spatharakis, "Cycle of St. Mamas." For an image of St. Mamas mounted on a lion in a 13th-century church in Syria (Mar Saba in Eddé al-Batrun), see Immerzeel, "Holy Horsemen," 34–35. For examples and a discussion of the portrait of St. Mamas in Byzantine churches, see Gerstel, "Byzantine Village Church," 172–77.

218. Marava-Chatzinikolaou, *Ἅγιος Μάμας*, 67–70, 79–80.

219. The area of Morphou, the center of Mamas's cult, belonged to the Lusignan court. Moreover, two churches of the 15th/16th century (the Gothic church in Potamia and the Franco-Byzantine church close to ancient Dali in the region of Potamia/St. Sozomenos, which also belonged to the court) are dedicated to St. Mamas—if this dedication goes back to the time of their foundation. See Enlart, *Gothic Art*, 194–201; Nicolaïdès and Vanderheyde, "Topographie cultuelle chrétienne," 254–55, 260.

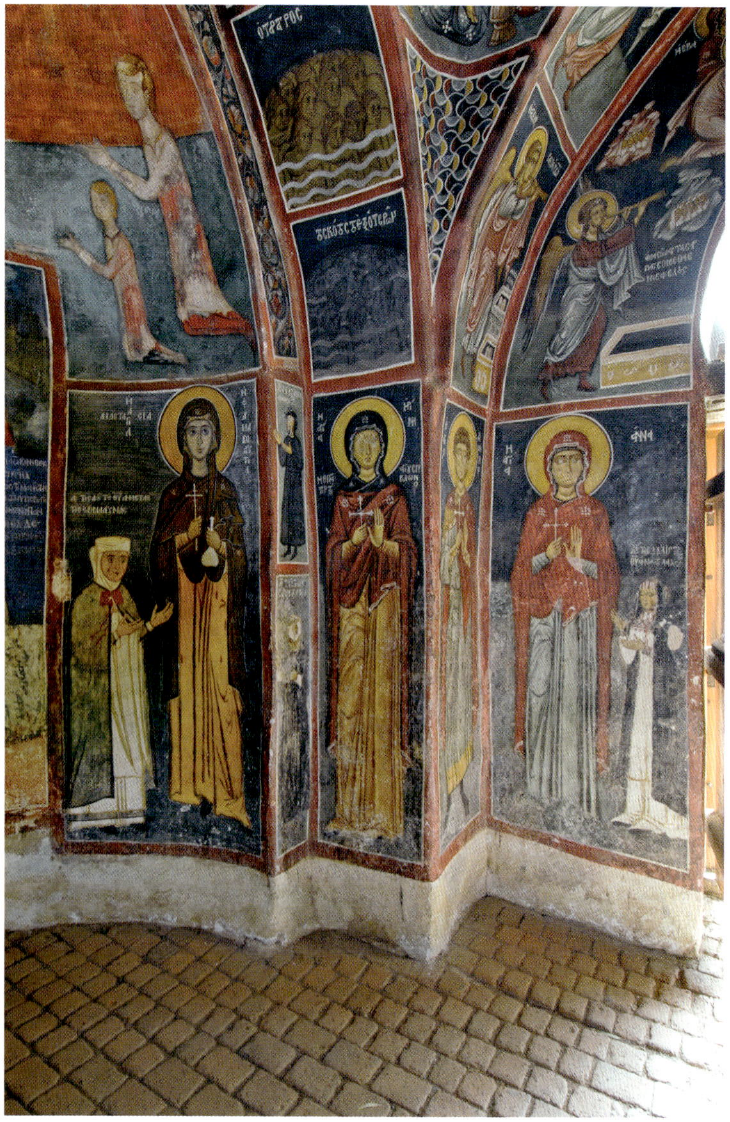

FIG. 5.34 Narthex, south conch and west wall. St. Anastasia with donor, monk Kallinikos (above) and lay supplicant Basileios (below), St. Irene, St. Demetrios, St. Anna with donor (photo courtesy of G. L. Carr)

his legendary capacity in Cyprus to cure people as well as animals, for Machairas and other medieval sources relate that the *myron* (fragrant oil) issuing from his tomb on his feast day was a cure for wounds and a medicine against many illnesses.[220] Thus the placement of Mamas's figure opposite the image of Anastasia Pharmakolytria in the southern conch of the narthex of Asinou is not likely to have been accidental.

To the right of the thirteenth-century figure of St. Anastasia is a unique representation of St. Irene, the daughter of St. Spyridon, η / ἁγί/α / Ἡρί/νη / η θιγά/τιρ τοῦ / αγίου Cπυ/ρίδων/ος = ἡ ἁγία Εἰρήνη ἡ θυγάτηρ τοῦ ἁγίου Cπυρίδωνος (Figs. 5.19, 5.34).[221] Her maphorion is bicolored, brown for the part over the body and dark blue for the part covering the head. In her right hand she holds a cross, the traditional attribute of the martyr. The only source about her is the seventh-century *Life* of St. Spyridon, bishop of Trimythus in the fourth century. A certain man entrusted his valuables to Irene before he left for a journey. On his return, he found her dead and he greatly feared that his property was lost. The bishop went to his daughter's grave and called her back to life so that she could indicate to him where the treasure was hidden. The story is also included in the synaxarion of the Constantinopolitan church and in the Menaion on the feast day of St. Spyridon, 12 December. This time it is a woman who has entrusted her money to Irene. And finally, the story of Irene is also mentioned in two odes (fourth and eighth) of the same day.[222] Irene is otherwise unattested in monumental painting.[223] She was probably chosen for inclusion in the narthex of Asinou not only for her being a local saint but because she is linked to death and resurrection, in accordance with the iconographic program of the narthex.

The next figure is St. Demetrios (ὁ / ἁγι/ος / Δι/μή/τρι/ος), one of the most popular saints in the entire Byzantine world and among its Christian neighbors, celebrated on 26 October (Figs. 5.1,

220. Marava-Chatzinikolaou, *Ἅγιος Μάμας*, 77, 82, 149, 151, 154.

221. Hackett, *History*, 382–83; Delehaye, "Saints de Chypre," 262; Eustratiades, *Ἁγιολόγιον*, 125.

222. Delehaye, *Synaxarium*, col. 303; *Menaion*, 12 December, 473, 475–76; *Κύπρια Μηναῖα*, 12 December, 99–104.

223. In the index of Stylianou and Stylianou, *Painted Churches*, no other portrait of her is mentioned.

5.34).[224] Thessalonike was his principal cult center.[225] He was also widely venerated in Cyprus, where four localities were named after him. Moreover, an encomium of St. Neophytos the Recluse was dedicated to him.[226]

St. Demetrios is painted in many Cypriot churches from the early twelfth to the early sixteenth centuries. One of the earliest examples occurs in St. John Chrysostom at Koutsovendis (ca. 1100), where the saint is represented in court dress.[227] In most cases, however, he is depicted in armor, either mounted or, more often, on foot, as in St. Anthony at Kellia (mid-thirteenth century).[228] His fourteenth-century image in the narthex of Asinou, as a martyr wearing the mantle and embroidered tunic of a dignitary, is rare and follows an old tradition going back to early Christian times, when Demetrios was depicted dressed as a consul, in accord with his Vita. John Cotsonis has shown, on the basis of sphragistic imagery, that Demetrios's transformation to a military saint occurred in Thessalonike in the tenth century and became very widespread from the eleventh century on.[229] In the Palaiologan period, when Demetrios was especially widely venerated, he was rarely depicted as a civil dignitary, although he continued to be clad in tunic and mantle in his biographical scenes.[230]

St. Anna (η / ἁγί/α / Ἄννα) is depicted next to St. Demetrios on the west wall of the narthex (Figs. 5.1, 5.19, 5.34). Daughter of the priest Mathan and mother of the Virgin Mary, Anna was as popular in Cyprus as she was elsewhere in the Byzantine world.[231] Five localities in Cyprus are named after her, and one of her arms was shown in 1485 to the Dominican friar Felix Fabri in a Latin church dedicated to her in a village near the foot of Stavrovouni.[232] St. Anna is depicted in a great number of Cypriot churches, either in scenes belonging to the Mariological cycle, such as the Birth of the Virgin, or paired with her husband, Joachim.[233] Isolated images of her among other saints, however, are rare. In Cyprus, besides the narthex of Asinou, she appears in this way only on the outer west wall (now inside the later narthex) of the church of St. Mamas at Louvaras (1495).[234] In the narthex of Asinou, St. Anna is represented holding a cross, although she was not a martyr. It seems that she had acquired the cross as an attribute by the middle

224. *BHG* 1:152–65; *BS* 4:556–65; Delehaye, *Synaxarium*, cols. 163–66; Lemerle, *Miracles de Saint Démétrius*. On the iconography of the saint see Xyngopoulos, *Ἅγιος Δημήτριος*; Grabar, "Nouveau reliquaire"; Walter, "St. Demetrius"; idem, *Warrior Saints*, 67–93; Papamastorakes, "Ιστορίες και ιστορήσεις," 222–28; Smirnova, "Iconographie de Saint Démétrios." On Demetrius's cult in the Balkans and Russia, see Obolensky, "Cult of St. Demetrius"; Tapkova-Zaimova, "Culte de St. Démétrius"; Djordjević, "Der heilige Demetrios"; Smirnova, "Culte et image."

225. Cormack, *Writing in Gold*, 50–94; Mentzos, *Προσκύνημα του Αγίου Δημητρίου*; Bakirtzis, "Culte de Saint Démétrius."

226. Delehaye, "Saints de Chypre," 267; Laourdas, "Βυζαντινὰ καὶ μεταβυζαντινὰ ἐγκώμια," 49–55, 122–25; *Ἁγίου Νεοφύτου συγγράμματα*, 317–26.

227. Mango, "Koutsovendis," 89, fig. 143; see index in Stylianou and Stylianou, *Painted Churches*, for other examples.

228. Spanou, "Τέχνη στη μητροπολιτική περιφέρεια Κιτίου," 40, fig. 25.

229. Cotsonis, "Contribution of Byzantine Lead Seals," 463–79.

230. Walter, "St. Demetrius," 174–75, fig. 4. An image of St. Demetrios clad in civil garments, in imitation of the early Christian mosaic representations of the saint, is painted in the homonymous church of Thessalonike, ca. 1220–30: see Tsigaridas, "Τοιχογραφία του Αγίου Δημητρίου." Cf. Chatzidakis, *Mystras*, fig. 21, where St. Demetrios is dressed very similarly to the saint in Asinou.

231. *BHG* 1:44–45; *BS* 1:1269–95; Delehaye, *Synaxarium*, cols. 29, 288–91, 841–42. On the iconography, see Kleinschmidt, *Heilige Anna*; Lafontaine-Dosogne, *Iconographie de l'enfance de la Vierge*, vol. 1, passim.

232. Hackett, *History*, 458; Delehaye, "Saints de Chypre," 266; Meinardus, "Relics," 23.

233. Stylianou and Stylianou, *Painted Churches*, see index. For the images of Anna and Joachim in the naos of Asinou, see below, p. 225.

234. Stylianou and Stylianou, *Painted Churches*, 254.

Byzantine period.[235] Equally standard in art is the red of her maphorion.

St. Anna, who was associated with fertility and childbearing,[236] must have been the personal choice of the homonymous commissioner of the image, Anna Lachana (see below, p. 188). As well as being the object of private devotion, St. Anna, as mother of the Virgin, was also venerated for her role in preparing the incarnation and thus as a symbol par excellence of the salvation of humankind through the incarnate Christ. These symbolic, theological attributes of St. Anna are repeatedly underlined in the texts of the services of 9 September (Synaxis of Joachim and Anna), 9 December (Conception of St. Anna) and 25 July (her Dormition), as included in the Menaia.[237] In this context, a picture of St. Anna commissioned to express private piety is formally assimilated into the salvific program of the narthex.

Nine other saints—five male and four female—as well as the archangel Michael are painted in the northern part of the narthex. St. John of Damascus (ο ἅγι/ος / Ιω(άννης) / ὁ Δαμα/σκινος = ὁ ἅγιος Ἰωάννης ὁ Δαμασκηνός),[238] depicted on the south face of the northeast respond, is next to the Virgin of the Deesis with his head slightly turned toward her (Fig. 5.28). Dressed as a monk, in a *pallion* over the inner tunic, *koukoullion* (hood), and cloak (μανδύας), he has an *analabos* (scapular) hanging in front of his body and a turban on his head. Part of his face is obliterated, but traces of the raised decoration on his halo are still visible. He points toward the Virgin with his right hand and holds an inscribed scroll with his left.

Well known as a writer of theological works, John of Damascus (ca. 675 to ca. 749 or 753/54) was also a distinguished hymnographer and contributed significantly to the formulation of the Oktoechos or Parakletike.[239] The Orthodox Church celebrates his memory on 4 December. In the monumental painting of Cyprus, he occurs *en buste* in a medallion in the bema of Panagia tou Arakos at Lagoudera (1192) and in the church of Panagia Amasgou at Monagri (first quarter of the thirteenth century).[240] He is depicted in the bema of Asinou on the triumphal arch in the thirteenth-century layer opposite the Sacrifice of Isaac (see below, p. 218). In the fourteenth century, full-length images of him were painted on what was once the east wall of the narthex at Lagoudera and in the northwestern part of the central vessel in the church of the Holy Cross at Pelendri.[241] Relics were kept in the church of St. George in Limassol.[242]

In the narthex of Asinou, the text written on the open scroll of John of Damascus reads: Πηαν σει / ἑπάξοϊ/ō̃ν ὁδὴν / ἡ εἱμετέ/ρα προσΐ̄σι = Ποίαν σοι ἐπάξιον ᾠδὴν / ἡ ἡμετέρα προσοίσει. This is the beginning of a canon to the Theotokos sung on Sunday morning in the first mode (ἦχος α′). It is also included as a theotokion in the matins of 12 May, which is the feast day of Epiphanios, bishop of Cyprus.[243] The full text, clearly referring to the incarnation, is: ποίαν σοι ἐπάξιον ᾠδὴν, / ἡ ἡμετέρα προσοίσει ἀσθένεια; / εἰ μὴ τὴν χαρμόσυνον, / ἣν Γαβριὴλ ἡμᾶς ἐμυσταγώγησε·/ χαῖρε Θεοτόκε, παρθένε Μῆτερ ἀνύμφευτε (What praiseworthy

235. Mouriki, *Nea Moni*, 148–49, pls. 67, 69. In the naos of Asinou, St. Anna also holds a cross.
236. Gerstel, "Painted Sources for Female Piety," 96–98.
237. *Menaion*, 9 September, sticheron (p. 106): "Ἰωακεὶμ καὶ Ἄννα πανηγυρίζουσιν τὴν ἀπαρχὴν τεκόντες τῆς ἡμῶν σωτηρίας, τὴν μόνην Θεοτόκον," sticheron (p. 107): "τὴν Θεοτόκον βλαστήσαντες, ἐξ ἧς ἡ σωτηρία τῷ κόσμῳ ἀνέτειλε," ode 1 (p. 108): "σωτηρίας πάσης ἀρχηγοί, ὁ μακαριώτατος Ἰωακεὶμ καὶ ἡ Ἄννα," etc.
238. *BHG* 2:17–18; *BS* 6:732–40.
239. Arranz, "Grandes étapes de la liturgie byzantine," 54.
240. Nicolaïdès, "Étude iconographique," [1996], 30–32, fig. 30; Boyd, "Monagri," 314, fig. 46. On the iconography of the hymnographers, see N. P. Ševčenko, "Five Hymnographers at Nerezi"; Bakalova, "Hymnography and Iconography" (with previous bibliography).
241. Stylianou and Stylianou, *Painted Churches*, 184, 230; Zarras, *Holy Cross*, fig. 33.
242. Meinardus, "Relics," 32.
243. *Παρακλητικὴ ἤτοι Ὀκτώηχος ἡ Μεγάλη*, 46; Eustratiades, *Θεοτοκάριον*, 53; *Menaion*, 12 May, 85; cf. Follieri, *Initia Hymnorum*, 3:334.

ode will our weakness offer to you [other] than the cheerful one into which Gabriel initiated us? Rejoice, You who gave birth to God, Virgin, unmarried Mother).

The image of John of Damascus at Asinou is associated with the Virgin in many ways: visually, since he looks and points toward her; textually, through the words on his scroll alluding to the incarnation, and contextually, through his reputation as a great hymnographer of Mary. Among the works considered authentically his are one sermon dedicated to the Nativity of the Virgin and three sermons on her Dormition. He also wrote many hymns in honor of the Theotokos, which are included in liturgical books.[244] Twenty-one canons dedicated to the Virgin have been published in the *Theotokarion* of Sophronios Eustratiades.[245]

Further connotations link John of Damascus to the iconographic program of the narthex at Asinou. Certain of his hymns are included in the funerary service (ἀκολουθία τοῦ ἐξοδιαστικοῦ), which took place in the narthex of a Byzantine church.[246] In addition, during vespers on the eve of 4 December, the date of his commemoration, the ecclesiastical hymns include several invocations asking him to intervene for the salvation of our souls.[247] Most interesting is the ninth ode of the orthros of 4 December, containing an appeal to John of Damascus to intervene through his hymns praising the orders of the saints: the Virgin, the Forerunner, the apostles, the prophets, the ascetics, the wise teachers (hierarchs), the just, and the martyrs—i.e., all those who are visually included in the program of the narthex.[248] Thus John of Damascus is related not only to the Virgin but also to the intercessory role of the Deesis and the funerary connotations of the whole program of the narthex. At the same time, his image serves as a pendant to the praying figure of the homonymous saint John the Baptist, painted opposite him on the south respond next to Christ in the Deesis (see above, p. 157).

On the west face of the northeast respond, next to St. John of Damascus, is St. Sozomenos (ὁ / ἅγι/ος / Cο/ζώ/με/νος = ὁ ἅγιος Cωζόμενος), dressed as a monk and with a raised halo (Figs. 5.28, 5.30). The hagiographical tradition on St. Sozomenos is confusing, because three saints with this name are mentioned in texts relevant to Cyprus. It is possible that all three should be identified with a single saint with different cult centers on the island. St. Sozomenos Eleemosynarios or Eleemon is included among the three hundred Alaman saints.[249] Another St. Sozomenos is mentioned among saints of Karpasia in the synaxaria and in services written in 1733 by the monk Akakios.[250] A third saint of the same name is

244. PG 96:661–80, 699–762. For a discussion of the works of John of Damascus and their authenticity, see Beck, *Kirche und theologische Literatur*, 476–86; Nasrallah, *Saint Jean de Damas*, 137–60; Mitchel, *Mariology of Saint John Damascene*. For his liturgical hymns, see Nasrallah, *Jean de Damas*, 152–55.
245. Eustratiades, *Θεοτοκάριον*. According to a 14th-century typikon, a theotokion of Damaskenos should be sung in the *lite*, a service celebrated in the narthex of monastic churches: Jerusalem, Patr. Libr. 309, Dmitrievskij, *Opisanie*, 3:201, ll. 1–3. John of Damascus is, moreover, linked to the Virgin through a miraculous healing. According to the version of his *Life* written by John Chrysostomites, the 12th-century Patriarch of Jerusalem, John of Damascus's amputated arm was fixed "in the previous harmony" thanks to a miracle-working icon of the Virgin. See Kazhdan and Maguire, "Byzantine Hagiographical Texts," 3, 14; PG 94:457A–C.
246. PG 96:1368–69; Goar, *Euchologion*, 428–29 (ἀκολουθία νεκρώσιμος εἰς κοσμικούς). The Canon for the Deceased, PG 95:247–83, is not considered authentic and should instead be attributed to Michael Synkellos. See Beck, *Kirche*, 483; Nasrallah, *Jean de Damas*, 157.
247. *Menaion*, 4 December: "Ἱκέτευε τοῦ σωθῆναι τὰς ψυχὰς ἡμῶν" and "Πρέσβευε Χριστῷ τῷ Θεῷ σωθῆναι τὰς ψυχὰς ἡμῶν" (pp. 361–62).
248. Ibid. "Ἁγίων τὰ τάγματα, ὑμνολογήσας Ὅσιε, τὴν ἁγνὴν Θεοτόκον, Χριστοῦ τὸν Πρόδρομον, αὖθις Ἀποστόλους, Προφήτας σὺν Ἀσκηταῖς, σοφοὺς Διδασκάλους, Δικαίους καὶ Μάρτυρας, ἐν ταῖς τούτων νῦν αὐλίζει σκηναῖς" (p. 369).
249. See above, p. 161, and Kyrris, "Three Hundred Alaman Saints," 215.
250. Spyridakis, Papacharalampous, and Klerides, "Ἅγιοι," κθ′–λβ′ and 101–12. See also below, n. 256.

believed to have lived as a hermit close to Potamia before the tenth century, probably at the time of the Arab invasions of the late seventh century.[251] His fusion with St. Sozomenos Eleemon, also a victim of the Arab conquests, is thus explicable. His *asketerion* containing his grave has been preserved in a cave near Potamia.[252] Of the three fresco layers there—the oldest probably going back to the tenth or eleventh century—the third includes scenes from the life and miracles of St. Sozomenos. This has been attributed to the second quarter of the fourteenth century, close in date to the cycle of 1332/33 at Asinou. It is interesting to note that the prosopographic features of the eponymous saint in this layer are identical to those of St. Sozomenos at Asinou. Moreover, the style of the third layer, as has been pointed out by Athanasios Papageorgiou, is very close to that of the frescoes in the narthex of Asinou.[253] It seems that the renovation of the painted decoration of his cave in the second quarter of the fourteenth century was decisive for the diffusion of his cult in Cyprus. In fact, his image occurs very frequently in Cypriot churches thereafter, for example in the southeastern compartment of St. Nicholas of the Roof at Kakopetria (after mid-fourteenth century), in the church of the Holy Cross of Agiasmati at Platanistassa (1494), and at Galata in the church dedicated to him (1513) and in that of the Virgin (1514).[254]

St. Sozomenos of Potamia is celebrated on 21 November, the day of the Presentation of the Virgin in the Temple, a fact that explains his association with the Virgin, as Andréas Nicolaïdès and Catherine Vanderheyde have pointed out.[255] In addition, a service written in his honor praises him for his healing abilities and repeatedly asks him to intervene for the salvation of the faithful.[256] St. Sozomenos may well have been depicted in the narthex of Asinou not only as a miracle-working local saint and for his association with the Virgin but also because of the derivation of his name from the verb *σώζω* = save, which links him directly to the redemptive character of the program of the narthex.[257]

Following Sozomenos, to the east of the north door of the narthex, is the ARCHANGEL MICHAEL (ο αρχ(άγγελος) / Μιχ(αήλ)) in imperial garb and standing on a cushion (Figs. 5.28, 5.35). His image is one of the most impressive in the narthex.[258] In

251. Machairas, *Recital*, 1:30, §32; 70, §77; Delehaye, "Saints de Chypre," 252; Stavrobouniotes, "Άγιοι τής μητροπολιτικής περιφερείας Μόρφου," 215.
252. Stylianou and Stylianou, *Painted Churches*, 511–14; Papageorgiou, "Λαξευτά ἀσκητήρια καί μοναστήρια," 47–52. Nicolaïdès and Vanderheyde, "Topographie cultuelle," 252–54.
253. Among the six monastic figures of the first layer, now exhibited in the Museum of the Foundation of Archbishop Makarios III in Nicosia, there is a portrait of St. Sozomenos: see Papageorgiou, "Λαξευτά ἀσκητήρια καί μοναστήρια," 48, pl. 21. On the stylistic affinities between the third layer and the 14th-c. murals of the narthex of Asinou, ibid., 52.
254. Stylianou and Stylianou, *Painted Churches*, 71, 88, 95, 216. See also an icon from the monastery of St. John Chrysostom at Koutsovendis (late 15th c.), Talbot Rice, *Icons of Cyprus*, 168, 266–67, no. 139.
255. Nicolaïdès and Vanderheyde, "Topographie cultuelle," 254.
256. *Κύπρια Μηναῖα*, 21 November, 183–95, with bibliography; Klerides, "Άγιος Σωζόμενος." A service for St. Sozomenos of Karpasia, celebrated on 20 November, is included in the 18th-century text of Akakios: Spyridakis, Papacharalampous, and Klerides, "Άγιοι," 101–12. The text of this service is completely different from the akolouthia of St. Sozomenos of Potamia. St. Sozomenos's life is not included in the synaxarion of the Constantinopolitan church or in the Menaia.
257. For a similar concept with regard to the inclusion of SS. Polykarpos and Therapon among other hierarchs in church programs, probably on the basis of the power of their name to guarantee a rich crop or healing, see Gerstel, "Byzantine Village Church," 177–78; see also Safran, "Art of Veneration," 185.
258. On the iconography, see Lamy-Lasalle, "Archanges en costume impérial"; Maguire, "Murderer among the Angels"; Jolivet-Lévy, "Note sur la représentation"; cf. Parani, *Reconstructing the Reality of Images*, 42–50. Michael in imperial *loros* is a popular image on lead seals from the 10th century onward: see Cotsonis, "Contribution of Byzantine Lead Seals," 437–47. On the diamond pattern of Michael's *suppedium*, see Hadermann-Misguich, "Tissus de pouvoir."

his right hand he holds a staff, which forms a lance at its lower end and culminates at its upper end in a finial in the shape of a double lily, reminiscent of a scepter. The lower part of his *loros* merges into the embroidered hem of his tunic in a misunderstood rendering of the archangels' attire.[259] Traces of a raised halo are visible. Serious damage in the area of the left arm reveals an earlier fresco layer where the same subject was depicted at a larger scale. One can still see traces of the left wing, segments of the gemmed *loros*, and parts of the purple dalmatic studded with ivy leaves. Pigment analysis has shown that these fragments belong to a phase closer to the paintings of 1332/33 than to the murals of the twelfth century (see below, pp. 363–64). Thus, this early image of the archangel was probably one more ex-voto preceding the renovation of 1332/33.

Michael is very widely venerated in the Orthodox world.[260] According to the ecclesiastical calendar he is celebrated on 8 November (Synaxis ton Asomaton), as well as on 1 September (Joshua) and 6 September (the Miracle at Chonae). His cult was very widespread in Asia Minor, where it probably incorporated ancient cults. In Constantinople there were twenty-four churches dedicated to him, a number of which were connected to imperial patronage.[261]

Toponyms, churches dedicated to him, and numerous depictions in wall paintings and icons make clear Michael's popularity in Cyprus. Ten localities are named Ἀρχάγγελος and two Μιχαὴλ Ἀρχάγγελος or Ἅγιος Μίχαλος. At least six churches dedicated to Archangel Michael preserve their murals. Moreover, St. Neophytos the Recluse dedicated a panegyric (no. 3) to him.[262]

The archangel Michael, like the other archangels and angels, is mainly a minister of God who praises him unceasingly in heaven and is a messenger of his will on earth. But many other qualities are attributed to him, either by the official church and ecclesiastical hymnography or by popular belief. Michael is considered preeminently a protector of

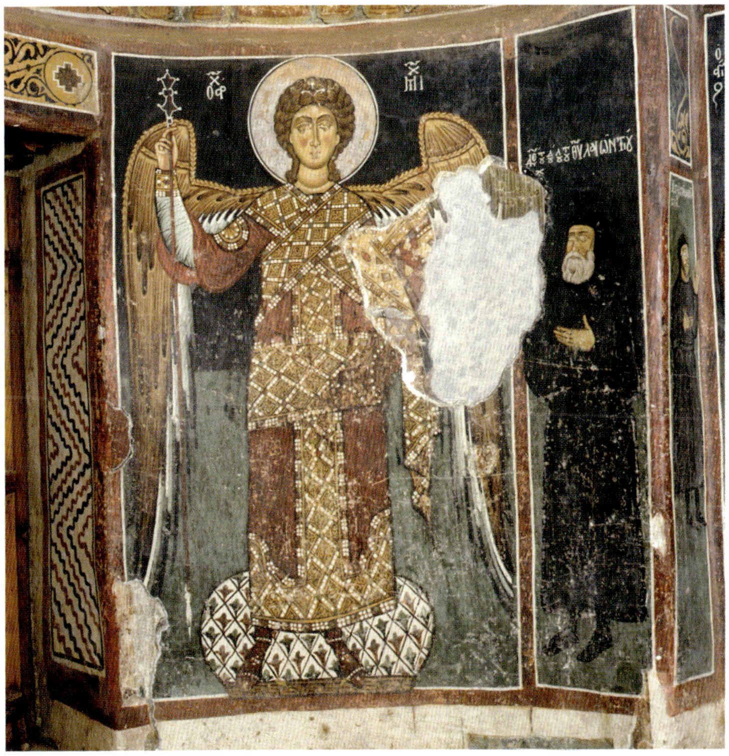

FIG. 5.35 Narthex, north conch. The archangel Michael and the monk Leontios (photo courtesy of courtesy of the Leventis Foundation and the Archaeological Research Unit, University of Cyprus, No. 006417)

259. For a correct rendering of the archangel's garments, see the figure of Michael in Panagia tou Arakos at Lagoudera, Nicolaïdès, "Étude iconographique," fig. 79.
260. J. Michl and T. Klauser, "Engel," *RAC* 5:243–351; Tatić-Djurić, *Bild der Engel*; Rohland, *Erzengel Michael*; D. I. Pallas, "Himmelsmächte, Erzengel und Engel," *RBK* 3:44–47; Martin-Hisard, "Le culte de l'archange Michel"; Peers, *Subtle Bodies*, 157–93.
261. On the diffusion of Michael's cult in Asia Minor and the possible fusion with Attis, see Mango, "St. Michael and Attis." On his cult in Cappadocia, see Jolivet-Lévy, "Culte et iconographie." On his cult in Syria, Canivet, "Michaelion de Huarte." On the churches in Constantinople, see Janin, *Les églises et les monastères*, 337–51; idem, "Sanctuaires byzantins de St. Michel"; Rohland, *Erzengel Michael*, 131–34; Jolivet-Lévy, "Culte et iconographie," 193.
262. Delehaye, "Saints de Chypre," 269; Stylianou and Stylianou, *Painted Churches*, passim; Papageorgiou, *Icons of Cyprus* [1992], figs. 13, 46, 50, 57, 66, 114; *Ἁγίου Νεοφύτου συγγράμματα*, 125–34.

the faithful against evil powers and a guardian of churches.[263] In this function he is depicted either in the narthex, as in the church of St. Nicholas of the Roof at Kakopetria (late thirteenth–early fourteenth century),[264] or close to or facing the entrance doors of churches, sometimes greater than life-size. Among Cypriot churches, the following examples may be mentioned: Panagia tou Arakos (1192, on the south wall opposite the entrance), Archangel Michael at Kato Lefkara (late twelfth–beginning of thirteenth century, traces to the right of the door on the south wall), St. Herakleidios in the monastery of St. John Lampadistes at Kalopanayiotis (ca. 1265–80, on the west wall, north of the entrance door), and the Panagia at Moutoullas (1280, on the north wall, opposite the south entrance door).[265] While regarded as a miracle-working healer, Archangel Michael is also associated with the cult of the dead, and many funerary chapels were dedicated to him.[266] He is, furthermore, connected with the hymn of the dying (εἰς ψυχορραγοῦντας) and is regarded as ψυχοπομπός, i.e., the companion of souls.[267] Moreover, Michael, like the other angels, is esteemed as an intercessor to God for humankind. The hymns included in the Menaion at 8 November often appeal to him to intercede for the redemption of the souls of the deceased.[268] In iconography the archangels often form part of the Great Deesis and are always depicted as part of the heavenly court in scenes of the Last Judgment, as they are in the vault of Asinou's narthex (see above, pp. 133–35). In all of these capacities, Michael takes a meaningful place in the narthex at Asinou.

To the west of the north door are the figures of the twin brothers Cosmas and Damian (ὁ / ἅγι/ος / Κοσ/μ/ας and ὁ / ἅγι/ος / Δα/μι/ἀνὸς), who are identically dressed and who each hold a medicine box in the left hand and a lancet in the right (Figs. 5.19, 5.28; for their images in the naos, see below, pp. 251, 254). The hagiographical traditions concerning the lives of SS. Cosmas and Damian became so complex that the tenth-century synaxarion of the Constantinopolitan church mentions three pairs of brother-doctors with their names. All were celebrated as *anargyroi* (unmercenary), because they practiced their profession without accepting money.[269] Their feast days were on 17 October, 1 July, and 1 November.

The twins that scholars now regard as the original pair were probably born in Arabia, went to Syria to study medicine, and suffered martyrdom

263. Xyngopoulos, "Ἀρχάγγελος Μιχαήλ"; Dölger, "Justinians Engel"; Tatić-Djurić, "Archanges gardiens."
264. Stylianou and Stylianou, *Painted Churches*, 66.
265. Nicolaïdès, "Étude iconographique," 111–12, fig. 79; Papageorgiou, "Ἐκκλησία τοῦ Ἀρχαγγέλου," 225, pl. 38; Young, "Byzantine Painting," 199–201; Mouriki, "Moutoullas," 198, fig. 17.
266. Mango, "St. Michael," 47ff.; Bakalova, "Cycle of the Holy Archangels," 217–18. On the funerary connotations, see *RAC* 5:249–50 (J. Michl); Stichel, *Verhältnis von Text und Bild*, 39; Rohland, *Erzengel Michael*, 31–32; Grabar, *Martyrium*, 1:87–88, 97.
267. Ἀνδρέα Κρήτης, Ἀκολουθία εἰς ψυχορραγοῦντα, Goar, *Euchologion*, 585–87; H. Leclercq, "Les anges psychopompes," in *DACL* 1–2:2130–41; Cumont, "Les vents et les Anges"; Heiser, *Engel im Glauben der Orthodoxie*, 176–86; Meinardus, "Erzengel Michael als psychopompos." Cf. a sticheron in the vespers of 6 September, "Μιχαὴλ . . . ἐν ὥρᾳ, Ἀρχάγγελε, τῇ τοῦ θανάτου σὺ πάρεσο βοηθός," *Menaion*, 6 September, 65. In the *Apocalypse of Anastasia*, it is Michael who leads the nun Anastasia to the other world: see Baun, *Tales from Another Byzantium*, 402–3. In iconography Michael sometimes appears holding the scales of the deceased, as, for example, on an icon in the Museo Civico in Pisa (end of 13th c.), Lazarev, *Storia*, 323, fig. 446.
268. *Menaion*, 8 November. *Lite*, stichera idiomela (pp. 77–78), "[Μιχαὴλ] . . . πρεσβεύει σωθῆναι τὰς ψυχὰς ἡμῶν." ". . . διὸ πρεσβεύσατε, σωθῆναι τὰς ψυχὰς ἡμῶν." ". . . ἵνα πρεσβεύῃ ἀπαύστως ὑπὲρ τῶν ψυχῶν ἡμῶν," etc.
269. (a) The pair from Arabia beheaded under Diocletian and Maximian, commemorated on 17 October; (b) the pair from Rome stoned to death in 284, commemorated on 1 July; and (c) the sons of Theodote from Asia Minor who died in peace, commemorated on 1 November: see Delehaye, *Synaxarium*, cols. 144–46, 792, 185–86. For the hagiographical tradition and cult of the *anargyroi*, see Deubner, *Kosmas und Damian*; Rupprecht, *Vita et miracula*; Festugière, *Saints Côme et Damien*, 83–213; *BHG* 1:126–36; *BS* 4:223–37; Wittman, *Kosmas und Damian*.

under Diocletian.[270] A revival of their cult occurred in Palaiologan times when Theodora, widow of Michael VIII, restored one of their churches and when the deacon Maximos, sometime after 1305/6, rewrote and supplemented their miracles for the Kosmidion, an early Christian monastery and healing shrine near Blachernai, which was dedicated to them and often mentioned in Palaiologan sources.[271]

Images of SS. Cosmas and Damian appear very frequently in the painted churches of Cyprus from the eleventh and twelfth centuries (St. Anthony at Kellia, Panagia tou Arakos at Lagoudera, Christ Antiphonetes at Kalogrea) through the sixteenth;[272] still earlier is the example of an icon from the church of Panagia Chrysaliniotissa in Nicosia attributed to the tenth century.[273] Their effigies appear, moreover, in a steatite reliquary diptych, now in the museum of the cathedral at Mdina in Malta, which has been assigned to a Cypriot workshop of the first half of the fourteenth century.[274] Relics of the two saints were kept in the Cypriot monasteries of Machairas, of Kykkos, and of the Chrysorroiatissa in the district of Paphos, and a panegyric (no. 18) of St. Neophytos was dedicated to them.[275]

In the Menaia, SS. Cosmas and Damian are praised as healers of bodies and souls.[276] Their placement next to the scene of the Anastasis at Lagoudera (1192) or on both sides of a tomb niche in the cave church of Palaia Enkleistra at Kouklia (after 1442) seems to corroborate their association with curing souls and securing redemption.[277] Thus the images of Cosmas and Damian take up themes introduced by the late thirteenth-century panel of Anastasia Pharmakolytria, sharing with her the same connotations of healing and salvation that resonate throughout the iconographic program of the narthex. Moreover, the capacity of the Holy Anargyroi to heal animals as well as humans, related to the rural milieu of the monastery church at Asinou,[278] responds contextually to the image of St. Mamas and harmonizes with the hippiatros inscription of the late twelfth-century St. George fresco (see above, pp. 82–83, 161–64).

Three female saints—Marina, Eudokia, and Paraskeve—are depicted next to the Anargyroi. St. Marina (ἡ / ἁγί/α / Μα/ρί/ν/α) (Figs. 5.19, 5.28), a third-century martyr from Antioch in

270. *BS* 4:223–24; Mango, "Cult of Saints Cosmas and Damian," 190.
271. On the church dedicated to SS. Cosmas and Damian, built ca. 480 outside the city wall near Blachernai, see Janin, *Églises*, 286–89; Mango, "Cult of Saints Cosmas and Damian," 189–92. On the Kosmidion in the Palaiologan period and Maximos, see Talbot, "Healing Shrines," 7–9; eadem, *Metaphrasis*. On the saints' veneration beyond the capital in the East and the West, see Esbroeck, "Diffusion orientale"; idem, "Légende 'romaine'"; Falla Castelfranchi, "Culto e immagini."
272. On the iconography of SS. Cosmas and Damian, see David-Danel, *Iconographie des saints médecins*; Skrobucha, *Kosmas und Damian*; cf. Xyngopoulos, "Ἀνάγλυφον τῶν Ἁγίων Ἀναργύρων." For a discussion on the iconography of all medical saints known as *anargyroi*, see Koukiares, "Ζεύγη τῶν Ἁγίων Ἀναργύρων"; Abp. Damianos of Sinai, "Medical Saints," 42–44. For middle Byzantine Cypriot examples, see Nicolaïdès, "Étude iconographique," 125–26; Stylianou and Stylianou, *Painted Churches*, 171, 184, 436, 472; for later examples, ibid., 136, 215, 222, 244, 273, 320, 328, 346, 379, 431; Gabelić, "Kophinou," 149.
273. Papageorgiou, *Icons of Cyprus* [1992], 9, figs. 4, 4a.
274. See note 8, above.
275. Delehaye, "Saints de Chypre," 290–91; Meinardus, "Relics," 26–27; Galatariotou, *Making of a Saint*, 264; *Ἁγίου Νεοφύτου συγγράμματα*, 347–50.
276. *Menaion*, 1 November, Sticheron idiomelon in vespers (p. 5): "θεράποντας ἰατροὺς ψυχῶν τε καὶ σωμάτων," Ode 3 and 5 in matins (pp. 6, 8): "σωμάτων τε καὶ ψυχῶν ὡς ἰατρεύοντες πάθη," "τῆς ψυχῆς καὶ τοῦ σώματος θεραπεύοντες νόσους," kathisma in matins (p. 7): "ἰατρεῖον τῶν ψυχῶν," sticheron idiomelon of Theophanes in matins (p. 14): "ἰατρεύοντες τὰ πάθη τῶν ψυχῶν καὶ τῶν σωμάτων ἡμῶν," stichera of Oktoechos (p. 15): "ἰατρεῖον τῶν ψυχῶν καὶ τῶν σωμάτων ἡμῶν." Similar expressions occur in the Menaion of 1 July as well as in the Cypriot Menaia.
277. Nicolaïdès, "Étude iconographique," 126; Stylianou and Stylianou, *Painted Churches*, 398.
278. Delehaye, *Synaxarium*, col. 792: "ἀνθρώποις καὶ κτήνεσι παρέχοντες τὰς ἰάσεις." *Menaion*, 1 November, automelon in vespers (p. 3): "ἀνθρώποις τε καὶ κτήνεσι τῆς εὐεργεσίας μετέδωκαν."

Pisidia, was tortured, imprisoned, and beheaded for her faith during the reign of Diocletian (d. 305). Her Vita is included in the synaxarion of the Constantinopolitan church, while her relics were sheltered in a monastery outside Constantinople and removed to Venice in 1213. In the West she is venerated as St. Margaret.[279] The Orthodox Church celebrates her memory on 17 July. In Byzantine iconography she is usually represented dressed in a red maphorion and holding the cross of martyrdom, as at Asinou, while she is occasionally depicted slaying Satan.[280]

Sometimes confused with this Marina was a second virgin-martyr with the name of Marina (alias Marinos) who lived in Syria in the fifth century. While still a child she entered the monastery Deir el-Qannoubine in the Qadisha Valley, today in Lebanon, with her widowed father. After his death she remained in the monastery disguised in male garments. Accused of having relations with a young woman who bore a child, she preferred not to deny the act, and by hiding her sex she was consequently submitted to the most severe penitence. She was greatly admired and venerated when, after her death, the monks discovered her secret. St. Marina of Syria appears more rarely in Byzantine art than does Marina of Pisidia, and her Vita is not included in the synaxarion of the Constantinopolitan church.[281] Images of the two homonymous saints are depicted on the columns of the Basilica of the Nativity in Bethlehem (ca. 1160), where they bear Greek and Latin inscriptions, thus revealing the importance of their cult in the Crusader Levant in both eastern and western religious contexts.[282]

St. Marina of Pisidia was highly venerated not only in the Crusader states and Sinai but also in Cyprus, where at least nineteen locations are named after her.[283] St. Neophytos the Recluse delivered an encomium in her honor on her feast day in a church dedicated to her, while relics of St. Marina were kept in the monasteries of Kykkos, Machairas, and Koutsovendis.[284] St. Marina is often depicted in Cypriot churches from the thirteenth century onward. Among the earlier images are those on the south wall of the church of the Panagia at Kophinou (twelfth–thirteenth century), the west wall at Moutoullas (1280), and on the southwest pier at St. Herakleidios in the monastery of St. John Lampadistes at Kalopanayiotis (ca. 1265–80).[285] In churches of the fourteenth through the sixteenth centuries, St. Marina is often depicted on the west wall next to St. Paraskeve.[286] Moreover, the popularity of St. Marina on the island is revealed by the number of icons, especially Vita icons, that have come down to us. Most notable are the Vita icon of ambiguous date in the Byzantine Museum of the Bishopric of Paphos, two thirteenth-century Vita icons of St. Marina—including the very well-known example from Pedoulas (ca. 1280)—now in the Museum of the Foundation of Archbishop Makarios III, and one from the church of St. Marina

279. Usener, *Acta S. Marinae et S. Christophori*, 15–46; *BHG* 2:84–86; *BS* 8:1150–65; Delehaye, *Synaxarium*, col. 825.
280. Ross and Downey, "Reliquary of St. Marina"; Lafontaine-Dosogne, "Un thème iconographique."
281. *BHG* 2:83; *BS* 8:1165–70; Patlagean, "Femme déguisée en moine."
282. Kühnel, *Wall Painting*, 105–12, fig. 74, pl. 30/51; Folda, "Saint Marina Icon," 107–9, 118, nn. 5, 6, and 53.
283. Folda, "Marina," 116ff. On the chapel dedicated to St. Marina attached to the north side of the church of St. Catherine and on a number of Crusader icons of St. Marina of Pisidia at St. Catherine's monastery on Mount Sinai, ibid., 117, figs. 109–11, nn. 50–51. For Cyprus, see Delehaye, "Saints de Chypre," 267.
284. Delehaye, "Saints," 278. For extracts of the encomium, see Tsiknopoullos, "Ἐγκώμιον εἰς Μαρῖναν"; idem, "Ἅγιοι τῆς Κύπρου," 160–61. On the relics, see Meinardus, "Relics," 34 (for Kykkos and Machairas); Mango and Hawkins, "Report on Field Work," 334, n. 58 (for Koutsovendis).
285. Gabelić, "Kophinou," 146–47, fig. 2; Mouriki, "Panagia at Moutoullas," 107, figs. 25–26; Young, "Byzantine Painting," 205–6; Connor, "Female Saints," 217, fig. 7. For images in other Cypriot churches, see Mouriki, "Cypriot Saints," 252–53.
286. Stylianou and Stylianou, *Painted Churches*, 96, 218, 254, 273; Connor, "Female Saints," 218–21, figs. 8, 9, 11, 27.

at Kyperounda.[287] St. Marina's triumphal victory over Satan serves as a model of salvation for the faithful, and this aspect of her life may offer the link to the iconographic program of the narthex.[288]

The image of St. Eudokia (ἡ / ἁγί/α / Εὐ/δο/κί/α, Fig. 5.19) is rare, if not unique, in Cypriot monumental painting.[289] Of the three saints with this name who are celebrated in the Orthodox church, the St. Eudokia at Asinou should probably be identified with the third-century martyr born in Helioupolis (Baalbek) and commemorated on 1 March. Her life is included in the synaxarion of the Constantinopolitan church.[290] A woman of extreme beauty, Eudokia first led the life of a prostitute; when she later converted to Christianity, she began a new life of austere penance. Her Vita includes resurrection miracles, and this link to resurrection, as well as the emphasis on penitence and redemption in the Menaion on her feast day of 1 March,[291] accord well with the salvific content of the narthex program. It may well be these associations that led to the inclusion of this rarely depicted saint in the cycle of Asinou's narthex.

St. Paraskeve (ἡ / ἁγί/α / Παρα/σκ(ε)βΐ = ἡ ἁγία Παρασκευή) holds before her chest a medallion with a bust of the dead Christ in the type of the Man of Sorrows (Figs. 5.28, 5.36). A cross is painted behind the figure of Christ and on both sides of his head can be read the sigla Ι(ησοῦ)ς Χ(ριστό)ς. The red striations on this figure were made by candle flames and attest to the fact that it was venerated intensively.

Born and martyred in second-century Rome, she was named Paraskeve, i.e. Friday, because she was born on a Friday. Her Vita is included in the synaxarion of the Constantinopolitan church. Her cult was widespread not only in Byzantium but also in southern Italy, where she is known by the name of Venera or Veneranda.[292]

This iconographic type, St Paraskeve holding the icon of the Man of Sorrows before her, is regarded as the allegorical personification of Good Friday.[293] It was very popular in late

287. Papageorgiou, *Icons of Cyprus* [1992], 8–9, fig. 2; idem, *Ιερά Μητρόπολις Πάφου*, 147, fig. 91; Sophocleous, *Icons of Cyprus*, 75, no. 1a (this icon has been dated to the 7th–9th century [?] but is probably later); Papageorgiou, *Ιερά Μητρόπολις Πάφου*, 55, fig. 34; Mouriki, "Thirteenth-Century," 36–37, figs. 37, 43; *Ἱερὰ Μητρόπολις Μόρφου*, 134. Sophocleous, *Icônes de Chypre*, 74–75, 195, no. 98. See also a 13th-c. icon of St. Marina (?) from Panagia Amasgou at Monagri: Sophocleous, *Icônes de Chypre*, 156–57, 243–44, no. 227.

288. Moreover, there is a local tradition in Cyprus that she was capable of curing insomnia. See Talbot Rice, *Icons of Cyprus*, 167.

289. See Stylianou and Stylianou, *Painted Churches*, Index.

290. Delehaye, *Synaxarium*, cols. 498–99. See also *BHG* 1:183–84; *BS* 5:145–47. The other two saints under the same name are the Athenian Eudokia Augusta, married to Theodosios II in 421 (feastday 13 August), see Delehaye, *Synaxarium*, col. 890; and the martyr Eudokia, who suffered in Persia in the 4th c. (feastday 4 August), ibid., col. 868, 31. For the saints honored by the Orthodox Church under the name of Eudokia, see Gerstel, "Saint Eudokia," 700–701.

291. Latyšev, *Menologii Anonymi Byzantini*, 1:158–65. *Menaion*, 1 March, *Synaxarion* (pp. 5–7). Relics belonging to her or to Eudokia Augusta were kept in the Kykkos monastery. See Meinardus, "Relics," 29.

292. *BHG* 2:170–72; *BS* 10:328–32; Delehaye, *Synaxarium*, cols. 344–45. For the meaning of the name, the different saints Paraskeve, and their iconographies and attributes, see Walter, "Portrait of Saint Paraskeve." For the homonymous saint in Epibatai (10th c.?), whose feastday is 14 October and who became very popular in the Balkans under the name of Petka, see Zeses, "Ἁγία Παρασκευή"; Bakalova, "Vie de sainte Parascève"; Popović, *Pod okriljem svetosti*, 271–93, 354–56 (English abstract). For St. Paraskeve, born in Ikonion and venerated in Russia, see Koukiares, *Κύκλος τοῦ βίου τῆς ἁγίας Παρασκευῆς*, 118–27. See also Onasch, "Paraskeva-Studien."

293. She was already associated with the allegorical figure of Good Friday in the middle Byzantine period. St. Paraskeve holding the instruments of the Passion is illustrated in the second oration for Easter in the Homilies of Gregory of Nazianzus (Paris. gr. 510, fol. 285r), dated to 879–83. See Der Nersessian, "Illustrations of the Homilies," 201–2, pl. 3; Young, "Byzantine Painting," 202; Gerstel, "Female Piety," 100; Brubaker, *Vision and Meaning*, 205, fig. 29. Cf. Pallas, *Passion und Bestattung*, 200–201.

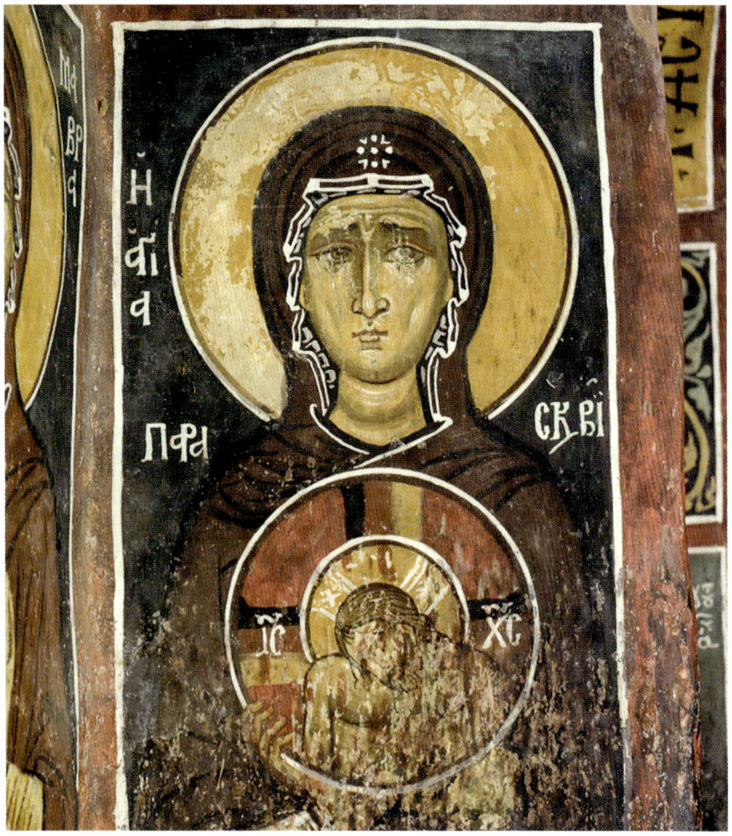

FIG. 5.36 Narthex, northwest respond. St. Paraskeve and Man of Sorrows (photo courtesy of the Leventis Foundation and the Archaeological Research Unit, University of Cyprus, No. 006321)

medieval Cypriot art: among the earliest examples are those in the churches of St. Herakleidios in the Monastery of St. John Lampadistes at Kalopanayiotis (ca. 1265–80), and of the Holy Cross at Pelendri (mid-fourteenth century); it also appears on icons.[294] Moreover, relics of St. Paraskeve are kept in the monasteries of Kykkos, Machairas, and St. Barbara, and nine Cypriot sites are named after her.[295]

In the Menaion at 26 July, the date of St. Paraskeve's commemoration, an appeal is made to her several times, especially in the Vespers service, to intercede with Christ on the Day of Judgment to save the souls of the faithful.[296] An indication of her role on the Day of Judgment is her inclusion in the tenth-century *Apocalypse of Anastasia*, where she appears, among others, before the throne of the Almighty as an accuser of the sinful.[297] The belief in St. Paraskeve's efficacy in intercession and the connection with the services of Good Friday and Christ's death—both through her name and through the iconography of the Man of Sorrows—link her portrait to the iconographic context of the narthex.

Images of SS. Timotheos and Mavra (ο αγι(ος) / Τη/μόθε/ος and η / ἁγί/α / Μά/βρ/α) share the framed rectangle on the west wall of the narthex, just north of the entrance door (Figs. 5.19, 5.28). They are shown glancing toward one another. Timotheos, depicted as a beardless youth holding a closed codex and a cross, was an ecclesiastical reader (τῶν ἱερῶν βίβλων ὑφηγητής) in a town

294. Stylianou and Stylianou, *Painted Churches,* 86, 96, 298, 231, 337; Young, "Byzantine Painting," 201–3, 392; Connor, "Female Saints," 219–21, figs. 12, 15, 23, 27; Papageorgiou, *Icons of Cyprus* [1992], 63, fig. 41; idem, *Ιερά Μητρόπολις Πάφου*, 175, fig. 111; Mouriki, "Cypriot Saints," 253–54, fig. 21. For Cypriot images of St. Paraskeve, see also Triantaphyllopoulos, "Τέχνη στὴν Κύπρο," 627–28.

295. Meinardus, "Relics," 37; Delehaye, "Saints de Chypre," 267.

296. *Menaion*, 26 July, at Vespers (p. 224): Παρασκευὴ πανένδοξε, τοὺς τὴν ἄθλησιν τὴν σὴν ἑορτάζοντας ἀξίως, αἴτησαι ῥυσθῆναι πειρασμῶν καὶ θλίψεων, ταῖς πρὸς Θεὸν πρεσβείαις σου, καὶ τῆς μελλούσης κρίσεως.... (p. 225): Παρασκευὴ ἀοίδιμε καὶ νῦν πρέσβευε τὸν Σωτῆρα τῶν ὅλων λύσιν δοῦναι ὀφλημάτων τοῖς ἐν πίστει ἐπιτελοῦσι τὴν μνήμην σου.... ἱκέτευε τοῦ σωθῆναι τὰς ψυχὰς ἡμῶν. It should be noted that in the Menaion there is no connection whatsoever of St. Paraskeve to Good Friday.

297. Baun, "Middle Byzantine 'Tours of Hell'," 47; eadem, *Tales from Another Byzantium*, 403, 405–6, §12–14, 25–28. According to an ambiguous fourteenth-century Slavic text of her vita, St. Paraskeve is considered a protector of cultivations and animals, a quality that links her to the agricultural environment of the monastery of Asinou and to St. Mamas depicted in the south conch of the narthex. See Subotić, *Sveti Konstantin i Jelena,* 92; Koukiares, *Κύκλος τοῦ βίου τῆς ἁγίας Παρασκευῆς*; Abp. Damianos, "Medical Saints," 47–48.

of Upper Egypt; hence the holy book is his attribute. He refused to obey the command of Arrianos, prefect of the Thebaid, to burn the sacred books, and was consequently tortured and put to death along with his new bride, Mavra, in the year 286. Their Vita is included in the synaxarion of the Constantinopolitan church, where there is no mention of any connection with Cyprus; they are commemorated on 3 May.[298]

According to Cypriot tradition, however, Timotheos and Mavra were martyred in Cyprus. The center of their cult is a monastery close to Koilani, where the water of the *hagiasma* (holy water fountain) is considered a remedy against fever.[299] Relics of St. Mavra are kept in the monastery of Machairas and five localities are named after her.[300]

St. Mavra is depicted in Cypriot monumental painting either alone, as on the west wall of the church of the Panagia at Moutoullas (1280), or, in most cases, together with her husband Timotheos, as in the narthex of Asinou and in a large composition surrounded by scenes of their martyrdom on the south wall of their monastery church at Koilani (late fifteenth century). Moreover, a thirteenth-century icon of Timotheos and Mavra is exhibited in the Ecclesiastical Museum of Koilani.[301]

The fourteenth-century sanctoral cycle of the narthex of Asinou—with its archangel, its eight male saints, and its six female saints—incorporated into its circuit both the late twelfth-century figure of St. George on horseback and the late thirteenth-century panel of St. Anastasia Pharmakolytria. At the same time, it covered over certain older murals, which presumably represented—at least partially—the same subjects, as attested by the traces of an archangel under the fourteenth-century figure of Michael. Female saints, though fewer in number and relegated to the western part of the narthex, are nonetheless equal in importance to male saints, thanks to the conspicuous panels of SS. Anastasia and Anna with their respective devotees. As usual, the majority of the saints of the fourteenth-century phase are celebrated between September and December.

Aside from the universal Byzantine saints, such as Demetrios, Anna, and Marina, the sanctoral cycle of the narthex embraces a number of saints who, although known in Byzantine iconography and included in the synaxarion of the Constantinopolitan church, are associated with the Cypriot hagiographical tradition and with local cult centers. Mamas, Timotheos, and Mavra belong to this group. In addition, SS. Sozomenos, George Machairomenos, and Irene, daughter of the Cypriot bishop Spyridon, represent purely local saints. The choice of local saints contrasts sharply with the saints represented in the naos, most of whom are well-known and widely venerated figures (see Chapter 6). This selection in the narthex seems to reflect the preferences of the donors—monastic and lay—whose portraits are distributed among the saints' images. Lay donors in particular seem to have a predilection for homonymous saints (thus Anastasia, George, and Anna). It is interesting to note, furthermore, that, despite the monastic character of the foundation and the dominant monastic patronage, only two monastic saints—Sozomenos and John of Damascus—are depicted. Another significant feature of the sanctoral cycle in the narthex at Asinou is the inclusion of saints who are venerated by both Greeks and Latins, such as George, Mamas, Paraskeve/Veneranda, and Marina/Margaret.

Themes of physical and spiritual restitution appropriate to a funerary and redemptive context stand out. The choice of St. Mamas, the protector of

298. *BHG* 2:306; *BS* 12:496–97; Delehaye, *Synaxarium*, cols. 649–52.
299. Hackett, *History*, 397–98; Delehaye, "Saints de Chypre," 272. On the monastery church, see Stylianou and Stylianou, *Painted Churches*, 236–37. On the *hagiasma* see Kyprianos, *Ἱστορία*, 528.
300. Meinardus, "Relics," 35; Delehaye, "Saints de Chypre," 267.
301. Mouriki, "Moutoullas," 196, fig. 24; eadem, "Cypriot Saints," 251–52. Stylianou and Stylianou, *Painted Churches*, 236; Papageorgiou, *Icons of Cyprus* [1992], 33, fig. 19; Sophocleous, *Icons of Cyprus*, 86–87, 147–48, no. 21; idem, *Icônes de Chypre*, 64–65, 189, no. 84.

sheep, reflects the agricultural milieu of the monastery church at Asinou. But at the same time, Mamas was regarded in Cypriot legend as a healer of people, and so is linked—along with the Holy Anargyroi and St. Anastasia, preeminent healers of body and soul—to the salvific context of the narthex cycle. Soteriological connotations are expressed, as well, by two female saints whose representation is rare, if not unique: both Irene, daughter of Spyridon, and Eudokia are associated with resurrection miracles. The funerary character of the program is corroborated by the depiction of the archangel Michael, the chief companion of souls (ψυχοπομπός), and by the mourning figure of St. Paraskeve, related to Good Friday and to Christ's passion, death, and burial. Moreover, the depiction of female saints in Byzantine narthexes reflects, according to Sharon Gerstel, actual customs and rites taking place in the narthex and should be linked to the involvement of women in the lamentation of the dead.[302]

In sum, the entire choir of saints depicted in the lower zone of the narthex—male and female, universal and local—with John the Baptist and John of Damascus at their head, join their intercessions to the prayers of the Virgin and address them to Christ Eleemon for the salvation of the donors who are painted among them and of the entire congregation.[303]

Inscription and Donor Portraits

Dedicatory Inscription

The dedicatory inscription is located on the lintel over the entrance door from the narthex to the naos (Figs. 5.37, 3.11). Over sixty percent of it is destroyed. The lintel is heavily layered: one can see the bare wooden beam itself, a first layer of plaster, which once covered the beam and displayed a pattern of painted roundels from the twelfth century (see below, p. 192), and a second layer of plaster on which the dedicatory inscription is painted. The inscription consists of two lines; it is painted in white uncial characters on red ground. It is in prose and has spelling mistakes in about fifteen percent of the preserved syllables. The text runs as follows:

> Ἀνιστ[ορήθη . . .] ẹν τῆς αὐτις μονῖς κ(αὶ) Θεοφιλου [. . .] κ(αὶ) κινοῦ / λαοῦ [. . .] οτερ [. . .] κ(αὶ) τάχα ἡστοριόγράφου ἵπο πονο(υ) τρ [. . .] ἀμὴν⁝ / ἔτο(υς) ,ϛω/μα / ινδ(ικτιῶνος) α = Ἀνιστ[ορήθη . . .] ἐν τῆς αὐτῆς μονῆς κ(αὶ) Θεοφίλου [. . .] καὶ κοινοῦ λαοῦ [. . .] οτερ[. . .] καὶ τάχα ἱστοριογράφου ὑπὸ πόνου τρ[. . .] ἀμὴν, ἔτους ,ϛω/μα' ἰνδικτιῶνος α'.

> It was repainted . . . of this same monastery and of Theophilos . . . and the common people . . . and so-called painter through the pains (labor) . . . amen. In the year 6841 [= 1332/33], first indiction.[304]

Accents and breathings are systematically indicated. There are few minuscule letters, for example α in the indication of the date.

Punctuation: three dots, one on top of the other, after amen.

Ligatures: L.1: αν, στ, τη, αυ, ου; L. 2: ου, στ, γρ, τρ, αμην.

Abbreviations: ϗ = καὶ

The inscription, although preserved only fragmentarily, includes some important information.

- L. 1. Ἀνιστορήθη: It refers to a repainting.
- L. 1. Μονῆς. It testifies that the church functioned as a monastery in the fourteenth century.
- L. 1/2. Θεοφίλου καὶ κοινοῦ λαοῦ: Among those who commissioned the repainting, the name of Theophilos and a reference to the common people have been preserved.
- L. 1. The Bucklers in 1933, when the inscription was better preserved, had read an eta

302. Gerstel, "Female Piety," 99–103.

303. On the belief in the intermediary function of the images of the saints as formulated by the iconophiles and established after Iconoclasm, see Maguire, *Icons of their Bodies*, 138–39.

304. Stylianou and Stylianou, "Donors and Dedicatory Inscriptions," 104–5; Kalopissi-Verti, "Painters," 145, fig. 9.

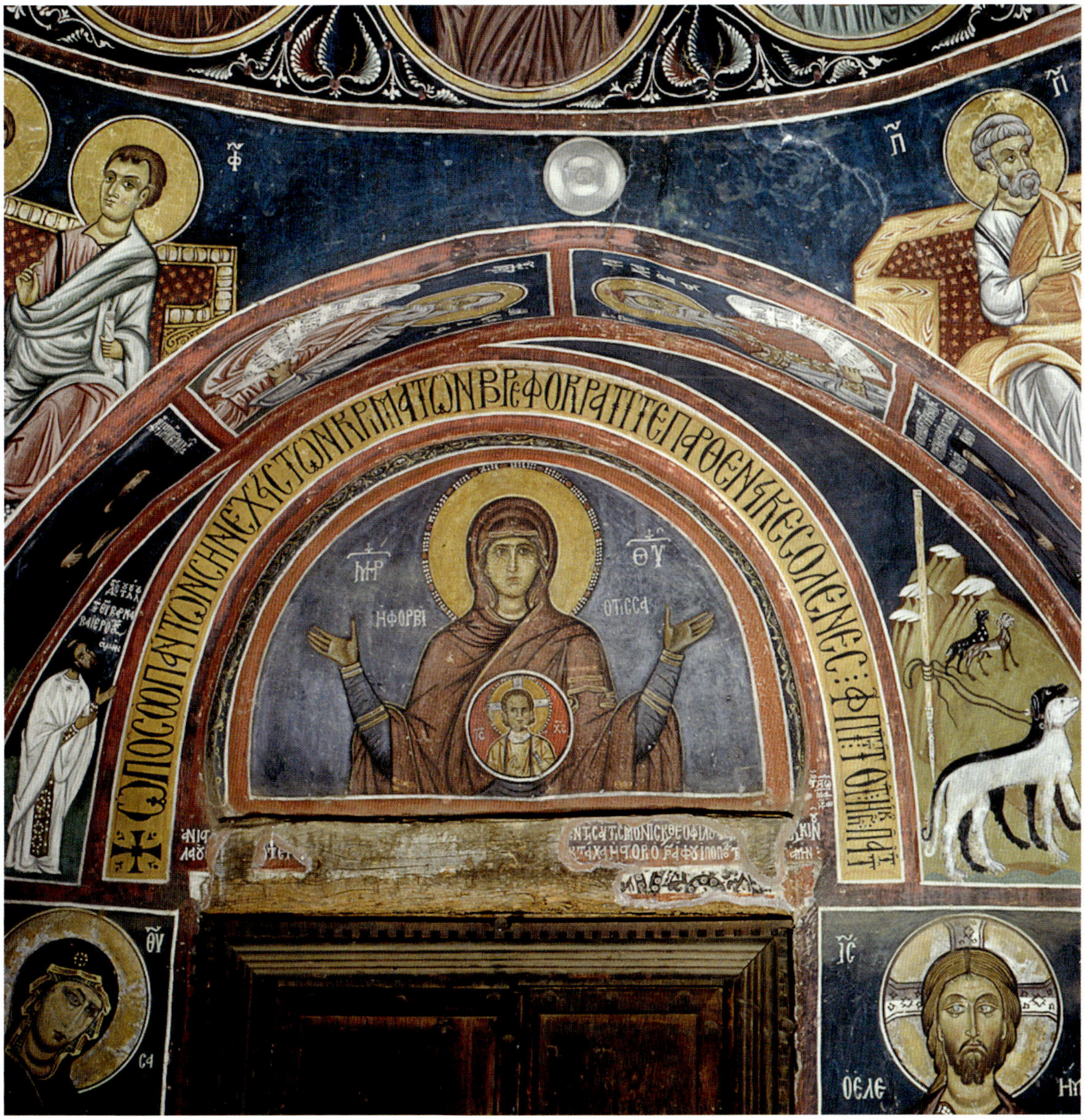

FIG. 5.37 Narthex, east lunette. Virgin Phorbiotissa and Dedicatory Inscription. East wall: the priest-monk Barnabas on the left, hounds and mouflons on the right. Face of arch: inscription (photo courtesy of the Leventis Foundation and the Archaeological Research Unit, University of Cyprus, No. 006393)

after Theophilos, which they completed as ἡ[γούμενος] (abbot).[305] However, the inscription accompanying Theophilos's portrait, which is preserved in a very good condition, does not mention that he was an abbot (see below, p. 182). Nor is there any mention of an abbot with the name of Theophilos in the fourteenth-century obituaries noted in the Synaxarium Par. Gr. 1590, possessed by the monastery of Panagia Phorbiotissa.[306]

- L. 2. Ἱστοριογράφου: The name of the painter was apparently cited but has not been preserved.

305. Buxton et al., "Church of Asinou," 336.

306. Darrouzès, "Notes", 86. See above, pp. 17–18, 25–27.

The date of completion of the wall paintings is recorded with smaller letters in the right margin: 6841 = A.D. 1332/33.

The Theophilos named in the inscription can probably be identified with the deceased monk by the same name who is depicted in a prominent position over Christ Eleemon on the south part of the soffit of the eastern arch (Fig. 5.40, discussed below, pp. 181–82). As we learn from church inscriptions, it was common practice in the late Byzantine period for a priest or monk to take the initiative in founding or renovating a church, followed by groups of predominantly lay people. Small-scale portraits of the most prominent of the "common" people mentioned in the inscription are painted among the figures of saints (below, pp. 179–90, 207). Thus the narthex of Asinou represents a typical example of collective patronage. It is not unique in Cyprus. Paris. gr. 301, a Gospel Lectionary of 1204 from the church of St. Epiphanios at Kouboukleia (today Kouklia) near Paphos, contains on folio 316v a marginal note that assigns the commissioning of the codex to the initiative of a monk with the help "of the Christian people" (του χ(ριστ)ωνυμ(ου) λαοῦ).[307] A later example of collective patronage is attested in the dedicatory inscription of the church of St. Sozomenos at Galata (1513), where fourteen donors—a church lector and notary (anagnostes and nomikos), two priests, and eleven lay people—are recorded.[308] A number of lay people are also portrayed in the church of the Holy Cross at Pelendri, but they contrast with the portraits in Asinou in that, where the supplicants at Asinou (with the exception of Theophilos) were all living, those at Pelendri were mostly deceased, in all likelihood victims of the Black Death that struck Cyprus in the year 1347 or 1348.[309]

The existence of many comparable examples of dedicatory inscriptions revealing collective patronage in the late Byzantine period reflects the historical and socioeconomic conditions of late medieval agrarian communities.[310] These examples are found mostly in village churches, both in the Byzantine provinces and in regions under Latin rule. In the Byzantine Morea, for example, a certain number of dedicatory inscriptions preserved in rural churches show that several individuals or families together contributed to the foundation or renovation of churches or monasteries.[311] The number of collaborators—clerical, monastic, and lay—ranged from four to perhaps more than thirty. As in the case of Asinou, the initiative in founding a church often belonged to priests or monks, who were supported by laypersons. Moreover, there are instances in which the most significant donors are registered by name and the rest of the sponsors are referred to collectively and anonymously; the expression "and the rest of the villagers" (καὶ τῶν λοιπῶν τῆς χώρας) in the inscription on the south aisle of St. Nicholas at Platsa in the Messenian Mani (1348/49) is a typical example.[312] A close parallel to Asinou, both linguistically and contextually, occurs in the inscription of the church of St. John the Baptist at Megale Kastania in the Messenian Mani, dating from around the middle of the thirteenth century, where it is stated that the church was founded by the *prokritoi*, i.e., the most prominent inhabitants

307. Constantinides and Browning, *Dated Greek Manuscripts*, 103–6.

308. Stylianou and Stylianou, "Donors and Dedicatory Inscriptions," 84–89. Moreover, the church of St. George at Choulou in the district of Paphos includes several inscriptions, as yet unpublished, beginning with the words δέησις τοῦ δούλου / τῆς δούλης τοῦ Θεοῦ . . . (supplication of God's servant), pointing to a patronage pattern based on the collaboration of a number of individuals, both monastic and lay.

309. Stylianou and Stylianou, "Donors and Dedicatory Inscriptions," 107–9, no. 7; eidem, *Painted Churches*, 223–32; Zarras, *Holy Cross*, 19. On the Black Death, see Edbury, *Kingdom of Cyprus*, 15, 159.

310. On collective patronage in villages and in the countryside in the late Byzantine period, see Kalopissi-Verti, "Church Foundations"; eadem, "Collective Patterns."

311. For the dedicatory inscriptions of the Palaiologan Peloponnese, see Feissel and Philippidis-Braat, "Inscriptions du Péloponnèse," 312–57; Kalopissi-Verti, *Dedicatory Inscriptions*, 65–82.

312. Feissel and Philippidis-Braat, "Inscriptions du Péloponnèse," 334–35, no. 73.

of the village, and the common people (κοινὸς λαός).[313] A characteristic example in Cyprus occurs in the first fresco layer of the apse in the church of the Holy Cross at Pelendri, sponsored in 1178 by the priest George and other priests and by (the people) of the village Πελέτρηον.[314]

Of the Latin-held provinces, Crete offers a particularly high percentage of rural churches with a collective patronage scheme, mainly dating from the fourteenth and the first half of the fifteenth century. The donors, inhabitants of the same village, are often relatives. The closest parallel to the narthex of Asinou is offered by certain churches in Crete where the dedicatory inscriptions are complemented by donor portraits, such as St. George at Kometades Sphakion (1313/14), Archangel Michael at Kabalariana in Kantanos Selinou (1327/28), Panagia at Kakodiki Selinou (1331/32), and St. Anna at Anisaraki in Kantanos Selinou (1352).[315]

References to the painter in late Byzantine foundation or dedicatory inscriptions occur mostly in churches of the periphery and under particular conditions,[316] namely, when painters are themselves sponsors of the entirety or of part of the wall paintings of a church; when the commissioners of murals do not rank very high in the social echelon; and when a fresco decoration is supported by collective patronage, as in the narthex of Asinou. Typical examples in this last category are found in the Byzantine province of Mesa Mani/Peloponnese, as in the churches of the Holy Anargyroi at Kepoula (1265) and of the Archangel Michael at Polemitas (1278).[317] The painters' names are also encountered in several churches of Venetian-ruled Crete dating from the fourteenth and the first half of the fifteenth century, and in the church of St. Nicholas at Maritsa (1434/35) in Rhodes, governed at that time by the Hospitallers.[318]

The earliest example in Cyprus of a painter mentioned in a foundation inscription occurs in the apse of the church of the Holy Cross at Pelendri, which was painted in the year 1178 by a monk whose name has not survived.[319] There are further references to painters in church inscriptions of the Lusignan and Venetian periods in the Cypriot countryside, such as Leontios the Deacon, mentioned in an inscription in the exterior lunette over the north entrance door to the church of Panagia tou Arakos, Lagoudera (see below, pp. 202, 204–5, 229 n. 60, and 310); the painter from Constantinople—presumably a refugee in the wake of 1453—who was cited but whose name has not been preserved in an inscription painted above the south door of the narthex of St. Herakleidios at Kalopanayiotis; and the painters Philippos Goul and Symeon Axentes, named in church foundation inscriptions of the fifteenth and sixteenth centuries.[320]

Donor portraits

No fewer than ten donor portraits painted in the narthex, including monks, laymen, and laywomen, seem to represent the monastic community and

313. Drosogianni, *Σχόλια στὶς τοιχογραφίες*, 5, 196–99, 216–24; Kalopissi-Verti, *Dedicatory Inscriptions*, 65–66, no. 17.
314. Stylianou and Stylianou, *Painted Churches*, 507–8, figs. 302–4; Zarras, *Holy Cross*, 15, fig. 8.
315. Gerola, *Monumenti Veneti*, Kometades: 4:472–73, no. 2; 2:334, no. 27, pl. 11, 1; Kabalariana: 4:453–54, no. 28; 2:333, no. 19, pl. 10, 3–4; Kakodiki: 4:462–63, no. 41; 2:330, no.14; Anisaraki: 4:451–52, no. 26; 2:333, no. 20; Xanthaki, "Ο ναός της Αγίας Άννας," 83–85. For the donors at Kabalariana, see Lymberopoulou, *Church of the Archangel Michael*, 204–17, figs. 28–29, 50–53.
316. Kalopissi-Verti, "Painters," 145–47.
317. Eadem, *Dedicatory Inscriptions*, 67–69, no. 19; 71–75, no. 21.
318. Eadem, "Painters," 145 and n. 35. Christophoraki, "Χορηγικές μαρτυρίες," 461, n. 94 (with previous bibliography).
319. See above, n. 314. On the inscription of the painter Theodoros Apseudes in the Enkleistra of St. Neophytos (1183), see Mango and Hawkins, "Hermitage," 182–83; for a further discussion, see Panayotidi, "Role of the Donor."
320. For the painter at Kalopanayiotis see Papageorgiou, *Μονή του Αγίου Ιωάννου*, 37, fig. 28; for Philippos Goul, see Stylianou and Stylianou, "Donors and Dedicatory Inscriptions," 110–12 (St. Mamas at Loubaras, 1455; Holy Cross of Agiasmati at Platanistassa, 1466); for Symeon Axentes, ibid., 116–19 (St. Sozomenos, 1513; Archangel or Panagia Theotokos, 1514; both at Galata).

the most prominent of the "common people" (κοινὸς λαός) mentioned in the inscription of the year 1332/33. In addition, the portraits of Anastasia Saramalina and the anonymous Latin devotee with her sons, although they belong to earlier phases of painting (see above, pp. 115–22, 124–30), have been incorporated contextually into the dominant program of 1332/33. All fourteenth-century donors are represented full-length, though on a smaller scale than the figures of saints. They stand with raised arms in the typical gesture of supplication, praying to their patron saints or, more often, to the great intercessors depicted on the east wall—the Virgin Phorbiotissa, the Virgin Eleousa, and St. John the Forerunner—to intervene with Christ for the salvation of their souls.

With the exception of the priest-monk Barnabas, painted high on the east wall beside the panel of Panagia Phorbiotissa, and the two monks—Theophilos and Germanos—depicted in the soffit of the eastern arch, all male donors, monastic and lay alike, are enclosed in separately framed panels among the saints of the lower zone. In most cases, one of their hands raised in prayer overlaps the red band of the frame, integrating their petition into the space of the narthex. It is interesting to note that—with the exception of Kallinikos—monks were placed by preference either on the east wall, close to the Virgin Phorbiotissa and the Deesis, or on the walls of the north half of the narthex, that is, in the part where Paradise and the Just are depicted. By contrast, laypersons are depicted in the south part of the narthex, where the scenes of Hell are located. Female donors, although limited in number and belonging to different phases, are given a special distinction, for they are depicted within the same panel as their patron saint. The Latin supplicant kneels before her main protector, the Virgin, and the local devotees Anastasia and Anna stand with their patron saints.

The inscriptions that accompany the donor figures are written in white uncial characters on green ground.[321] They begin with the word δέησις, meaning supplication or prayer, followed by the expression "servant of God" and the name of the supplicant.

Monks Barnabas the hieromonk (monk who is also a priest) and the monk Theophilos (secondarily also the monk Germanos) seem to be the most eminent among the monastic patrons, as deduced from their conspicuous placement on both sides of the entrance door next to the dedicatory inscription and the twelfth-century fresco of the Virgin Phorbiotissa, the patron of the church, and at the same time above the Deesis. The priest-monk Barnabas, painted on the east wall of the narthex in a narrow triangular space to the left of the Phorbiotissa, lifts his head toward the Virgin and raises his hands in prayer (Figs. 5.37, 5.38). He is tonsured and dressed in a white *sticharion* and a white *phelonion* with small black crosses around the neck. The cuffs *(epimanikia)* and the *epitrachelion* are embroidered with gold and ornamented with pearls. His inscription reads: δε(ησις) του δούλου / τοῦ θ(εο)υ Βαρνά/βα ἱερο(μον)αχ(ου) / ἀμῆν = δέησις τοῦ δούλου τοῦ θεοῦ Βαρνάβα ἱερομονάχου, ἀμήν (prayer of the servant of God Barnabas priest-monk, amen).

According to the typika, white is specified for priests' vestments worn during services of the feast day of the Holy Cross (14 September), for Vespers of Holy Saturday, for Matins of Easter Sunday, and for the whole period between Easter and the Ascension, even for burials.[322] If the white color of Barnabas's vestments is associated with the time between Easter and the Ascension, and thus linked to the Resurrection, it may be deduced that the use of this color implies the salvation of humankind through the death of Christ on the cross and his resurrection. It thus conforms with the funerary character of the narthex and probably alludes to the deceased monk Theophilos painted on the opposite side.

White phelonia and white sticharia are worn by the two donor-priests depicted in the scene of the Second Coming in the narthex of St. Herakleidios

321. With the exception of the inscriptions accompanying the monks Barnabas, Theophilos, and Germanos, painted on a blue ground.

322. Papas, *Geschichte der Messgewänder*, 75.

in the monastery of St. John Lampadistes at Kalopanayiotis (after the mid-fifteenth century) and by the priest Basileios, who donated the church of the Archangel Michael at Pedoulas in Cyprus (1474).[323] A priest-monk clad in a white phelonion and a white sticharion is the donor of a thirteenth-century icon of St. George in the monastery of St. Catherine at Sinai.[324] Furthermore, white sacerdotal vestments occur in representations of donor priests in churches of Venetian-occupied Crete from the fourteenth to the beginning of the sixteenth century.[325]

Priests in Byzantium had been tonsured since the sixth century.[326] The ring of hair that remained around the tonsured part of the head was believed to recall Jesus's crown of thorns.[327] In art the tonsure is seen mostly on deacons and occasionally on priests and bishops. Among Cypriot examples one might single out the two kneeling supplicant priests in the narthex of St. Herakleidios and the four monks and one bishop on a mid-fourteenth-century icon at Sinai that has been recently attributed to a Cypriot workshop.[328]

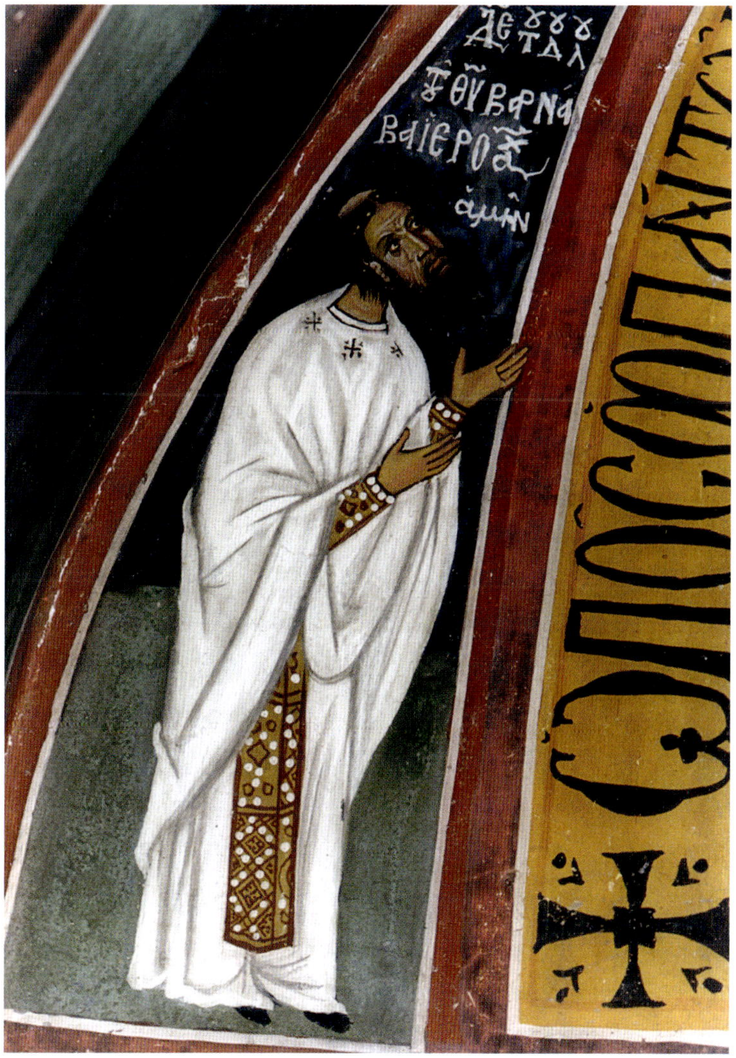

FIG. 5.38 Narthex, east wall. The priest-monk Barnabas (photo courtesy of S. Kalopissi-Verti)

Painted conspicuously in the southern soffit of the eastern arch, next to the entrance, the monk THEOPHILOS is also mentioned in the dedicatory inscription as main donor supported by the common people (Fig. 5.40; see above, pp. 176, 178). Though his body is slightly turned aside, toward the

323. Stylianou and Stylianou, *Painted Churches*, 306–7, 331, fig. 196; Cholet, "Jugement dernier," 107–15. For a color plate of the priest at Pedoulas, see Connor, "Female Saints," pl. 24; Papageorgiou, *Μονή του Αγίου Ιωάννου*, fig. 31.
324. Soteriou and Soteriou, *Εἰκόνες*, 1: fig. 167, 2:149–51; Mouriki, "Portraits de donateurs," 112, no. 7.
325. Gerola, *Monumenti Veneti*, 2:330–31, no. 14, fig. 381 (Panagia in Kakodiki Selinou/Chania, 1331/32); 334, no. 30, pl. 11.3 (St. John the Evangelist in Margarites Mylopotamou/Rethymnon, 1383); 337, no. 43, pl. 13.2 (Panagia in St. Paraskeve, Amari/Rethymnon, 1516); Spatharakis, *Dated Byzantine Wall Paintings*, 207–10, fig. 181 (St. Anna in Anisaraki, Kantanos Selinou/Chania).
326. John Lydus, *De Mensibus*, 4.46 (p. 82, ll. 4–6 in Bekker edition); Ralles and Potles, *Σύνταγμα*, 2:352–54; *DACL* 15:2430–35 (H. Leclercq); Alivizatos, "Κουρὰ τῶν κληρικῶν"; Papaevangelou, *Διαμόρφωση*, 79ff, 89ff.
327. Symeon of Thessalonike, PG 155:873. Cf. Koukoules, *Βυζαντινῶν βίος καὶ πολιτισμός*, 4:355.
328. For Kalopanayiotis, see Stylianou and Stylianou, *Painted Churches*, 295, fig. 176; Papageorgiou, *Μονή του Αγίου Ιωάννου*, 22, fig. 12; for the icon, see Evans, *Byzantium, Faith and Power*, 360–61, no. 219 (with bibliography); for its attribution to a workshop active in Cyprus in the mid-14th c., see Drandaki, *Pilgrimage to Sinai*, 41, n. 51. For other examples in Byzantine painting, see Moutsopoulos and Demetrokalles, *Γεράκι*, 111–19.

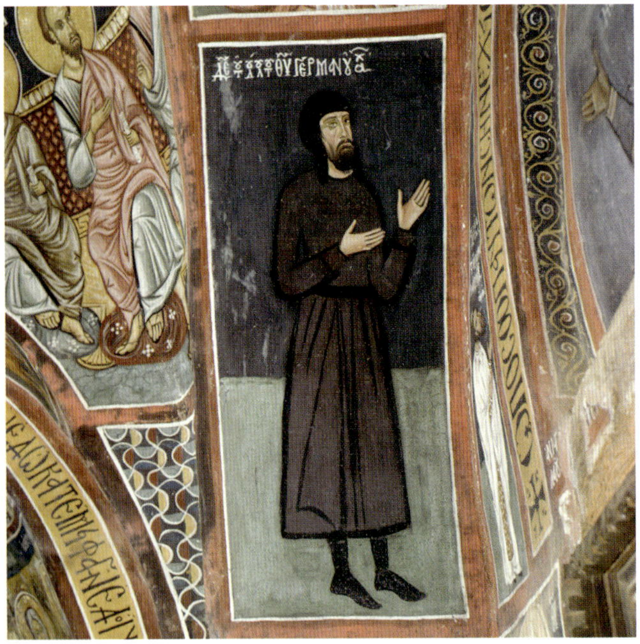

FIG. 5.39 Narthex, soffit of east arch, north side. The monk Germanos (photo courtesy of the Leventis Foundation and the Archaeological Research Unit, University of Cyprus, No. 006423)

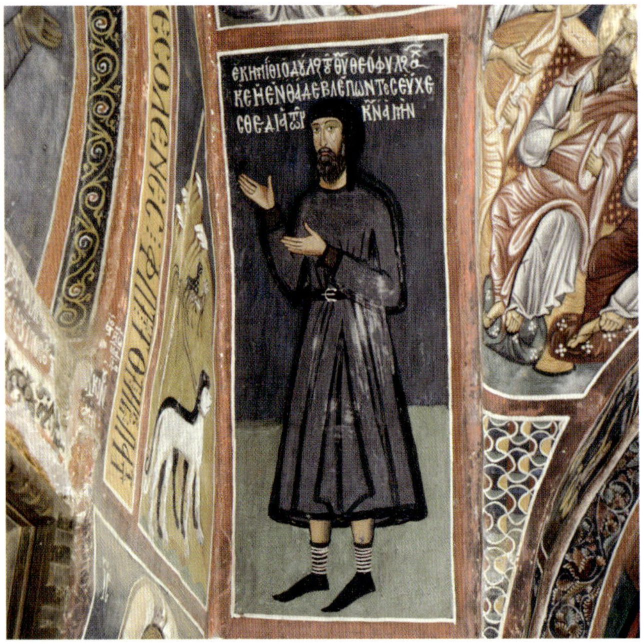

FIG. 5.40 Narthex, soffit of east arch, south side, and part of the east wall. The deceased monk Theophilos, the hounds and mouflons (photo courtesy of the Leventis Foundation and the Archaeological Research Unit, University of Cyprus, No. 006424)

Virgin Phorbiotissa depicted in the lunette under the arch, he glances at the spectator. He wears a dark gray tunic and a brown undergarment, the cuffs of which are visible. Two triangles where the edges are folded back show that the tunic had a vertical opening in front running from the waist to the hem. The tunic is unusually short, revealing part of the legs and the boots. The boots are black and have white straps around the ankles. The tunic is girdled with a black belt fastened with a metallic buckle. Theophilos wears a black *koukoullion* on the head. The inscription above his head declares that the monk Theophilos is deceased: ἐκημῖθι ὁ δοῦλος τοῦ θ(εο)υ Θεόφυλος (μον)αχ(ὸς) / κὲ ἡ ἐνθάδε βλέπωντες εὔχε/σθε διὰ τῶν / κ(ύριο)ν ἀμὴν = ἐκοιμήθη ὁ δοῦλος τοῦ θεοῦ Θεόφιλος μοναχὸς καὶ οἱ ἐνθάδε βλέποντες εὔχεσθε διὰ τὸν κύριον, ἀμήν. (The servant of God Theophilos the monk is dead, and those who look at this pray to the Lord, amen.)

In connection with the figure of the monk Theophilos, an iconographic subject that seems very peculiar for an Orthodox church is painted on the south part of the east wall, between the figures of the Virgin Phorbiotissa and Theophilos. Two mouflons stand in a landscape against steep hills and two hounds are tied to a spear in the foreground (Figs. 3.11, 5.30, 5.37). All animals turn to the right, while the hounds raise their heads staring intently toward Theophilos as if to their master (pp. 184–85).

The monk GERMANOS is depicted in the north part of the soffit of the eastern arch, the pendant to Theophilos (Fig. 5.39). Turned toward the figure of the Panagia Phorbiotissa, his head is covered with a black *koukoullion* and he wears a brown, girdled tunic over a brown undergarment, the cuffs of which are visible. A triangular fold seems to indicate that the tunic had an opening in front.

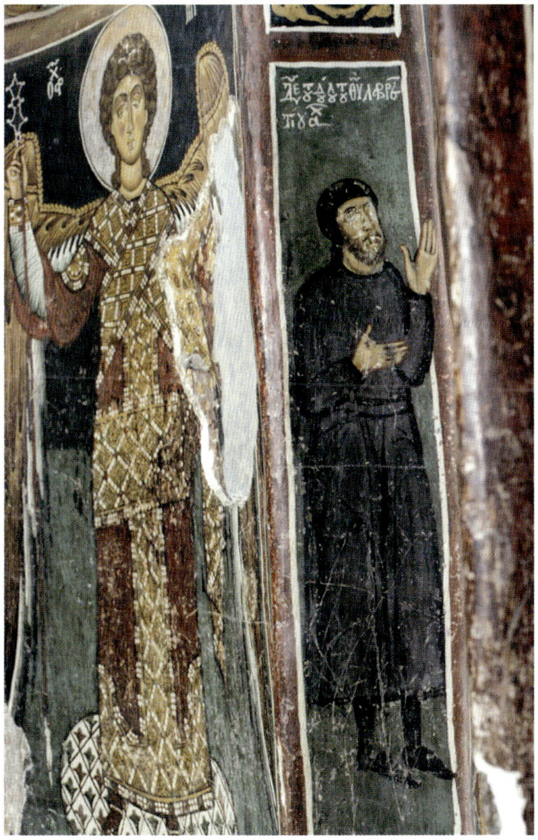

FIG. 5.41 Narthex, north-east respond. The monk Laurentios (photo courtesy of the Leventis Foundation and the Archaeological Research Unit, University of Cyprus, No. 006418)

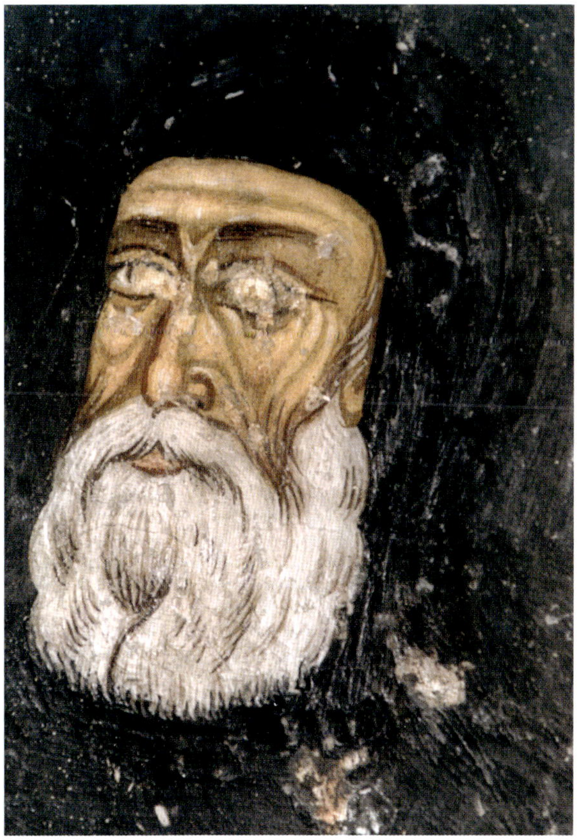

FIG. 5.42 Narthex, north conch. The monk Leontios (photo courtesy of S. Kalopissi-Verti)

The tunic is relatively short, allowing most of his black boots to be seen. The accompanying inscription reads: δε(ησις) τοῦ δούλου του θ(εο)ύ Γερμανοῦ (μον)αχ(οῦ) = δέησις τοῦ δούλου τοῦ θεοῦ Γερμανοῦ μοναχοῦ (prayer of the servant of God Germanos the monk).

The monks Laurentios and Babylas are painted on the east and west responds of the north arch, respectively. Laurentios, standing next to St. Sozomenos, is turned to the east toward the Virgin Phorbiotissa (Figs. 5.28, 5.41). He wears a dark-gray girdled tunic that is short enough to allow the high black boots to be seen. The *koukoullion* is also black. Babylas, painted between SS. Marina and Eudokia, is also turned to the east and is clad in a dark gray tunic and a black hood (Fig. 5.28). The paint that depicts his face is almost completely abraded. The accompanying inscriptions read: δε(ησις) του δούλου του θ(εο)ὐ Λαβρε(ν)/τίου (μον)αχ(οῦ) = δέησις τοῦ δούλου τοῦ θεοῦ Λαυρεντίου μοναχοῦ (prayer of the servant of God Laurentios the monk); and δέ(ησις) του δούλου του / θ(εο)υ Βαβίλα (μον)αχ(οῦ) = δέησις τοῦ δούλου τοῦ θεοῦ Βαβύλα μοναχοῦ (prayer of the servant of God Babylas the monk).

The monk Leontios stands in a narrow framed space in the north conch next to the figure of the archangel Michael (Figs. 5.28, 5.30, 5.35, 5.42). He is dressed in the usual dark gray tunic with girdle, black hood, and black boots. He is painted as an old man, with a thick white beard and many wrinkles on his face. Above his head is the inscription: δέ(ησις) του δούλου του θ(εο)υ Λαιῶντίου /

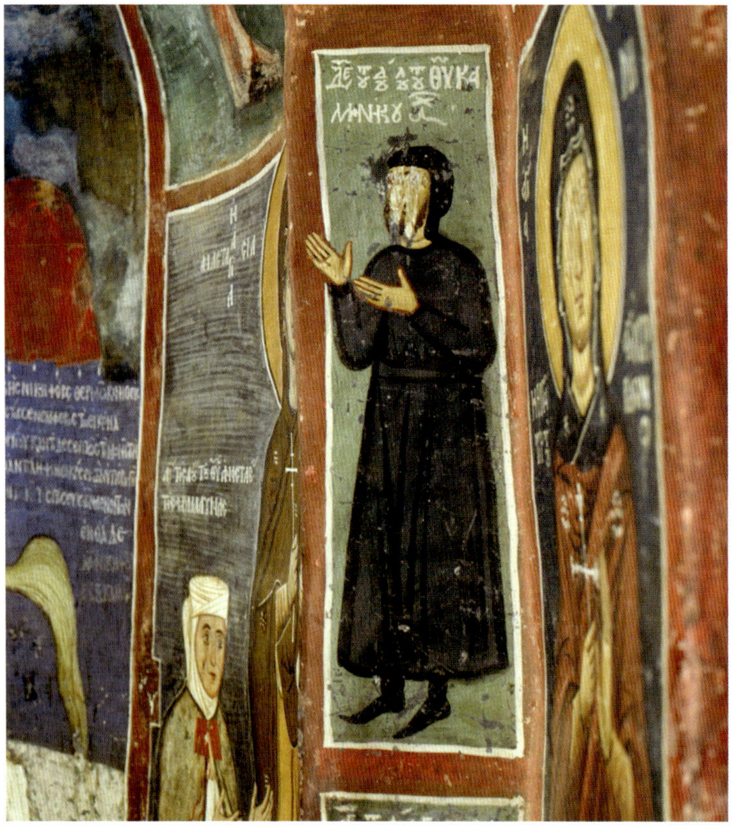

FIG. 5.43 Narthex, south-west respond. The monk Kallinikos (photo courtesy of the Leventis Foundation and the Archaeological Research Unit, University of Cyprus, No. 006420)

(μον)[α]χ(οῦ) = δέησις τοῦ δούλου τοῦ θεοῦ Λεοντίου μοναχοῦ (prayer of the servant of God Leontios the monk). In contrast to all the other monks, Leontios turns not eastward, toward the Virgin Phorbiotissa, but toward the image of the archangel Michael. Addressing his prayer to the archangel, Leontios forms a separate votive ensemble like the panels of Anastasia Saramalina and Anna Lachana, although he is not included within the same frame. The preference of an aged monk to accompany the archangel might be connected with Michael's function as psychopompos.[329]

Finally, the monk KALLINIKOS is depicted on the west respond of the south arch, above the figure of the lay supplicant Basileios and between the saints Anastasia Pharmakolytria and Irene (Figs. 5.1, 5.43). Kallinikos is the only monk who is depicted in the south bay of the narthex, where the lay donors are. Turned to the east, he is dressed in the usual monastic garments: dark-gray girdled tunic, black *koukoullion,* and black boots; his face is abraded. The accompanying inscription reads: δε(ησις) του δούλου του θ(εο)υ Κα/λληνήκου (μον)αχ(οῦ) = δέησις τοῦ δούλου τοῦ θεοῦ Καλλινίκου μοναχοῦ (prayer of the servant of God Kallinikos the monk).

Of all the supplicant figures in the narthex, Theophilos alone is explicitly identified as deceased. He differs in neither posture nor gesture from the other, living supplicants. The long, sleeved tunic and the girdle around the waist had, along with such garments as the mantle and the *analabos,* been part of the vestments of a monk since the beginnings of Christian monasticism, as can be seen in descriptions and representations of early Pachomian and Antonian monastic vestments.[330] These garments still belong to the basic monastic attire today. The shortness of Theophilos's tunic, however, and the peculiar opening in its front do not conform to either western or Byzantine monastic clothing. Stella Frigerio-Zeniou has interpreted them as appropriate for horsemen.[331] She regards features like the hunting dogs and the mouflons painted on the east wall, the profession of the curer of horses mentioned in the inscription of St. George in the south conch, and the likely derivation of the Virgin's epithet φορβιώτισσα from either φορβειά (harness) or φορβή (pasture) as indications that the monks of Asinou in the fourteenth century raised and trained horses for hunting.

329. See Weissbrod, *Hier liegt der Knecht,* 58–61. Cf. above, pp. 133, 168–70, 176.

330. On monastic vestments, see Oppenheim, *Mönchskleid,* 89–212; on their black color and on the girdle, ibid., 71–78, 174–84. See also Innemée, *Ecclesiastical Dress,* 90–133.

331. Frigerio-Zeniou, "Μονὴ τῶν Φορβίων," 191–99. For a relatively short monastic garment in Crusader context, see the figure of St. Leonard of Limoges on a 12th-century icon in St. Catherine's monastery depicting six saints: Folda, *Art of the Crusaders,* 461–62, pl. 10.19.

Metallic buckles like the one on Theophilos's belt have come to light in Syria and Palestine from the Crusader period, especially from excavations of thirteenth-century layers.[332] The type of *koukoullion* worn by Theophilos and the other monks is paralleled in pictorial evidence from the eastern Mediterranean and the Balkans in the late medieval period.[333] Black boots with white straps around the ankles occur in Byzantium, in the West, and in the Crusader East in secular contexts.[334] Hunters, farmers, and soldiers wear them; examples appear in the naos of Asinou itself, in the fourteenth-century scenes of the Betrayal and the Via Crucis (Figs. 6.43, 6.44).

It is true that the garments of the monks depicted in the narthex of Asinou differ from those usually represented in figures of monastic saints or of living monks.[335] There are many peculiarities, such as the short tunic worn by Theophilos, Germanos, and Laurentios; the opening in the front of the tunics of Theophilos and Germanos; and the strapped boots of Theophilos. It seems that the monks depicted at Asinou wear the everyday clothing that facilitated their working activities. Apparently unique, as well, is the depiction in a prominent place—on the east wall next to the Phorbiotissa—of mouflons and of hounds who stare attentively at Theophilos in a way that seems to mirror the special relationship between hounds and master. All these components are certainly not incidental, and they beg an explanation. Frigerio-Zeniou's interpretation may point in the right direction, but written sources offer no confirmation.[336] Could the composition including Theophilos, the mouflons, and the hounds represent *in abstracto* a hunting scene in remembrance of a favorite activity of the deceased monk?[337] The rural milieu of the monastery of Asinou favors a connection between its monks, agrarian and hunting activities, and the breeding of livestock and horses.

Laypersons A male lay donor named Georgios is depicted full-length, standing in a narrow, framed space on the east respond of the south arch next to his eponymous patron saint, St. George Machairomenos (Figs. 5.1, 5.44, 5.45). He turns toward the saint and raises his arms in prayer. He is dressed in a dark blue-green overcoat that falls just above the ankles. The overcoat has a brown lining that is visible in the front opening, in the sleeves, and at the neck, where it folds back to form the two triangular parts of a collar. Under the coat Georgios wears a dark-blue tunic (cotte) with long tight sleeves closed with buttons—five white buttons on each sleeve. He wears black shoes with long, slightly raised ends. He has a brown moustache and a short beard; a white headdress covers his curly hair, which is rolled at the ends under his ears

332. Brosh, "Between East and West," 268–69, figs. 3 and 4. A metallic buckle with circular bulges on each of the front angles exactly like those on Theophilos's belt has been found in a grave of the 13th century in Sémur, Yonne/France. See Viollet-le-Duc, *Encyclopédie médiévale*, 2:464–65, fig. 3A on 465.

333. On the icon of St. George in St. Catherine's monastery (13th c.), see Soteriou and Soteriou, *Εἰκόνες*, 1: fig. 167, 2:149–51; Mouriki, "Portraits de donateurs," 112, no. 7. In St. George at Kometades Sphakion, Crete (1314), see Gerola, *Monumenti Veneti*, 2:334, no. 27, pl. 11, 1. In Archangel Michael in Thari, Rhodes (1506), see Bitha, "Ενδυματολογικές μαρτυρίες," 2:436, fig. ιζ', pl. 174a. In Markov Manastir (1376–81), see N. P. Ševčenko, *Life of Saint Nicholas*, 315, fig. 36.13.

334. Spatharakis, *Illustrations of the Cynegetica*, 198, figs. 39–41, 50, 70, etc.; Boucher, *Histoire du costume*, 182, fig. 330, Bibl. Nat. ms. fr. 146, fol. 34, end of the 13th c.

335. See, for example, the twelfth-century monk's figure in St. Nicholas of the Roof at Kakopetria, in Stylianou and Stylianou, *Painted Churches*, 62–65, fig. 25.

336. Gilles Grivaud (above, p. 27) finds Frigerio-Zeniou's assumption plausible, although according to the Assizes of Jerusalem, stud farms were an exclusive privilege of the king or the landlords.

337. For a hunting scene in funerary context, now destroyed, which was depicted in the narthex of the Panagia at Monochoro of Galia Kainouriou, Crete (1345), representing the donor Georgios Mousouros and two attendants on horseback, see Gerola, *Monumenti Veneti*, 2:339, no. 52, pl. 17, 1; 4:544, no. 11–12; Mylopotamitaki, "Παρατηρήσεις," 1:143.

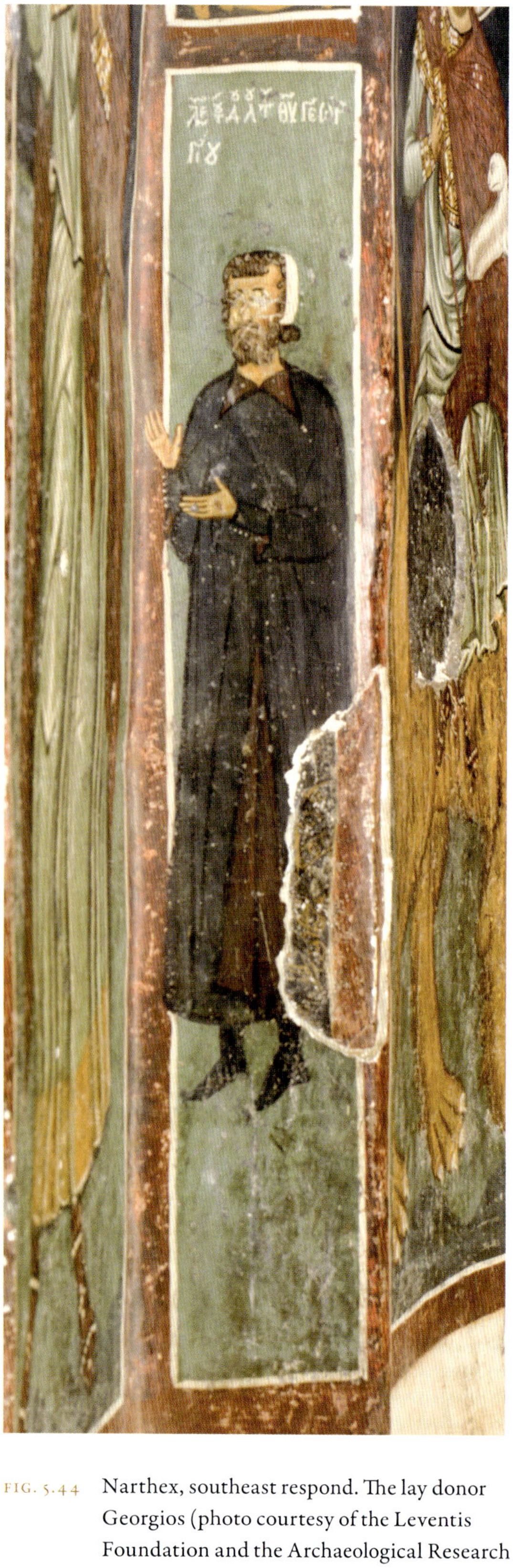

FIG. 5.44 Narthex, southeast respond. The lay donor Georgios (photo courtesy of the Leventis Foundation and the Archaeological Research Unit, University of Cyprus, No. 006421)

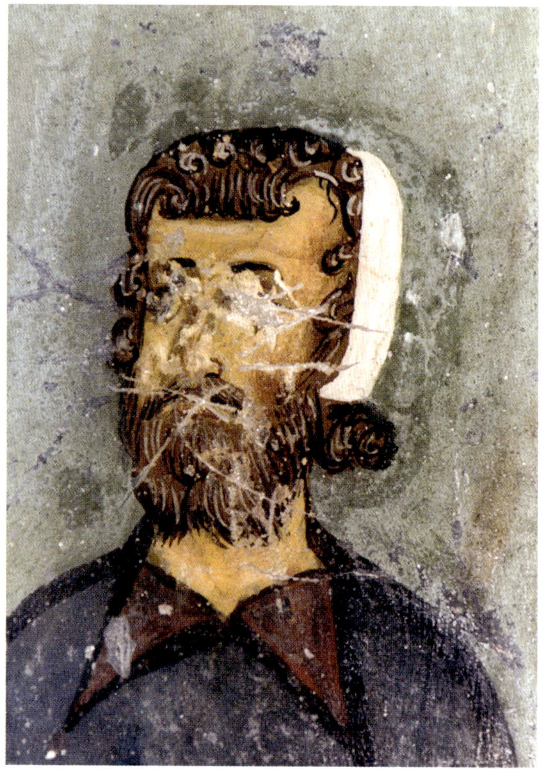

FIG. 5.45 Narthex, southeast respond. The lay donor Georgios, detail (photo courtesy of S. Kalopissi-Verti)

and forms a fringe on the forehead (Fig. 5.45). The accompanying inscription reads: δέ(ησις) του δουλου του θ(εο)υ Γεῶρ/γίου = δέησις τοῦ δούλου τοῦ θεοῦ Γεωργίου (prayer of the servant of God Georgios).

Basileios Drakocheres (ὁ Δρακοχέρης), another male donor, is represented full-length on the west respond of the south arch, between St. Anastasia and St. Irene (Fig. 5.1). He is turned to the east with arms raised in prayer. Although in a poor state of preservation, he seems to be clad, like Georgios, in a long, dark blue overcoat. The white cuffs of the cotte are clearly visible. The short brown beard, rolled hair, and white coif also seem to be very similar to those of Georgios. The accompanying inscription reads: δε(ησις) του δούλου του θ(εο)υ Βα̣/ς̣ιλϊου του Δρακ̣ο/[χ]έ[ρη][338] = δέησις τοῦ

338. The reading of Basileios's surname is based on the notes of Ihor Ševčenko when he visited Asinou in 1966.

δούλου τοῦ θεοῦ Βασιλείου τοῦ Δρακοχέρη (prayer of the servant of God Basileios Drako[ch]e[res]).

The garments of the male donors follow western fashion as it was introduced to Cyprus by the Crusaders in the thirteenth century. The triangular endings of the collars, encountered also in the figure of the donor Ioannes in the church of the Panagia at Moutoullas (1280; Fig. 5.3), are in accord with western practices.[339] Buttons to hold the cuffs tight had been popular in Western Europe since the end of the thirteenth century.[340] Shoes with very long pointed ends reflect a fashion predominant in the West from the mid-fourteenth to the mid-fifteenth century.[341] The hairstyles and headdresses of both Georgios and Basileios follow the French and Italian trends of the thirteenth century and the first half of the fourteenth century. The hair is rolled outward, behind the head at the height of the ears, while a large lock of hair called *dorelot* or fringe is traced on the forehead.[342] Both male donors wear the headdress known as the coif. It is a kind of *bonnet,* a close-fitting cap consisting of two white linen pieces of equal size, sewn together and bound by narrow straps under the chin. In combination with the hairstyle described above, it was common in France and Italy during the thirteenth and fourteenth centuries.[343] The coif was sometimes worn under a hat or a cap, as in the case of Michael Katzouroumpos, donor of St. Demetrianos at Dali (1317).[344]

The coif was in fashion in the eastern Mediterranean world, as shown in thirteenth-century manuscripts produced in the scriptorium of Acre, in thirteenth–fourteenth-century illuminated manuscripts of Armenian Cilicia, and

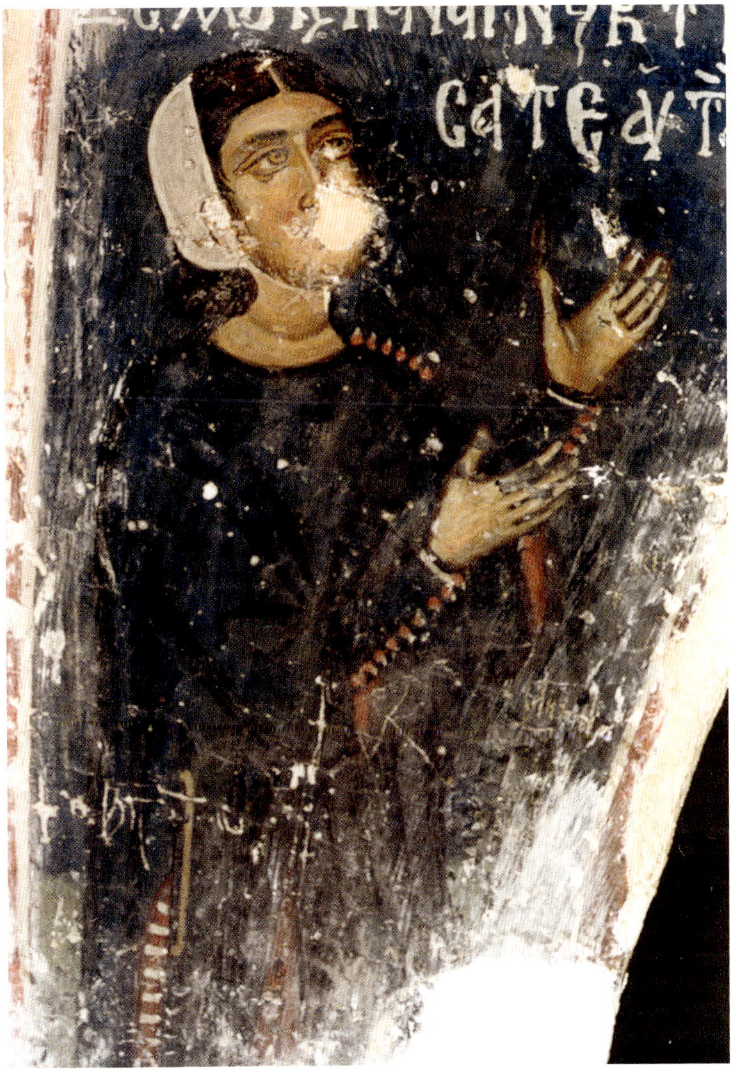

FIG. 5.46 Pelendri, church of the Holy Cross, central vessel. The deceased supplicant Basileios (photo courtesy of S. Kalopissi-Verti)

339. Mouriki, "Moutoullas," 181–83, fig. 11. For a color plate, see Stylianou and Stylianou, *Painted Churches*, 324–25, fig. 192. For the triangular collar endings in the West, see Houston, *Medieval Costume*, 82, figs. 139, 214.
340. Pinasa, *Costumes*, 77, 175, fig. 302.
341. Boucher, *Histoire du costume*, 198, 203; Pinasa, *Costumes*, 101. However, shoes with long pointed ends were well known in Byzantium and were called μακρυμύτικα. See Koukoules, *Βυζαντινῶν βίος καὶ πολιτισμός*, 4:407–8; Parani, *Reconstructing the Reality*, 71.
342. Viollet-le-Duc, *Encyclopédie médiévale*, 497, figs. 10, 12; Pinasa, *Costumes*, 97–98.
343. In French it was called *cale*; when it did not have straps tied under the chin it was called *coiffe*. See Boucher, *Histoire du costume*, 184, pls. 8, 14; Pinasa, *Costumes*, 85, 97, 99; *Giotto e i Giotteschi*, figs. 50, 52, 55, 67, 70, 165, etc. See also Greenhill, *Incised Effigial Slabs*, 1:201, fig. 23 (ca. 1275), 2: pl. 25a (1307).
344. Stylianou and Stylianou, *Painted Churches*, 425–26, fig. 256.

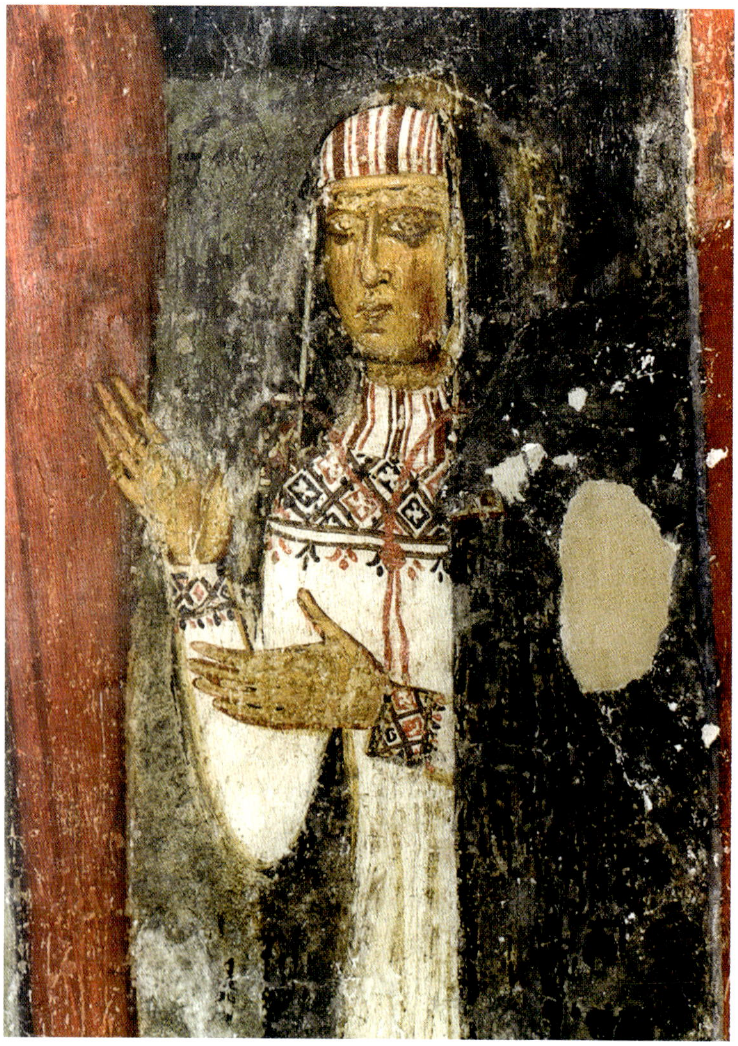

FIG. 5.47 Asinou, narthex, west wall. The donor Anna Lachana (photo courtesy of S. Kalopissi-Verti)

5.46) in the central vessel, Leon Skouleas in the north vessel, and the male figure in the lunette of the western entrance—as well as by the male figure identified with John Lusignan (d. 1375) in the Doubting Thomas scene in the north vessel of the same church.[346]

Finally, in the panel with St. Anna, the homonymous donor, ANNA LACHANA, is turned toward her patron saint, raising her arms in supplication (Figs. 5.34, 5.47). The woman wears a long white dress that clings to her upper body and has long, tight sleeves. The cuffs and collar are painted to simulate beautifully woven black and red geometrical patterns, rhomboid motifs enclosing crosses within a network. A long black mantle falls from the top of the head and is loosely held together under the neck with two knotted red ribbons sewn on red patches, the paint of which is now abraded. A headdress made of white cloth woven with parallel red bands covers her hair and neck tightly. Under this headdress, another, transparent one (or maybe just a band) is faintly perceptible on the lady's forehead. The accompanying inscription reads: δέ(ησις) της δουλις του / θ(εο)υ Ἀννα(ς) του Λαχαν̣ὰ = δέησις τῆς δούλης τοῦ θεοῦ Ἄννας τοῦ Λαχανᾶ (prayer of the servant of God Anna of Lachanas).[347]

Anna's garments follow local tradition. The ribbons sewn on rectangular patches (or a brooch) holding the mantle together are also seen in the figure of the donor Anastasia Saramalina (above, p. 118; Figs. 5.2, 5.4). A similar headdress with in donor portraits painted in churches of Crete.[345] In Cyprus it is worn by the donor Ioannes on the icon of St. John the Baptist from the church of the Panagia at Moutoullas (ca. 1280), by the fourteenth-century supplicant in the narthex of St. Nicholas of the Roof at Kakopetria (Fig. 5.9), by the deceased men depicted in the church of the Holy Cross at Pelendri (mid-fourteenth century)—Basileios (Fig.

345. Buchthal, *Miniature Painting*, pls. 118b, 128c, 129b–c; Der Nersessian, *Miniature Painting*, 2: fig. 642; Gerola, *Monumenti Veneti*, 2:333, 335, 384, nos. 22, 36, 50, pls. 9.4, 12.1, 15.2.

346. For the icon from the church at Moutoullas, see Vocotopoulos, "Three Thirteenth-Century Icons," 167–71, figs. 7, 9, 10, and color plate 12. The author reasonably identifies the figure of Ioannes on the icon with Ioannes Gerakiotes, donor of the church of Panagia at Moutoullas, where the icon was placed. For Kakopetria, see Stylianou and Stylianou, "Ναὸς τοῦ Ἁγίου Νικολάου τῆς Στέγης," 132–36, fig. 9; Kalopissi-Verti, "Church Inscriptions as Documents," 85, fig. 5. For Pelendri, see Stylianou and Stylianou, "Donors and Dedicatory Inscriptions," 107–9, fig. 9, 10; eidem, *Painted Churches*, 231–32; Zarras, *Holy Cross*, 19, 49, figs. 43–44.

347. For a possible connection of Anna to the rich Nestorian Lacha family at Famagusta, see above, p. 27.

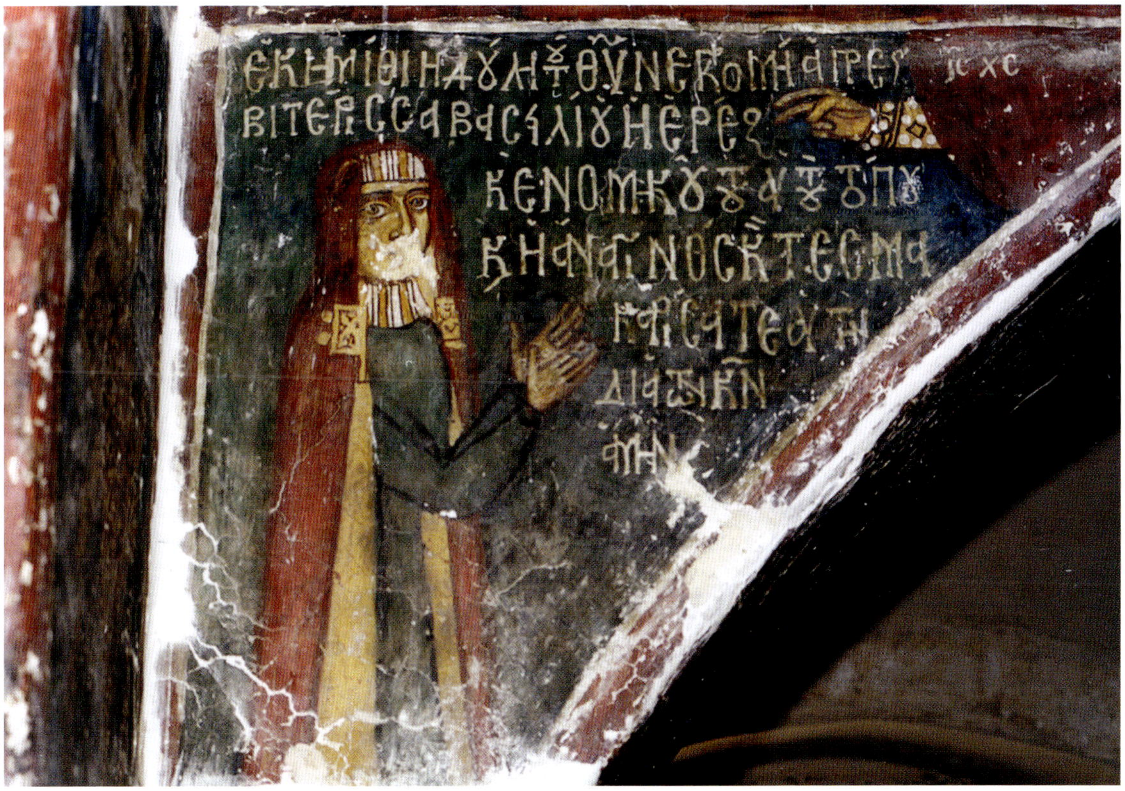

FIG. 5.48 Pelendri, church of the Holy Cross, central vessel. The deceased supplicant Nenkomia (photo courtesy of S. Kalopissi-Verti)

woven patterns is worn in the same way by the figure of a deceased woman—Nenkomia, the priest's wife (Fig. 5.48)—in the church of the Holy Cross at Pelendri (third quarter of the fourteenth century).[348] The garment itself and the ornamental weaving obviously represent a local fashion. Decorative weaving is occasionally depicted in Cypriot wall paintings, as in the white veils worn by the donor's daughters in the church of the Archangel Michael at Pedoulas (1474) and on the veil falling behind St. Helena's crown in the narthex of the katholikon of the monastery of St. John Lampadistes at Kalopanayiotis (third quarter of the fifteenth century).[349] The representation of ornamented woven textiles conforms with the late medieval predilection for depicting contemporary fabrics, not only in lay scenes, like donor portraits, but also in religious contexts; at the same time, it reflects the flourishing craft of weaving in Cyprus. The type of woven ornaments seen in the garment of Anna have continued until modern times in Cyprus, especially in the village of Phyte (Φύτη) in the province of Paphos; hence these woven textiles are known as φυθκιώτικα.[350]

A network of rhombuses enclosing crosslike motifs, like that on Anna's garment, occurs again in the lining of the mantle of St. Margarita in a thirteenth-century Vita icon of the saint in the

348. Stylianou and Stylianou, "Donors and Dedicatory Inscriptions," fig. 9; Zarras, *Holy Cross,* fig. 13.

349. For Pedoulas, see Stylianou and Stylianou, *Painted Churches*, 331, fig. 196; Semoglou, "Portraits chypriotes de donateurs," 495–96; for a color plate, see Connor, "Female Saints," fig. 24; For Kalopanayiotis, see Papageorgiou, *Μονή του Αγίου Ιωάννου*, fig. 40.

350. Papademetriou, *Κυπριακές Εθνογραφικές Συλλογές*, 41, fig. on 43. For striped, woven silk textiles, like the one in Anna's headdress, see ibid., fig. on p. 42.

Pinacoteca Provinciale of Bari.[351] The icon is associated with a stylistic trend developed in the eastern Mediterranean world that exhibited both eastern and western traits. Like the other features noted above, similar woven patterns of rhombuses enclosing different motifs survived in the Cypriot folk art of weaving until recently.[352]

Looking back over the portraits of the supplicants, one realizes that the inscriptions accompanying the seven monks depicted in the narthex provide no information about the hierarchical structure and offices within the monastic community. However, the hierarchical placement of these portraits within the iconographic program of the narthex clearly indicates that the most significant individuals were the priest-monk Barnabas, depicted on the east wall, and the monks Theophilos and Germanos, painted in the soffit of the east arch. The garments of the lay donors, on the other hand, show that they belonged to the local elite; evidently they represent the more prominent members among the "common people" mentioned in the dedicatory inscription and probably those who contributed most substantially to the mural decoration of the narthex.

With regard to the theological context of the supplicants included in the iconographic program of the narthex, one may note that all portrayed monks and lay persons, by raising their hands in prayer, join their entreaties to the supplications of the depicted saints, the Virgin Eleousa, and John the Forerunner in a Great Deesis addressed to Christ, who is represented on the east wall next to the entrance door. Consequently, the intercessory and soteriological context of the narthex is expressed by the totality of the saints' figures and the donors' portraits.[353]

351. *Βυζάντιο ως Οικουμένη*, 298–300 (with previous bibliography).

352. Papademetriou, *Λαϊκή τέχνη της Κύπρου*, 11–14, 18–19, 20–21.

353. For a discussion on how ktetors incorporated themselves into church salvation programs, see Teteriatnikov, "Private Salvation Programs."

Crosses with Cryptograms

Each jamb of the western door of the narthex bears a three-barred cross, painted in brown on a white background, with the crown of thorns woven around the middle bar. Cryptograms are written on both sides of the vertical bar.

Crosses with legends and acronyms are often painted in churches.[354] Due to their prophylactic-apotropaic function against evil powers, crosses are often placed close to doorways or passageways. An epigram of Theodore Stoudites is addressed to a cross that guards the entrance to a church.[355] Crosses with cryptograms also occur in the bema, often on the altar side of the screen.[356]

Painted crosses with cryptograms are well known in churches of Cyprus. Besides the naos and narthex of Asinou (see below, pp. 257–60, and Figs. 6.30, 6.32, 6.34), examples survive in the Enkleistra of St. Neophytos (1183), the Panagia tou Arakos in Lagoudera (1192), the Panagia at Moutoullas (1280), and the Holy Cross near Platanistassa (1494).[357]

The cryptograms written around the crosses in the narthex of Asinou point to the significance of

354. Walter, "IC XC NI KA," has surveyed the representation of the cross accompanied by legends and acronyms in different media—coins, manuscripts, minor objects, churches—and investigated its origins and functions. For an older bibliography, see Frolow, "IC XC NI KA"; Babić, "Croix à cryptogrammes." See also Mutafov, "Epigrafikata na svetija krŭsti." On the apotropaic function of the crosses with cryptograms, see Gabelić, "Linearno slikarstvo Sisojevca." On the relations of epigrams and the holy cross, see Hörandner, "Das byzantinische Epigramm."

355. PG 99:1796b, no. 47; Speck, *Theodoros Studites Jamben*, 199–200; Walter, "IC XC NI KA," 213.

356. On the placement of foliate crosses with apotropaic inscriptions in the sanctuary and on the reverse side of bilateral icons, see Gerstel, "Alternate View," 146–47.

357. Mango and Hawkins, "Hermitage," 162–63; Nicolaïdès, "Panagia Arakiotissa à Lagoudéra" [1993], 132–34; Mouriki, "Moutoullas," 183; Stylianou and Stylianou, *Painted Churches*, 210, pl. 120. In the church of the Panagia tou Arakos, crosses painted on the jambs of the north and south doors are accompanied by epigrams referring to the qualities of the cross: see Rhoby, *Byzantinische Epigramme*, 326–29, nos. 226–29.

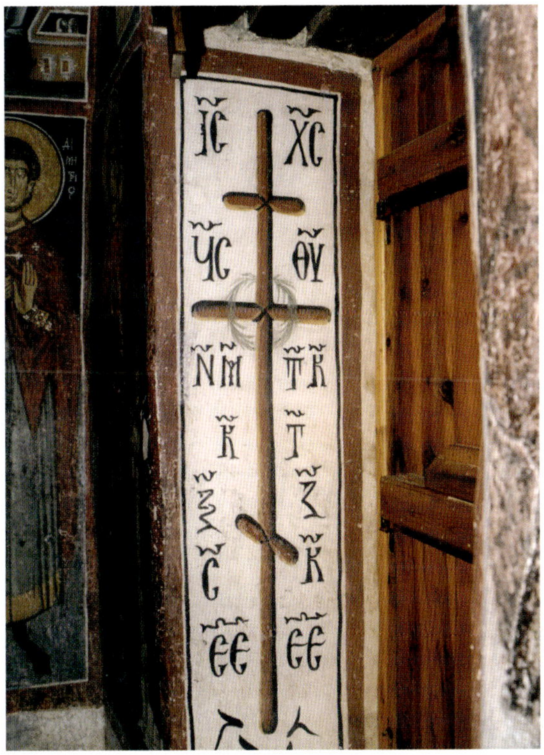

FIG. 5.49 Narthex, south jamb of west door. Cross with cryptograms (photo courtesy of S. Kalopissi-Verti)

TABLE 5.1 Transcription and translation of Fig. 5.49

IC	XC	Ἰ(ησοῦ)ς Χ(ριστό)ς	Jesus Christ;
YC	ΘY	υ(ἱό)ς θ(εο)ῦ	Son of God;
N M	T K	ν(όμος) Μ(ωϋσέως), τ(όπος) κ(υρίου)	Moses' Law, Place of the Lord;
K	T	κ(ρανίου) τ(όπος)	Skull's Place;
Ξ	Z	ξ(ύλον) ζ(ωῆς) *or* ξ(ύλον) ζ(ωοποιόν)	Wood of Life; *or* Life-Giving Wood;
C	K	σ(ωτηρία) κ(όσμου)	Salvation of the World;
E E	E E	Ἑ(λένης) ε(ὕρημα) ἐ(λέους) ἔ(ρεισμα) *or* Ἑ(λένη) ε(ὗρεν) ἐ(λέους) ἔ(ρεισμα) *or* Ἑ(λένη) ε(ὗρεν) ε(ὕρημα) ἐ(λέους)	Helena's Discovery, the Staff of Mercy; *or* Helena Found the Staff of Mercy; *or* Helena Found the Discovery [that gives] Mercy.

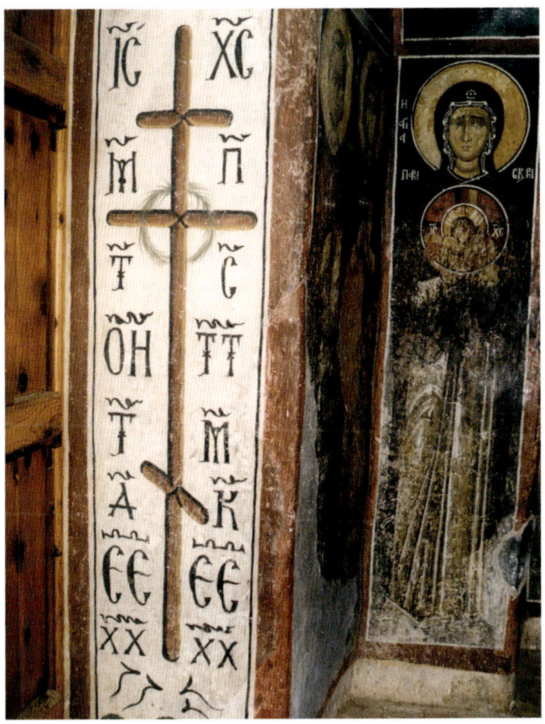

FIG. 5.50 Narthex, north jamb of west door. Cross with cryptograms (photo courtesy of S. Kalopissi-Verti)

TABLE 5.2 Transcription and translation of Fig. 5.50.

IC	XC	Ἰ(ησοῦ)ς Χ(ριστό)ς	Jesus Christ;
M	Π	μ(αρτύρων) π(ίστις)	Faith of Martyrs;
T	C	τ(ίμιος) σ(ταυρός)	Holy Cross;
O H	T T	ο(. . .) η(. . .) τ(ίμιος) τ(ύπος)	[. . .] Holy Type;
T	M	τ(όπος) μ(αρτυρίου)	Place of Martyrdom;
Δ	K	δ(ίκαιος) κ(ριτής) *or* δ(ικαία) κ(ρίσις)	Just Judge; *or* Fair Judgement
E E	E E	Ἑ(λένης) ε(ὕρημα) ἐ(λέους) ἔ(ρεισμα) *or* Ἑ(λένη) ε(ὗρεν) ἐ(λέους) ἔ(ρεισμα) *or* Ἑ(λένη) ε(ὗρεν) ε(ὕρημα) ἐ(λέους)	Helena's Discovery, the Staff of Mercy (*or variants as above*);
X X	X X	Χ(ριστός) χ(άριν) Χ(ριστιανοῖς) χ(αρίζει) or Χ(ριστός) Χ(ριστιανοῖς) χ(άριν) χ(αρίζεται) *or* Χ(ριστός) χ(άριν) χ(αρίζει) Χ(ριστιανοῖς)	Christ Grants Grace to the Christians.

the cross as a symbol of Christ's sacrifice (T M) and charity (E E E E), and as a sign of the faith of the martyrs (M Π). Cryptograms on both crosses also emphasize the salvific and eschatological functions of the cross (Ξ Z, C K, Δ K, and X X X X).

Decorative Patterns

Decorative Patterns of the Late Twelfth-Century Layer

Juxtaposed roundels on brown ground, inspired by marble revetments, are preserved under the figure of Christ (Fig. 5.30) on the east wall and under the image of St. George in the south apse (Figs. 5.1, 4.1, 4.6). The large interior medallion is black in most cases and is encircled by a white ring. A black (rarely white) sawtooth ornament runs along the circumference. In one case there is a pattern consisting of small black circles along the circumference (see Fig. 4.6 for reconstructed drawing). This decorative motif is used throughout the dado zone in the church of Panagia tou Arakos at Lagoudera (1192).[358] It also occurs in different parts of the Enkleistra of St. Neophytos near Paphos, dated to the last decades of the twelfth century.[359] Moreover, it is interesting to note, as Ioanna Kakoulli illustrates (pp. 317–19), that the plaster of the dado zone bearing this ornament on the east wall is the same as the dado plaster under the image of St. George, and that this entire ornamental zone and St. George belong to the same phase, namely, the late twelfth century.

The half roundels on white ground consist of two concentric, studded semicircles enclosing radially placed split-palmette motifs. Portions of this pattern, which imitates textile decoration, are preserved under the dedicatory inscription on the east lunette (Figs. 5.37, 3.11). A more-or-less similar motif is visible to the right of the image of the lay donor Georgios (Fig. 5.44). The closest parallels have been observed in the church of the Holy Apostles at Perachorio (1160–80).[360]

An oblique wavy band between parallel lines is painted in red ocher on white ground. It is visible on the dado zone under the left foot of John the Baptist (Fig. 5.1). Similar motifs occur in twelfth- and thirteenth-century Cypriot churches, for example in the dado zone of the west wall of the naos at Asinou (layer of 1105/6; Fig. 6.15), in the panel of the two donor monks in the apse of St. Herakleidios in the monastery of St. John Lampadistes (twelfth century), in the cell and bema of the Enkleistra of St. Neophytos near Paphos (ca. 1180), and in the church of Panagia Amasgou at Monagri (ca. 1275–1300).[361]

The comparanda assembled above, particularly for the first two motifs, and the evidence of the subsequent fresco layers lead one to date these decorative patterns, all lying beneath the paintings of 1332/33, to the twelfth century and, more precisely, to its last decades, together with the panel of St. George.

Decorative Pattern of the Late Thirteenth-Century Layer (ca. 1300)

A foliate scroll design on black ground decorates the archivolt of the south semidome framing the panel of the Virgin della Misericordia and the Latin supplicants (Figs. 5.1, 5.6). This design is bordered by white lines and red bands and consists of curved stalks ending in half leaves with rounded blossoms in between and continuous loops that enclose five-leafed flowers. Red, green, and gray alternate on the leaves and the half leaves. Very characteristic are the short white stems ending in buds that decorate the edges of the leaves. The whole decorative band gives the

358. Nicolaïdès, "Étude iconographique," figs. 9, 10, 18–20, 22, 67, 77, 79, 80, 90 for roundels with a sawtooth pattern; figs. 18, 67, 79, 90 for roundels with small circles in the surrounding white ring.
359. Mango and Hawkins, "Hermitage," figs. 82 (cell), 110 (refectory), 118 (cave of St. John).

360. Megaw and Hawkins, "Perachorio," 336, fig. 44, semi-roundels next to the east recess; fig. 42, full roundels on the valance of the bed of the Virgin in the Dormition. See also above, p. 95.
361. Stylianou and Stylianou, *Painted Churches*, fig. 176; Papageorgiou, *Μονή του Αγίου Ιωάννου*, fig. 12; Mango and Hawkins, "Hermitage," figs. 52, 60, 82, 100; Boyd, "Monagri," 315, fig. 49.

impression of an elaborate, three-dimensional, multicolored ornament.

Stalks with half leaves forming wavy lines or circles that enclose flowers, the flowers consisting of five broad leaves in different colors and placed atop each other, are common in Byzantine miniatures of the middle and late periods.[362] Similar patterns occur in twelfth-century illuminated manuscripts from the scriptorium of the Holy Sepulcher and in Armenian miniatures of the thirteenth century.[363] Moreover, the characteristic white stems with dots on the edges of the leaves, abstract imitations of curled leaves with white contour lines in more realistic paintings, are seen in twelfth-century miniatures of the Latin Kingdom of Jerusalem, in late thirteenth-century miniatures from Acre, and in great abundance in the illuminated manuscripts of Armenian Cilicia in the late twelfth and thirteenth centuries.[364]

Analogous motifs in Byzantine monumental painting are more rarely encountered.[365] White stems ending in dots decorate leaf patterns in the church of St. John Chrysostom at Koutsovendis (ca. 1100).[366] A flower-leaf motif that could be considered a remote ancestor of the one in the narthex of Asinou is painted in the churches of the Holy Anargyroi in Kastoria and of St. George at Kurbinovo (1191), while it occurs later in a more simplified version, closer to that of Asinou, in Staro Nagoričino (1318).[367] Stylized stemmed dots on trefoils are encountered in monumental painting in regions of the Byzantine Empire under Latin control.[368]

Although certain parallels exist in Byzantine monumental painting, the Crusader context of the panel framed by this decorative motif makes it seem more likely that miniatures created in scriptoria of the Crusader states or of Armenian Cilicia in the twelfth and thirteenth centuries inspired the painter.

Decorative Patterns of the Layer of 1332/33

A sequence of THREE CRENELLATED LOZENGES OR STEPPED CROSSES enclosed in an equal number of interconnected circles, on ocher yellow ground, appear on the panel painted on the lintel of the north door (Figs. 5.28, 5.29). The crosses are outlined in white and filled alternately with black, green, and brown. The circles are precisely drawn with a compass. Black arabesque motifs fill the background. The motif of the stepped crosses, half or full, is very common in the Byzantine world in general and Cyprus in particular.[369] Exact parallels in design and coloring occur in the naos of Asinou (see below, p. 248; Fig. 6.25), in the layer dated to the first half of the fourteenth century in the church of Panagia Amasgou at Monagri, and in the church of St. Nicholas of the Roof at Kakopetria (fourteenth century).[370]

362. Frantz, "Byzantine Illuminated Ornament," 55–59 ("Sassanian palmette"). On floral motifs in middle Byzantine illuminated manuscripts and the so-called "Blütenblattstil", see Weitzmann, *Byzantinische Buchmalerei*, 22–32. On foliate and floral patterns of the late Byzantine period, see Lepage, "Ornementation végétale fantastique."

363. Buchthal, *Miniature Painting*, pls. 36, 37, 43; Folda, *Art of the Crusaders*, pl. 27; Der Nersessian, *Miniature Painting*, 2: figs. 129, 153, 167, 330, etc.

364. Buchthal, *Miniature Painting*, pls. 30h, 32b; Folda, *Crusader Manuscript Illumination*, fig. 22; Der Nersessian, *Miniature Painting*, 2: figs. 21, 36, 40, 47–48, 114, 132, 134–36, 310, etc.

365. Winding leaves with white stems ending in buds, painted in a free manner, occur in the columned churches of Göreme at Cappadocia (3rd quarter of 11th c.); see Restle, *Byzantine Wall Painting*, vol. 2, figs. 167, 168, 182, 185, 187–89, 210, 211, 216, 232, 243.

366. Mango, "Koutsovendis," figs. 54, 57, 58.

367. Pelekanides and Chatzidakes, *Καστοριά*, 32; Hadermann-Misguich, *Kurbinovo*, 304–5, figs. 114, 116, 158; Grozdanov and Hadermann-Misguich, *Kurbinovo*, fig. 20; Millet, *Peinture du Moyen Age*, 3: pl. 119, fig. 3.

368. For example, in the church of the Dormition at Oxylithos in Euboea (ca. 1300), see Emmanuel, *Τοιχογραφίες τοῦ Ἁγ. Δημητρίου*, 152, pl. 78.

369. Janc, *Ornamenti fresaka*, figs., 1–10, 218, 220–24, 227–32, 374; Megaw and Hawkins, "Perachorio," 340, fig. 52.

370. Boyd, "Monagri," 326, fig. 65; the motif in the church of St. Nicholas of the Roof (in the southwestern compartment) is unpublished.

A FOLDED-RIBBON OR ZIGZAG PATTERN, on black ground, between red bands surrounds the image of the Pantokrator in the vault (Fig. 5.11). It consists of a double band: one alternately red and yellow ocher, the other white and red. Three white dots fill in the triangular spaces formed between the zigzag design and the red bands framing it.

The folded-ribbon motif is commonplace in Byzantine art from early Christian times onward. It was widespread throughout the Byzantine world and in Cyprus in the Komnenian and Palaiologan periods.[371] It should be noted that in the two twelfth-century examples on Cyprus, at Perachorio and Lagoudera,[372] the bands are shaded to give an impression of perspective, whereas the folded ribbons in the narthex of Asinou create a flat and purely decorative effect.

POLYCHROME DOUBLE AXES fill the lower parts of the pendentives of the vault (Figs. 5.1, 5.13, 5.14, 5.18, 5.19, 5.23, 5.25, 5.27, 5.28, 5.30, 5.34). The main body of the axe is black, the wavy outlines white; the semicircular endings of the axes are alternately red and orange-yellow for the horizontal elements, blue and gray for the vertical.

Widespread in western European painting of the Carolingian and Romanesque periods and in Byzantine art of the Komnenian and Palaiologan periods,[373] the double-axe pattern is popular in Cypriot churches, especially for the decoration of spandrels and soffits, from the late thirteenth century to the first decades of the fifteenth. Thus, it is painted over the southeast window of the dome in the church of Panagia Chryseleousa at Strovolos (ca. 1275–80), above the apse in the cave hermitage of St. Sozomenos at Potamia (ca. 1300–1330), in the central vessel of the church of the Holy Cross at Pelendri (ca. 1350–75), in the naos of Asinou in a more careless way (see below, p. 301; Figs. 6.37, 6.42), in the north crossarm of the church of St. Nicholas of the Roof (fourteenth–fifteenth century), and in the Latin Royal Chapel at Pyrga (1421).[374]

FLORAL MOTIFS against black ground appear in the spandrels of the medallions in the vault (Figs. 5.11, 5.12). White, heart-shaped linear patterns enclose floral trefoils comprising three pointed leaves, the first in red and brown, the middle in blue and red, the third in gray and brown-red. All three leaves have white dots on stems along their edge. The extensions of the white lines forming the heart motifs end in two half leaves, again colored with two hues; their circumference is studded with white dots on stems. Red circles interrupt the heart-shaped lines. Very similar patterns, painted less carefully, occur in the fourteenth-century layer of the naos (see below, p. 247; Figs. 6.23, 6.24).

This rare floral pattern seems to be a more simplified and schematized version of the foliate scroll design on the archivolt of the south conch. A floral design in the soffit over the northeast window of the dome in the church of Panagia Chryseleousa at Strovolos, near Nicosia (ca. 1275–1300), includes half leaves with the characteristic white dots on stems along their edge.[375]

371. On the pattern, its origins in antique tradition, and its dissemination, see Hadermann-Misguich, *Kurbinovo*, 296–98. For late Byzantine examples, see Janc, *Ornamenti*, figs. 100–104, 113; the closest parallel, i.e., a double ribbon with three dots in the triangular spaces, is encountered in the church of the Virgin at Studenica, ibid., fig. 100; see also Emmanuel, *Τοιχογραφίες τοῦ Ἁγ. Δημητρίου*, 151–52. For examples in Cyprus, see Young, "Byzantine Painting," 210; Papageorgiou, "Paintings in the Dome," 147–54, figs. 1, 2, 5.

372. Megaw and Hawkins, "Perachorio," figs. 2, 12, 56; Nicolaïdès, "Étude iconographique," fig. 36.

373. O'Connor, "Double-Axe Motif"; Hadermann-Misguich, *Kurbinovo*, 298–99, fig. 155; for Palaiologan examples in Serbia, see Janc, *Ornamenti*, figs. 168, 170; for examples in the Peloponnese, see Drandakes, *Βυζαντινὲς τοιχογραφίες*, 388–91, fig. 27; Chassoura, *Peintures murales byzantines*, 245–46, fig. 62; Hirschbichler, "Crusader Painting," 15, fig. 5.

374. There are very few published pictures of the pattern in Cypriot churches. See Papageorgiou, "Strovolos," 153, fig. 1; Soteriou, *Βυζαντινὰ μνημεῖα*, pl. 94a.

375. Papageorgiou, "Strovolos," 153, fig. 14. For a similar floral motif, including the characteristic white dots on stems, in the church of the Taxiarches at Desphina on Mt. Parnassos (also dated to 1332), see Soteriou, "Τοιχογραφίαι τοῦ βυζαντινοῦ ναΰδρίου," 179, fig. 3.

A TENDRIL OR RINCEAU DESIGN, alternately in green, ocher, and dark red on black ground is painted (a) on a narrow zone of the east wall, to the right of Christ Eleemon (Fig. 5.30); and (b) on rectangular compartments above the monks Laurentios and Babylas (Figs. 5.28, 5.29) in the north conch and above the lay donor Georgios in the south conch (Fig. 5.1). The tendril design, especially in its vermiculated arabesque form, is a common decoration in Byzantine monumental and miniature painting from the tenth century onward. It was very popular in the twelfth century, especially in its last decades, all over Byzantium and in Cyprus and continued to occur in monuments of the thirteenth and fourteenth centuries.[376]

An ocher-yellow TENDRIL DESIGN painted against a black ground (Figs. 5.37, 3.11) appears on the soffit of the arch over the lunette where the Virgin Phorbiotissa is depicted. It is a simplified variant of the tendril or rinceau design. It also occurs and is similarly painted in a late thirteenth-century illuminated manuscript from the scriptorium at Acre.[377]

A CHEVRON DESIGN consisting of superimposed wavy lines alternately in black and red on white ground is painted on the jambs of the north door (Fig. 5.35) and on the soffit over the west door (Fig. 5.22). It also occurs on the dado zone of the naos (see below, pp. 237, 246; Figs. 6.16 and 6.22 among others). It is a very simple pattern found in every period of Byzantine art.

Style

The dominant stylistic characteristics of the paintings of 1332/33 in the narthex of Asinou are linearity, a two-dimensional rendering of the figures, standardization of forms, and muted colors. On the figures, contour lines, hair, and facial features are drawn with fine linear brushstrokes. The vertical folds of the garments, shaded in darker tones of the local color, fall in parallel lines from under the waist to the hem on both sides of the left, standing leg (Fig. 5.33). A small V-shaped fold immediately under the right knee, nested in a longer fold of the same shape, lends definition to the knee, while five oblique folds are formed on the right thigh. Highlights are rendered in a light hue of the garment's local color and in pure white. This treatment of the drapery is standardized in pretty much all of the frontally standing figures.

The modeling of the flesh portions of the figures is also formulaic. The outlines are drawn in black or brown (Fig. 5.59). Over the ocher that underlies the entire face is an olive green layer that is left visible to define the shaded parts of the face close to the contour, around the eyes, on both sides of the nose, and under the mouth. The green shading may be darkened with brown brushstrokes. The flesh of the young faces is modeled in tones of ocher; sparse highlights are rendered with fine white lines, and the cheeks are enlivened with reddish touches. The faces of the aged figures are modeled in much the same way, but dense olive green and brown linear brushstrokes are added on the forehead and the cheeks to denote wrinkles (Figs. 5.42, 5.63). The exposed parts of the body, such as feet and hands, are modeled using similar effects: brown or black outlines, olive green and brown shading, flesh in tones of ocher, and white highlights.

The rendering of the faces is very uniform, especially among the young saints. Young female saints, such as Marina, Eudokia, Anna, and Mavra (Figs. 5.19, 5.28), look almost identical. Some differentiation in expression is conveyed through variations such as greater or lesser arching of the eyebrows, as in the images of the prophets Isaiah and Zechariah (Figs. 5.31, 5.32), or through frowning, as in the figures of SS. Paraskeve and John the Forerunner (Figs. 5.36, 5.63). Distinct nuances, however, in the rendering of prosopographical features do stand out in the modeling of the faces of the donors. The face of the priest-monk Barnabas is characterized by a rather painterly modeling; the stylized wrinkles of the monk Theophilos's face give the impression of a man of spare build; the faces of the monks

376. Hadermann-Misguich, *Kurbinovo*, 303; Megaw and Hawkins, "Perachorio," 341–42; Kalopissi-Verti, *Kirche der Hagia Triada*, 229–30.
377. Folda, *Crusader Manuscript Illumination*, figs. 7, 92, 171, etc.

Laurentios, Germanos, and Leontios clearly reflect men of different age and physiognomy. The rendering of Anna Lachana's face reveals the fresh complexion of a young maiden (Figs. 5.38–42, 5.47).

Distinctions may also be noted between the saints of the lower zone of the walls and the figures in the upper parts of the narthex. Although they share the main stylistic devices, hastier drawing and a more summary modeling characterize the figures of the upper zones. This distinction, a common practice in Byzantine monumental painting, does not point to a different painter but rather to a more concise handling of the minor figures or of those placed farther from the beholder. It should be noted, however, that the very same modeling, attentive drawing, and graduated coloring seen in the saints' images of the lower zone of the narthex is encountered in the major figures of the upper zones, especially the Pantokrator, the Virgin, and the archangels Michael and Gabriel painted in the central vault of the narthex (Figs. 5.53, 5.54, 5.67).

In most of the wall paintings in the narthex, the background comprises two zones, a low green section alluding to the earth and an upper dark blue area implying the sky or heaven (Figs. 5.1, 5.19, 5.28, 5.30, 5.38–40).[378] Accordingly, the medallion of the Pantokrator in the vault is dark blue (Fig. 5.11), whereas most of the donors are painted against a full green background (monks Laurentios, Babylas, Kallinikos, and layman Georgios; Figs. 5.28, 5.41, 5.43, 5.44). The angels in the vault are painted in medallions with alternating blue and red backgrounds, alluding to heaven and light, respectively.[379]

Indications of landscape—such as hills, waves, and trees—and of animal life—such as the birds and fish in the scenes of Paradise and of the personified Earth and Sea—are rendered in a very stylized and repetitive manner (Figs. 5.28, 5.29). The scant indications of buildings, such as the door to Paradise, are painted in an abstract and conventional way, which is closer to the middle Byzantine than to the Palaiologan tradition. The wooden thrones of the apostles in the pendentives, with their grained wood and conspicuously sculpted legs, are realistically painted; in fact, certain elements, such as the ornamented colonettes of the throne in the southwest pendentive (Fig. 5.14), seem to imitate contemporary woodwork.[380] The rendering of perspective is conventional, with lines converging toward the beholder, as in the thrones of the Patriarchs in Paradise (Fig. 5.29), or to different points within the same composition. Despite the occasional use of perspective, the sense of depth is restricted and, overall, the compositions give the impression of flatness.

Technical details of the wall paintings in the narthex of Asinou—plaster, preliminary drawing, incised guide lines, pigments, order of coloring—were first studied by David Winfield in 1968.[381] In addition, Ioanna Kakoulli in Chapter 7 points, among other things, to the use of lime plaster rich in organic fibres (probably chaff and hemp), to the identification of plaster joins *(pontate* and *giornate)* following the outline of the scenes, and to the coexistence of the two mural techniques: fresco for the base colors, and secco for the modeling, highlights, background, and gilding.

The wall paintings of the narthex that are dated by inscription to the year 1332/33, and those in the second layer of the naos, which are undated, have several stylistic features in common, as shown by Annemarie Carr (pp. 300–306). In addition, they share much the same ornamental vocabulary. Moreover, in both spaces the technique of pastiglia haloes—a common practice in Cypriot art—has been applied with the same patterns of intersecting circles, though the circles differ in size (see below, pp. 301–2).

378. According to Ioanna Kakoulli's analysis, azurite applied in vertical brushstrokes over a black layer was used for the blue of the background. See below, p. 343.
379. Wunderlich, *Bedeutung der roten Farbe*, 96–97; Lehmann, "Dome of Heaven," 2, n. 8, and p. 11; Mouriki, "Thirteenth-Century Icon Painting," 25.

380. They are comparable to the wooden ornaments of the door preserved between the narthex and the naos in St. Nicholas of the Roof at Kakopetria.
381. Winfield, "Byzantine Wall Painting Methods," 61–139, passim.

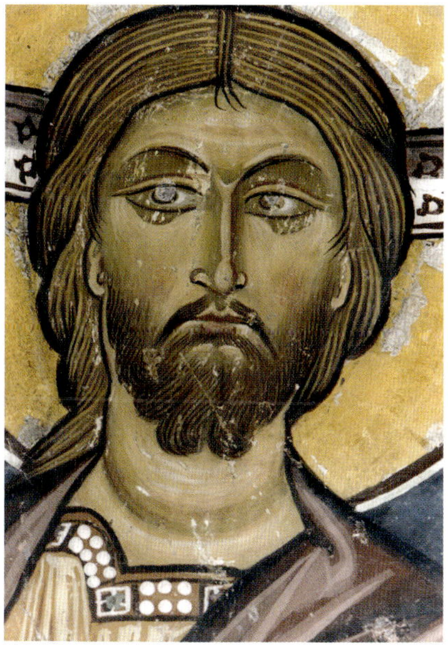

FIG. 5.51 Narthex, east wall. Christ Eleemon (photo courtesy of S. Kalopissi-Verti)

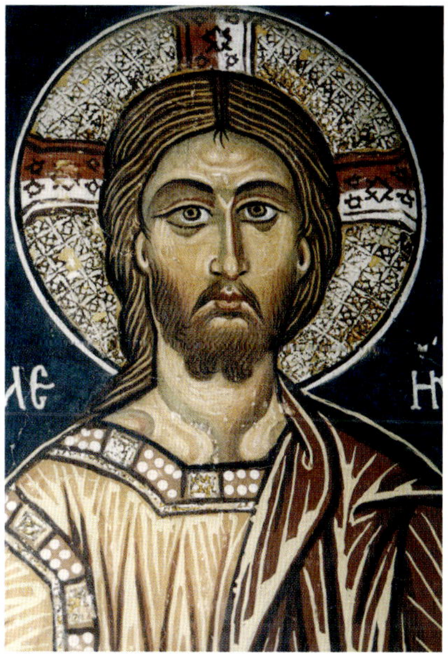

FIG. 5.52 Naos, south bema respond. Christ Eleemon, detail (photo courtesy of S. Kalopissi-Verti)

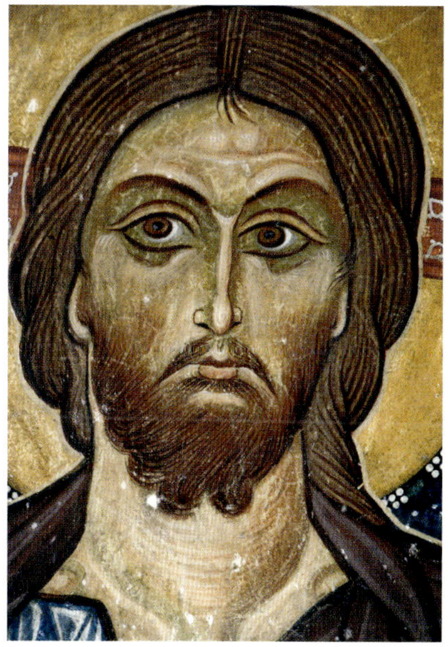

FIG. 5.53 Narthex, vault. The Pantokrator, detail (photo courtesy of S. Kalopissi-Verti)

However, as Annemarie Carr analyzes, certain differences in the role of line and of color may be noted between the paintings of the narthex, especially those in the lower zone, and the murals of the naos (see below, pp. 304–6) . If we compare, for example, the figure of Christ Eleemon next to the door of the narthex (Fig. 5.51) with the equivalent image on the south bema respond in the naos (Fig. 5.52), we may note in the first example that the basic ocher color of the flesh is paler and yellower, the lines are very fine and carefully drawn, the modeling is very subtle, and the whole impression of the face is flat. By contrast, the figure of Christ in the naos is distinguished by more vivid coloring and uses a reddish brown ocher. Despite the linear features shared with the image of Christ in the narthex, the modeling here is more pronounced and the expression more animated. The figure of Christ on the bema respond resembles the image of the Pantokrator (Fig. 5.53) in the vault of the narthex more than it does that of Christ Eleemon on the east wall, both because of the choice of brownish rather than yellowish colors and because of the shape of the eyes, which is distinguished by the stronger curve of the upper eyelid and the full circle of the iris.

Fine linearity and subtle modeling—based on delicately graduated yellowish ocher and olive green—characterize the figure of the Virgin in the vault of the narthex (Fig. 5.54). By contrast, the Mother of God on the south wall of the naos (Fig. 5.55) is painted with lively brownish-red colors, and its modeling is based more on colors than on lines, which are drawn in a rather careless way. Furthermore, if one compares Adam in the composition of the Last Judgment in the narthex (Fig. 5.56) with Adam in the scene of the Resurrection in the naos (Fig. 5.57), it is possible to contrast the dominant role of line in modeling the former with the latter's leading role of color laid in larger, more casual strokes. One may note in particular how the white of each eyeball is placed. In the case of the figures of the narthex, it is painted next to the iris, carefully following its contour; in the images of the naos it is a vague touch or stroke, which sometimes overlaps the outline of the iris, as in the figure of Adam.

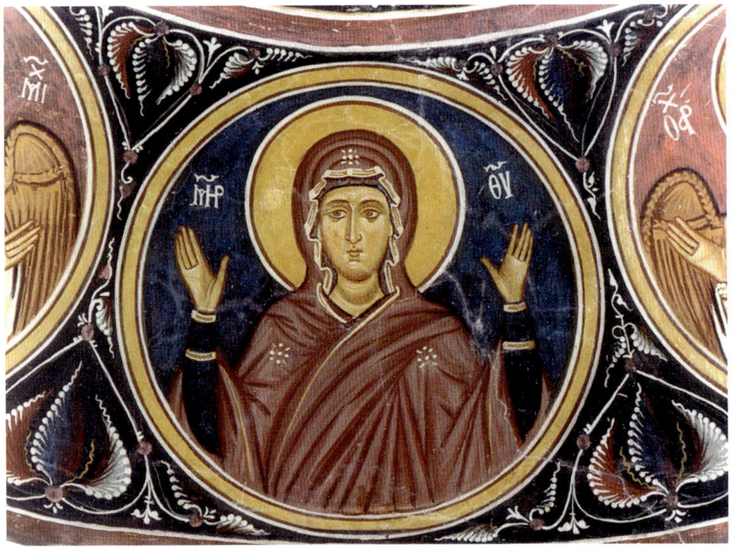

fig. 5.54

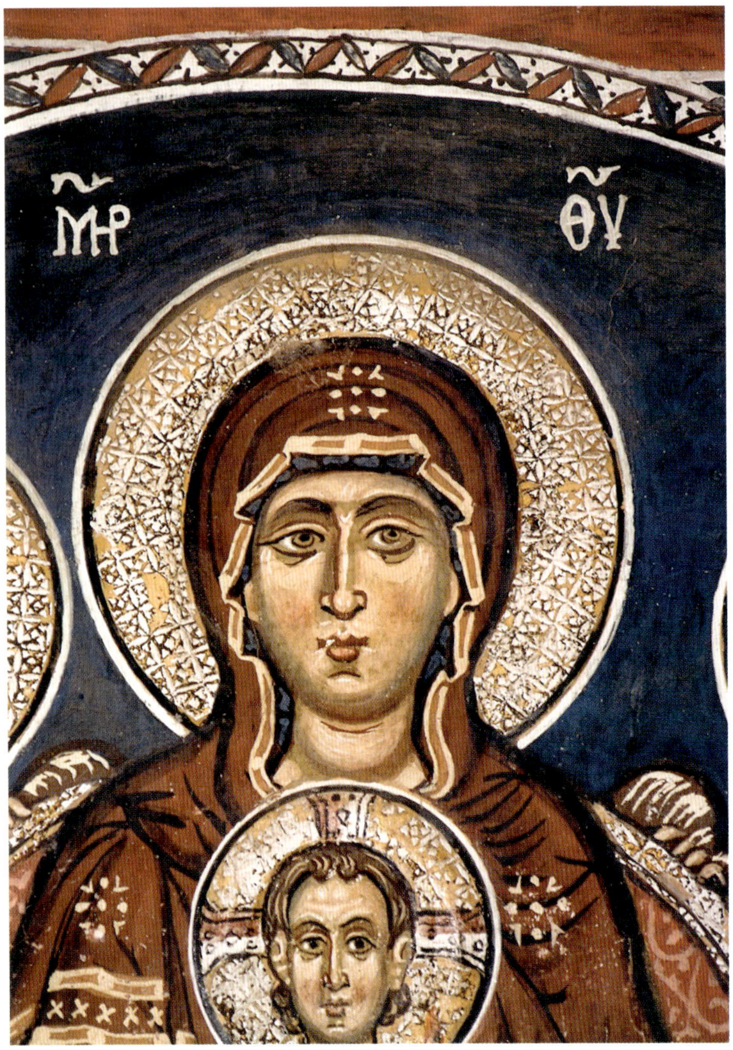

fig. 5.55

FIG. 5.54
Narthex, vault. Roundel of the Virgin (photo courtesy of S. Kalopissi-Verti)

FIG. 5.55
Naos, south wall. The Virgin, detail (photo courtesy of S. Kalopissi-Verti)

In sum, the stylistic differences between the paintings of the narthex—where yellowish ochers are used in conjunction with a very well-defined linearity—and the frescoes of the naos—characterized by an intensive colorism—result in a meditative calmness for the images in the narthex, whereas those in the naos have a more animated effect. In certain figures of the narthex, however, such as the archangel Michael and the Personifications of Earth and Sea, the choice of intensive colors, in particular the reddish-brown ochers, brings them closer to those in the naos. As Annemarie Carr shows, these figures bridge the stylistic differences between the fresco decoration of the narthex and that of the naos (see below, pp. 305–6).

The frescoes of the narthex of Asinou (1332/33) belong to a group of wall paintings that continue the so-called maniera cypria of the previous century (see above, pp. 121–22). This trend, rooted in the high-quality art of the Komnenian era, developed in Cypriot painting during the thirteenth century, at a time when relations with Constantinople decreased and the impact of the art of Crusaders and refugees from the Levant, mainly Syrians and Cilician Armenians, assumed a major role. The dominant features of this trend include a decorative linearity, a two-dimensional rendering of bodies and draperies, and a rather flat facial modeling in subdued tones: ocher for the flesh with reddish touches on the cheeks and light green for the shading. A standardized way of rendering the eyes has also been noted: a curved red outline for the upper eyelid; black pupils in brown irises outlined with black that are almost completely visible, resulting in a staring gaze; and white brushstrokes repeating the curve of the iris on the eyeballs.

FIG. 5.56
Narthex, west wall. Detail of the Last Judgment, head of Adam (photo courtesy of S. Kalopissi-Verti).

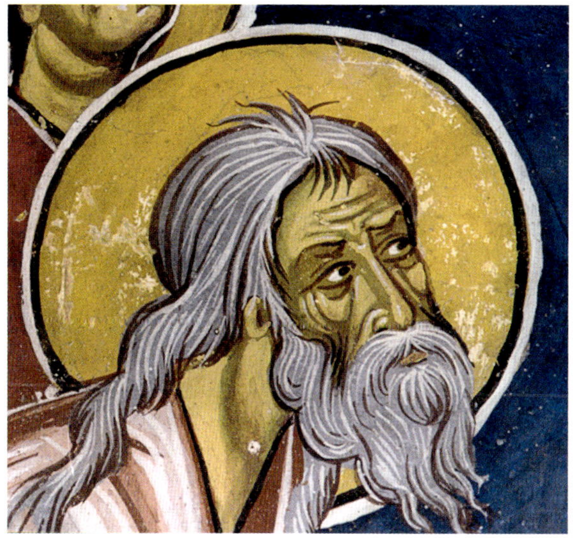

This trend was practiced in both icon painting and monumental art. For example, the icon of the Virgin Kykkotissa from the church at Asinou, now in the Museum of the Foundation of Archbishop Makarios III (Fig. 5.58),[382] is a typical panel of the maniera cypria. If one compares this panel with the figures of the young saints in the lower zone of the narthex at Asinou (Fig. 5.59), several common features become apparent, such as the ocher hues of the flesh, the light green shading along the contours of the face and around the facial features, and the red touches on the cheeks. The modeling of the eyes—with the curved red contour of the upper lid, the crescent-shaped lower lid, and the round, almost completely visible light brown iris with a black outline and with a small black pupil—are also very similar. Moreover, the parallel white highlights at the corner of the eyes, above and below the lips, and on the chin and the neck, are also comparable. The two works are stylistically very similar and look nearly contemporary, as though painters of the same workshop had executed them. It is evident that the master of the paintings of the narthex of Asinou in the year 1332/33 adheres closely to and continues the stylistic principles of the icon, dated, as generally accepted, in the last decades of the thirteenth century.

In monumental painting the fresco decoration of the church of the Panagia at Moutoullas, dated to 1280, is the most frequently cited example of the maniera cypria.[383] If one compares the figure of Christ painted on the templon of the Panagia at Moutoullas (Fig. 5.60) or the icon of Christ from the same church[384] with Christ Eleemon in the narthex of Asinou (Fig. 5.51), one may observe

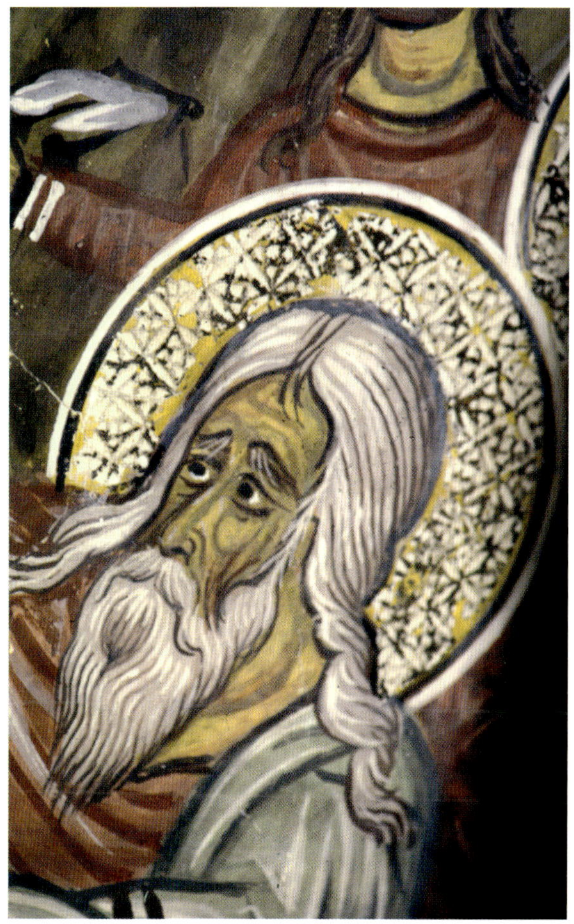

FIG. 5.57 Naos, central bay, north lunette. Detail of the Anastasis, head of Adam (photo courtesy of S. Kalopissi-Verti)

382. Papageorgiou, *Icons of Cyprus* [1992], 55, fig. 35; cf. above, pp. 120–21 and below, p. 200.
383. Mouriki, "Moutoullas," 171–213.
384. Mouriki, "Moutoullas," 191, fig. 29; Papageorgiou, *Icons of Cyprus* [1992], 46, fig. 28.

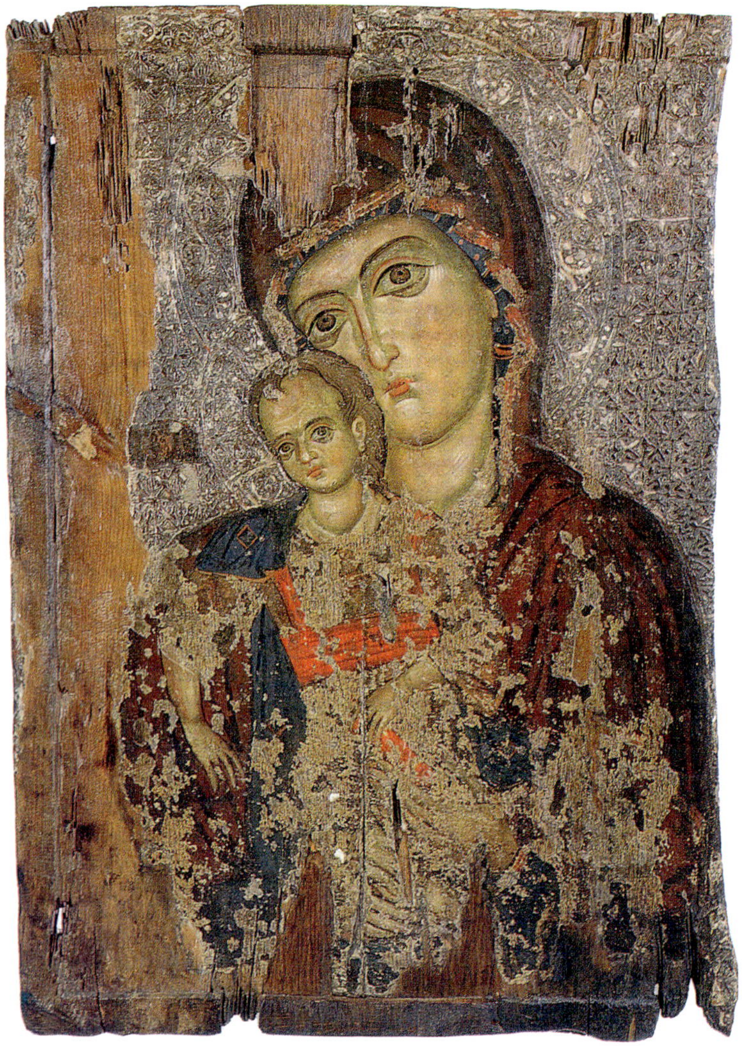

FIG. 5.58 Museum of the Foundation of Archbishop Makarios III, icon of the Virgin Kykkotissa from the church of Asinou (photo courtesy of the Byzantine Museum, Archbishop Makarios III Cultural Foundation, Nicosia)

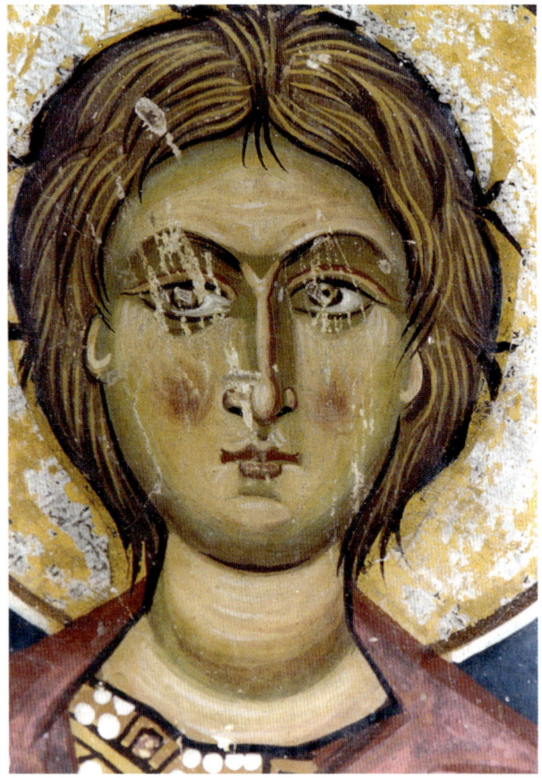

FIG. 5.59
Asinou, narthex, south conch. St. Mamas, detail (photo courtesy of S. Kalopissi-Verti)

that all three figures share certain linear characteristics, although the "rolling eyes" give the images of Christ at Moutoullas a more staring gaze. There are further examples of thirteenth-century monumental painting showing the same features, such as a group of frescoes in St. Herakleidios in the monastery of St. John Lampadistes at Kalopanayiotes (ca. 1265–80), the wall paintings in the church of the Transfiguration at Sotera Famagusta (1280–1300), and the late thirteenth-century fresco layer in the church of Asinou itself, as exemplified by the figures of the Panagia Pantanassa in the apse and of Anastasia Pharmakolytria and her devotee in the narthex (Figs. 5.2, 6.8, 6.9).[385] This thirteenth-century Cypriot trend continues to develop after the turn of the century. The frescoes of St. Demetrianos at Dali, dated by an inscription to 1317, and the third phase in Panagia Amasgou at Monagri, dating to the first decades of the fourteenth century, may be considered the link between the fresco decoration of the church of the Panagia at Moutoullas (1280) and the wall

385. Young, "Byzantine Painting," 144–245; Mouriki, "Thirteenth-Century Icon Painting," 37, figs. 39, 42; A. Papageorgiou in *ARDAC* 1989, 29–30, figs. 11–12; for Asinou, see above, pp. 115–22, and below, pp. 215–16.

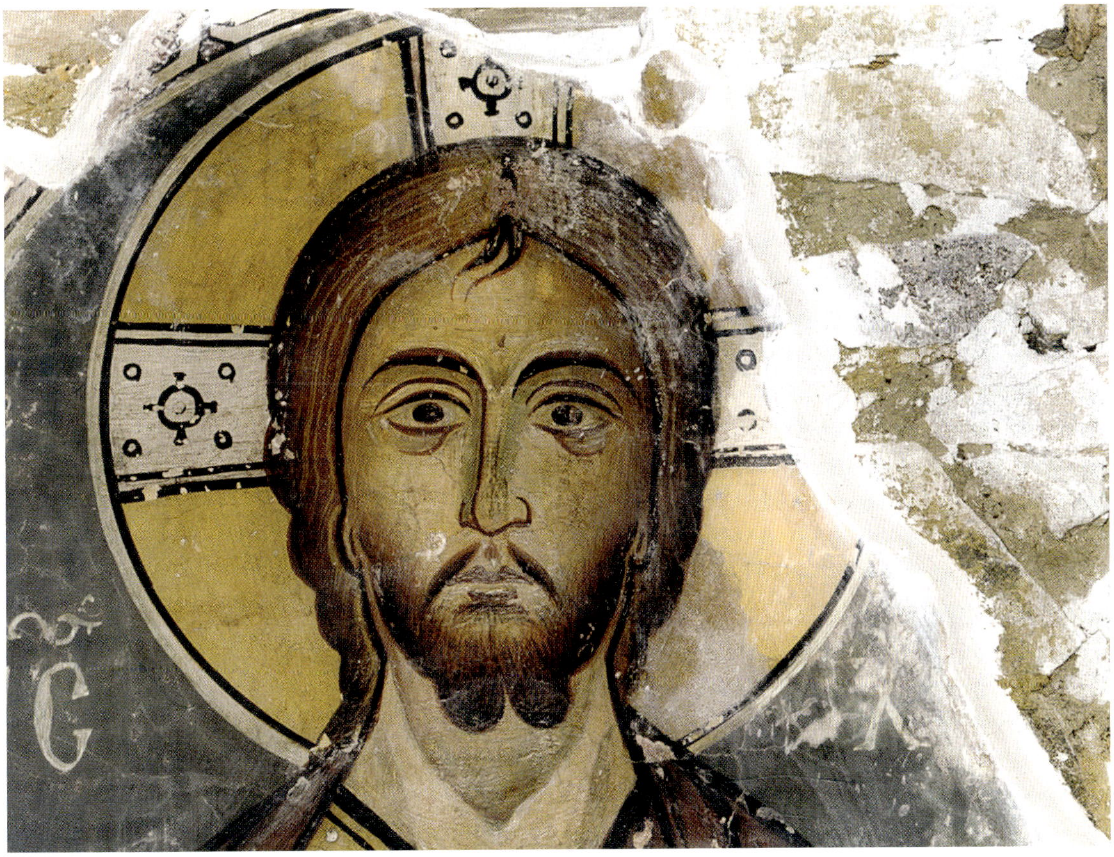

FIG. 5.60 Moutoullas, church of the Panagia, screen. Christ, detail (photo courtesy of S. Kalopissi-Verti)

paintings of the narthex at Asinou (1332/33).[386] At the same time, the two early fourteenth-century monuments illustrate new artistic developments. The linear trend, which adheres to the prevailing style of the thirteenth century on the island, coexists with a new current that reflects the Palaiologan artistic evolution in a provincial version; this places more emphasis on painterly and volumetric values.

The closest stylistic affinities to the wall paintings of the narthex of Asinou may be noted in the fresco decoration of four Cypriot churches: the old narthex of Panagia tou Arakos at Lagoudera, St. Sozomenos at Potamia, Holy Cross at Pelendri, and St. Marina at Pyrga. Of this group, the frescoes in the narthex of Asinou are the only ones that have been firmly dated in 1332/33; the dating of the other wall paintings thus depends on their greater or lesser kinship to Asinou.

The few figures that are preserved on the east wall of the space that once functioned as the narthex of the church of Panagia tou Arakos at Lagoudera (Fig. 5.61) present a close kinship to the murals of the narthex at Asinou in the rendering of the folds, the modeling and coloring of the faces, and the shapes of the eyes and ears. They also share finer details, such as the decorative bands of the *analaboi* and the mantles, the shape of the stars decorating the shoulders, and the letterforms of the inscriptions. These frescoes in the old narthex of Lagoudera have been associated with repair work in the naos and with the Mother of God Panachrantos painted in

386. Stylianou and Stylianou, *Painted Churches*, 425–27; Boyd, "Monagri," 323–27, figs. 54–63. For the development of this stylistic trend in Cyprus during the 14th century, see Carr, "Art," 311–12.

the exterior lunette over the north entrance door to the church.[387] The inscription written above the figure of the Virgin, excerpted from a heirmos by Georgios Sikeliotes, includes the name of the painter, Leontios the Deacon.[388] The close kinship—stylistic and palaeographic—between the murals of the old narthex of Lagoudera and those of the narthex of Asinou have been stressed by David and June Winfield, who have attributed them to the same school.[389]

St. Sozomenos is a cave church near Potamia, southeast of Nicosia.[390] If we compare, for example, the figure of St. Paul of Thebes in St. Sozomenos (Fig. 5.62) with that of St. John the Baptist in the narthex of Asinou (Fig. 5.63), we may note very close similarities in the shape and modeling of the face, the shape and rendering of the eyes, the concerned glance, the contracted eyebrows, and the linear rendering of hair and beard. Moreover, the identical shape of the crosses held by the saints and the identical form of the letters and ligatures in the inscriptions point to a very similar date for the two fresco ensembles and probably to the same painter, as Athanasios Papageorgiou has suggested.[391]

Close affinities may also be noted with part of the mid-fourteenth-century painted decoration of the church of the Holy Cross at Pelendri,[392] in particular with the paintings of the western part of the central vessel and with the apse fresco, which has been removed to reveal the original layer of the late twelfth century (1178). The figures of St. Paul at Pelendri (Fig. 5.64) and in the southeast pendentive of the narthex of Asinou (Fig. 5.65), for example, share many common features in the linear rendering of the wrinkles and the beard, in the drawing of the arched eyebrows, and in the rendering of the eyes. In addition, the images of the archangels in the apse of Pelendri (Fig. 5.66) and those in the vault of the narthex

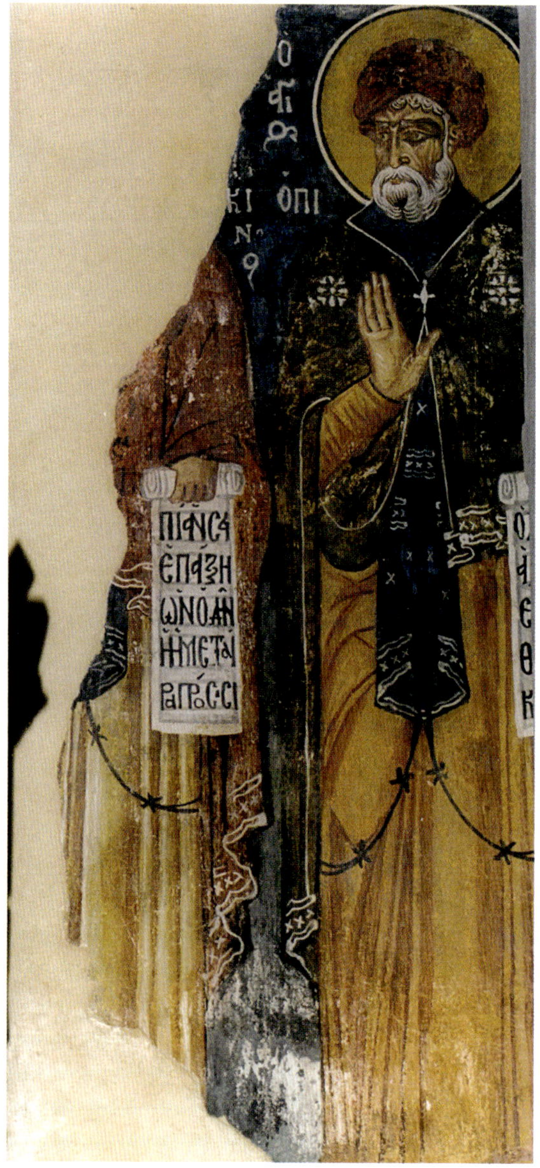

FIG. 5.61 Lagoudera, church of the Panagia, old narthex. The poet Kosmas (photo courtesy of S. Kalopissi-Verti)

387. Winfield and Winfield, *Panaghia tou Arakos at Lagoudhera*, 68–69, 329–35, figs. 8, 300–303.
388. The inscription was first published by C. Mango in the appendix to Winfield, "Lagoudera: First Preliminary Report," 379–80, figs. 8–9.
389. Winfield and Winfield, *Panaghia tou Arakos at Lagoudhera*, 69.
390. Papageorgiou, "Λαξευτά ἀσκητήρια," 47–52, pls. 22–27.
391. Ibid., 52.
392. Stylianou and Stylianou, *Painted Churches*, 223–32, 507–8; Carr, "Byzantines and Italians," 345–47; Christoforaki, "Cyprus Between Byzantium and the Levant."

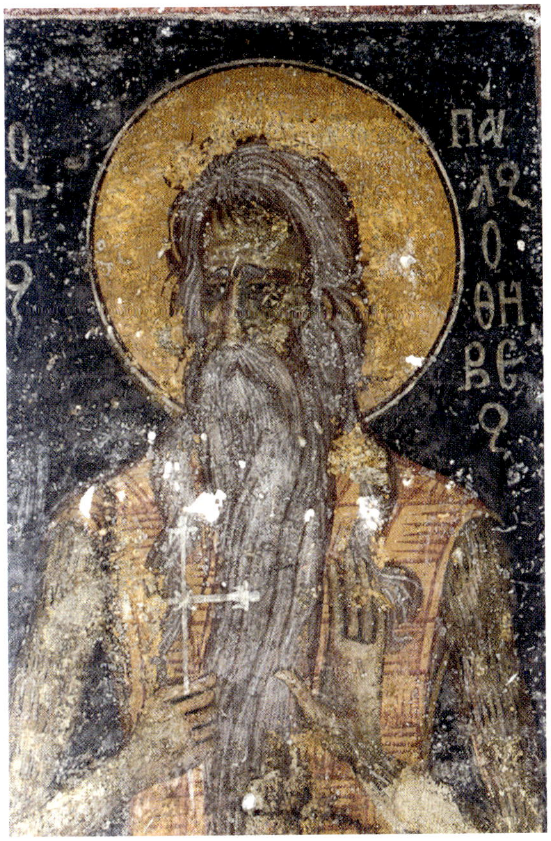

FIG. 5.62 Potamia, cave church of St. Sozomenos. St. Paul of Thebes, detail (photo courtesy of S. Kalopissi-Verti)

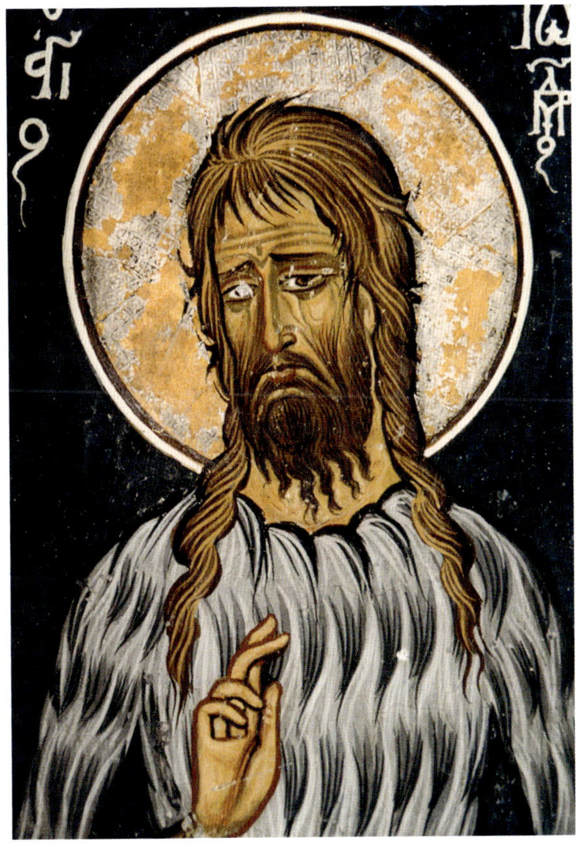

FIG. 5.63 Asinou, narthex, south-east respond. St. John the Baptist, detail (photo courtesy of S. Kalopissi-Verti)

at Asinou (Fig. 5.67)—although the coloring at Pelendri is more vivid—share similarities in the physiognomic type, the modeling of the face, the rendering of the features, the shading of the facial contours, the use of reddish spots on the cheeks, and the fork-shaped endings of the lips.

The two churches—Panagia at Asinou, a monastic church, and Holy Cross at Pelendri, probably a parochial church—seem to reflect very similar social contexts, as indicated by the collective character of the patronage revealed in their dedicatory inscriptions and their donor portraits, in which a large number of figures wear the same style of clothing.[393] Furthermore, certain rare representations of saints in both churches, such as that of St. George Machairomenos, and certain motifs, such as the shape of the cross held by saints, the metallic discs, the double-axe motif, as well as the identical lettering, bring out the close relationship of the two fresco decorations to one another. In addition, the stronger colors and looser execution evident in the scenes of the upper zones of the central vessel at Pelendri reveal the coexistence of the same two

393. For Asinou see above, pp. 185–90. For Pelendri, see Stylianou and Stylianou, *Painted Churches*, 223; eidem, "Donors and Dedicatory Inscriptions," 107. The dedicatory inscription in Pelendri includes the epithet εὐλαβέστατοι, usually referring to priests (no names are preserved), while in the lunette above the western entrance door a lay couple is painted; moreover, there are several portraits within the church, mostly of deceased persons.

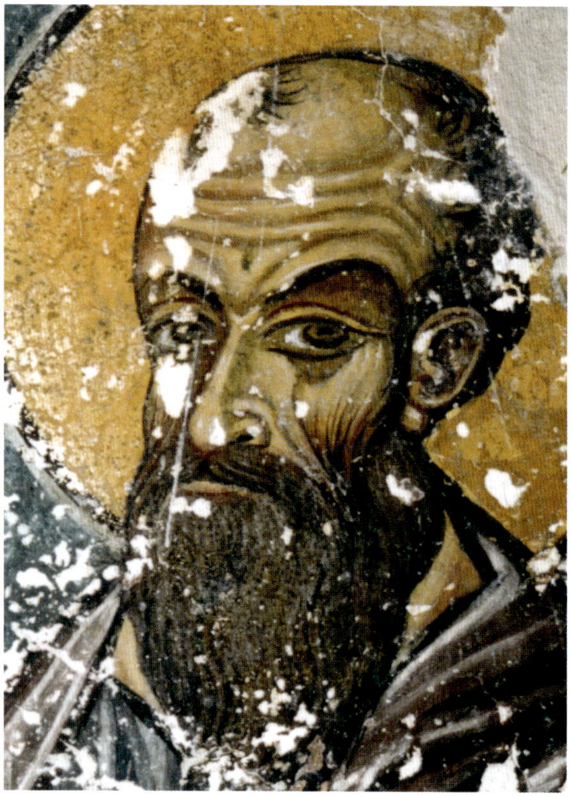

FIG. 5.64 Pelendri, church of the Holy Cross, central vessel. St. Paul, detail (photo courtesy of S. Kalopissi-Verti)

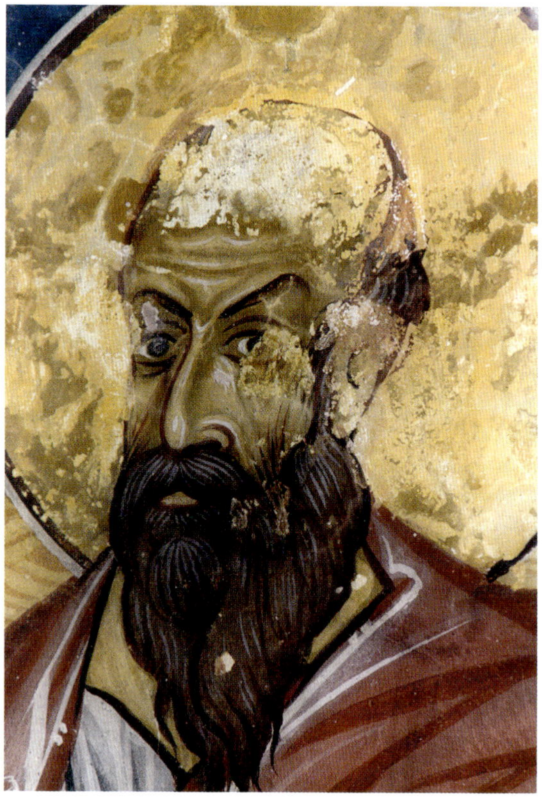

FIG. 5.65 Asinou, narthex, southeast pendentive. St. Paul, detail (photo courtesy of S. Kalopissi-Verti)

different modes of painting that became apparent in contrasting the narthex and the naos of Asinou (see above, pp. 197–98 and below, pp. 308–9).

Furthermore, certain wall paintings preserved in the single-aisled, domed church of St. Marina at Pyrga, such as the figure of St. Polycarp, share features not only with the frescoes at Pelendri, as has already been noted,[394] but also with the murals of the other churches in the group of monuments under discussion, in elements such as the linear contours and the shapes of the ears and the eyes. The rendering of the face in other figures at Pyrga is more painterly, however.[395]

The group of monumental ensembles discussed above, closely linked through the style of the frescoes and the lettering of the inscriptions, points to an industrious local workshop, active in a relatively wide area south of Nicosia from the Troodos Mountains to the Potamia Valley and further south to Pyrga in the decades shortly before and during the mid-fourteenth century. The inscription in the narthex of Asinou offers a fixed date for the activity of the workshop in 1332/33. The inscription in Lagoudera preserves the name of one of the painters, Leontios the Deacon, whereas the name of the painter once included in the dedicatory inscription at Asinou has not been preserved. David

394. Spanou, "Τέχνη στη μητροπολιτική περιφέρεια Κιτίου," 46–48, fig. 27.

395. Spanou, "Τέχνη," 48, fig. 28. Furthermore, Annemarie Carr (below, p. 249) points to a fresco of the Virgin in the church of the Hodegetria in Arediou which bears similarities with the paintings of Asinou; see M. Loulloupis, in *ARDAC* 1991, 18, pls. 1–2.

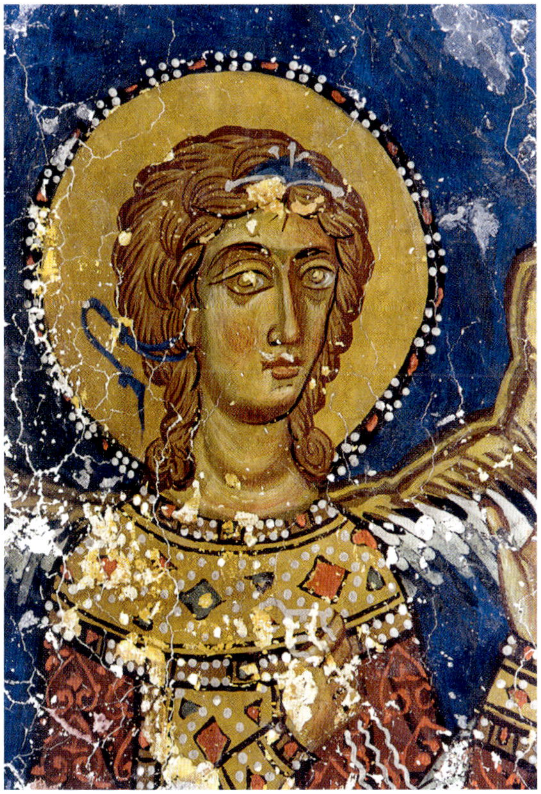

FIG. 5.66 Pelendri, church of the Holy Cross, apse. Archangel, detail (photo courtesy of S. Kalopissi-Verti)

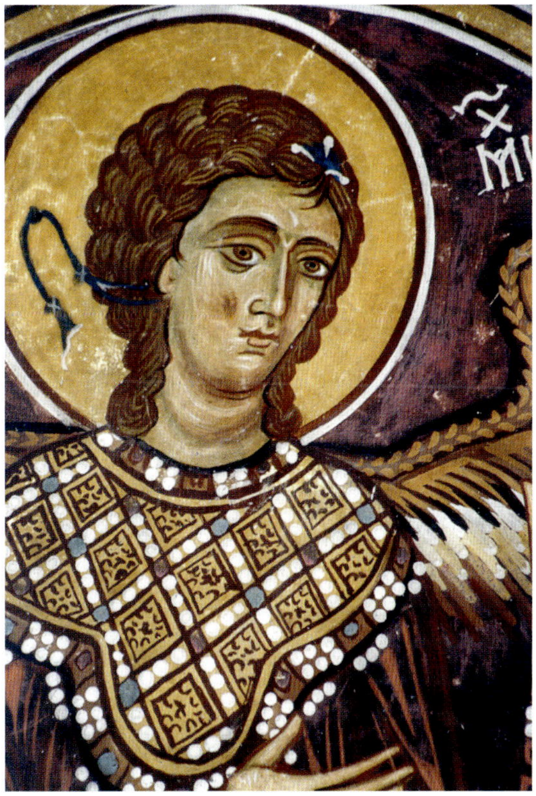

FIG. 5.67 Asinou, narthex, vault. Archangel Michael, detail (photo courtesy of S. Kalopissi-Verti)

Winfield has associated the frescoes of the Asinou narthex and naos with the painter Leontios, and Annemarie Carr identifies him with the master of the paintings of the naos (see below, p. 310). In any case, the painters engaged in the workshop attested in the above-mentioned fourteenth-century Cypriot churches, as well as in the narthex and naos of Asinou, whether they laid more emphasis on linear or on coloristic values in their paintings, were trained in the local Cypriot tradition, deeply rooted in the late twelfth century and simplified during the thirteenth century. Only occasionally did they reflect features of the artistic trends that developed in the great centers of their time.

The continuation of the linear trend, as attested in the Asinou narthex, may be traced further in the fourteenth-century layer of frescoes in the lower zones of the narthex and the western part of the naos in St. Nicholas of the Roof at Kakopetria.[396] A comparison between the images of Christ Eleemon in the narthexes of the two churches, at Kakopetria (Fig. 5.68) and at Asinou (Fig. 5.51) shows that at Kakopetria the linear devices are more stylized; in addition, the very arched eyebrows and the rolling eyes lend the face a more intense and vivid expression. Moreover, the letters of the inscriptions differ from those at Asinou. Although the Kakopetria frescoes share linear components with the wall

396. Stylianou and Stylianou, *Painted Churches*, 72–75. Features of the 14th-century linear style occur also in certain figures of the Royal Chapel at Pyrga (1421); see Enlart, *Gothic Art*, 325–34; Stylianou and Stylianou, *Painted Churches*, 428–32; Papageorgiou, *Βασιλικό παρεκκλήσι*. These figures have been recently attributed to a phase prior to 1421; see Spanou, "Τέχνη στη μητροπολιτική περιφέρεια Κιτίου," 49–50.

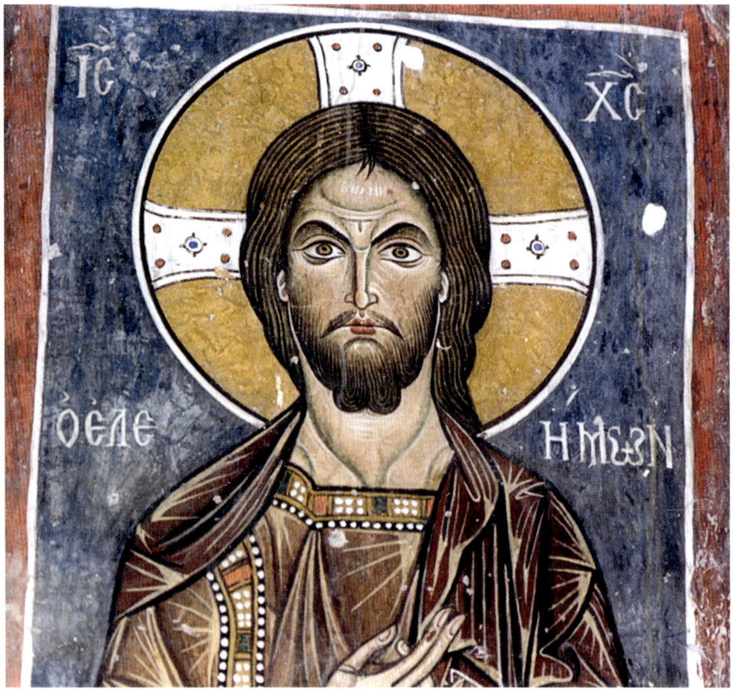

FIG. 5.68 Kakopetria, Church of St. Nicholas of the Roof, narthex. Christ Eleemon, detail (photo courtesy of S. Kalopissi-Verti)

paintings of the narthex at Asinou, they seem to be chronologically and stylistically more distant from them than those of Pelendri and Lagoudera. They should probably be dated to the third quarter of the fourteenth century.

The decorative linearity and the two-dimensional quality of the linear current, traced in the narthex of Asinou and in the other fourteenth-century monuments of Cyprus discussed above, contrast with contemporary stylistic developments in the leading centers of Byzantium—Constantinople, Mistras, Thessalonike, Mt. Athos—and in Serbia. The Cypriot painting lacks the innovative pictorial devices and the painterly and volumetric qualities of the contemporary Palaiologan style. Metropolitan Palaiologan style is represented in the fourteenth-century painting of Cyprus only in certain murals and icons produced after the middle of the century.[397]

In summary, the fresco decoration in the narthex of Asinou adheres to the local Cypriot trend of the thirteenth century. This trend had resulted from the historical conditions that prevailed on the island from the end of the twelfth century, namely, the occupation of Cyprus by the Crusaders and its alienation from metropolitan artistic developments. The same local trend persisted in a cluster of monuments during the first half of the fourteenth century, reflecting the taste of monastic and lay patrons and viewers in the setting of the Cypriot countryside.

The Narthex in Sum

The narthex was added to the naos of Asinou sometime during the twelfth century, probably to serve the liturgical or funerary needs of the monastery (see above, p. 54). It incorporated the fresco of the Virgin Phorbiotissa in the lunette of the entrance door, which belonged to the original paintings of 1105/6. The narthex was first decorated, though possibly only partially, in the 1180s. The date is implied by the roundels and the split-palmette pattern visible in the dado zone of the east wall, on the lintel of the doorway to the naos, and under the donor Georgios, as well as by the cult image of St. George, painted after the door opening in the south apse was walled in. While the decorative patterns were covered by the paintings of 1332/33, the fresco of St. George remained intact and was respectfully integrated in the fourteenth-century decorative program. Regarded as one of the finest examples of monumental painting in Cyprus from the late twelfth century, it bears witness to the high quality of this layer.

The narthex was fully or partly renewed in the late thirteenth century, when restoration work was undertaken in the bema and the naos. The panels of St. Anastasia the Pharmakolytria with her devotee Anastasia Saramalina—and, subsequently, of the Virgin of Mercy commissioned by Latin supplicants—belong to this restoration project

397. For a survey and discussion of the stylistic developments in Cypriot art of Orthodox and Latin patronage in the 14th century, see Carr, "Art," 310–28 (with bibliography).

(ca. 1290–1300). Moreover, the traces of an archangel, presumably also a votive, that are visible under the fourteenth-century Archangel Michael can be assigned on the basis of technical analysis to a phase preceding, yet close to, the renovation of 1332/33.

The large renovation program of the year 1332/33, undertaken by the monastery with the support "of the common people," as the dedicatory inscription says, gave the narthex a coherent program without changing its votive character. While covering certain parts of the prior mural decoration that had worn away, it skillfully and harmoniously incorporated all of the previous paintings that were in good condition. Thus, besides the Virgin Phorbiotissa in the lunette (1105/06), which received repainting, the votive images of St. George (final quarter of the twelfth century) and of St. Anastasia and the Virgin of Mercy (ca. 1290–1300) were integrated with great respect.

The dominant scene of the Last Judgment and the Deesis, essential components of the fourteenth-century program, are soteriological in character, and may be linked to the funerary, intercessory, and commemorative services performed in the narthex,[398] and possibly to burials.[399] The lateral apses of the narthex of Asinou, typical of Cypriot monastic churches in the twelfth century, may have served as an abbreviated form of the lateral chapels used to enlarge the available space for the performance of these rites.[400] The two monumental inscriptions that run along the head of the north and the east arches are associated contextually with the principal iconographic subject of the narthex, the Last Judgment, revealing an interplay of text, imagery, and space.[401]

The therapeutic and salvific content of the narthex decoration is further underlined by the depiction in the lower zone of saints such as Cosmas and Damian and Anastasia Pharmakolytria, regarded as preeminent healers of body and soul, and of other saints, such as Eudokia and Irene (daughter of the Cypriot bishop Spyridon), who have been linked to resurrection miracles. Certain of the saints' figures seem to have functioned as cult icons in their own right, revealing the deep devotion of the worshippers. Thus, the great votive of St. George was supplied with lateral sconces[402] and the Christ in the medallion held by St. Paraskeve bears traces of candle flames. Saints and supplicants together join their prayers in a Great Deesis addressed to the Virgin Paraklesis, inscribed Eleousa, and to John the Baptist, to intervene with Christ for their salvation. Christ, labeled Eleemon, responds benevolently by blessing the worshippers. Thus the Virgin, to whom the church is dedicated

398. On the funerary functions of the narthex and on burial practices and services, see Bache, "Fonction funéraire du narthex," 25–28; Ivison, "Mortuary Practices in Byzantium"; Kyriakakis, "Byzantine Burial Customs"; Fedwick, "Death and Dying"; Galadza, "Evolution of Funerals for Monks." On commemorative services for the dead performed in the narthex of Serbian churches, see Ćurčić, "Twin-Domed Narthex," 342. On the depiction of the Last Judgment, the preeminent eschatological subject, in the narthex, see Tomeković, "Contribution à l'étude," 140–41. On other symbolic interpretations of the narthex, see above, n. 190 and Gerov, "Narthex as Desert."

399. Ambiguous information about two plundered tombs in the narthex of Asinou was reported by Peristianes, *Μονογραφία*, 8. Recent electromagnetic research has revealed a rectangular pit in the center of the narthex, which could possibly be interpreted as a grave; I owe this information to Andréas Nicolaïdès. However, it was not possible to make a trial trench. For graves in the narthex of other Cypriot churches, see Mango, "Koutsovendis," 67; Stylianou and Stylianou, "Ναὸς τοῦ Ἁγίου Νικολάου," 130–36. Burials in the narthex are a commonplace in the middle and late Byzantine period; they are found mainly in monastic churches, both in urban centers and in provinces: Ousterhout, *Architecture of the Kariye Camii*, 98–99; Teteriatnikov, "Burial Places," 147–48; eadem, *Liturgical Planning*, 167–73.

400. On the narthexes in Cyprus, see Papageorgiou, "Narthex of the Churches," 442–44; idem, Chapter 2, n. 65. On the function of the lateral chapels in middle Byzantine churches, see Chatzidakis-Bacharas, *Hosios Loukas*, 109–18; Sinkević, *Church of St. Panteleimon at Nerezi*, 15–19; cf. Ćurčić, "Architectural Significance."

401. On the inscription on the head of the east arch, see above, p. 77; Savage, "Interrelationship," 101.

402. Correspondence between David Winfield and Annemarie Weyl Carr, 3 March 2011.

and who is represented twice on the east wall of the narthex—as orant with the eponym Phorbiotissa, and as Paraklesis interceding with Christ—plays a key role in mediating with Christ for the salvation of the donors painted among the saints.

Iconographically, the Last Judgment adheres in its details to middle Byzantine tradition; at the same time it shares certain characteristics with the art that developed in the eastern Mediterranean world after the Crusades, revealing an artistic language shared across confessional boundaries and rooted in a common background. In addition, its amalgamation with the image of the Pantokrator in the vault surrounded by angels, which simulates the iconography of the central dome, confers upon the narthex space the aura of a naos. Moreover, the Deesis on the east wall, though itself part of the composition of the Last Judgment, also alludes to the recurrent iconographic program of threshold spaces and entry walls, establishing a liminal zone which serves as a threshold between narthex and naos. The same iconography is repeated on the screen, the threshold between naos and bema.

The range of saints depicted in the lower zone displays the multiple contexts present in the program of the narthex. Certain saints, such as Mamas, Timotheos and Mavra, George Machairomenos, and Irene are linked to Cypriot hagiographical tradition and to local cult centers; others, like Mamas, Marina, Paraskeve, and George, are equally venerated by both Greeks and Latins. In addition, the retention of the Latin votive, with its western Madonna della Misericordia, Latin postures, and European garments, alongside the votives of Orthodox monks and local lay devotees, reveals a harmonious symbiosis and interaction of the two cultures. The fact that monks accepted and showed respect to a Latin votive probably points to the need of the small monastery in the Troodos Mountains to be protected and supported by the local Latin lords.

The array of patrons' portraits in the thirteenth- and fourteenth-century layers—male and female, monastic and lay, Greek and Latin—reveals that the narthex was used by both the monastic and lay communities and that the people portrayed were both patrons and viewers. The prominence of women as sponsors in the narthex in the thirteenth and fourteenth centuries—being included in separate panels together with their patron saints—not only reflects female private devotion but also implies that the legal status of widowhood allowed women to manage their own property (see below, p. 367).

Stylistically, the late thirteenth-century painter of St. Anastasia has been identified with the artist of the thirteenth-century phase in the bema, a phase that has been linked in some way with the artistic tradition of the Christian communities of the Levant. The fourteenth-century painter of the narthex, on the other hand, a skilled and active member of a workshop attested in a cluster of monuments in the rural milieu of the Troodos Mountains and the plain south of Nicosia in the second quarter to mid-fourteenth century, essentially continues the maniera cypria as it had developed on Cyprus in the previous century.

The narthex of Asinou preserved its votive character through the ages. The coherent program of 1332/33, determined by its monastic patrons, assimilated local traditions. Adjusted to the available space, it challenged beholders to view it spatially. Conservative in iconography and style in accord with the agrarian setting of the monastic foundation, the church was open to Latin interaction. Asinou, initially an aristocratic private foundation, soon became a monastic church that hosted the private devotion of large groups of local worshippers, not only monks but also lay men and women—the common people (κοινὸς λαός) as recorded in the dedicatory inscription of the narthex.

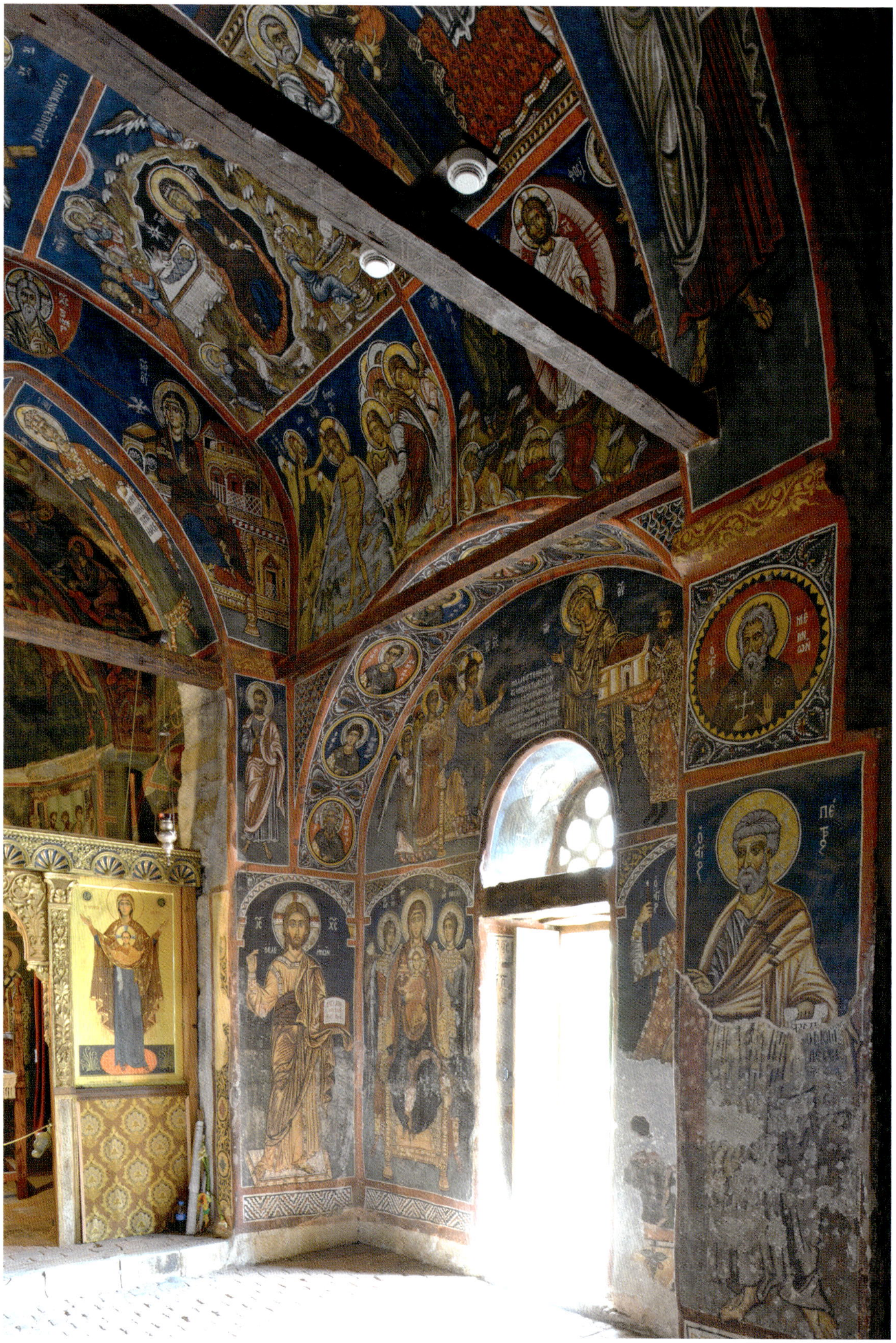

The church of Panagia Phorbiotissa: the south side of the central bay (photo courtesy of G. L. Carr)

CHAPTER SIX

The Murals of the Bema and the Naos: The Paintings of the Late Thirteenth and Fourteenth Centuries

Annemarie Weyl Carr

This chapter returns from the narthex to the interior of the church of the Panagia Phorbiotissa to examine the frescoes of the late thirteenth and fourteenth centuries in the bema and naos. These are the areas frescoed by the Asinou Master in 1105/6. They had not, however, survived the centuries unscathed. As detailed in Chapter 2, one or more structural failures in the eastern end, most probably in the thirteenth century, had demanded the introduction of new masonry into both the bema and the naos. The apse was replaced with a new, deeper conch and supporting responds, their masonry encasing the original triumphal arch and the wall below. In the naos, the responds defining both the eastern and the western periphery of the central bay were thickened, and pointed transverse arches were thrown from them across the bay beneath the vault, reinforcing the thin, semicircular transverse arches. Because the eastern face of the new eastern transverse arch and the western face of the western arch were never painted, their bare masonry remains, revealing clearly the contrast between the voussoirs of the initial transverse and the rougher stones of the reinforcing ones (Figs. 6.1, 2.29). By stages, however, the remaining surfaces of the new masonry were covered with imagery. First to be painted were the apse conch, its triumphal arch (but curiously not the responds supporting it), and the inner faces of the two western responds in the naos. This first phase of the new painting, here assigned to the late thirteenth century, opens our discussion.

The Late Thirteenth-Century Paintings in the Bema and the Naos

The responds were frescoed on shallow beds of plaster with full-length figures of the Apostle Princes (Figs. 6.2, 6.3), Peter on the south and Paul on the north.[1] Only

1. On the iconography of the Apostle Princes see in particular Weitzmann, *St. Peter Icon*, and, for monumental wall painting in Cyprus, Nicolaïdès, "Étude iconographique," 114–16.

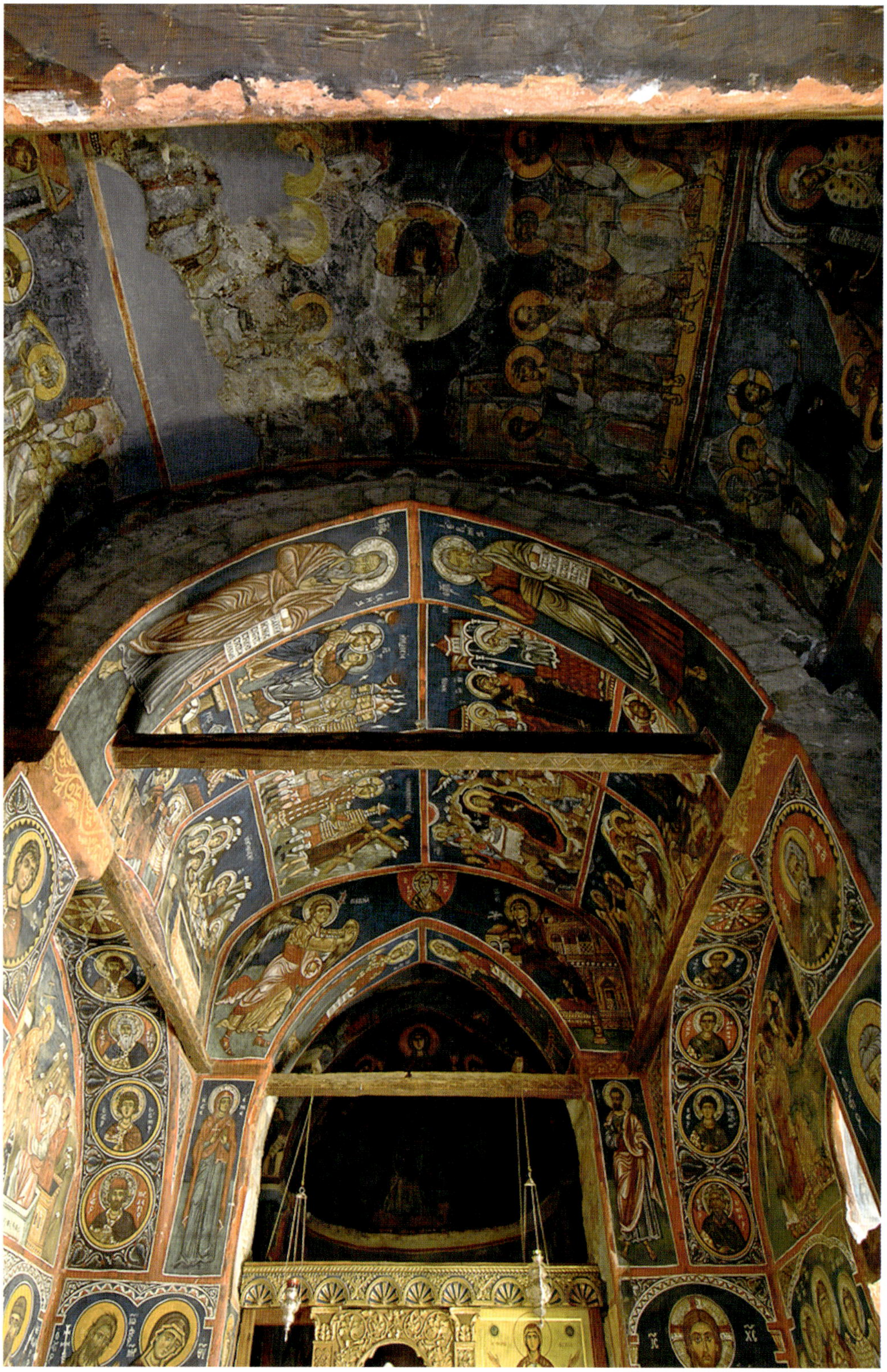

FIG. 6.1 Naos vault from the west: Pentecost and scenes of the life of Christ. The west side of the western transverse arch, unpainted in the fourteenth century, still shows the stepped lozenges painted on the thinner, original transverse arch (photo courtesy of G. L. Carr)

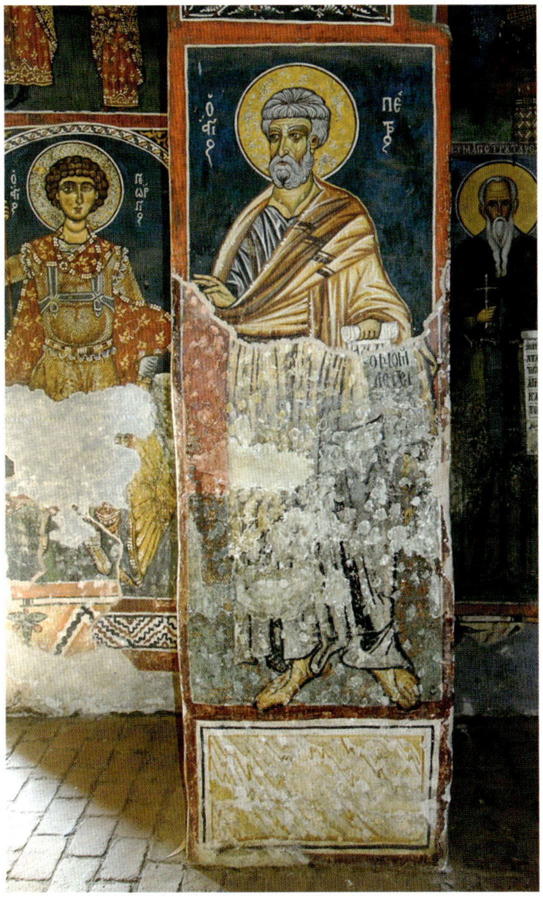

FIG. 6.2 Naos, central bay, south respond: St. Peter (photo courtesy of G. L. Carr)

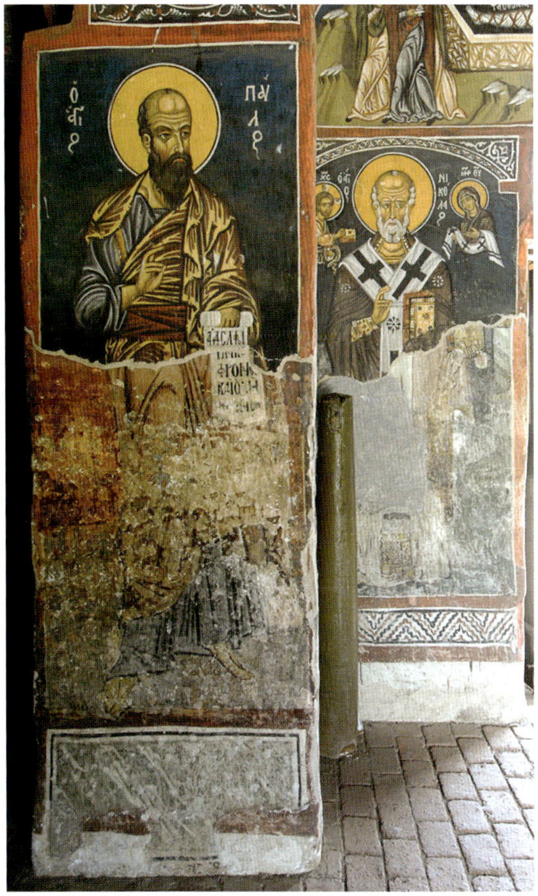

FIG. 6.3 Naos, central bay, north respond: St. Paul (photo courtesy of G. L. Carr)

the lower portion of these original figures is visible today; both were overpainted when the whole central bay was refrescoed in the fourteenth century, and the upper portion of each figure is still masked by those fourteenth-century images.[2] The figures stand before red grounds. Both wear gray chitons, Peter under an ocher himation and Paul under a pink one. The folds of their garments cluster at their feet, which are sandaled and which project over the bottom frame. Both hold open scrolls: one can still see the words ὁ νόμο(ς) λέγει τ[αῖς . . .] on Peter's scroll and φρονει καὶ ὁ μὴ [. . .]ων on Paul's.

The apse conch shows, against a gray-blue ground, the full-length MOTHER OF GOD (Μ(ήτ)ηρ / Θ(εο)υ η παντά/νασσα) orant between the archangels, who stride toward her with bare hands extended in veneration; MICHAEL (ο αρχ(άγγελος) Μιχ(αὴλ)) stands on her right, GABRIEL (ο αρχ(άγγελος) Γαβριῆλ) on her left (Fig. 6.4). The triumphal arch is dominated by the Sacrifice of Isaac, distributed in four vignettes: the ram tied to a tree; the flaming altar (Fig. 6.5); Abraham (ο πρ(οφή)της Αβραὰμ) halting the sacrifice as an angel, labeled ἄγγελος κ(υρίο)υ, commands him Ἀβρααμ / Ἀβραάμ μη επιβάλης τὴν / χείραν σου

2. A letter from David Winfield to Paul Underwood on 3 August 1966 presents arguments for removing the 14th-century half-figures, both on aesthetic grounds and because of the historical value of the figures they conceal. But he also notes that their plaster is very thin, and in the event the 14th-century layer was left in place.

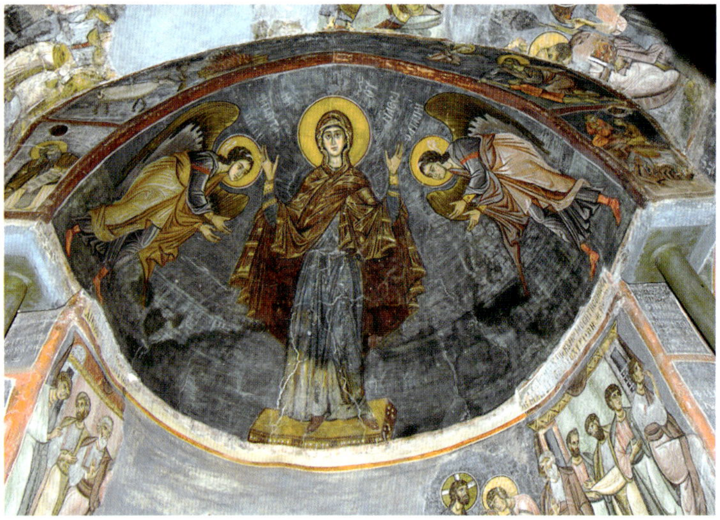

fig. 6.4

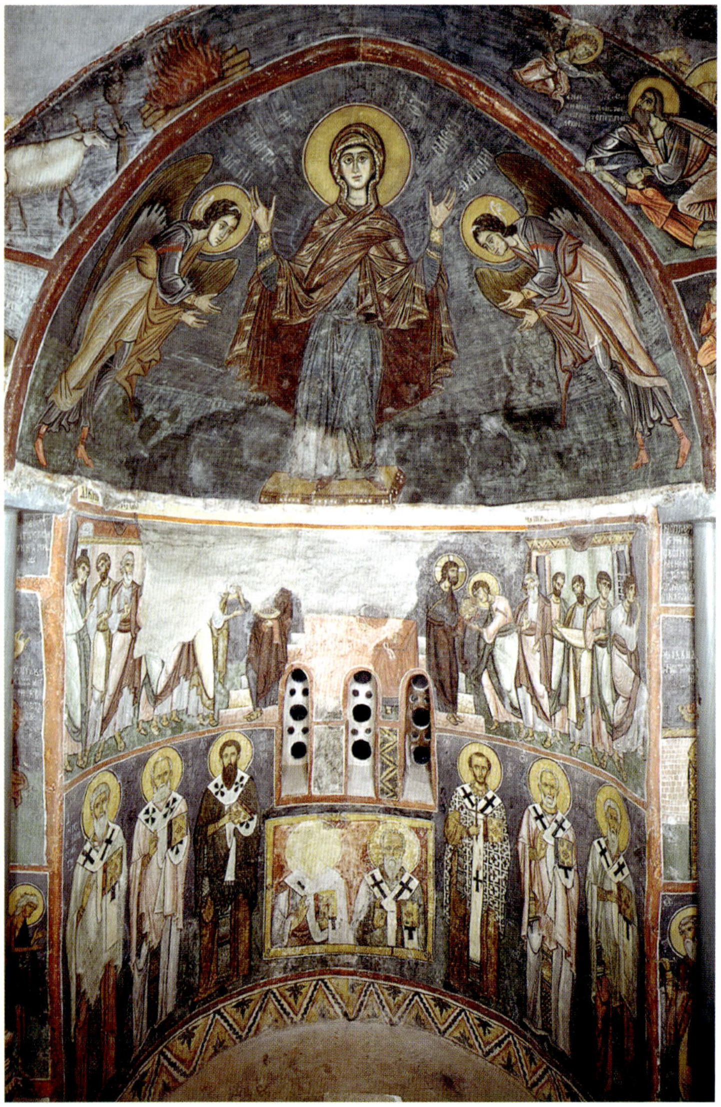

fig. 6.5

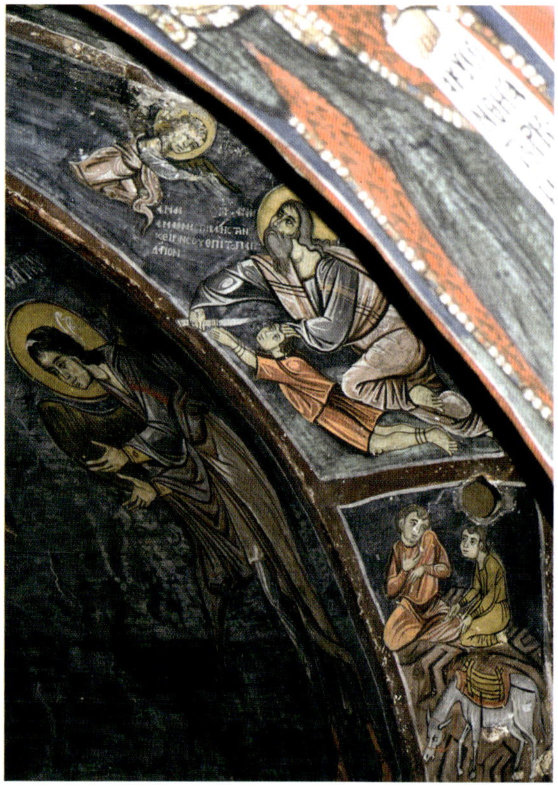

fig. 6.6

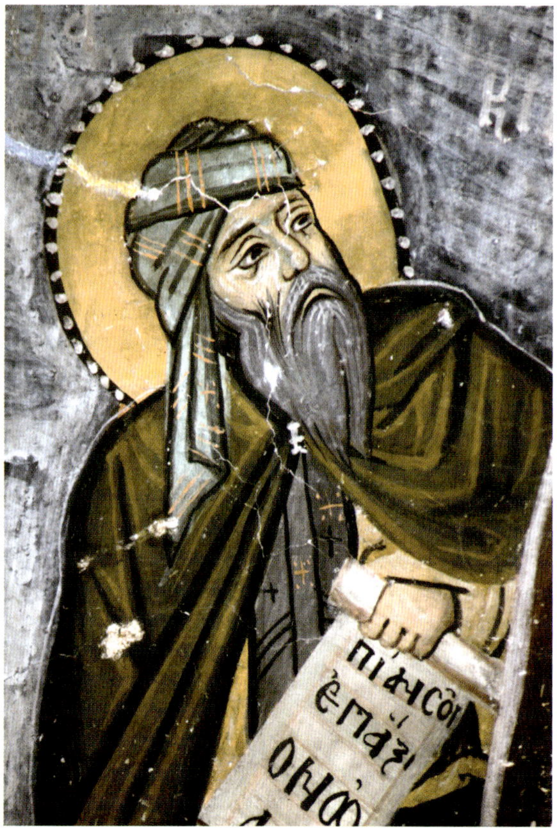

fig. 6.7

FIG. 6.4

Apse and triumphal arch: The Mother of God between archangels; St. John of Damascus; four elements of the Sacrifice of Isaac (photo courtesy of G. L. Carr)

FIG. 6.5

Apse and triumphal arch: Sacrifice of Isaac, Mother of God between archangels, Communion of the Apostles, Church Fathers. Partially visible behind pipes: 1105/6 Annunciation, SS. Mary of Egypt and Zosimas (photo courtesy of Dumbarton Oaks, BF.T.As.B.1.1)

FIG. 6.6

Triumphal arch, south side: Sacrifice of Isaac, two youths waiting with the donkey (photo courtesy of A. W. Carr)

FIG. 6.7

Triumphal arch, north side: St. John of Damascus (photo courtesy of A. W. Carr)

επὶ το παι/δάριον, or, "Abraham, Abraham, do not lay your hand on the boy" (excerpted from Gen. 22:11–12); and two youths with the grazing donkey (Fig. 6.6). On the north side of the arch is the three-quarter-length figure of St. John of Damascus (Fig. 6.7), gazing upward to the sacrifice and holding an open scroll inscribed πίαν σõι / ἐπᾶξι/ον ὠ/δῆν ("What praiseworthy ode . . . to you"), the beginning to the same text that he carries in the narthex (Fig. 5.28; pp. 166–67).

The paintings in the apse and on the triumphal arch have been associated—on stylistic grounds by Sophia Kalopissi-Verti (p. 120) and technical grounds by Ioanna Kakoulli (p. 341)—with the fresco of St. Anastasia Pharmakolytria (Poison-Curer) and her devotee, Anastasia Saramalina, in the narthex. The kinships are so clear that the two must be assigned to the same hand and so to the same date, in the final quarter of the thirteenth century (Figs. 6.8, 6.9). The figures of Peter and Paul on the responds are not so closely akin either in style or in technique to the frescoes of the apse and Anastasia (see p. 341), and, as Athanasios Papageorgiou has argued, it is not entirely clear that the responds they occupy were built at the same time as the new apse (see above, pp. 60–65). Nonetheless, the figures present a number of features that do associate them with the paintings of the apse and the Anastasia panel: apse and Apostles employ very similar letterforms in their inscriptions; they share the practice of sketching the figures with incisions in the still-damp plaster; and a comparison of the lower bodies of the four standing saints—Peter, Paul, the Mother of God, and Anastasia (Figs. 6.2–4, 5.2)—brings out close kinships in their unhighlighted drapery folds, their mobile postures emphasizing the free leg, and the distinctive triangular swath of drapery that swings around from behind to enfold the ankle of that leg. On this basis, it is unlikely that the Apostles were painted at a date significantly different from that of the apse and the Anastasia fresco. Whether in sequential campaigns as funds became available, or at much the same moment by two hands, they belong to the same late thirteenth-century phase of painting.

Only a very small portion of one figure is still visible from the original, twelfth-century painting on the wall behind the responds bearing Peter and Paul. This is the crown of the head of the figure behind St. Peter. Its hair is thick and brown, indicating a young man, and thus not St. Peter. The thirteenth-century paintings, then, did not repeat the original imagery. Rather, they altered the original program to conform to what seems in the interim to have become a standard pattern of Cypriot programs, placing Peter and Paul on piers facing each other across the naos. Though the pairing of Peter and Paul on either side of a door can be traced back deep into Byzantine custom, it is only at Lagoudera in 1192, and in the nearly contemporary church of Christ Antiphonetes at Kalogrea, that one first finds them facing each other across the naos as they do at Asinou.[3] The same pattern was repeated in the

3. Nicolaïdès, "Étude iconographique," pls. 2, 3; fig. 18. At Perachorio, Peter and Paul stand side by side on the south wall of the naos (Megaw and Hawkins, "Church of the Holy Apostles at Perachorio," 335, fig. 36), but

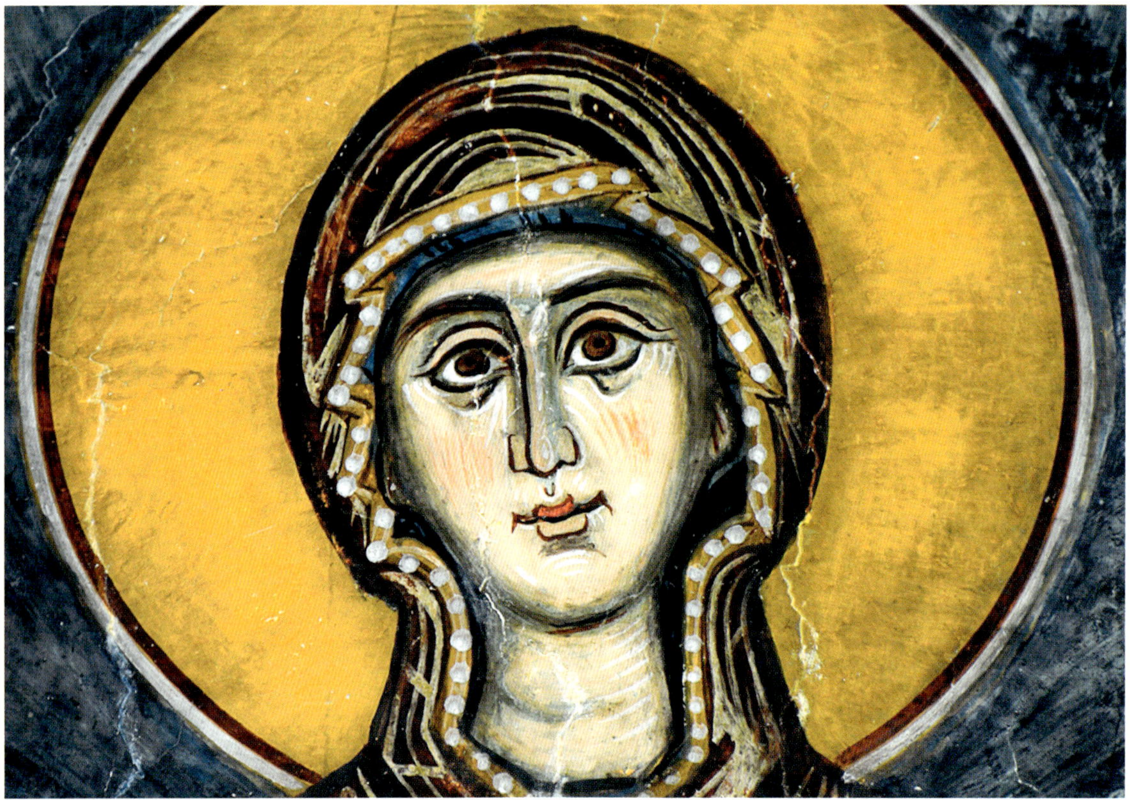

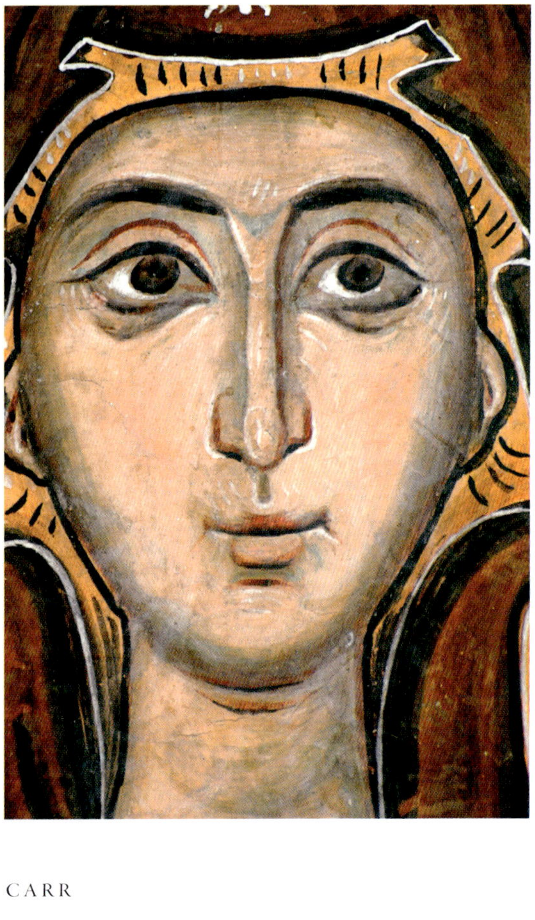

FIG. 6.8

Apse. Detail, face of the Mother of God (photo courtesy of G. L. Carr)

FIG. 6.9

Narthex: Panel with St. Anastasia Pharmakolytria. Detail, face of St. Anastasia (photo courtesy of G. L. Carr)

little church of the Panagia at Moutoullas of 1280,[4] and at much the same date in the church of the Transfiguration of the Savior, Sotera. At Sotera and Moutoullas the saints stand against red grounds, as they do at Asinou. In Lagoudera, Sotera, and Moutoullas, again as in Asinou, they hold open and

---

the effect is very different from their placement across from one another.

4. Mouriki, "Wall Paintings of the Church of the Panagia at Moutoullas," 195.

inscribed scrolls,[5] an exceptional feature that makes the Cypriot examples stand out.[6] Peter and Paul at Asinou, then, bespeak a decision not to replicate the twelfth-century program but to bring Asinou into accord with thirteenth-century Cypriot currents. This willingness to depart from the twelfth-century scheme should make us cautious as we proceed to analyze other aspects of Asinou's repainting.

The apse and the triumphal arch also depart from the twelfth-century themes, though they retain the poetic inscription of Nikephoros Ischyrios at the base of the apse (Figs. 3.6, 3.7, 6.4 and pp. 77–79). The Virgin orant was a long-established apse motif; the earliest surviving middle Byzantine example on Cyprus is in the eleventh-century apse at St. Nicholas of the Roof (τῆς Στέγης).[7] Nonetheless, a range of factors suggests that the original fresco in the Asinou apse showed the Mother of God orant with a medallion of Christ on her breast. Not only does the Virgin with the medallion appear in the Asinou Master's own fresco over the west door at Asinou (Fig. 3.11), and in his later apse at Trikomo,[8] but it figures in six of the nine surviving Cypriot apses of the twelfth and thirteenth centuries.[9] The Virgin appears without a medallion in only one, at

5. At Moutoullas and Asinou the scrolls are now illegible; at Lagoudera (Nicolaïdès, "Étude iconographique," 115) and at Sotera, Peter carries an inscription from 1 Peter 2:11 ("Beloved, I urge you as aliens and exiles to abstain from the desires of the flesh that wage war against the soul"), and Paul carries a lection based on Galatians 5:22–23 ("But the fruit of the Spirit is love, joy, peace, patience, kindness, generosity, faithfulness, gentleness, self-control..."). Later, at the Holy Cross, Pelendri, Peter and Paul carried scrolls, but the texts are not clear.

6. Peter and Paul are rarely shown with an inscribed scroll before the Palaiologan period, and the texts vary. At the Protaton Monastery on Mount Athos, there is a late 12th-century full-length icon of St. Peter holding a long open scroll, but unfortunately the scroll is too abraded to read: see Karakatsanis, *Treasures of Mount Athos*, 62, no. 2.5. A late 12th-century instance of Peter with a scroll in the church of St. Peter near Novi Pazar is noted by Constantinides, *Wall Paintings of the Panagia Olympiotissa*, 1:241, citing Djurić, *Byzantinische Fresken in Jugoslawien*, fig. 23. A number of Palaiologan examples follow the type apparently initiated in the Protaton (Constantinides, *Wall Paintings of the Panagia Olympiotissa*, 2:215a), in which Peter holds a scroll that sits upright and slightly open in his hand like a modified codex: see Peter at the Panagia Olympiotissa itself (ibid., 2:98), and the icon of St. Peter in the British Museum (Buckton, *Byzantium*, 205–6, no. 222). These figures display the text of 1 Peter 2:11 (see preceding note). A 16th-century icon on Cyprus of this type from the church of the Kourdaliotissa, Kourdali, displays the words "You are Christ the son of the living God": see Hadjichristodoulou and Papaioakeim, "Φορητὲς Εἰκόνες," 143, pl. 30. Weitzmann, *St. Peter Icon*, 40, figs. 47–48, cites a late 16th-century pair of icons in which Peter holds a scroll inscribed with 1 Peter 1:3 ("Blessed be the God and Father of our Lord Jesus Christ!"); and Paul holds a codex inscribed with 1 Cor. 13:1 ("If I speak in the tongues of mortals and of angels, but do not have love, I am a noisy gong or a clanging cymbal"). The figure of Paul in the church of St. Nicholas Orphanos in Thessalonike holds a half-open codex with words inside, but the words are too damaged to decipher: Tsitouridou, *Ὁ ζωγραφικὸς διάκοσμος τοῦ Ἁγίου Νικολάου*, 203, fig. 103.

7. Stylianou and Stylianou, *Painted Churches*, 55. Archangels appeared also in the Church of the Holy Trinity, Koutsovendis, around 1100, though the figure of the Mother of God there is lost: see Mango, "Monastery of St. Chrysostom at Koutsovendis," 75.

8. Stylianou and Stylianou, *Painted Churches*, 488; Hein et al., *Cyprus*, fig. 168. The apse at Trikomo repeats almost verbatim the inscription of Nikephoros Ischyrios in the apse at Asinou, omitting only the patron's name, reinforcing the belief that the iconography there repeated that of Asinou. The apse of the church of the Apsinthiotissa showed the Virgin with the medallion on her breast between two archangels, but it was repainted in the 14th century: see Papageorgiou, *Christian Art*, 397.

9. The six are at Trikomo, Perachorio, Kalogrea, Lysi, Rizokarpasso, and Moutoullas. For the Apostles' church, Perachorio, see Megaw and Hawkins, "Church of the Holy Apostles," fig. 12; for the church of Christ Antiphonetes, Kalogrea, see Stylianou and Stylianou, *Painted Churches*, 472 and figure 283; for St. Themonianos, Lysi, see ibid., 492 and fig. 299; for St. Mavra, Rizokarpasso, see Chotzakoglou, "Βυζαντινή αρχιτεκτονική," 2: fig. 523 or Nicolaïdès, *Η κομνήνεια και υστεροκομνήνεια*, fig. 42; for Moutoullas see Mouriki, "Wall Paintings of the Church of the Panagia," fig. 2.

the Enkleistra of St. Neophytos.[10] Such a change is not necessarily surprising: in neither St. Nicholas of the Roof nor the Holy Cross, Pelendri—where both an earlier apse and its later overpainting survive—does the later composition repeat the original one.[11] More notable in Asinou's case is the fact that, in contrast to the placement of SS. Peter and Paul on the responds, the new image was not one that had become current in Cyprus in the intervening period.

The composition on the triumphal arch above the apse is even more rare. The triumphal arch joins two themes, the SACRIFICE OF ISAAC and the single figure of ST. JOHN OF DAMASCUS (Figs. 6.4–7). It might best be seen as a composite, the figure of John simply filling the space not used by the larger theme of the Sacrifice. But the two may have been designed to function together. As an independent figure, St. John had been a comparative latecomer to mural programs, his first dated appearance occurring in 1192 at Lagoudera in Cyprus.[12] There, as in Asinou, he is on the triumphal arch, bearing words from one of his troparia to Christ that can be seen to relate, as Nancy Ševčenko points out, to the Mandylion (the towel imprinted with Christ's face) just above him.[13] His next appearance on Cyprus is here at Asinou, and his placement on the triumphal arch probably echoes Lagoudera. In this case, however, he bears the opening of a canon to the Theotokos identified by Kalopissi-Verti that honors the Virgin and her Annunciation: "What praiseworthy ode will our weakness offer to you [other] than the cheerful one into which Gabriel initiated us? Rejoice, you who gave birth to God, Virgin, unmarried Mother."[14] After appearing on the triumphal arch at Asinou, John of Damascus recurs in the narthex at Asinou, the narthex at Lagoudera, the central vessel at Pelendri, and the naos at Monagri, all by painters whose style is similar to the one used at Asinou, and in each case the saint bears the same text as the one seen at Asinou.[15] As Kalopissi-Verti

10. This is at the Enkleistra of St. Neophytos: see Mango and Hawkins, "Hermitage of St. Neophytos," figure 60. The apse there is exceptional, for the Virgin is also the central figure in the scene of the Ascension. The remaining two 12th-century apses are at Lagoudera, with an enthroned Virgin between archangels (Nicolaïdès, "Étude iconographique," fig. 6), and at St. Solomone, Paphos, with archangels flanking a now-illegible figure of the orant Mary: see Young, "Iconography and Date," 99. The orant Virgin without the medallion becomes frequent in the 14th century, when she appears in the overpainted apse at St. Nicholas of the Roof (Stylianou and Stylianou, *Painted Churches*, 58); in the overpainted apse at the Holy Cross, Pelendri (see above, p. 202, fig. 5.66); and in the apse in St. Sozomenos, Potamia: see Papageorgiou, "Λαξευτά ασκητήρια," 49 and fig. 23. Apses of the 15th century, however, all return to the image of the Mother of God with the medallion on her breast: see SS. Kerykos and Ioulitta, Letympou (Karageorghis, *A. G. Leventis Foundation*, 35, fig. D; Stylianou and Stylianou, *Painted Churches,* 471); the Archangel church, Pedoulas, of 1474 (Stylianou and Stylianou, *Painted Churches*, 339 and fig. 204); St. Herakleidios, Kalopanayiotis (ibid., 302; and Myriantheas, *Μελέται*, fig. 8, color pl. 9); St. Mamas, Louvaras, by Philip Goul in 1495 (Stylianou and Stylianou, *Painted Churches*, 245); and the church of Agiasmati, Platanistassa, also by Goul, probably in 1494 (ibid., 206 and fig. 122). The apse of St. Mamas, Sotera Famagusta, is reproduced in G. Soteriou, *Βυζαντινὰ μνημεῖα*, pl. 106. The Virgin with the medallion is thus a particularly consistent preference.

11. See preceding note.

12. On John of Damascus see above, pp. 166–67; N. P. Ševčenko, "Five Hymnographers"; Ovcharova, "Holy Hymnographers"; Sinkević, *Church of St. Panteleimon*, 63; and Nicolaïdès, "Étude iconographique," 31.

13. N. P. Ševčenko, "Five Hymnographers," 66–67. John's text varies. At Nerezi it is taken from his Second Canon, sung at Matins on Christmas Day. He holds a different passage from his Christmas Canon at Studenica forty-four years later. I am indebted to Nancy Patterson Ševčenko for her fine inventory of the inscriptions in images of John of Damascus.

14. See above, pp. 166–67.

15. For the narthex at Asinou, see above, pp. 166–67; for Lagoudera, see Stylianou and Stylianou, *Painted Churches*, 184; for Pelendri, see ibid., 230; for Monagri, see Boyd, "Church of the Panagia Amasgou, Monagri," 314, fig. 46. On their relation to the painters of Asinou, see above, pp. 200–205, and below, pp. 306–9. John bears the same inscription in the 15th-century apse painting at St. Kerykos and Ioulitta, Letympou, where he and Kosmas kneel with long, sinuous scrolls of hymnic praise

has pointed out, this text was sung as a theotokion at Matins on the feast day of the venerated Cypriot saint, Epiphanios, and was thus surely familiar to monastic communities on the island. This connection between image and rite may explain the use of this text in mural paintings. It is first used at Asinou, however, and here it figures in a place often adorned with the scene of the Annunciation; indeed, it replaces the Annunciation originally flanking the apse. Moreover, the theme of the Annunciation that St. John invokes here has a history of association with the Sacrifice of Isaac that will emerge as the imagery of the Sacrifice is explored just below. It suggests that the figure of St. John bearing this particular text was invented for the program here at Asinou. His image is unlikely to have replicated an early twelfth-century original, for, as noted, St. John is not attested in mural painting of that date.

The Sacrifice of Isaac, in turn, is a powerful theme with a history reaching deep into Jewish, Christian, and Muslim antiquity.[16] It is among the earliest themes in Hebrew Scripture that Christians linked typologically with the Eucharist,[17] and its Eucharistic content surely explains its use on the triumphal arch at Asinou.[18] Among the most powerful aspects of the original twelfth-century program at Asinou had been its apse program, which was a rich visual meditation upon the Eucharist, in the person of Mary.[19] The Sacrifice takes up this theme, though in a fiercer, more patriarchal mode that contrasts starkly with the original iconography.

For all the scene's longstanding Eucharistic association, evidence of its use in middle Byzantine monumental painting is meager, especially in the bema. Of the ten known middle Byzantine examples, seven are located in the naos. Three of these are subsumed in Old Testament narrative cycles,[20] two are independent votive panels,[21] and the remaining two—in Hagia Sophia in Kiev and in the Virgin's church at Samari—are located at the west of the naos in conjunction with scenes of the Three Hebrews in the Furnace and the Hospitality of Abraham.[22] The eighth example adorns a niche in the eastern passageway to the north church at the church of St. John the Baptist at Güllü Dere, Cappadocia (913–920), a unique placement associated with the adjacent tomb.[23] Only twice does the scene occur in the bema itself: at Hagia Sophia, Ohrid (1037–52),

at the feet of a standing Mother of God with Christ in a medallion on her breast.

16. See esp. Finney, "Abraham and Isaac"; Weitzmann and Kessler, *Dura Synagogue*, 156–57.

17. Woerden, "Sacrifice of Abraham," 214–20; van Loon, *Gate of Heaven*, 131–39 passim.

18. It had been introduced by the 4th century into the Liturgy, and continued to be cited in the liturgies of St. Basil and St. James, though not in that of St.John Chrysostom: see *Divine Liturgy*, 20.

19. See Carr, "Iconography and Identity," 140–41. The bema was painted with scenes of the Virgin's life—her Birth, her Presentation, and the Annunciation—and the apse conch most probably showed her orant with the bust-medallion of the Christ-child on her breast. Her birth marks the advent of the flesh that God would assume in his salvific mission, as emphasized by the epigram accompanying the image (p. 73). The Presentation, in turn, sees that flesh consecrated to its sacred use. As the "perfect gift," Mary is paralleled in the Presentation with the Eucharistic loaf, often called the "Panagia," the perfect matter offered to receive God. Above her Presentation the Asinou Master showed her fed in the Temple by an angel; "angel's bread" is a frequent metaphor for the Eucharist. The Annunciation then sees Mary imbued with God, and in the apse she stands "radiant with God within" (Pentcheva, *Icons and Power*, 153) like the Eucharist itself.

20. These are at the Cappella Palatina in Palermo (Demus, *Mosaics of Norman Sicily*, figure 34), the Duomo in Monreale (ibid., figure 105), and the church of the Savior at Nereditsa (Lazarev, *Old Russian*, 126–27).

21. The cave church of St. John, Çavuşin (7th to 9th century), and Ballı kilise in Soğanlı (before 1051): see Jolivet-Lévy, *Les Églises byzantines de Cappadoce*, 38, 255.

22. For Kiev, see Lazarev, "Regard sur l'art," 233–36 and figs. F, G, and H. Along with the Three Hebrews and Philoxenia, the Sacrifice is accompanied by the Last Supper and the Wedding at Cana, a combination so Eucharistic in content that Lazarev proposes that the royal family must have received communion in the western tribune before it. For Samari, see Grigoriadou-Cabagnols, "Décor peint," 179; Skawran, *Middle Byzantine Fresco*, 166.

23. Jolivet-Lévy, "Les programmes iconographiques," 255.

where it figures with other theophanic scenes from the Old Testament in a rich program flanking the Communion of the Apostles;[24] and in the prothesis of the church of the Savior, Megara (ca. 1200), where it appears with Abraham's Hospitality and Moses with the Burning Bush.[25] In the course of the thirteenth and fourteenth centuries the scene of the Sacrifice of Isaac can be found in the bema, but no more frequently than in the naos, in the narthex as a votive image, or in one of the side chapels among the miracles of the archangels.[26] Only in the fifteenth century does it finally settle with regularity in the area of the prothesis.[27]

On Cyprus the Sacrifice of Isaac follows much the same pattern. Before being adopted at Asinou, this theme had appeared in two earlier churches, in both cases at the western end: at St. Anthony, Kellia, an eleventh-century fresco of the Sacrifice on the southwest pier of the naos was overpainted with the same scene in the twelfth or thirteenth century;[28] and at St. Herakleidios, Kalopanayiotis, the Sacrifice was incorporated in the program of the western arm of the naos in the 1270s, close in date to the one at Asinou.[29] It reappears only in 1474 in the Archangel church at Pedoulas, but from that point it becomes truly standard, recurring in the bema of church after church, most often paired with the Hospitality on either side of the apse.[30] As in Byzantium at large, then, so also in Cyprus the theme is not frequent until the fifteenth century, when it takes its place in the bema with regularity. Until then, its customary location was in the naos; it never appears on the triumphal arch.

24. Hamann-MacLean and Hallensleben, *Die Monumentalmalerei*, figs. 20–21.
25. Grigoriadou, "Peintures murales," figs. XV a, XV b; Skawran, *Middle Byzantine Fresco*, 175, fig. 322.
26. See Church no. 2 in Gülşehir of the late 13th century, where it appears in the niche that served as a prothesis (Jolivet-Lévy, *Les Églises byzantines de Cappadoce*, 238); the Virgin's church, Studenica, where it is in the north porch (Millet, *La peinture du Moyen Âge*, 1:37, 2); Arilje (1296), where it is on the east wall of the narthex (ibid., 2: figs. 83, 1–3); Gračanića (1318), where the Sacrifice appears in the bema with Gideon's Fleece, the Tabernacle, Abraham Inviting the Angels to His House, the Hospitality, and Wisdom Building Her House (Petković, *La peinture serbe*, 2: fig. 34); on the prothesis side of the apse in the Peribleptos in Mistra (Millet, *Monuments byzantins de Mistra*, fig. 113, 3); and the church of John the Baptist at Garipas, Mylopotamos on Crete, of the early 14th century, where it is on the westernmost part of the south wall (Spatharakis, *Byzantine Wall Paintings*, 183, n. 3). Yet later, Papadopoulos-Kerameus, *Manuel d'iconographie chrétienne*, cites it among the scenes illustrating the parable of the man hiring workers (p. 117) and again, among the miracles of the archangels (p. 174).
27. See note 30 below for examples in Cyprus; good examples in Crete are seen in Spatharakis, *Byzantine Wall Paintings*: Agia Trias, Agia Trias of ca. 1400 (p. 37), where it is above the prothesis; St. Constantine, Artos, church of St. George, 1401, where it is on the north side of the bema over the niche that served as the prothesis (p. 50 and fig. 24); St. George in Ano Viannos, with the Sacrifice on the north bema wall (p. 95 n. 41); and Roustika, church of the Panagia (1391), where the Sacrifice is on the lower part of the north half of the bema vault (p. 182 and fig. 243).
28. Stylianou and Stylianou, *Painted Churches*, 434 and pl. 260; Hein et al., *Cyprus*, 134, pl. 137.
29. Carr, "Holy Sepulcher," 485–86.
30. For Pedoulas, see Stylianou and Stylianou, *Painted Churches*, 339. In the late 15th century it appears on the northwest pendentive of the western dome at St. Paraskeve, Yeroskipos (Stylianou and Stylianou, *Painted Churches*, 385); at St. Mavra, Koilani, in the northeast bema recess balancing the Hospitality in the southeast bema recess (ibid., 237); and on the north wall of the bema at St. Mamas, Louvaras, facing the Hospitality on the south wall. In the 16th century it is seen at St. Sozomenos, Galata, paired with the Hospitality flanking the apse (ibid., 88); at the Archangel-Theotokos church, Galata, on the north bema wall facing the Hospitality (ibid., 96); at the Holy Cross church, St. Eirene, on the south bema wall (ibid., 152); at the church of the Transfiguration of the Savior, Palaichori, on the north bema wall facing the Hospitality on the south bema wall (ibid., 273 and fig. 164); on the north bema wall in St. Christina, Askas (ibid., 290); on the north bema wall of the Holy Cross church, Palaiomylos (ibid., 344); at the church of the Mother of God, Kaminaria, on the north bema wall facing deacon saints on the south bema wall (ibid., 348); and at St. Nicholas, Galataria, on the north side of the bema vault balanced by the Hospitality (ibid., 405).

The appearance of the Sacrifice of Isaac in the bema at Ohrid shows that the theme did exist in the repertoire of middle Byzantine sanctuary images before Asinou's initial adornment, and the sheer sophistication of the program at Ohrid links it with a metropolitan origin rather than a regional one.[31] Thus the Sacrifice at Asinou might be understood as an element of the original program, painted above the Annunciation on the now-lost triumphal arch of the original church, and repeated in the late thirteenth century. Two factors militate against this conclusion. One is architectural: the original triumphal arch was too narrow for an image of the Sacrifice over the apse. The other factor concerns the placement of the scene. Though the Sacrifice of Isaac would eventually take a regular place on the bema wall or vault, this was still centuries beyond 1105/6, and there was no Byzantine tradition of placing it on the triumphal arch.

A vigorous tradition of mural painting existed that did place the Sacrifice of Isaac on the triumphal arch in the twelfth and thirteenth centuries. This was not centered in areas dominated by the Byzantine Church, however. Four examples from the late twelfth and thirteenth centuries survive in Coptic churches in Egypt: in St. George at Deir Seifein, Old Cairo; in St. Mark at Abu Makar and the Virgin's church at Deir al-Baramus, both in the Wadi al-Natrun; and at St. Anthony on the Red Sea, signed by the painter Theodore in 1232/33.[32] In these churches the Sacrifice joined a small repertoire of further Old Testament scenes in the spandrels of the dome in the *haikal*—the sanctuary space before the apse. The scenes emphasize either theophany, especially Moses receiving the Law, or the Eucharist: the Eucharist as sacrifice in the scenes of Abraham and Jephthah; the Eucharist as the communion of bread and wine in scenes of Abraham and Melchizedek. The various versions of the Sacrifice of Isaac differ in details, but each is so composed that the figure of Abraham appears to look toward the apse as he turns to respond to the divine command to save his son. Thus all of them link his sacrifice to the apse and so to the Eucharistic rite. At Abu Makar, he turns at the same time to the Annunciation, which borders the apse itself, joining the Old Testament theophanies with the Sacrifice of Isaac on one side and the figure of Moses receiving the Law on the other.

In addition to the four Coptic examples, the Sacrifice appears on the triumphal arch in three Syrian churches of the thirteenth century: in Mar Girius at Raskida, Mar Yakub at Qara, and Mar Tadros at Bahdeidat.[33] The scenes accompanying it at Raskida no longer survive; in both Qara and Bahdeidat, it flanks Moses Receiving the Law,

31. On the program at Ohrid, see Epstein, "Political Content."

32. On St. George see van Loon, *Gate of Heaven*, 4, 22–30, figs. 23–26, who dates it between 1168 and 1189. A date early in the second quarter of the 13th century is proposed by Hunt, "Christian-Muslim Relations," 118. The scene of the Sacrifice of Isaac is on the east side of the octagon of the haikal, in essence on the triumphal arch of the apse. On Abu Makar see van Loon, *Gate of Heaven*, 4, 30–59, figs. 47–48, who attributes it to the mid-12th century; Leroy, *Les peintures des couvents*, pls. 35–36. Moving around the spandrels of the haikal's octagon from the northwest face, one finds: Jacob's ladder (NW), Abraham's sacrifice (N), Annunciation to Mary (NE), Moses receiving the Law, and Aaron (E), Annunciation to Zacharias (SE), Abraham and Melchizedek and Isaiah's mouth purified (S), Job (SW), and two prophets (W). On St. Anthony, see van Loon, *Gate of Heaven*, 4, 91–107; Bolman, *Monastic Visions*, 66, fig. 4.32; van Moorsel, *Les peintures du monastère*, 1:35–36, 2: pls. 9–10. Here the Sacrifice flanks the apse on the south side of the haikal in the chapel of Benjamin, and is signed by the painter Theodore in 1232/33; the scene balances Jephthah's sacrifice of his daughter. On the church of the Mother of God in Deir al-Baramus in the Wadi al-Natrun, see van Loon, *Gate of Heaven*, 4, 65–74, figs. 83–85. This was probably painted in the 13th century; here the Sacrifice is on the north spandrel of the triumphal arch, balancing the scene of Melchizedek's offering to Abraham in the south spandrel.

33. On Raskida see Nordiguian and Voisin, *Châteaux et Églises*, 407, fig. on p. 263; Dodd, *Medieval Painting*, 273, fig. 14.9. On Qara see Westphalen, "Das Kloster Mar Yakub," 111. On Bahdeidat see Nordiguian and Voisin, *Châteaux et Églises*, 216–17, fig. 254; Dodd, *Medieval Painting*, 56–58, pl. 78.

and in Bahdeidat the two Old Testament theophanies stand above the figures of Mary and Gabriel in the Annunciation. Finally, an eighth example, though of ambiguous date, is surely relevant here. The apse of the monastery church at Sinai contains two encaustic mural paintings (assigned to the seventh century by Kurt Weitzmann) that show the Sacrifice of Isaac and the Sacrifice of Jephthah's Daughter.[34] The same two scenes were paired in 1232/33 in the haikal of St. Anthony on the Red Sea. The parallel is so striking that Lucy-Anne Hunt has proposed a thirteenth-century date for the paintings at Sinai, as well.[35] Though her attribution is speculative, her link of the two monuments is not. Whatever their date, the scenes at Sinai surely prompted the pairing of Abraham and Jephthah at St. Anthony, and may have helped to shape the programs of the Coptic haikals more broadly.

In a manner not paralleled in Byzantium itself, but widespread on the mainland, the Sacrifice of Isaac is found recurrently on the threshold of the apse in the decades before the scene was introduced on the triumphal arch at Asinou. The scene at Asinou seems best interpreted as a reflection of this vigorous tradition. In four cases—Deir al-Baramus, Mar Yakub at Qara, Mar Girius at Raskida, and Mar Tadros at Bahdeidat—the Sacrifice is on the triumphal arch itself; in all cases it appears in conjunction with Old Testament Eucharistic types, and in both Abu Makar and Bahdeidat, it is joined with the Annunciation. At Asinou, too, the Annunciation is present, evoked by the hymn of John of Damascus. Joining Eucharistic typology with the Annunciation at the threshold of the apse, the triumphal arch at Asinou emerges as a condensed version of the program seen at Abu Makar and above all at Bahdeidat.

The union of the Annunciation and Old Testament typology that characterizes these programs has been linked to a feature of Syriac theological language.[36] As studied by Sebastian Brock,[37] a single word, *aggen,* overshadow, is used in a significant cluster of cases to translate what in Greek is a range of different words for divine action. The word is employed in certain Old Testament events of divine protection including the covenant with Abraham and Moses on Sinai, in the Annunciation narrative in Luke 1:35, and in the Epiclesis in the Eucharist itself. The recurrent use of this word thus unites these themes in a way not paralleled in Greek expression, and so unlikely to arise from it. The programs cited here adorn both Melkite and Miaphysite churches; they are not creed-specific. But they point to a visual tradition that belongs to the eastern Christian more than the Byzantine world.

The alignment of Asinou with these monuments is significant. Not only does the Sacrifice of Isaac not repeat the earlier, twelfth-century program but it also turns to a very different source of inspiration. Rather than to the traditions of Byzantium and its Orthodox Christianity, the choice and placement of the Sacrifice of Isaac look to the contemporary, often non-Chalcedonian monuments of the east Christian mainland. This reorientation is readily associated with the historical conditions of Cyprus in the thirteenth century, when the island's powerful cultural bond with Byzantium had been broken by the destruction of its archon class, the emigration of the painters they sponsored, and the savaging of Constantinople in the Fourth Crusade.[38] The alignment of Cyprus with the mainland in the thirteenth century has been emphasized in many studies during the decades since Doula Mouriki showed the bonds of what she called the "maniera cypria" with stylistic and ornamental motifs in mainland monuments, above all Mar Tadros

34. Weitzmann, *Monastery of Saint Catherine,* 52–54, pls. 77–78.
35. Hunt, "Christian Art in Greater Syria and Egypt."

36. Carr, "Iconography and Identity," 127–51.
37. Brock, "Passover, Annunciation, and Epiclesis"; idem, *Bible in the Syriac Liturgy,* 94.
38. See Carr, "Art," 285–310, with earlier bibliography, especially Mouriki, "Thirteenth-Century Icon Painting"; eadem, "Wall Paintings of the Church of the Panagia"; Papageorgiou, "Ἰδιάζουσαι βυζαντιναὶ τοιχογραφίαι," 206–12.

at Bahdeidat.[39] Two factors, however, make the Sacrifice of Isaac at Asinou especially informative.

In the first place, the direction of movement in the composition's use is notable: the painter at Asinou drew upon an iconographic tradition that was not native to Cyprus, but was disseminated along the lines of interchange between Syria and Egypt—often, no doubt, by way of Sinai. This is not an instance of Cypriot tradition traveling eastward to the mainland Crusader States; it is assimilation by Cyprus of a tradition already widely established on the mainland.

In the second place, the wide establishment of this tradition helps to define what the "mainland" means. Features reaching Cyprus during the thirteenth century are usually identified as Crusader. Of the parallel monuments discussed above, however, Bahdeidat alone is in the Crusader States. The Sacrifice of Isaac owes less to the Crusaders than to the east Christian communities. The latter reached far beyond the Crusader States, which hugged the merest verge along the sea. There is nothing especially Crusader in the scene of the Sacrifice. The "mainland" that Cyprus interacted with in the thirteenth century was larger than the Crusader States, and its emissaries reached Cyprus not as invaders from abroad but as immigrants from indigenous east Christian communities. The conditions that fostered this immigration were particular to the thirteenth century, and the imagery of the apse and triumphal arch at Asinou, too, marks a special interlude in the building's history. The mingling of mainland with Byzantine traditions that characterized this interlude, however, would continue to color Cypriot painting, as the somewhat later, fourteenth-century painting in the naos shows.

39. Mouriki, "Thirteenth-Century Icon Painting"; eadem, "Wall Paintings of the Church of the Panagia." For recent bibliography on the relation of Cyprus and the mainland, see Immerzeel and Hélou, "Icon Painting in the County of Tripoli"; Carr, "Perspectives on Visual Culture," 58–63; Folda, *Crusader Art in the Holy Land*, 97–104, 305–45; idem, "Figural Arts in Crusader Syria and Palestine."

The Fourteenth-Century Paintings in the Naos

Some five or six decades after the apse and piers at Asinou were frescoed, the entire central bay of the naos was sheathed anew in mural painting (Intro. Fig. 2). The date of this campaign is debated; arguments favoring a date in the 1340s will be presented later in this chapter. The images cover the walls, the vault, and the inner faces of the responds and transverse arches in a coherent carpet of color. The engulfing warmth of this painting still has a powerful effect on visitors and plays a major role in the church's appeal.

It is hard to overemphasize how radically the space of Asinou's twelfth-century naos had been altered by the intervening structural changes. Especially in the central bay, the vault had sagged from its semicircular form to a flatter curve, and the divisions between bays had become far more emphatic. The original transverse arches—semicircular like the vault—had projected only minimally from the vault's surface, creating little interruption, and had tapered into its thickness by the time they reached its base. Thus no shafts ran up the walls, and frescoes of the Evangelists seated between decorative buildings were spread across unbroken surfaces that are now cut by the responds. Even at the eastern perimeter of the naos, the masonry of the bema responds projected by only 76 rather than the current 98 cm from the wall on either side, bearing a templon beam even slightly lower than the present one. Thus only the barest projections broke the view from one end to the other of the building's simple, loaf-like space. Above the templon beam, apse and bema vault spread wide before the viewer's gaze with much the same monumental breadth that is seen today in the Dormition on the western wall (Fig. 2.25). The original space at Asinou might be compared to Giotto's Arena Chapel in Padua, with its deliberately simple, barrel-vaulted space and broad, unbroken surfaces. By contrast, the projection of the responds and above all of the transverses, which support thick diaphragm arches, breaks the naos into a cadenced sequence of spaces, and the pointed shape of the arches imposes a vertical accent upon the easy breadth of the original. These interventions transform the western bay into a shadowed pause before the symphonic burst of color in the central bay, and screen the bema from view. Only the gentle glow of Mary's face, perfectly placed in the curvature of the apse, emerges from the eastern penumbra to close the vista.

In designing their imagery, the fourteenth-century painter(s) exploited the new shape of the building. Their work can be investigated in two portions. One portion, on the transverse arches and responds, covers masonry not present in the original church, where there is no clear trace of thirteenth-century painting other than the figures of Peter and Paul. This imagery must have been newly conceived in the fourteenth century. The other portion, on the barrel vault and the walls, covers surfaces that had borne paintings in the early twelfth century, and so poses questions of how the new imagery relates to the earlier paintings

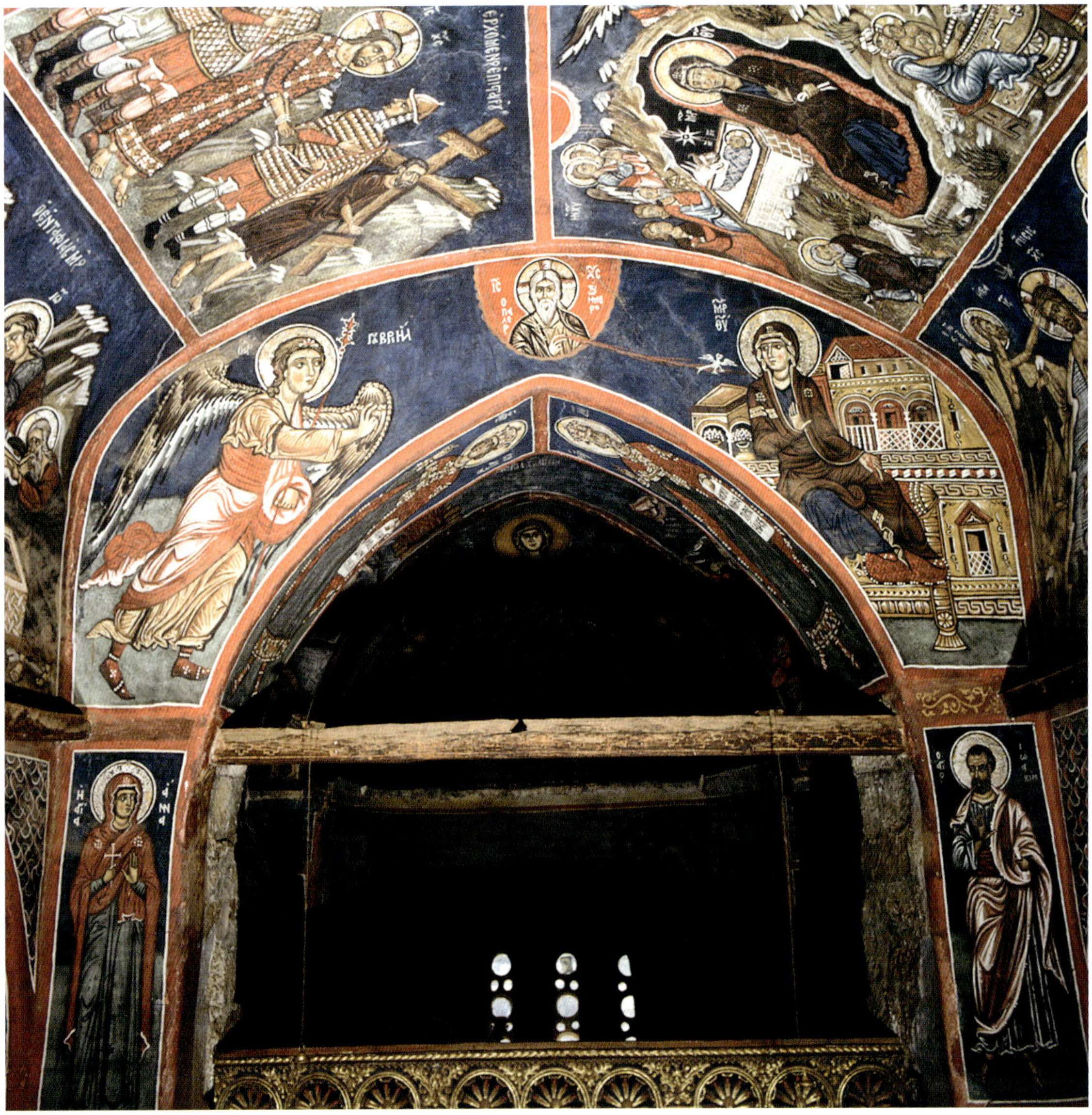

FIG. 6.10 Naos, eastern transverse arch: Annunciation with the Ancient of Days; SS. Anna and Joachim (photo courtesy of the Leventis Foundation and the Archaeological Research Unit, University of Cyprus, No. 006269)

in theme and iconography. We will examine first the imagery of the transverses, and then turn to the paintings on the vault and on the walls.

The Transverse Arches

The most prominent of the new surfaces, the western face of the bema arch, received the scene of the ANNUNCIATION (Fig. 6.10). From a hot red arc of heaven at the apex of the composition, the Ancient of Days (Ι(ησοῦ)ς / Χ(ριστό)ς / ὁ / πα/λε/ος / τῶν / ημε/ρων) releases the dove of the Spirit toward Mary (Μ(ήτ)ηρ / Θ(εο)ῦ), who sits before ornate architecture enhanced by a pot of flowers—the first Cypriot instance of a motif pervasive in the West. Gabriel (ὁ ἀρχ(άγγελος) Γαβριῆλ) strides toward her. Figures of the Virgin's parents stand on the supporting responds just below: Anna (ἡ / αγί/α / Α/νν/α) to the north and Joachim (ὁ / ἅγι/ος Ι/ώ/α/κῆμ) to the south. The Annunciation was a standard theme for the bema opening. Asinou's original Annunciation scene, concealed in the thirteenth century, had lain inside the bema (Fig. 6.11), but programs from Koutsovendis onward had placed the scene outside, on the bema arch. The painter's deliberate evocation of dynamic, twelfth-century drapery forms underscores the scene's traditionalism. Nonetheless, the expansive surface, emphatic colors, and exuberant gestures give it a wholly novel prominence. In a way unparalleled in the early twelfth-century program, where she dominated the bema, this scene announces Mary's integration into the visual program of the naos.

Mary's parents take their place below the Annunciation to affirm the true humanity of the flesh Christ assumed at the incarnation. They had long been linked with the Annunciation on Cyprus: at Trikomo, scenes of the annunciation to Joachim and Anna lie just above Gabriel and the annunciate Virgin on either side of the bema opening; at Asinou itself in 1105/6, scenes of Mary's childhood flanked the Annunciation in the bema. But the composition on the bema arch reflects late Byzantine conventions, as exemplified especially clearly in a program recurrent on bema arches in contemporary Crete, in which medallions of Anna and Joachim lie below the Annunciation with the Mandylion at the apex.[40] As Stella Papadaki-Oekland points out, the program's components can be traced back well into the twelfth century, but the composition itself was first seen in 1290/91.[41]

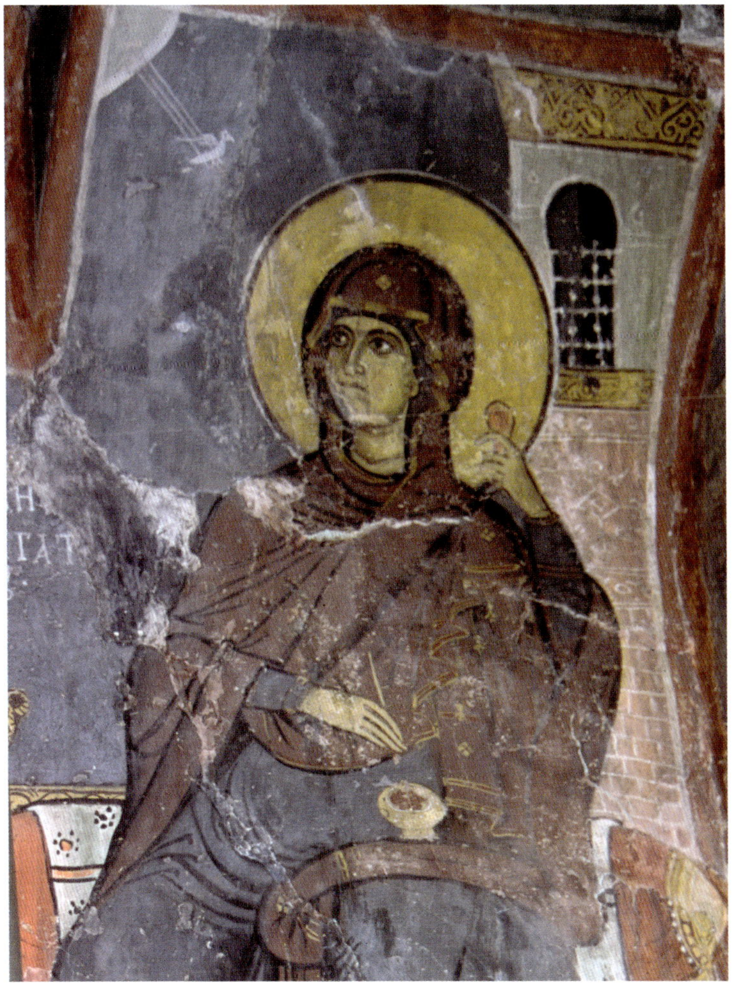

FIG. 6.11 Bema, east wall: Virgin and dove from the 1105/6 Annunciation (photo courtesy of A. W. Carr)

40. Papadaki-Oekland, "Το Άγιο Μανδήλιο," 283 n. 2, gives a list of the churches that display this combination of themes. The earliest example she cites is in the church of St. George, Sklavopoulou-Selinou, of 1290–91 (ibid., fig. 1)

41. Thus the Cathedral of the Transfiguration, Mirozhsky Monastery, Pskov (1156) displays the Mandylion and Keramion on the east and west arches

Far less conventional is the ANCIENT OF DAYS; one expects instead the Mandylion.[42] Christ Emmanuel had figured prominently in Annunciations on Cyprus,[43] but this is the first instance there of the mature God,[44] and it is the first appearance of the Ancient of Days on Cyprus altogether. A Byzantine tradition that linked the Ancient of Days to the Annunciation can be traced to the early twelfth century, when it appears for the first known time in the magnificent Ustyug icon in the Tretyakov Gallery in Moscow.[45] In these images God appears twice, once in an arc of Heaven as the Ancient of Days and once in the form of the infant Christ; in the Ustyug icon the infant hovers as a mirage on his mother's torso. This image can be traced sporadically through the thirteenth century in wall paintings in Greece.[46] Seen fully intact at St. Nicholas, Agoriane (around 1300),[47] it shows a thick ray descending toward Mary from the Ancient of Days, bearing a pod in which one can discern the faint figure of the infant Christ. With Agoriane we approach the era of Asinou, whose Annunciation seems to be the next step in this iconographic tradition.

The Ancient of Days is based on a description in Daniel 7:9–14 of the almighty judge, who gives dominion to the Son of Man when he comes on the clouds of heaven to govern the earth. Depicted in art with the cross-halo and labeled as Jesus Christ, he conveys the eternal oneness of Christ with the Father.[48] His presence in the Annunciation emphasizes God's participation in the incarnation from before the beginning of time; the dual images, ancient and infant, show that the incarnate and mortal Son is, at the same time, the eternal and pre-existent Father. At Asinou, however, the child Christ is not visible, and the belief in God's mortal humanity is visualized by the inclusion of his Mother's parents. What issues instead from the Ancient of Days is the dove. The dove had a long tradition in Annunciations on Cyprus, running back to the Annunciation of 1105/6 at Asinou itself (Fig. 6.11), the earliest Byzantine mural painting of the Annunciation to include it.[49] An image of the Spirit, it brings a Trinitarian message, showing the full participation of the Trinity in the incarnation.[50]

---

supporting the central dome, and medallions of Joachim and Anna on the north and south arches, thereby uniting the sign of God's human visibility with the sign of the human conception of his one mortal parent (Papadaki-Oekland, "Το Άγιο Μανδήλιο," 286), while the 12th-century church of St. Nicholas in Megale Kastania in Mesa Mane adorns the triumphal arch with medallion figures of Emmanuel, Joachim, and Anna, joining the incarnational aspect of Christ with figures of his mother's parents (ibid., 291, fig. 4, erroneously cited as fig. 2 in the text). From the time of St. George, Sklavopoulou-Selinou, this conjunction of themes was joined on the triumphal arch with the Annunciation.

42. Gerstel, *Beholding the Sacred Mysteries*, 70 n. 14, with a list of churches in which the Mandylion appears in the Annunciation.

43. He appears most strikingly as a full-length figure in the Annunciation of 1183 at the Enkleistra, perhaps reflecting the youthful Christ in the 11th-century mosaic of the Annunciation in the Holy Sepulchre in Jerusalem: Mango and Hawkins, "Hermitage," fig. 72; Wharton, *Art of Empire*, 89. He then appears as a bust in a medallion at Lagoudera (Nicolaïdès, "Étude iconographique," figs. 18, 62).

44. The mature Christ is rare in Annunciations, though he appears in a medallion in the prothesis vault in the 10th-century Ballı kilise in Cappadocia, and in 1201 on the bema arch at Palaiomonastero at Vrontamas: see Varales, "Παρατηρήσεις για τη θέση του Ευαγγελισμού," 206 n. 45, 215, fig. 5; Drandakes, "Πόκος ή νεφέλη," fig. 1. At the church of the Anargyroi in Kastoria, of the late 12th century, the figure of Christ above the Annunciation is white-haired, though not labeled "Ancient of Days": see Pelekanides, *Καστοριά*, pl. 14a.

45. Salko, *Early Russian Painting*, figs. 182–85. Lidov and Sidorenko, *Miraculous Image*, 6, give the inscription as "Jesus Christ Thrice Holy Ancient of Days."

46. See Drandakes, "Πόκος ή νεφέλη," 258–67. Variants appear in 1201 at Palaiomonastero in Vrontamas, Lakedaimon, in the roughly contemporary church of St. Theodore in Tsopakas, and around 1300 in St. Nicholas at Agoriane in Lakonia.

47. Emmanuel, "Οι τοιχογραφίες του Αγίου Νικολάου."

48. McKay, "Eastern Christian Exegetical Tradition"; in *ODB* 1:438, s.v. "Christ: Types of Christ. Ancient of Days."

49. Kitzinger, "Descent of the Dove," 104.

50. Ibid., 99–115.

In conjunction with the Ancient of Days, however, the Trinitarian inflection is problematic: as the Stylianous have noted, the emanation of the Spirit from a figure uniting Father and Son awkwardly smacks of the *filioque*, the Latin emendation of the Creed saying that the Spirit proceeds from the Father *and the Son*, rather than from the Father alone.[51] The use of the dove and the Ancient of Days in the Annunciation, not only at Asinou, but later at St. Nicholas of the Roof near Kakopetria and St. Mamas at Louvaras,[52] indicates that the image did not arouse concern, perhaps lending support to Chris Schabel's contention that the *filioque* was not an abiding issue in Lusignan Cyprus.[53] Nonetheless, the dove disrupts the visual and theological structure of the tradition seen in the Ustyug icon and in Greek churches, and makes it likely that the figure of the Ancient of Days in Asinou was adopted for other reasons. These become apparent when we turn to the imagery of the facing transverse.

The figures on the western transverse (Figs. 2.25, 6.12) at Asinou are more subdued in color and smaller in scale than those of the Annunciation and so do not at once invite visual association with it. Thematically, however, the two arches are paired. Both are devoted to the incarnation in the person of Mary, and both draw on Old Testament imagery to place that event beyond time. As the Annunciation with the Ancient of Days presents the incarnation rooted in the depths of eternity, so the western transverse presents the incarnation rooted in the depths of prophecy.

The east face of the west arch shows the Mandylion centered above two Old Testament prefigurations of the incarnation: Moses with the Burning Bush and Ezekiel with the Closed Door. The Mandylion, looped in thick swags over painted hooks and identified on the fabric as Ι(ησοῦ)ς / Χ(ριστὸ)ς / το / ἅγι/ον / Μαν/δί/λη/ω(ν), assumes its draped, late Byzantine form, but displays the face of Christ in the old, middle Byzantine way familiar on Cyprus, in which the clavicles break the pure circle of the halo. Moses is labeled ὁ πρ(ο)φ(ή)τ(η)ς / Μο/ϊ/σῖς; the bush is identified as ἡ βά/τος, and contains a half-length orant Mary with the sigla Μ(ήτ)ηρ / Θ(εο)ῦ. Ezekiel, labeled ὁ πρ(ο)φ(ή)τ(ης) / Ἡἐ/ζε/κι/ῆλ, carries a scroll in his left hand that reads ηδου η / πύλι κ(αι)/-κλισμ/ενη και / ουδις δι, based on Ezekiel 44:2: Καὶ εἶπε Κύριος πρός με, ἡ πύλη αὕτη κεκλεισμένη ἔσται, οὐκ ἀνοιχθήσεται, καὶ οὐδεὶς μὴ διέλθῃ δι' αὐτῆς, ὅτι κύριος ὁ Θεὸς τοῦ Ἰσραηλ εἰσελεύσεται δι' αὐτῆς, καὶ ἔσται κεκλεισμένη, that is, "The Lord said to me: This gate shall remain shut; it shall not be opened, and no one shall enter by it; for the Lord, the God of Israel, has entered by it; therefore it shall remain shut." The closed door, labeled ἡ πύλι, frames Mary accompanied by her sigla, Μ(ήτ)ηρ Θ(εο)ῦ. SS. Kerykos and Ioulitta occupy the responds, Kerykos on the south and his mother on the north (Figs. 6.27, 6.29).

The Mandylion, displaced from the eastern arch, assumes a place unique in Cypriot church

51. Stylianou and Stylianou, *Painted Churches*, 68, 127. The imagery of God in Lusignan Cyprus deserves study, as several images have seemed distinctive, shaped or even misshaped by local relations with Christians of other creeds. One is the Preparation of the Throne at St. Herakleidios in Kalopanayiotis, questioned by Gkioles, "Οἱ λειτουργικὲς πηγὲς τῆς Ἀνάληψης," 521. Another is the Christ in the Palaia Enkleistra near Kouklia, questioned by Stylianou and Stylianou, *Painted Churches*, 397. A third is the Melismos at the Archangel church, Kato Lefkara and St. Solomone, Paphos, interpreted in relation to the Latins by Christoforaki, "Displaying the Liturgy."

52. For St. Nicholas, see Stylianou and Stylianou, *Painted Churches*, 68; for Louvaras see ibid., 254, and *Annual Report of the Chief Antiquities Officer for the Year 1960* (Nicosia, 1961), fig. 6. At St. Nicholas he holds a scroll inscribed "I shall come to save the world." The Ancient of Days appears in other Cypriot churches after its advent at Asinou, but not in the Annunciation: at the apex of the western wall in the central vessel at the Holy Cross, Pelendri; above the "ἄνωθεν οἱ προφῆται" at the Panagia Podithou, Galata; above the scene of the Crucifixion at the church of the Holy Cross of Agiasmati; and in a now much-damaged image of the Trinity in the monastery church of St. Neophytos. On the Panagia Podithou, see Frigerio-Zeniou, *L'art "italo-byzantin"*, 30, fig. 51; on the Holy Cross of Agiasmati, see Argyrou and Myrianthefs, *Church of the Holy Cross*, figure on p. 17.

53. Schabel, "Religion," 195–98.

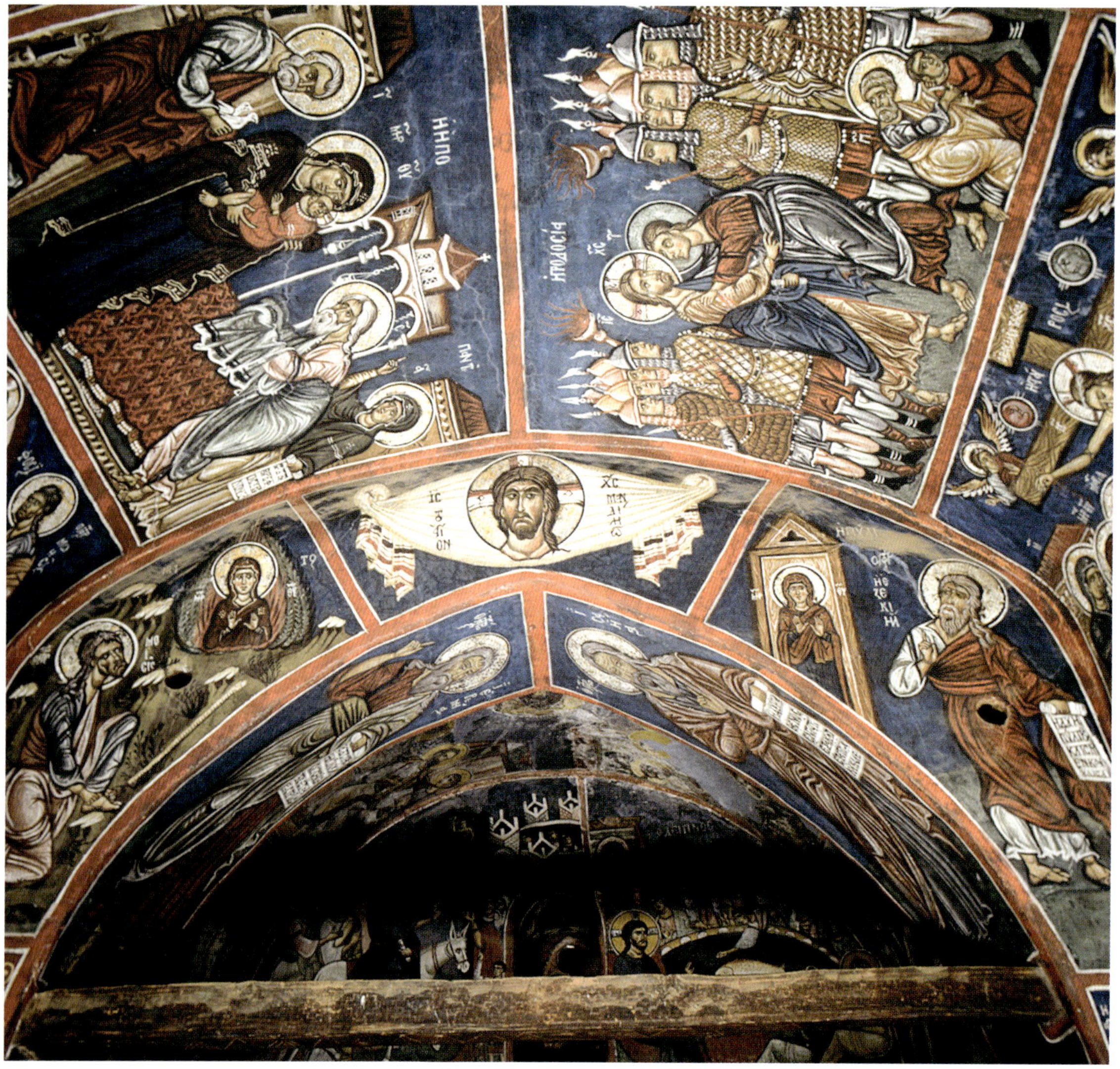

FIG. 6.12 Naos, western transverse arch: Mandylion; Moses with the Burning Bush; Ezekiel with the Closed Gate (photo courtesy of the Leventis Foundation and the Archaeological Research Unit, University of Cyprus, No. 006315)

programs.[54] It was clearly determined by the scenes just below it. The Mandylion was the visible proof of God's incarnate being, the sign of his incarnate visibility.[55] Moses' experience of the burning bush on Sinai was known as his ὅραμα, his vision.[56] Here at Asinou, in gazing at the bush, his face is turned equally to the Mandylion hovering above it, as if one vision glossed the other. Ezekiel, too—his biblical text modified to include the vocative ἰδοῦ, "behold!"—turns to the image of the door and so

54. It figures otherwise over the bema, as at Lagoudera, or over a door, as at Kato Lefkara: see Nicolaïdès, "Étude iconographique," 35–37, fig. 34; Papageorgiou, "Ἡ ἐκκλησία τοῦ Ἀρχαγγέλου," 221–22, giving other Cypriot examples. See also Stylianou and Stylianou, *Painted Churches*, 521, s.v. Holy Handkerchief. It had occupied the east face of the western transverse in other regions: see Kitzinger, "Mandylion at Monreale."

55. On the subject of the Mandylion see articles in Kessler, *Holy Face*.

56. Frigerio-Zenio, *L'art "italo-byzantin"*, 71.

toward the fabric that displayed God's corporeal visibility. The Mandylion confirms the prophets' visions and links them to the Annunciation.

The appearance of the two prefigurations at Asinou is something of a surprise. Pervasive as they are in the liturgical offices of the Marian feasts,[57] especially the Annunciation, the Old Testament prefigurations of Mary assume a significant role in monumental art only late, in the decades between 1260 and 1320.[58] They cluster in the decades leading up to this Asinou fresco,[59] and the two themes chosen at Asinou were among the most standard: the bush and the gate occur in almost all cases. At the same time, however, they are concentrated in churches of very high social prominence, with donors of notable cultural pretension. In the rural churches of Greece, the islands, and Cyprus, such sophisticated imagery was exceptional. On Cyprus one must wait for a full century to find images comparable to those at Asinou,[60] in the fifteenth-century mural of Jeremiah gesturing to a figure of the Virgin and Child looming from a circuit of city walls in the north overdoor at St. Mavra in Koilani or, later still, in the mid-sixteenth-century, Italo-Byzantine scenes of Moses and the Burning Bush over the apse images of Mary in the Panagia Podithou and the so-called Latin Chapel at St. John Lampadistes.[61] Thus the program on the transverses at Asinou is singular. It clearly does not reflect middle Byzantine precedents on the island, and one wonders what its sources might have been.

Two factors may cast some light on this question. First, the fourteenth century did see the beginning on Cyprus of what became in time a fertile allegorical imagery of Mary and the prophets. It was first manifest in the form of the Tree of Jesse, showing Mary as the highest flower of the genealogical tree sprung from David's father, Jesse. Jesse's royal issue are aligned along the tree trunk; they are then joined in the tree's branches by prophets bearing on open scrolls their predictions of the incarnation. Only one Jesse Tree in Cyprus is as early as the fourteenth century; it fills the western wall of the

57. Babić, "L'image symbolique," 147–48, discusses the liturgical uses of Ezekiel 44:2 itself or its image of the sealed door. Chatzidakis, "Τοιχογραφίες στὴ Μονὴ τῆς Ἁγίας Αἰκατερίνης," 212, discusses the liturgical uses of the burning bush. See also Taylor, "Historiated Tree of Jesse," 166, on the burning bush.

58. The classic study on the iconography of the Old Testament prefigurations of Mary is Der Nersessian, "Program and Iconography of the Frescoes of the Parecclesion." Before the Palaiologan period, she cites the depictions of the prefigurations in the marginal Psalters, the Kokkinobaphos manuscripts (Vatican. gr. 1162 and Paris. gr. 1208), and the beautiful icon of the Virgin surrounded by the prophets with images of their prefigurations at Mount Sinai. Patterson [Ševčenko], "Byzantine Frescoes at Pherrai," 142–43, suggests that the Virgin was surrounded by her Old Testament ancestors in the dome of the northwest angle chamber in the church of the Kosmosoteira monastery.

59. These include the north porch at Hagia Sophia, Trebizond (see Talbot Rice, *Haghia Sophia at Trebizond*, 149–53, figs. 112–15); the narthex of the Peribleptos (St. Clement), Ohrid (Der Nersessian, "Program and Iconography," 314; Babić, "L'image symbolique," 145–46); the outer narthex of the church of the Holy Apostles in Thessalonike (Der Nersessian, "Program and Iconography," 315); the church of St. George, Staro Nagoričino (Todić, *Staro Nagoričino*, 227, fig. 27; Babić, "L'image symbolique," fig. 2); the exonarthex of the Bogorodica Ljeviška in Prizren (fine drawings in Panić and Babić, *Bogorodica Ljeviška*, drawings 29–30), the Virgin's church at Peć (Der Nersessian, "Program and Iconography," 316), and the narthex at Lesnovo (ibid., 316; Gabelić, *Manastir Lesnovo*, 174–78).

60. There is a possible exception. The painter Leontios, who signed the image of the Mother of God Achrantos over the north door to Lagoudera in the 14th century, invoked her with an inscription that cites Habakkuk's prophecy of her: see p. 310 below.

61. The image at St. Mavra adjoins one of the Zoodochos Pege, tempting one to identify it as the Hagiosoritissa in the walls of Constantinople and to pair the two as Constantinopolitan miracle-working icons. The presence of Jeremiah, however, identifies the image as a prefiguration: on the image of Mary as a city, and especially the association of Jeremiah with imagery of her as the "living city of God," see Mouriki, "Αἱ βιβλικαὶ προεικονίσεις τῆς Παναγίας," 234–35, 242 n. 139 section δ'. The image is published in Taousianes, *Εκκλησίες και μοναστήρια*, 109, bottom. On the scenes of Moses see Frigerio-Zeniou, *L'art "italo-byzantin"*, figs. 63, 64, 129–32.

north vessel at the double church of the Holy Cross, Pelendri. This space contains the heraldic crest of Jean de Lusignan (+1375), brother of King Peter I (1359–1369) and lord of Pelendri, and it is assumed to have been adorned as a chapel of Latin rite in his lifetime, most probably for his own use.[62] Thus it may well be that the Jesse Tree at Pelendri was Jean's expression of pride in his royal lineage, and was a Latin import.[63] The theme had a Byzantine history as well as a Latin one, however,[64] and once in Cyprus, it took sturdy root, appearing in the fifteenth century in the churches of St. Herakleidios at St. John Lampadistes, Kalopanayiotis; Christ Antiphonetes at Kalogrea; and St. Themonianos, Lysi.[65] Thus the image implanted at Pelendri—at much the same time as Asinou's repainting—found a receptive environment, suggesting an interest in visualizing Mary's bond to Old Testament prophecy.

The other factor that sheds light on the sources of the composition at Asinou is the image of the burning bush (Figs. 6.12, 6.41). Unlike the image of the closed door, for which no persuasive iconographic parallel is known,[66] the imagery of the bush is not unprecedented. Its figure of Moses is indicative: the grizzled Moses with a thin beard is distinctive of the icons of Sinai.[67] It is to Sinai, too, that the image of the burning bush with Mary among its branches can be assigned, for it appears for the first time in a small cluster of thirteenth-century icons associated with Sinai.[68] The version at Asinou

62. Stylianou and Stylianou, *Painted Churches*, 231–32; Carr, "Byzantines and Italians," 345. On Jean's lordship of the fief of Pelendri, see Schabel, *Synodicum Nicosiense*, X.55.1.

63. Taylor, "Historiated Tree of Jesse," interprets the Serbian Jesse Trees in just this way, as reflecting pride in their donors' royal genealogy, and assigns to them, as well, a Latin origin. Papamastorakes, "Ενα εικαστικό εγκώμιο," reads into the Jesse Tree at the Mavriotissa in Kastoria a very similar message of genealogical pride.

64. See in particular Velmans, "L'arbre de Jessé en orient chrétien," who points out that the Jesse Tree was shown already in the 12th century in a small chapel in Tarsos, in the early 13th century in the Mytilene Gospels, at the Mavriotissa in Kastoria in 1259, and in the 1260s in the north porch at Hagia Sophia, Trebizond, all before it appeared for the first time in Serbia at Sopoćani. See also Milanović, "Tree of Jesse," who adds the Apostles' Church in Thessalonike and the Bogorodica Ljeviška in Prizren. I am indebted to Rossitza Roussanova Schroeder for showing me this article.

65. Stylianou and Stylianou, *Painted Churches*, 302 and fig. 180 for St. Herakleidios, and 481 and fig. 291 for Kalogrea. The latter painting was destroyed by art thieves in the decades after 1974; fragments of it are now on display in the Byzantine Museum in Nicosia. The Tree of Jesse at Lysi is known only from drawings of the church submitted to the director of the Menil Museum by art thief Ayden Dikman: see Carr and Morrocco, *Byzantine Masterpiece*, 10, fig. 7. Two further Jesse Trees on Cyprus from the 16th century, one at Xylophagou and the other in the so-called Latin Chapel at St. John Lampadistes, Kalopanayiotis, are in spaces that could possibly be associated with Latin use, for a heraldic crest is painted at Xylophagou, and the chapel in Kalopanayiotis is painted in Italo-Byzantine style: see Yerasimou, "Η αγιογραφική τέχνη στη Μητρόπολη Κιτίου," fig. 40, and Frigerio-Zeniou, *L'art "italo-byzantin"*, 104–18, color pls. 12–13, figs. 79, 82, 84–93. I believe, however, that there is no reason in either case to regard the space as Latin in function or message: see Frigerio-Zeniou, *L'art*, 202–3. Finally, in the 18th century, the Jesse Tree was painted in the cathedral church of St. John Bibi in Nicosia: see Papageorgiou, "Ὁ καθεδρικὸς ναὸς τοῦ Ἁγίου Ἰωάννου," 66.

66. Its singularity is not exceptional. As H. Belting notes in Belting, Mango, and Mouriki, *Mosaics and Frescoes of St. Mary Pammakaristos*, 109–10, no coherent stemma for the theme can be composed from the surviving examples in Constantinople and Serbia, for each is unique. The scene occurs in the Pammakaristos (ibid., figs. 108–10), at the Peribleptos (St. Clement) in Ohrid (Babić, "L'image symbolique," fig. 1), and at the Virgin's church, Peć (ibid., fig. 3).

67. See Mouriki, "Four Thirteenth-Century Sinai Icons," 337. All the pre-Palaiologan figures of Moses with a beard that are cited in Aliprantis, *Moses auf dem Berge Sinai*, are at Sinai, including the 6th-century mosaics of the Burning Bush and the Giving of the Law on the triumphal arch in the basilica (figs. 8, 79), a small icon of ambiguous date with the Burning Bush (fig. 23), and two icons by the painter Peter, studied by Mouriki (figs. 51, 54).

68. Collins, "Visual Piety," 106–13; Weitzmann, "*Loca Sancta*," 53–54. Collins lists, along with a 9th-century icon of the Ascension at Sinai in which a plant with red blossoms rises behind Mary (fig. 78), a late 12th-century

resembles most closely the images of the bush in two of the Sinai icons, including the upper frame of the famous diptych that pairs St. Prokopios with a figure of the Mother of God, an image that is often identified as a "Kykkotissa," the great miracle-working icon on Cyprus.[69] The connection that this diptych implies between Cyprus and Sinai is only underscored by the many visual parallels drawn by Doula Mouriki between Cypriot icons and those at Sinai, leaving little question but that ideas and images traveled readily between the two sites.[70]

Especially interesting in this regard is an icon of the burning bush from around 1200 that is now in the Greek Orthodox Patriarchate in Jerusalem.[71] This icon is among the very earliest to depict Mary as the bush. To either side of her are figures of Moses, first kneeling to remove his sandals and then standing with raised hands to receive the law. Moses' exclamation from Exodus 3:3—παρελθὼν ὄψομαι τὸ ὅραμα ("I will now turn aside, and see this great sight")—labels the image. Steep mountains flanking the bush in the background give the landscape the familiar three-peaked form of Sinai, and it is to Sinai that the panel's production has been attributed.[72] This said, the color scheme; the raised gesso of Mary's halo; the shape of Mary's face; the close kinship of Moses' fluttering drapery with the drapery pattern of the archangel Gabriel in the apse from St. Themonianos, Lysi: all show that the painter could equally well have been Cypriot. What makes this icon notable are the angel hovering over the bush and the spindle in Mary's right hand.[73] The angel belongs to the Old Testament story; he is mentioned in the text. When seen together with the Virgin's spindle, however, he becomes a reference to the Annunciation. The icon, in short, makes very much the same association between Old Testament prefigurations of Mary and the Annunciation that we see at Asinou.[74] The kinship of the iconography of Asinou's Moses with that on Sinai, and the kinships that link Sinai's icons to Cypriot works, point to Sinai as a likely source for Asinou's iconography of Moses with the Burning Bush. As Kristen Collins has pointed out, a comparable bond of the Annunciation and the Marian prefigurations had been made in the late twelfth-century apse at Deir al-Suriani in Wadi al-Natrun, Egypt, where the figures of Gabriel and Mary are flanked by four prophets bearing the texts of their prophecies on open scrolls. Among them are both Moses and Ezekiel with the texts seen at Asinou.[75] Thus the program developed for the transverse arches at Asinou seems

---

icon in Jerusalem (fig. 88), two 13th-century icons at Sinai—St. Catherine with the burning bush (fig. 85) and the notorious diptych with St. Prokopios and the Mother of God "Kykkotissa" that is discussed in note 69 below (figs. 86–87)—and two 14th-century icons at Sinai, one devoted solely to Moses at the burning bush and the other a triptych including that theme (figs. 95–97). Weitzmann, "*Loca Sancta,*" 53–54, figs. 50, 51, also reproduces Collins's figures 85 and 95 and cites the Prokopios diptych.

69. Asinou's burning bush is especially similar to those in the Prokopios diptych and the 14th-century triptych: Collins, "Visual Piety," figs. 96, 97. On the former, see most recently Vassilaki, *Mother of God*, 444–46, no. 71, entry by M. Aspra-Vardavaki; eadem, "Observations on a Thirteenth-Century Sinaitic Diptych," 89–98.

70. Mouriki, "Thirteenth-Century Icon Painting," 9–112.

71. Collins, "Visual Piety," 108, fig. 88; Garides, "Icônes du XIIIe et du XIVe siècles," 29, fig. 1, with earlier bibliography; see also the reproduction in color in Onasch and Schnieper, *Icons*, pl. p. 174.

72. Garides, "Icônes du XIIIe et XIVe siècles," 229.

73. First noted by Collins, "Visual Piety," 108.

74. In two widely separated instances, Isaiah had been shown on the bema arch in the scene of the Annunciation, bearing his prophecy about the rod of Jesse: in the mid-11th-century Saklı kilise in the Göreme Valley, Cappadocia, and in the late 12th-century St. Stylianos in Kastoria. These images make a similar association between prophecy and the Annunciation, but not by depicting the prophecy. On Saklı kilise, see N. Thierry, "Deux notes à propos du Mandylion," 17, figs. 4, 5; on Kastoria see Tsigaridas, "La peinture à Kastoria," 309–10, figs. 3, 4, 7.

75. Collins, "Visual Piety," 109, fig. 90. On this image see Hunt, "Fine Incense of Virginity." Two instances of Isaiah's integration into the scene of the Annunciation with his prophecy of the rod of Jesse are cited in note 74 just above.

to have owed a fundamental debt to the Syro-Palestinian mainland. As in the earlier program of the church's triumphal arch, regionally available images were used, but now to realize a modern, metropolitan Byzantine idea.

The theme of prophecy is carried further in the soffits of the transverse arches. Below the Annunciation are Mary's royal ancestors, DAVID AND SOLOMON (Figs. 6.37, 6.42, 2.29); below the scenes of prefiguration are Jeremiah and Isaiah (Figs. 6.13, 6.14). The upper zone of the church had traditionally been the place for prophets, and these are among the most frequently shown; at Lagoudera they stand together in the drum of the dome directly above the Annunciation, Isaiah and Jeremiah on the central axis and David and Solomon flanking them.[76] At Asinou, David (ὁ προφ(ή)τ(η)ς / Δα(βί)δ), on the south, holds a scroll reading ἄκουσο/ν θήγα/τερ κε / ἤδε κ(αὶ), words from (Ps. 44[45]:11[10], ἄκουσον θύγατερ καὶ ἰδὲ καὶ κλῖνον τὸ οὖς σου, or, "Hear, O daughter, consider, and incline your ear." Solomon (ὁ προφ(ή)τ(η)ς / Cο/λο/μ(ῶν)), on the north, displays ἡ σοφι/ά οικοδ/ώμεις / εν ἑαύ[τῇ], words from Prov. 9:1: ἡ σοφία ᾠκοδόμησεν ἑαυτῇ οἶκον, καὶ ὑπήρεισε στύλους ἑπτά, or, "Wisdom has built her house, she has set up her seven pillars." These are standard texts, frequently assigned to the two kings, but they mesh effectively when placed between Annunciation and naos. David's admonition suits both the Annunciation, in which the Word reaches Mary's ear, and the liturgy, in which it enters the church for attentive Christians. Solomon's invocation of wisdom's temple, in turn, refers both to the Virgin herself, who is the temple of the Logos, and to the church that Mary establishes through the incarnation.[77]

The prophets wear the *lacerna*—the cloak clasped over the chest—over jeweled tunics and red boots that look duly imperial; their high, flaring, crowns without *prependoulia*, however, are more reminiscent of the crowns of western monarchs than of the globed *kamelaukion* or the diadem of rounded plaques known in Byzantium.[78] Before jumping to the conclusion that they reflect the regalia of Cyprus's Latin rulers, though, it is useful to see how much more Gothic is the crown of King Janus in his portrait at Pyrga.[79] Rather than Gothic, the crowns at Asinou may be just the opposite: efforts in a Latin kingdom to recall Byzantine regalia.

The western arch bears ISAIAH AND JEREMIAH, who turn to face the Annunciation (Figs. 6.12–6.14). Jeremiah (ὁ προφ(ή)τ(η)ς Ἰ/έ/ρε/μή/ας), below the burning bush, proclaims οὗτος ο θ(εὸ)ς / ἡμῶν ού λ/ογισθίσε/τε ἕται/ρος πρὸς, from Baruch 3:36[35]: οὗτος ὁ θεὸς ἡμῶν, οὐ λογισθήσεται ἕτερος πρὸς αὐτόν, or, "This is our God; no other can be compared to him."[80] Thus he confirms that what is visible in and through Mary is the God of Scripture. Isaiah (ὁ προφ(ή)τ(η)ς Ἰ/σα/ή/ας) is below the closed gate, displaying the words ἠδοῦ ἡ παρ/θἕνος / ἐν γαστρῖ / ἕξει καὶ τ/έξετε ὑῶν / καὶ καλέ[σεις], from Isaiah 7:14: ἰδοὺ ἡ παρθένος ἐν γαστρὶ ἕξει καὶ τέξεται υἱόν, καὶ καλέσεις τὸ ὄνομα αὐτοῦ Ἐμμανουήλ, or, "Behold, a young woman shall conceive and bear a son, and shall call his name Immanuel." By far the most frequently cited of Isaiah's prophecies, this passage fits the closed gate in stressing Mary's virginity and divine pregnancy.

Below the scenes of the Burning Bush and the closed door, finally, are full-length figures of SS. KERYKOS AND IOULITTA (ὁ / ἅγι/ος / Κή/ρι/κ/ος, Fig. 6.29; η / αγι/α Ουλίττα, Fig. 6.27). The maternal figures of SS. Ioulitta and Anna face one another on the north (Figs. 6.1, 6.26, 6.27); Joachim

76. Nicolaïdès, "Étude iconographique," 44–47, fig. 18.
77. See Meyendorff, "L'iconographie de la Sagesse divine," 261: "L'image de la Sagesse venant habiter une maison terrestre et invitant les hommes à prendre part à son festin a donc été comprise comme une *image dynamique de l'Incarnation*, la maison représentant essentiellement le *réceptacle* de cet acte divin: la chair en général et, enfin, l'Église."

78. *ODB* 1:554, s.v. "Crown."
79. Stylianou and Stylianou, *Painted Churches*, fig. 258. This overtly Gothic circuit of points is seen in the crown of Solomon at Kakopetria (ibid., fig. 27). The type of crown at Asinou is also seen in the Jesse Tree at Pelendri.
80. Quoted from Komroff, *Apocrypha*, 234.

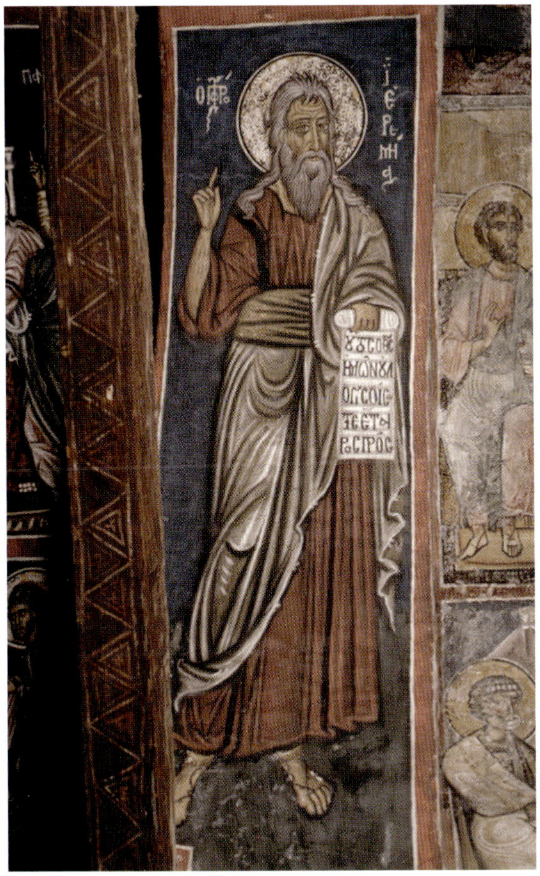

FIG. 6.13 Naos, western transverse arch, soffit: Prophet Jeremiah (photo courtesy of the Leventis Foundation and the Archaeological Research Unit, University of Cyprus, No. 006348)

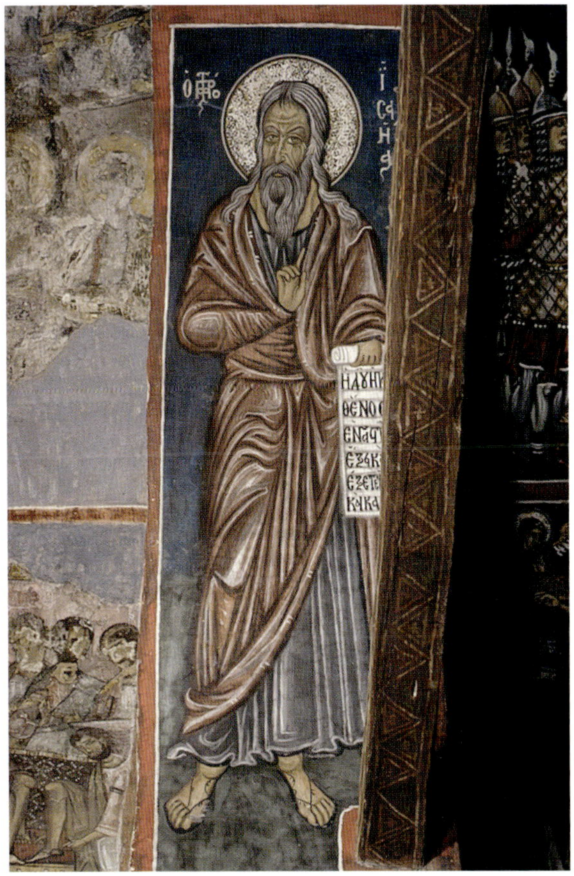

FIG. 6.14 Naos, western transverse arch, soffit: Prophet Isaiah (photo courtesy of the Leventis Foundation and the Archaeological Research Unit, University of Cyprus, No. 006369)

faces Kerykos on the south (Figs. 6.1, 6.28, 6.29). Kerykos and Ioulitta were venerated on Cyprus, as indicated by the imposing twelfth-century church in Letympou that is dedicated to them,[81] and their inclusion here may have been a deliberate effort to introduce locally favored saints into the courtly cycle chosen by the original patron. As mother and child,[82] however, they suggest a broader theme, of mothers with saintly offspring. Asinou's rich inventory of female saints has drawn scholarly attention,[83] but this has focused largely on the matrons and ascetics of the narthex, whose presence has been associated with the narthex's funerary function.[84] Aside from Thekla, included among

81. Papageorgiou, "Κηρύκου και Ιουλίττης Αγίων Εκκλησία"; Stylianou and Stylianou, *Painted Churches*, 414–18.
82. On Kerykos and Ioulitta as a mother-and-child theme, see Drewer, "Saints and Their Families," 261–62.

83. Connor, "Female Saints," 213–14 inventories the women saints included in the naos, turning later on 218–19 to those in the narthex.
84. Ibid., 219; see also Gerstel, "Painted Sources for Female Piety," 103: "The placement of female saints in close proximity to the dead, whether in the church narthex or flanking arcosolia, suggests that Byzantine monumental decoration responded to the important role of female vigil and female lamentation in the eternal life of the deceased." See also above, p. 207.

the monastics, the matrons of the naos are associated above all with their children: Helena with Constantine, Ioulitta with Kerykos, and Anna with Mary. Rather than of marriage and death, the women of the naos seem to speak of fertility and birth, thus underscoring the theme of Mary's own wondrous advent and saving pregnancy. Ioulitta and Kerykos take their place in this configuration of sacred parenting. It may also be significant that the young Kerykos is near Gephyra (Fig. 6.51), presented in the fourteenth-century overpainting as small in stature and thus probably understood as the donor's child.

The paintings on the transverse arches emerge as a coherent program dedicated to Mary and her role in the incarnation. With a force hard to imagine in the twelfth-century program, they embed Mary in the imagery of the central bay. This is in accord with Pelendri, the other major surviving naos program of the fourteenth century on Cyprus, in which the narrative of Mary's early life displaces the scenes of Christ's infancy as the visual image of the incarnation. The composition of the Annunciation and the use of the prefigurations, both attested in Byzantine monumental painting only in the Palaiologan period, make it clear that the painters were drawing on contemporary developments. At the same time, the union of Annunciation and prefigurations points to the Syro-Egyptian mainland, to which Cyprus was connected by pilgrimage, commerce, and monastic exchange.

The Ancient of Days and the Mandylion have been analyzed so far in conjunction with the Marian images that appear just below them. But they have a second function, as well: they provide the image of Christ that seems to be missing at the apex of the naos (Fig. 6.37). Whatever the original program of the central vault, the fourteenth-century decision to clothe it entirely with narratives left the naos without a culminating image of the Pantokrator. The apices of the transverses were used for this purpose. Both the Mandylion and the Ancient of Days had, in the course of the twelfth century, come to occupy places in the summit of monumental programs. Ernst Kitzinger, who analyzed this concept especially clearly, associated the proliferation of types of Christ in the upper zones of church programs with the mounting sensitivity during the Komnenian period to the relation of the persons of the Trinity to one another and to the natures of Christ.[85] The Mandylion had entered the upper zone of the main vessel for the first time in 1156 at Pskov.[86] There, where medallions of Joachim and Anna join the Mandylion and Keramion at the summits of the arches supporting the central dome, the Mandylion functioned as a visualization of God's incarnation. It figures most often in vertical sequences diagramming his descent into flesh. This is exemplified on Cyprus at Lagoudera, where it takes its place in the descending series of Christ images from the Pantokrator in the dome through the Mandylion and from Emmanuel to the Logos enthroned in the lap of Mary in the apse.[87]

The Ancient of Days, in turn, functioned as a visualization of Christ's coeternity with the preexistent Father. Rather than in the kind of vertical image sequences in which the Mandylion was used, it figured most effectively in horizontal constellations aligning multiple persons of God. Once again, this is clear already in its earliest instance in the vaults: the subsidiary domes at Nerezi of 1164, where Emmanuel, the Ancient of Days, the Pantokrator, and Christ the Priest occupy the four subsidiary domes, surrounding what, once again, must have been the Pantokrator in the main

85. Kitzinger, "Mandylion at Monreale," 575–602.
86. Ibid., 569; Lazarev, *Old Russian*, 101.
87. Nicolaïdès, "Étude iconographique," 35–37, and with particular clarity the diagram of Lagoudera's program in Stylianou and Stylianou, *Painted Churches*, fig. 101. Much the same vertical sequencing appears in programs such as that of St. Nicholas Kasnitzes in Kastoria, discussed by Gerstel (*Beholding the Sacred Mysteries*, 70, fig. 23), where the Mandylion occupies the eastern gable of the naos, forming a link between the heavenly realm of the Pantokrator and the Mother of God in the apse, or at the church of the Anastasis of Christ, Veroia, of 1315, where the Mandylion hovers between Christ at the apex of the eastern wall and the Virgin in the apse (ibid., fig. 49).

dome.[88] In the dome arches of Boiana in 1259, then, the Ancient of Days and the Mandylion were used together as paired components of the central dome: the Mandylion and Keramion on the east and west arches are balanced by the Emmanuel and Ancient of Days on the north and south arches.[89] The vertical sequence from celestial Pantokrator to incarnate visage in which the Mandylion customarily figures is integrated here with the horizontal constellation of multiple persons to which the Ancient of Days characteristically belongs. A comparable parity of Mandylion and Ancient of Days is seen at Asinou.

Often, as at Lagoudera,[90] in Nereditsa and Monreale,[91] or again in the domes of San Marco in Venice,[92] the different persons of God are aligned with the Preparation of the Throne. At Asinou, too, the Preparation of the Throne is painted at the apex of the vault over the western naos bay (Fig. 6.1). Being so aligned that it is read properly from the vantage point of the central bay and not from the western entrance, the Preparation of the Throne joins in the alignment of Christ figures.

In its equal deployment of the Mandylion and the Ancient of Days, and in their alignment with the Preparation of the Throne, the program at the apex of the naos at Asinou draws knowledgeably upon iconographic developments that had occurred in Byzantine monumental painting in the centuries since 1106. The components of Asinou's program differ, however, in one fundamental respect. In Asinou, the Ancient of Days and Mandylion are *the* images of Christ; in the other programs, they surround and complement the central and dominant figure of the mature Pantokrator. This dominant figure is absent at Asinou. Had there once been a focal figure of Christ? With this, the fourteenth-century transverses turn us to the abiding question that hovers over this bay: to what extent is the fourteenth-century imagery a reliable transcript of the original, twelfth-century program? The question becomes far more insistent as we turn to the frescoes known to have covered earlier images.

The Sanctoral Cycle

The murals on the walls and the vault of the central bay occupy surfaces painted in 1105/6. They fall into four categories of subject matter—the saints, the apotropaic crosses, the scenes of Christ, and the portrait of the donor—that will be discussed category by category and then integrated at the end of this chapter. We begin with the saints. Many of these figures can be shown to repeat the subjects used initially in the twelfth-century program. Thus their selection and grouping are illuminating above all for the original, twelfth-century campaign. Their forms and some of their subjects are new, however, and illuminate the circumstances of the fourteenth-century renovation.

At the threshold of the central bay, on the inner faces of the central naos piers are SS. Peter and Paul (Figs. 6.2, 6.3). They were painted initially in the thirteenth century, as discussed earlier, but were overpainted in the fourteenth. Only the upper portion of the fourteenth-century figures survives; the centimeter-thick bed of fourteenth-century plaster breaks off at waist level to reveal the late thirteenth-century surface with the saints' lower bodies. It is on the fourteenth-century layer that one sees the saints' names, ὁ / ἅγι/ος / Παύ/λ/ο(ς) and ὁ / ἅγι/ος / Πέ/τρ/ος, and the top of Paul's scroll, bearing the word ἀδελφοί (brothers) with which his

88. Sinkević, *Church of Saint Panteleimon at Nerezi*, 40–43. One sees this again at St. Stephen, Kastoria, of around 1200, where medallions of the Pantokrator, the Emmanuel, and the Ancient of Days run along the crest of the barrel vault over the naos (Pelekanides, *Καστορία*, fig. 89 b).
89. Grabar, *L'église de Boïana*, 35–36.
90. Stylianou and Stylianou, *Painted Churches*, fig. 101; Nicolaïdès, "Étude iconographique," 40.
91. On Monreale, see Kitzinger, "Mandylion at Monreale," 581. The Preparation of the Throne is on the vault between the Pantokrator in the apse and the Mandylion on the east face of the solea arch.
92. Demus, *Byzantine Mosaic Decoration*, figs. 6, 8, 9. Here the eastern dome displays the Emmanuel at its center, the central dome displays the mature Christ of the Ascension, and the western dome displays the Preparation of the Throne.

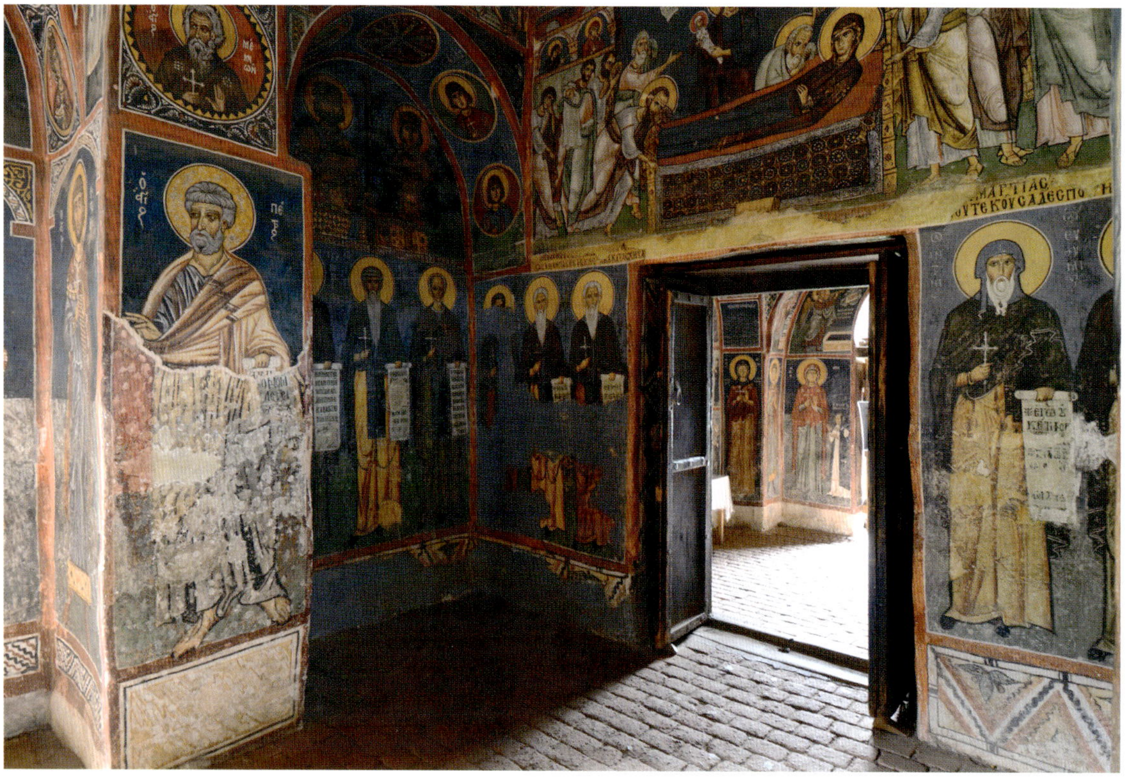

FIG. 6.15 West bay, view toward southwest: St. Peter, SS. Constantine and Helena, monastic saints, Dormition (photo courtesy of G. L. Carr)

lections often begin.[93] This layer repeats the imagery of the thirteenth-century figures, adopting their color scheme, their open scrolls, and probably also the texts upon the scrolls, but abandoning their red backgrounds in favor of the dark blue that unites the fourteenth-century program of painting as a whole. Peter and Paul are distinguished by their lay status from the saints of the western bay, who are dominantly monastic, and the slight turn of their bodies toward the bema links them with the central bay. Yet their apostolic status distinguishes them from the saints of this bay, too. They remain threshold figures (Fig. 6.15). Distinct in scale and differentiated by the pattern of the frame around them and dado below, they flank the entrance to the central bay but are not integrated into its circuit of saintly figures.

At the center of this circuit is the trio of Christ, the Mother of God, and John the Baptist on the bema responds (Figs. 6.16, 3.13). They illuminate both the twelfth- and the fourteenth-century program. Especially revealing is the figure of MARY. Labeled Μ(ήτ)ηρ Θ(εο)ῦ, she turns to her Son across the bema opening, holding a scroll with an eleven-line dialogue in which she pleads with him to redeem humankind, her words in black and his in red (see Chapter 3 for analysis). Mary's iconographic type, known as the Paraklesis, or Intercession, occurs also in the narthex, where much the same composition flanks the door to the naos (see Chapter 5 for analysis). It functions there, as Sophia Kalopissi-Verti says, to create a visual bond between the threshold to the church and the threshold to the bema.[94] The bond is particularly effective at Asinou because the figures on the bema responds, especially the figure of Christ, copy those

93. See notes 5 and 6 above.

94. See Kalopissi-Verti, "Proskynetaria of the Templon and Narthex."

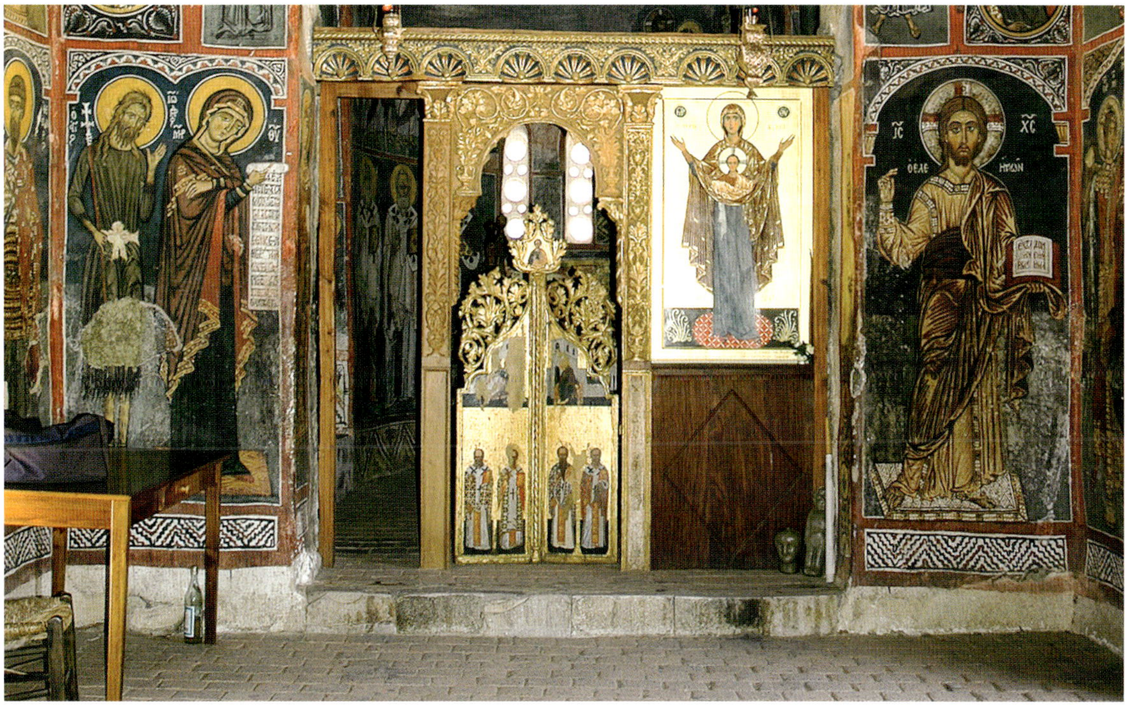

FIG. 6.16 Naos, bema responds: John the Baptist; Mother of God Paraklesis; Christ Eleemon (photo courtesy of A. W. Carr)

of the narthex (Figs. 6.16, 5.30). But whether this same composition could already have appeared on Asinou's bema responds in 1105/6 is problematic.

The figure of the scroll-bearing Mary was both ancient and widespread, as shown in Chapter 3. Used together in a coherent dramatic composition with the eleven-line dialogue and the full-length figure of Christ, however, it was conspicuously rare in monumental painting before the late twelfth century.[95] The composition appears for the first time in full at St. George, Kurbinovo, in 1191, and becomes frequent only thereafter.[96] On Cyprus, too, though it was possibly used at Perachorio, it appears clearly only in 1192 at Lagoudera; the other examples cited by Ševčenko are later.[97] An example as early as the cycle of 1105/6 at Asinou would stand out sharply.

95. Walter, "Further Notes on the Deësis," 166–67, sought an explanation for the chronology of its use in the typikon of 1136 for the church of the Mother of God Eleousa at the Pantokrator Monastery in Constantinople. This instituted a Friday-night memorial service for the dead with prayers of intercession (probably the "parakletikos kanon") and a procession to the imperial tombs bearing the "signon tes presbeias," presumably a large portable icon of intercession. Given the clearly intercessory role of the Virgin with the scroll, he suggested that this might have been the figure portrayed on the "signon tes presbeias," and that this icon was then reflected in the monumental images. On the Friday-night service, see N. P. Ševčenko, "Icons in the Liturgy," 55–56.

96. Hadermann-Misguich, *Kurbinovo*, 1:229–342; 2: figs. 116–18. The composition at Kurbinovo is anticipated shortly before 1156 by an unaccompanied figure of Mary with a now-illegible scroll at the Cathedral of the Transfiguration, Mirozhsky Monastery, Pskov (see Yamshchikov, *Pskov*, fig. 17), and a later 12th-century fresco at the church of the Anargyroi, Kastoria, with the Hand of God.

97. For Perachorio see Megaw and Hawkins, "Church of the Holy Apostles," 333, fig. 48. As I believe the figure on the facing bema pier at Perachorio was not Christ, but John the Baptist, I do not believe the Virgin held the scroll with her dialogue with Christ. For Lagoudera, see Nicolaïdès, "Étude iconographique,"

A version of very nearly this date may have existed, however, in the now-vandalized murals of the church of the Virgin Apsinthiotissa near Sychari on Cyprus.[98] Frescoed in the early twelfth century by a hand very close in style and iconography to the painter of Asinou, and partially overpainted later, the Apsinthiotissa included on its northern bema respond a full-length figure of Mary turned to her left and holding an inscribed scroll.[99] A corresponding image of Christ on the south respond is readily imagined. The scroll is no longer legible in surviving photographs. Nonetheless, the presence of this figure in the work of a painter closely related to Asinou makes it clear that a similar figure could also have been used at Asinou.

Glimpses of a lower layer of paint along Mary's back near her knees, with the colors that she wears, show that a figure of the Mother of God must have initially stood on the bema respond where the fourteenth-century one stands now (Fig. 3.13). This passage of paint, though it appears along the left edge of the fourteenth-century figure, at its back, must have belonged along the right edge of its original one, for it is only beneath her outstretched arms, where the maphorion parts to reveal her dress, that one finds its alignment of a passage of blue between two areas of red. This tells us that the early twelfth-century figure stood farther to the left than the present one, in accord with the fact that the initial twelfth-century respond was narrower than the present one. At some 50 cm from the north wall, the front of the figure would have been about 25 cm from the border of the pier, leaving room for a narrow scroll. On the basis of the figure at the Apsinthiotissa, it seems warranted to assume that the 1105/6 Virgin also bore a scroll at Asinou. It is suggestive in this regard that the inscription of the Virgin on the bema respond at Asinou is given in full, while the very similar figure in the narthex bears only a summary of the conversation. A truncated version may have been used in the narthex because the full text was readily available in the then-visible twelfth-century painting in the naos. As such, Asinou emerges as one of the very earliest instances of the Paraklesis composition. This casts valuable light on its original program. It was iconographically innovative. The elegance of the twelfth-century bema program, devoted to the Eucharist through the imagery of the body of Mary, has already been noted. The composition of the bema responds underscores the innovative character of the twelfth-century program.

A figure of CHRIST, in turn, surely occupied the south respond in the twelfth century, for the dialogue on the scroll of the Virgin Paraklesis requires his presence. It must, however, have been substantially rethought by the fourteenth-century painter. Christ's expansive gestures must have been adopted to fill the space of the broadened respond, but the figure as a whole imitates the full-length Christ in the narthex (Fig. 5.30). The Christ figure here echoes its color scheme; it is labeled Ι(ησοῦ)ς / Χ(ριστὸ)ς / ὁ ἐλε/ήμῶν, thus repeating the epithet "Eleemon," or "Merciful"; and it adopts both the open book and the inscription taken from the Gospel of John: ἐντολ(ὴν) καινην δείδομε ἡμην ἥνα α. . . . from John 13:34, ἐντολὴν καινὴν δίδωμι ὑμῖν, ἵνα ἀγαπᾶτε ἀλλήλους· καθὼς ἠγάπησα ὑμᾶς, or, "A new commandment I give to you, that you love one another; even as I have loved you. . . ." Although Christ adorns the south bema pier in a number of churches from the decades leading to Asinou's initial decoration, most famously in the Dormition church in Nicaea and at Daphni,[100] neither the epithet nor the open book occurs, and it is likely that these constitute fourteenth-century "modernizations" of the Christ figure of 1106. The inscription from John 13:34 had already been used in the late twelfth century on the bema pier at Kato

107–9, figs. 77–78; for the other Cypriot examples see above, p. 87 and note 53 in Chapter 3.

98. Winfield, "Hagios Chrysostomos," 289.

99. Chotzakoglou, "Βυζαντινή αρχιτεκτονική και τέχνη," 1:609, 2: fig. 441; Papageorgiou, *Christian Art*, 395–405.

100. For Nicaea, see Mango, *Brazen House*, 142–48, fig. 24; idem, "Date of the Narthex Mosaics." For Daphni, see Diez and Demus, *Byzantine Mosaics in Greece*, pl. 65.

Lefkara, and was still in use in the sixteenth century.[101] Its admonition to love one another was chosen probably as a message to monastic communities. This was appropriate for Asinou, which had served as a katholikon for nearly two centuries when the text was adopted in the narthex.

Though Christ and the Mother of God repeat twelfth-century figures, this is probably not the case with the figure of JOHN THE BAPTIST. There was no room for him either on the bema respond behind Mary, who stood closer than she does now to the north wall, or on the north wall itself, where surviving fragments of the original paint indicate the presence of a military saint. A miniature of 1054 in the Syrian Homs Lectionary shows the Baptist accompanying the pleading Mary and Christ,[102] making it clear that John had been associated with the Paraklesis composition well before 1105/6, in essence turning it into a Deesis.[103] A similar assimilation seems to have occurred in monumental painting on Cyprus, but only in the course of the later twelfth and thirteenth centuries. A Deesis probably occupied the bema piers at Perachorio, as A. H. S. Megaw has argued, but it was without the dialogue, for the Baptist—not Christ—balanced Mary.[104] At Lagoudera, in turn, the Baptist stands on the north wall adjoining the Virgin Paraklesis, but his scroll, bearing John 1:29, "Behold the lamb of God who takes away the sins of the world," is customarily read in conjunction with the Christ child in the arms of Symeon to his right. It is only in Kato Lefkara that John clearly joins the dialogue of Christ and his Mother, standing to Christ's left as she does to his right in a symmetrical Deesis, and displaying on his scroll Matthew 3:2: "Repent, for the kingdom of Heaven is at hand."[105] John bears the same text at Moutoullas, where he stands beside Mary, and again in the narthex of Asinou itself, where he flanks Christ, as at Kato Lefkara.[106] Thus it seems that the fourteenth-century designer, taking advantage of the broadened surface of the bema respond, decided to move the Mother of God to the right and to introduce behind her the figure of the Baptist, who had become a customary member of the group in the intervening century and a half. The addition of John, like the broad gesture of Christ, gives the composition an animation not paralleled in the narthex, and probably not present in the twelfth-century version, either.

The figures on the bema responds at Asinou illuminate both the innovative twelfth-century program and its adaptation in the fourteenth century, when the figure of John the Baptist and the text in Christ's book were introduced, and the image was animated. Precedent for both of the additions can readily be found in Cypriot programs, especially

101. Papageorgiou, "Ἡ ἐκκλησία τοῦ Ἀρχαγγέλου," 224. Rasolkoska-Nikolavska, "Le Christ Antiphonitis," 526, fig. 6, notes that a 16th-century icon of Christ Antiphonetes at Emba retains the inscription from John 8:12 that is usual for Christ Antiphonetes as if embroidered on Christ's collar, while his open book displays John 13:34. The text, then, had a sufficiently strong continuing relevance to require inclusion even when another text was deemed necessary.

102. Homs, Bibliothèque patriarchale, MS syriaque (unnumbered), 349v: see Leroy, *Les manuscrits syriaques*, 1:225. The figures of John, Mary, and Christ occupy successive full-page miniatures. Mary stands frontally but holds in her right hand an open scroll that reads: Τί, μήτηρ, αἰτεῖς; τῶν βροτῶν σωτηρίαν ("What do you ask, Mother?" "Mortals' salvation"). The inscription was unfamiliar to the Syrian scribe, who wrote as a "translation" of her inscription the words of Mary's Magnificat; nonetheless, he copied faithfully what was obviously a legible Greek model using the words seen in the canonical dialogue.

103. On this much-discussed theme see *ODB* 1:599–600, s.v. "Deesis," with earlier bibliography.

104. Megaw and Hawkins, "Church of the Holy Apostles at Perachorio," 333. They are surely right that the figure facing Mary was not Christ. What remains of the figure is merely a section of the right hand. This is held out from the body at hip level, lowered, with its fingers extended. Such a gesture cannot have belonged to Christ, who would have held his right hand in a gesture of speech.

105. Papageorgiou, "Ἡ ἐκκλησία τοῦ Ἀρχαγγέλου," 224–25. The painting on the north bema pier here has been destroyed, but it is hard to believe that the Virgin was not shown there with her open scroll.

106. Mouriki, "Wall Paintings of the Church of the Panagia," 191.

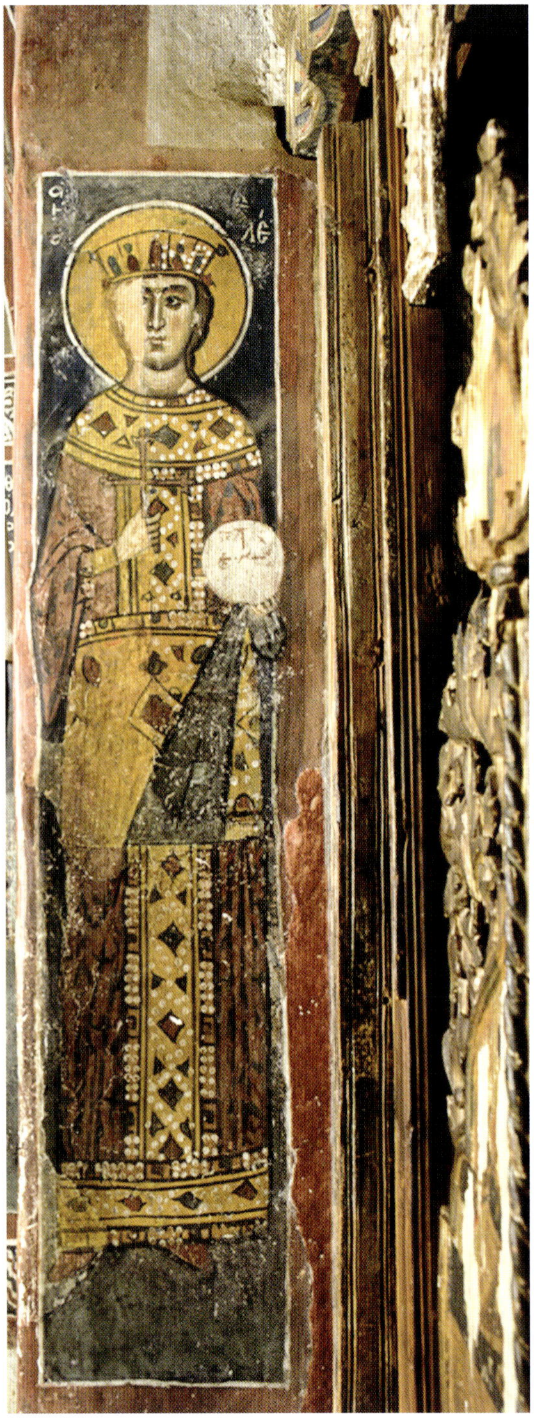

FIG. 6.17 Naos, south face of north bema respond: St. Helena (photo courtesy of the Leventis Foundation and the Archaeological Research Unit, University of Cyprus. No. 006328)

Lagoudera and Moutoullas. As a fourteenth-century program, the imagery is unexceptional; as conceived at the beginning of the twelfth century it was significant in its precocious adoption of the dialogue of Christ and his Mother.

Before leaving the bema responds one should address the female saint on the south face of the respond bearing the Baptist and Mary (Fig. 6.17). She is painted on masonry added in the thirteenth century and so cannot cover a painting of 1105/6. Her crown, loros, and red shoes show that she is an imperial saint, and her partially obliterated label, ἁ/γί/α / ε/λέ[. . .], identifies her as St. Helena. Helena's iteration here—she had already been painted in the west bay of the naos (Fig. 6.15)—is curious; so too is her lone appearance, given her customary pairing with Constantine and the emphasis in the naos on mother-child pairs. Helena is seen again without Constantine in two further churches of the Lusignan period in Famagusta, and it seems likely that she was singled out for her role in the legend of Cyprus's relics of the True Cross.[107] The Cross relics assumed particular prominence in Cyprus under the Lusignans, especially in 1340, just the period of this painting, when King Hugh IV used the Cross of Tochni—cut by Helena from the footrest of the True Cross—as a potent symbol in negotiating the relation of the crown to the Church

107. She appears in the apse of the Carmelite church, again with a white orb, and on the west wall of the Armenian church (Enlart, *Gothic Art*, 271, 288). On Helena at Asinou, see Connor, "Female Saints," 215–16. On the relics of the Cross, see Machairas, *Recital*, 1: §8 and §67–77. Helena was believed to have brought relics of both Christ's and the Good Thief's crosses to Cyprus, installing the latter on Stavrovouni, the "mountain of the Cross," and the former at the base of Stavrovouni at Tochni. Both the implantation of Benedictine monks on Stavrovouni and the theft and desecration of the Tochni relic by a Latin priest elevated Cypriot sensitivities to the relics. Helena's role in the history of Cyprus has a considerable bibliography of its own: see Kyrris, "Ελένη, αγία, και Κύπρος"; Menardos, "Ἡ Ἁγία Ἑλένη εἰς τὴν Κύπρον."

and people of Cyprus.[108] A marginal note cited in Chapter 1 (p. 26) confirms the attention given to the feast of the Cross at Asinou itself at this time.

Of the remaining seven saints encircling the central bay, five reveal traces of the twelfth-century figures, and all of them repeat the same subject with greater or lesser fidelity. Three are armed warrior saints: George; THEODORE STRATELATES (ὁ / ἅγι/ος / Θε/ὥδο/ρος / ὁ στρατι/λάτις), that is, Theodore the General;[109] and THEODORE TERON (ὁ / ἅγι/ος / Θε/ὥδο/ρ/ος / ὁ τήρων), or Theodore the Recruit.[110] The Theodores stand together (Fig. 6.18), as they often do, to the east of the north door. Like the other saints on the north wall at Asinou, their feast days—on 7 and 17 February respectively—were in winter. Traces of a red chlamys and an elaborately patterned legging on a lower layer of plaster under Theodore the Recruit show that a military saint occupied this place in the twelfth century, and there is little reason to doubt that then—as now—the Theodores stood here. Venerated throughout the empire with a fervor matched only—among warriors—by George and Demetrios,[111] the Theodores had long before acquired firmly codified images, the General with a strong, straight-nosed face, dark hair, and full, forked beard; the Recruit with shorter hair and a beard with just one point.[112] The straight, twelfth-century stocking shows that the initial Theodore the Recruit wore a short tunic and stood without moving. The later figures wear long tunics of a kind introduced in the eleventh century,[113] but used to particular effect as the saints assumed active postures from the middle of the twelfth century on, lending their wearers a dashing sartorial panache.[114] A vivid energy characterizes

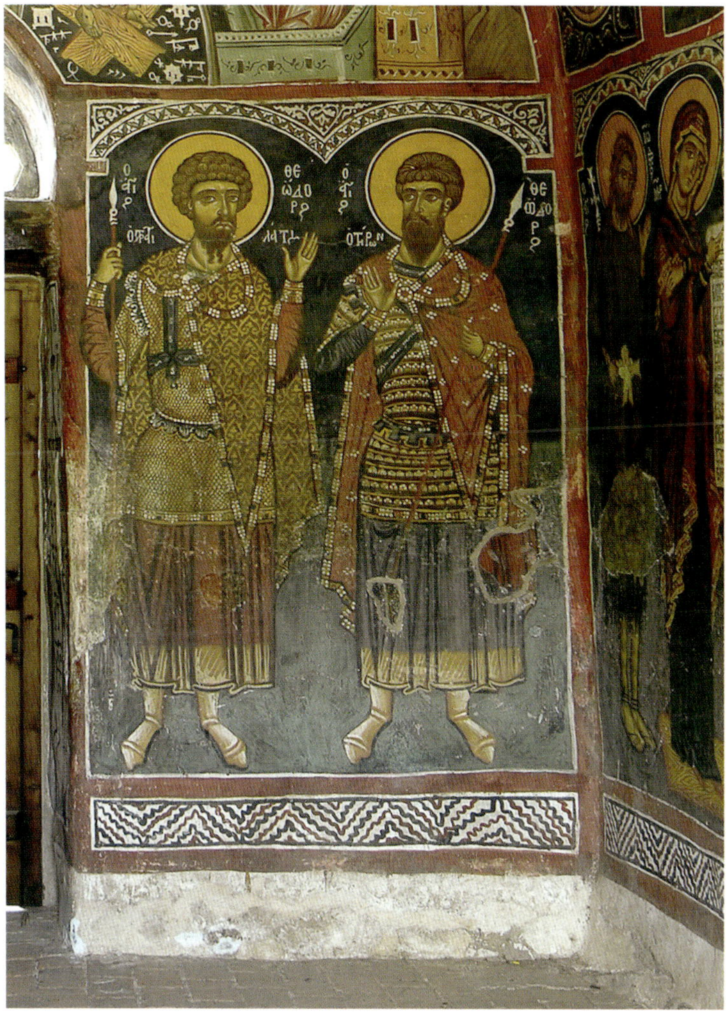

FIG. 6.18 Naos, central bay, north wall: SS. Theodore Stratelates and Theodore Teron (photo courtesy of G. L. Carr)

108. On the Cross of Tochni and its cult under the Lusignans, see Grivaud, "Grecs et Francs," 334–36; Carr, "Holy Icons: A Lusignan Asset?" 314–15.
109. Delehaye, *Synaxarium*, col. 451; *ODB* 3:2047.
110. Delehaye, *Synaxarium*, 11–82; *ODB* 3:2048–49.
111. On the warrior saints, see esp. Cotsonis, "Contribution of Byzantine Lead Seals," 437–73, with a table on p. 439 showing the chronological frequency on seals of fifteen military saints; Walter, *Warrior Saints*; Patterson [Ševčenko], "Byzantine Frescoes at Pherrai," 77–89; and on their clothing and gear, Parani, *Reconstructing the Reality of Images*, 149–55; Underwood, *Kariye Djami*, 1:249–61.
112. Maguire, *Icons of Their Bodies*, 20–24. For a cogent summary of the two saints' variously related cults, and their appearance—individually differentiated, or simply as "Theodore"—see Cotsonis, "Contribution of Byzantine Lead Seals," 448–57.
113. See St. Orestes in the northwest chapel at Hosios Loukas: Chatzidakis-Bacharas, *Les Peintures murales de Hosios Loukas*, pl. 11.
114. See SS. Demetrios, Theodore Teron, and Theodore Stratelates in Nerezi (Sinkević, *Church of Saint*

the two Theodores of the fourteenth century, too. Here, as in the figures on the bema responds, the fourteenth-century paintings are distinguished by their animation. This is enhanced by the ripple of the arches over their heads and the way Theodore Stratelates' raised hand rhymes with the raised hands of the Baptist and Mary on the bema respond to their left, linking them visually.

St. George (ὁ / ἅγι/ος / Γε/ώρ/γι/ος), the military saint par excellence,[115] stands on the south wall among Asinou's summertime saints (his feast is April 23) (Fig. 6.22). His cult on Cyprus is reflected nowhere more dramatically than in the magnificent mural icon in the narthex at Asinou (Fig. 4.1); he was venerated with equal enthusiasm by the island's Latin population,[116] and he appears in knightly guise on horseback in mural and portable icons, including Vita icons.[117] Given this prominence, the image beside Asinou's south door seems rather understated, with a mild youth in his short tunic. Except for the *maniakion* (jeweled ring) around his neck,[118] he has not been updated as the Theodores have, and though we can see in exposed passages that his original figure had elaborate stockings and jeweled boots, its poised, eleventh-century conception still echoes in his form.

Especially suggestive insight into the twelfth-century imagery is cast by St. Nicholas of Myra (Fig. 6.19), who stands to the west of the north door, and the figure beside him in the intrados of the north arch (Fig. 6.20). These two figures preserve extensive residues of their twelfth-century representations. The upper portion of Nicholas's fourteenth-century figure, labeled ὁ ἅγι/ος / Νι/κό/λα/ος, survives intact. Its dark phelonion and small flanking half-length figures of Christ (Ι(ησοῦ)ς Χ(ριστό)ς) proffering a book and the Mother of God (Μ(ήτ)ηρ Θ(εο)ῦ) presenting an omophorion conform to the saint's customary late Byzantine image. The plaster is abraded in the lower portion of the panel, revealing the vestiges of the twelfth-century figure. He, too, was a bishop, surely also Nicholas.[119] His pale pink garments conform as clearly to early twelfth-century figures of Nicholas as the dark phelonion does to later ones;[120] both this color and the way he holds his book to one side in

Panteleimon, figs. 57, 61–63) or St. Demetrios in the church of the Anargyroi, Kastoria (Pelekanides and Chatzidakis, *Kastoria*, 33, fig. 12).

115. On St. George and his imagery, see above, pp. 95–101 and notes 5–29 in Chapter 4. St. George's popularity is graphically illustrated by Cotsonis, "Contribution of Byzantine Lead Seals," 457–62, in the figures in Chart III on 393–97 giving George 445 seals, after Nicholas with 664, Michael with 503, and the two Theodores together with 446.

116. This could cut both ways: the saint chosen by the Orthodox as the patron of their splendid Gothic cathedral of St. George in Famagusta was, ironically, the same one used as the patron and emblem of the bank established by the Genoese to collect and administer the huge indemnity imposed on Cyprus after the war of 1373.

117. See the newly discovered Vita icon in the Pedoulas Museum (*Ἱερὰ Μητρόπολις Μόρφου*, 270–71, no. 13), and the 14th-century Vita icon from Philousa in the Byzantine Museum, Paphos (Papageorgiou, *Icons of Cyprus* [1992], pl. 53). See also the mural icons of George on horseback in the Aphendrika, Moutoullas, Pelendri, Sotera, Kakopetria, Emba, and St. George, Choulou.

118. Mouriki, "Four Thirteenth-Century Sinai Icons," 343–44 notes that the *maniakion* was exceptional except for SS. Sergios and Bakkhos, and barely known in the later Byzantine centuries. As she notes, it was used by the 13th-century painter Peter for his icon of St. Prokopios.

119. On the cult of St. Nicholas in Cyprus, see Triantaphyllopoulos, "Il culto e l'immagine di San Nicola a Cipro," 117–26.

120. He wears pink in the mid-12th-century mural icon in St. Nicholas of the Roof (Stylianou and Stylianou, *Painted Churches*, fig. 25), and at Lagoudera (Nicolaïdès, "Étude iconographique," fig. 80), both on Cyprus, and also in the mural icon at St. Nicholas Kasnitzes in Kastoria (Pelekanides and Chatzidakis, *Kastoria*, 59, fig. 11). Thereafter he is usually shown in a dark phelonion: see N. P. Ševčenko, *Life of Saint Nicholas*, contrasting the pale phelonion of cat. nos. 1 and 2 with the dark one in later examples. In portable panels, see the 10th-century icon on Sinai (Weitzmann, *Monastery of Saint Catherine*, no. B61; Evans and Wixom, *Glory of Byzantium*, 118, no. 65), the icon of about 1200 at Sinai (Mouriki, "Icons," 177, pl. 51) or the miniature mosaic icon in Kiev of about 1300 (Bank, *Byzantine Art in the Collections of Soviet Museums*, pl. 246).

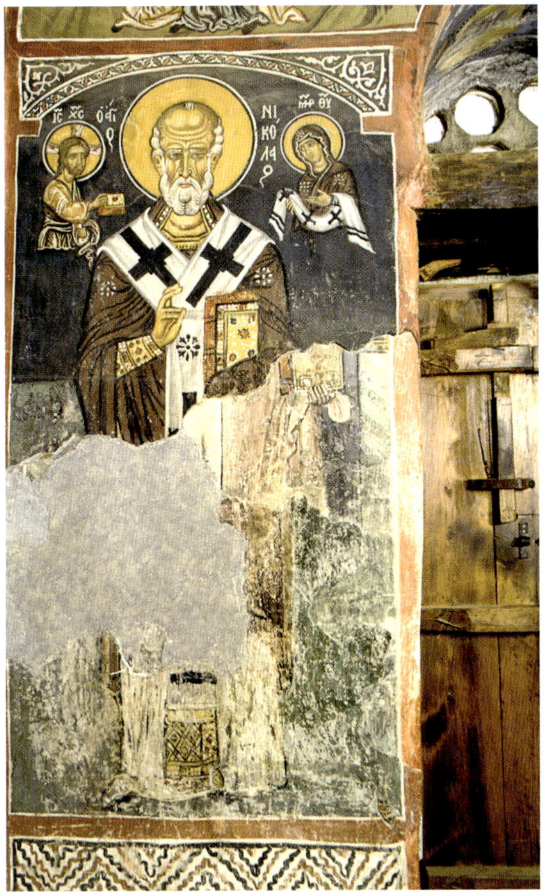

FIG. 6.19 Naos, central bay, north wall: St. Nicholas (photo courtesy of the Leventis Foundation and the Archaeological Research Unit, University of Cyprus, No. 006278)

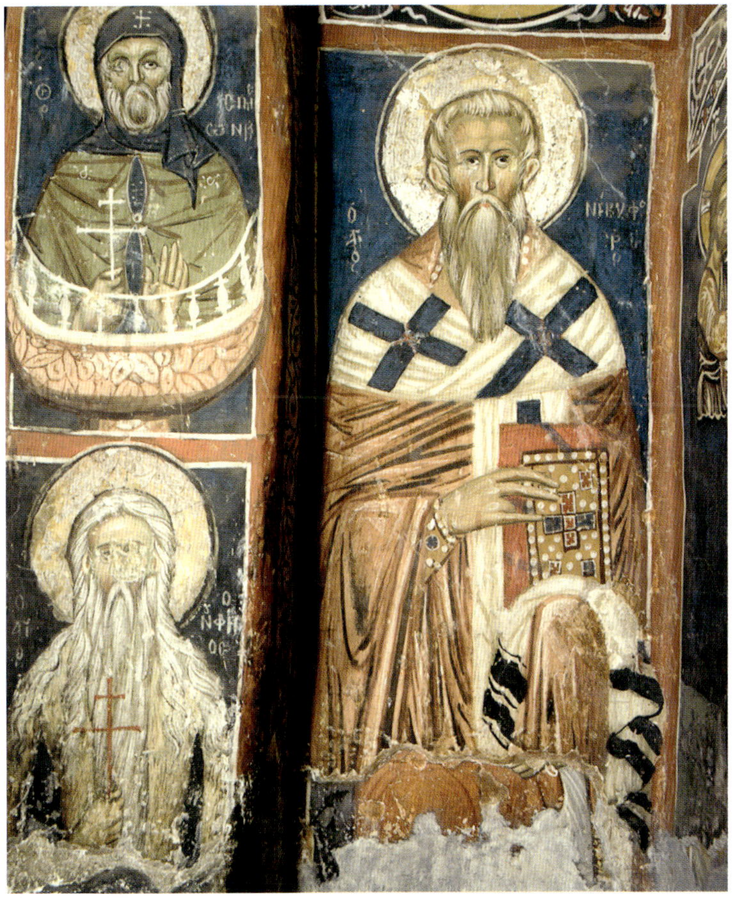

FIG. 6.20 Naos, central bay, east face of north respond: SS. Symeon Stylites, Onouphrios, and Nikephoros, with earlier saint under Nikephoros (photo courtesy of the Leventis Foundation and the Archaeological Research Unit, University of Cyprus, No. 006297)

an unveiled hand repeat precisely the iconography seen in the twelfth-century mural on the bema pier at Nicholas of the Roof, later echoed in the famous thirteenth-century icon of the saint with a Latin knight from the same church.[121] Two twisted, pale green columns bordered the twelfth-century panel, supporting an arch over Nicholas's head. The arch would have precluded the small figures of Christ and Mary, which—though first seen in the eleventh century—became customary only long after 1105/6. They seem to have been adopted into the imagery of St. Nicholas from the late ninth- or tenth-century *Vita compilata* of St. Nicholas of Sion, which relates that Christ and the Virgin appeared at the time of the saint's installation as bishop and presented him with the symbols of his office.[122]

121. Stylianou and Stylianou, *Painted Churches*, fig. 25; N. P. Ševčenko, "*Vita* Icon," 159–62, fig. 20; Folda, "Crusader Art in the Kingdom of Cyprus," 209–38 with earlier bibliography; and, above all, Papageorgiou, *Icons of Cyprus* (1992), pl. 32A; and N. P. Ševčenko, *Life of St. Nicholas*, 38 passim, no. 14.

122. N. P. Ševčenko, *Life of St. Nicholas*, 79, cites a mosaic icon on Patmos as the earliest surviving example of this motif in art: see Marava-Chatzinikolaou, "Η ψηφιδωτὴ εἰκόνα τῆς Πάτμου." If, as Ševčenko suspects, this episode

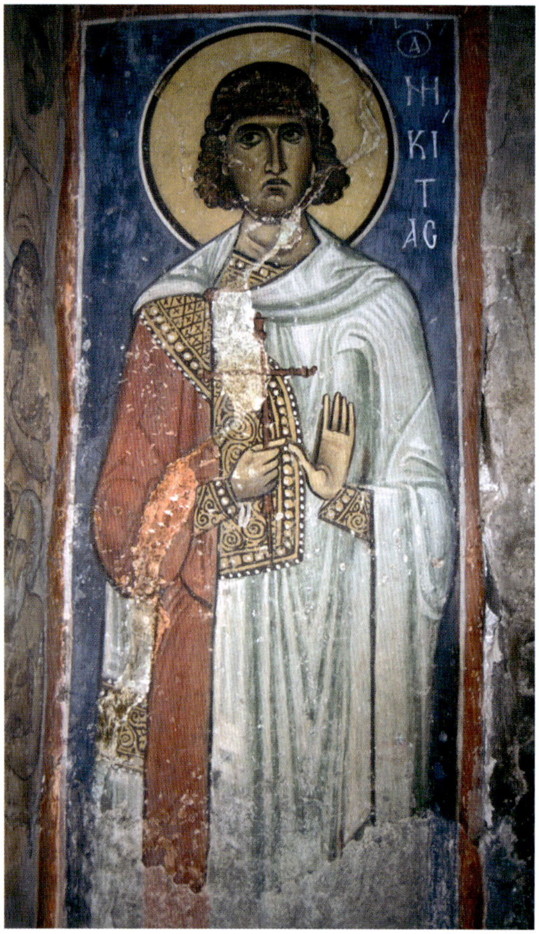

FIG. 6.21 West bay, west face of north respond: St. Niketas (photo courtesty of A. W. Carr)

Substantial twelfth-century portions of the saint just to the left, on the intrados of the north arch, also survive (Fig. 6.20). His red chlamys and pale gray chiton, exposing a fine edge of white fabric at the cuff, resemble closely those of St. Niketas on the western face of the same respond (Fig. 6.21) and suggest that he, too, was a courtly martyr. Two factors stand out about this figure. First, the surface on which it is painted was not enclosed in reinforcing masonry, as was the corresponding face of the south respond. The masonry added to the respond extends to the east of the intrados, leaving the intrados itself as a kind of recessed niche between respond and wall, but the recess was never filled. Second, the figure was overpainted not in the fourteenth century but only in the sixteenth. At that time, the east surface of the added masonry was painted with half-length figures of St. Symeon Stylites (ο (α)γ(ι)/ος Cιμε/ων β) and St. Onouphrios (ο / αγι/ος O/νουφρη/ος), and the courtly martyr on the intrados was covered with an elderly bishop identified as St. Nikephoros (ὁ/ αγι/ος Νίκυφο/ρ/ος), presumably, given his age, St. Nikephoros the iconophile patriarch.

Both the initial preservation of the figure on the intrados, and its substantially later replacement with St. Nikephoros, deserve attention. The iconophile bishop is rare in art and not seen elsewhere in Cypriot iconography.[123] While Symeon and Onouphrios are well-attested ascetic heroes who would have been readily understood in a monastic setting, it is harder to account for Nikephoros. The confident painterliness of the figure's style bespeaks familiarity with High Renaissance techniques exceptional even among Cyprus's Italo-Byzantine masters; nonetheless, it is hard to believe that the nascent Counter-Reformation sentiment that was turning contemporary European readers to Nikephoros's work could have prompted the

in the *Vita compilata* is based on visual images, one would have to postulate earlier examples in art. These figures may have acquired a particular significance on Cyprus, for the Monastery of the Priests (Agia Mone) in Paphos claimed to have the *epimanikia* given to Nicholas by the Virgin: see Hackett, *History*, 455.

123. Sacopoulou, *Asinou*, 84, identifies as Nikephoros the medallion bust of a bishop over the Birth of the Virgin on the north wall, but this identification is not adopted by either Winfield, *Asinou*, or Hadjichristodoulou, *Church of Our Lady of Asinou*, 14–17. Stylianou and Stylianou, *Painted Churches*, do not list him in their iconographic index, and the only reference to him in Jolivet-Lévy, *Les Églises byzantines de Cappadoce*, 324 n. 172, is made in order to reidentify a figure formerly regarded as representing him. An otherwise unidentified Nikephoros in one of the enamel medallions of the handled chalice of Romanos II in San Marco is identified as the iconophile patriarch by Buckton, *Treasury of San Marco*, 133; the Princeton Index lists a Nikephoros in Nereditsa, as well.

great iconophile's portrayal here. Rather, the patriarch may have been painted over a less readily recognizable saint of the same name. There were Saints Nikephoros other than the patriarch; the most prominent of them, martyred in Antioch under Valerian and Gallienus,[124] was shown in art as a brown-bearded youth with the long tunic and chlamys of a courtly martyr, very like the twelfth-century figure on the intrados.[125] His feast day on 9 February is in accord with the winter feasts of the other saints on the north wall. Thus he may have been the one who was represented in 1105/6. The likelihood that the youthful martyr Nikephoros stood beside St. Nicholas here is suggestive, because these are the names of the men associated with Asinou's foundation: the magistros Nikephoros named in three inscriptions and portrayed in the donor portrait, and the ktetor Nicholas cited in Paris. gr. 1590 (see above, pp. 17–20). The awkward recess between the added respond and the north wall may have been left deliberately to preserve the panel of St. Nicholas, which was set apart for special veneration by its frame of painted columns. Just to the left, in turn, was Nikephoros, bearing the name of the patron, and distinguished by its not being overpainted in the fourteenth century.

The figures discussed so far—Nikephoros, Nicholas, the Theodores, and George—can all be linked to subjects in the twelfth-century layer. The remaining two figures cannot. Alongside George, on the eastern face of the adjoining respond, is St. Eustathios (ο / ἅγι/ος / Εὐ/στά/θι/ος), celebrated on 20 September (Fig. 6.22). Eustathios occupies the place on the south respond that Nikephoros does on the north, but in Eustathios's case the recession between added masonry and intrados was filled in, burying all traces of the original painted surface. Abrasions in the lower portion of the saint's tunic, offering no glimpses of earlier painting, were colored in during the restoration of 1965–67. A courtly martyr most probably occupied the original intrados, at issue is his name. Eustathios, a Roman *stratelates* (general), was usually shown as a martyr,[126] but his inclusion here is mildly surprising. He appears in long cycles, especially in the Komnenian period, but he did not enjoy the selective popularity of the Theodores or George; nor was he a familiar figure in Cypriot art. It may be that he was included in the original program simply as one in the litany of recognized warriors—certainly the concentration of warrior saints is a feature of the twelfth-century imagery in the central bay. On the other hand, given the thirteenth-century obliteration of the original figure, Eustathios could have been chosen in the fourteenth century.

Eustathios seems to have had two personae. One, as a warrior triumphant over death, was developed especially in Cappadocia, where his

124. Delehaye, *Synaxarium*, col. 453.

125. Thus he is shown being martyred in the Menologion of Basil II and again in Moscow, Synodal Library 183, p. 32, and stands before his Vita on 9 February in Messina, Biblioteca Universitaria San Salvatore 27, 120r: see *Menologio Basilio II*, 387, and N. P. Ševčenko, *Illustrated Manuscripts of the Metaphrastian Menologion*, 76 and fiche 2C4–2C5. He is depicted standing among the saints near the bema in the Virgin's Church at Studenica: see Millet, *La peinture du Moyen-Âge*, 1: pl. 42 (1). He also figures in a roundel in Athos, Koutloumousiou 412.

126. Eustathios assumed a range of different iconographic guises. When shown with his family, as he is in El Nazar in the 10th century, he is gray-haired and patriarchal: see Restle, *Byzantine Wall Painting*, 2:20. In the early 11th century at Hosios Loukas, on the other hand, he is youthful with brown hair and a short beard—see Connor, *Art and Miracles*, figs. 18–19—while the mosaic cycles of Norman Sicily portray him as a mature, brown-bearded man dressed in the tunic and chlamys of the courtly martyr: see Kitzinger, *Mosaics of St. Mary's of the Admiral*, 296, fig. 76; idem, *I mosaici del periodo normanno*, fasc. 1, fig. 82. He is in elaborate full armor at St. Savior in Chora (Underwood, *Kariye Djami*, 1:257). His cult was especially developed in Cappadocia, where he is usually mature with brown hair and beard, armored in his hunting scenes and otherwise often in tunic and chlamys: see especially Jolivet-Lévy, "Hagiographie cappadocienne," and Thierry, "Vision d'Eustache." They list seventeen representations of the vision of St. Eustathios, and a number of standing portraits.

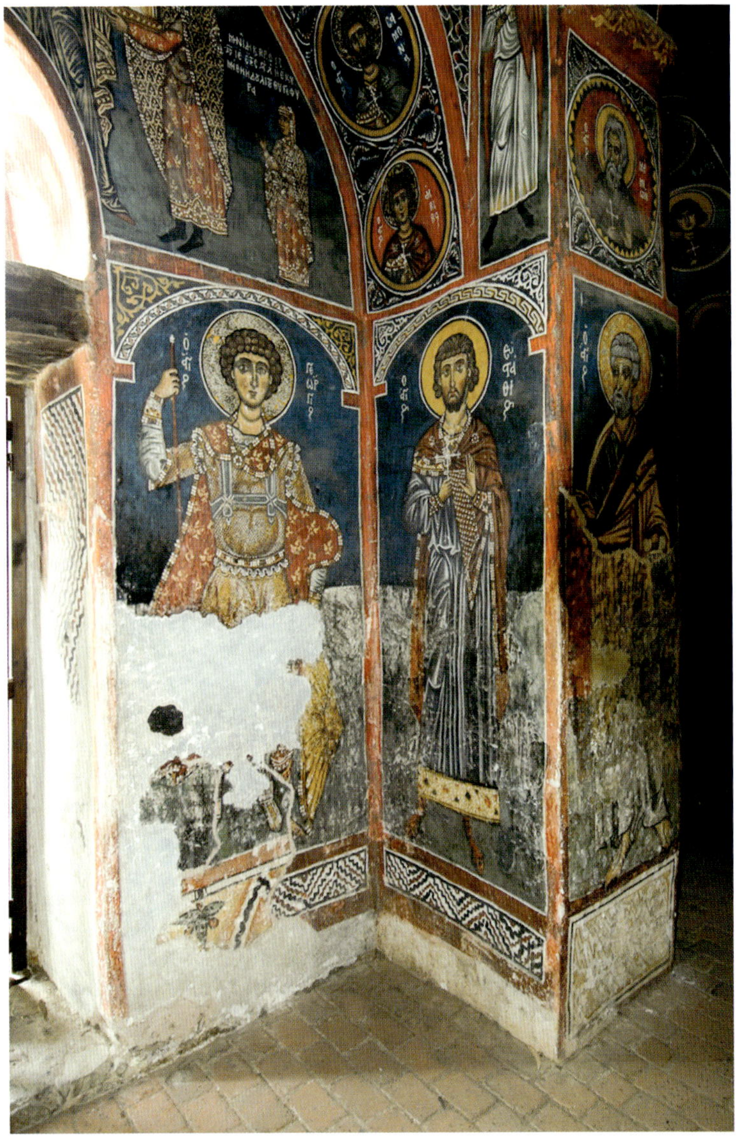

FIG. 6.22 Naos, central bay, south wall and respond: SS. George and Eustathios (photo courtesy of G. L. Carr)

figure is often linked with prayers for salvation at death, and where graffiti invoking repose cluster thickly around his icons.[127] There is no evidence that Cyprus shared in this cult, but it would accord well with the patron Nikephoros's anxious inscriptions about the salvation of his soul after death, which are gathered on the south wall not far from Eustathios. Eustathios's other competence was that of protector of livestock. Thus a ritual given in the euchologion on Holy Thursday and the Sunday after Easter known as the "exorcism of St. Tryphon" has the priest light a lamp before the icons of saints Tryphon, Eustathios, or Julian, all of whom were associated with animals, and recite certain prayers in the first person, in imitation of the miracle-worker Tryphon's response when he witnessed the destruction of plants and crops in his neighborhood.[128] These are followed by an exorcism that identifies seventeen reptiles and other creatures that infest vineyards, plants, and gardens.[129] A vivid bust of St. Tryphon (ὁ / ἅγι/ος / Τρί/φ/ῶν) was painted above St. Paul on the western transverse at Asinou, very probably as a new subject in the fourteenth century (Fig. 6.23). Across from him, just behind Eustathios, is a similar bust of St. Memnon (ὁ / ἅγι/ος / Μέ/μν/ῶν; Fig. 6.24). Tryphon, celebrated on 1 February, was often associated with healing saints, as he is at Asinou, where his image is just to the west of the martyrs of 11 November on the soffit of the north arch.[130] But on Cyprus Tryphon was significant above all as a defender against locusts.[131] So, too, was Memnon.[132] A hermit-monk and miracle-worker who was celebrated on 29 April, Memnon is vividly painted, with hoary locks and

127. See esp. Thierry, "Vision d'Eustache"; eadem, "Découvertes à la nécropole de Göreme."

128. Safran, "Art of Veneration," 189; Meester, *Rituale-benedizionale bizantino*, 266–67, 410, quoting the 1632 imprint of Goar. I am indebted to Linda Safran for making me aware of this ritual and its literature.

129. Jolivet-Lévy, *Les Églises byzantines de Cappadoce*, 43; eadem, *La Cappadoce médiévale*, 340.

130. In the northwest chapel at Nerezi the martyrs of Sebaste and the saints of 11 November are joined by St. Tryphon (see Sinkević, *Church of Saint Panteleimon*, 72–73), and again in Lagoudera, St. Tryphon follows the martyrs of 11 November (Nicolaïdès, "Étude iconographique," 132, figure 105).

131. Machairas, *Recital*, 2:72.

132. Delehaye, *Synaxarium*, 637, celebrated as a thaumaturgic saint on 29 April. On Memnon as a protector against locusts, see Machairas, *Recital*, 1: ¶40, 2:72.

FIG. 6.23
Naos, central bay, south face of north respond: St. Tryphon (photo courtesy of G. L. Carr)

FIG. 6.24
Naos, central bay, north face of south respond: St. Memnon (photo courtesy of G. L. Carr)

piercing gaze, but he is a unicum in the published cycles of Cyprus and known for no other special competence. This competence assumes significance, however, when one considers that the first recorded instance of a devastating plague of locusts on Cyprus occurred in 1351, near the date at which the naos at Asinou must have been painted.[133] This fact invites the conclusion that Eustathios, along with Memnon and Tryphon, was introduced to the cycle in the fourteenth century in response to a threat that must have been of acute concern to an agricultural community such as Asinou.

The final panel in this group, to the east of the south door, shows the MOTHER OF GOD in a round-backed throne, flanked by archangels and holding the Christ child suspended in a seated position above her lap (Fig. 6.25). Mother and Child are identified with their sigla, Μ(ήτ)ηρ / Θ(εο)ῦ and Ι(ησοῦ)ς / Χ(ριστό)ς; the archangels are labeled ὁ ἀρχ(άγγελος) / Μιχ(αήλ) to the left of Mary, and ὁ ἀρχ(άγγελος) / Γαβριῆλ to the right. Like that of St. Eustathios, this image offers no evidence of its twelfth-century precursor, though the elongation of the legs gives it a curious incoherence, as if a twelfth-century standing figure had been adapted to the enthroned composition. Areas of damage below Mary's right hand and across Gabriel's lower body create an interruption in the continuity of the surface. They revealed no traces of earlier painting, and were in-painted in the restoration of 1965–67.

133. See most recently Nikolaou-Konnari, "Η Κύπρος στις απαρχές της Τουρκοκρατίας," 221, noting the indications of a locust problem before the plague of 1351, and citing earlier literature.

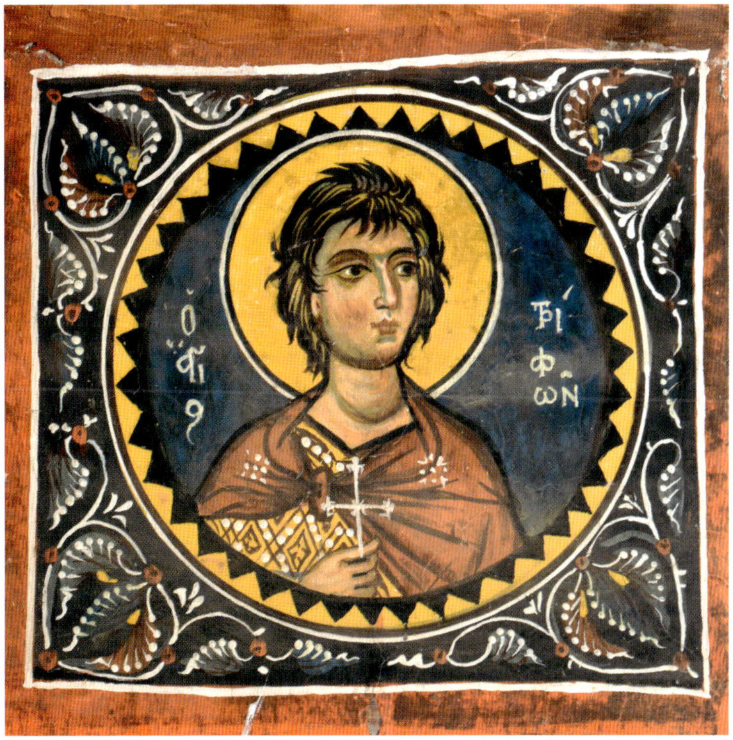

fig. 6.23

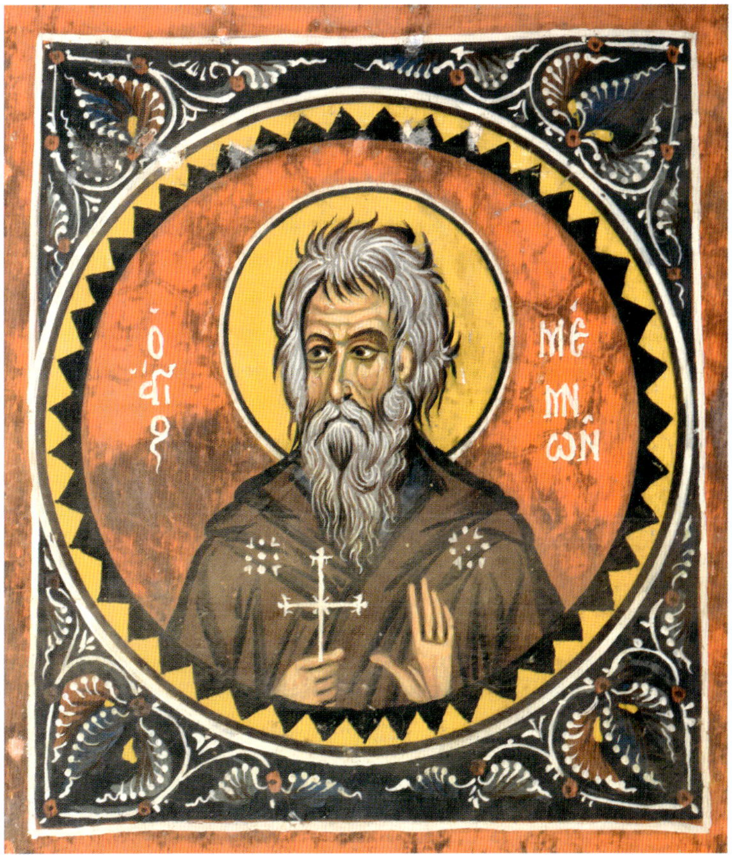

fig. 6.24

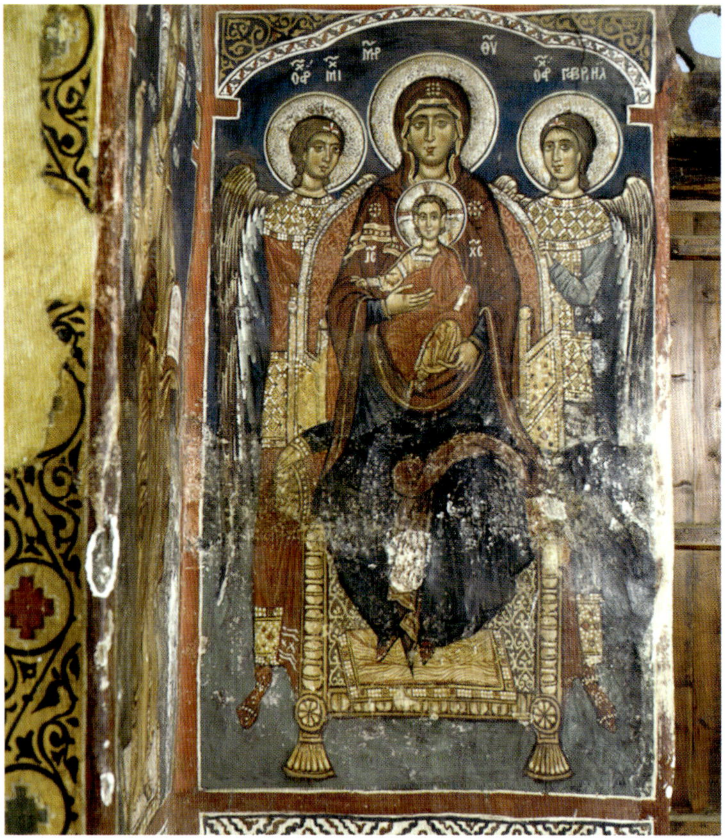

FIG. 6.25 Naos, central bay, south wall: Mother of God with Archangels Michael and Gabriel (photo courtesy of the Leventis Foundation and the Archaeological Research Unit, University of Cyprus, No. 006271)

The paint of Mary's legs as it resumes below the damage belongs to the fourteenth century, not the twelfth. Thus the figure seems to belong, elongation and all, to the fourteenth-century campaign.

The present panel functions as a proskynetarion icon, an icon for special veneration. It adjoins the large proskynetaria of Mary and Christ Eleemon offered for veneration on the bema responds and, in a sense, it duplicates the icon of the Virgin Paraklesis, offering a second icon of the Virgin for veneration but now in her role as patron of the church. Similar icons of the Virgin as patron had appeared in both Lagoudera and Moutoullas. At Lagoudera the fragment of a fresco displaying the enthroned Virgin between archangels was found beneath the paint layer of 1192 in the dado area of the wall that now displays the Arakiotissa.[134] Dated in the interval between the construction of the church—usually placed in the late twelfth century—and the frescoes of 1192, it resembled the icon at Asinou in both subject and location. It was replaced in 1192 with the icon of the standing Arakiotissa. A century later at Moutoullas a large mural icon of the Mother of God in a high-backed throne was painted beside the templon on the south wall.[135] From Moutoullas it is but a step to the similarly placed mural icon at Asinou. The sequence of similar icons at Lagoudera, Moutoullas, and Asinou is clear. Yet they pose a question: did the sequence actually begin at Asinou, in 1105/6?

The evolution of mural proskynetaria has been studied extensively by historians interested in the development of the templon as an armature for devotional images.[136] The installation of monumental icons flanking the entrance to the bema can be found sporadically from the tenth century onward, most often displaying Christ and the Mother of God, as in the well-known cases of Daphni or the Dormition church in Nicaea, but occasionally also showing a saintly patron.[137]

134. The use of a throne in this earlier image of the Virgin at Lagoudera might help to explain the presence of the throne in the currently-visible image of the Arakiotissa from 1192 in the same church.

135. Mouriki, "Wall Paintings of the Church of the Panagia," 191, fig. 10.

136. See in particular Gerstel, *Thresholds of the Sacred*; and Sinković, *Church of Saint Panteleimon*, 90–92; Walter, "New Look at the Byzantine Sanctuary Barrier"; Epstein, "Middle Byzantine Sanctuary Barrier"; Hadermann-Misguich, *Kurbinovo*, 1:217–18; Chatzidakis, "L'évolution de l'icône," 162–63 passim; Velmans, "Rayonnement de l'icône," 204–8 passim; Babić, "La décoration en fresques."

137. The most consistently cited example is the figure of St. Barbara on the south side of the now-broken templon in the Cappadocian church of St. Barbara, Soğanlı, of 1006 or 1021; see Restle, *Byzantine Wall Painting*, 3: fig. 433. Jolivet-Lévy ("Hagiographie," 214) suggests that the scene of the vision of St. Eustathios in the comparable space to the south of the bema opening in the 10th-century church at Tavşanlı in Cappadocia may indicate

Then, in the mid-twelfth century, the use of such proskynetarion figures increased dramatically. Churches with bema piers began to address the problem of including the patron saint without displacing either Christ or the Virgin; churches without bema piers experimented with placing proskynetarion icons on the walls beside the templon.[138] Eventually, in the fourteenth century, both problems would be resolved by the intercolumnar icons of the templon, as exemplified in 1318 by St. George, Staro Nagoričino, where figures of the Virgin Paraklesis and Christ flank smaller icons of St. George and the Virgin Pelagonitissa.[139]

A different solution emerged in Cyprus during the second half of the twelfth century. It is first seen at St. Nicholas of the Roof, Kakopetria: when the templon was renovated in the middle of the century, a monumental mural icon of St. Nicholas was painted on the east wall just to the south of the templon.[140] It adjoins and extends the templon. This idea was then applied at Lagoudera, first with the icon of the enthroned Virgin to one side of the templon, and then fully developed in 1192, when the large mural icon of the Virgin bearing the name of the church was incorporated into the sanctoral cycle on the south wall, adjoining the framed figure of Christ on the south bema pier. This pattern recurs at Moutoullas in 1280, and then again at Asinou. It is a pattern that evolves in, and accords with, developments in other parts of Byzantium during the second half of the twelfth century. To presume the presence of a monumental icon of the Virgin adjoining the bema responds at Asinou already in 1105/6 would anticipate this development by at least a half century. The use of the Virgin Paraklesis on the north bema respond in 1105/6 has already shown, however, that just such precocious developments did occur at Asinou. Thus it is impossible to say categorically that an image of Mary could not have been there earlier, though one might question its form.

In form, the existing image is conspicuously awkward, with its crowded angels and attenuated Virgin; the kinship of its throne to that of Christ in the donor panel just above it (Fig. 6.50) makes it clear that the current composition is a fourteenth-century one. It draws attention to the rarity with which Mary was shown enthroned in any part of the Byzantine church, except in the apse, before the late twelfth century.[141] The three examples that predate

that he was the patron saint of this space. Mango, "On the History of the Templon," points out that the icon of St. Artemios at the entrance to his chapel and to the stairs leading to his relic shrine must have constituted such an icon for special veneration already in pre-Iconoclastic times, but it is not clear whether it was a mural or a movable icon. Koutsovendis on Cyprus itself offers an interesting case: the church's dedication to the Trinity precludes a saint as patron, yet the large icon frame on the south bema pier seems to have displayed not Christ, but a figure wearing shoes: see Mango, "Monastery of St. Chrysostom at Koutsovendis," 78.

138. If placed flanking the bema, the saint of necessity displaces either Christ or Mary, as illustrated by Nerezi in 1164, where the standing Hodegetria and—rather than Christ—St. Panteleimon are portrayed in the specially sculpted arched frames on the bema piers (Sinkević, *Church of Saint Panteleimon*, 66, figs. 34, 49, 50). The best-known examples of churches without bema piers are in the Balkans: thus a monumental mural icon of SS. Cosmas and Damian on the south pier faces viewers approaching the bema at the church of the Anargyroi at Kastoria (Pelekanides and Chatzidakis, *Kastoria*, 30, fig. 7); the figure of St. Nicholas is framed in grand scale on the south wall of St. Nicholas Kasnitzes, Kastoria, facing a yet more monumental icon of Christ enframed by a painted arch on the north wall (ibid., 52, plan; 54, fig. 4; 59, fig. 11); a monumental icon of St. George on the north wall at Kurbinovo faces a similarly elaborately framed icon of Christ on the south wall (Hadermann-Misguich, *Kurbinovo*, 1:214–34; 2 figs. 114, 116); and the usage continues in the 13th century with St. Nicholas and Christ Evergetes at Boiana and St. Demetrios and the Mother of God at Varoš (ibid., 1:219).

139. Babić, "La décoration en fresques," pls. 24–25.

140. Stylianou and Stylianou, *Painted Churches*, 62–65, fig. 25.

141. Thus, the enthroned Hodegetria on the north bema pier at Samari belongs in the late 12th century, and the magnificent Virgin with archangels in the parekklesion at Patmos is from around 1200: see Grigoriadou-Cabagnols, "Décor peint," 188, fig. 7; and Orlandos, *Ἡ ἀρχιτεκτονικὴ καὶ αἱ βυζαντιναὶ τοιχογραφίαι*, pl. 2; Corrie,

1150 are the tenth-century tomb painting with the Virgin and Child on a high- and lightly lyre-backed throne at Eğri taş Kilisesi in Cappadocia; the enthroned Mother of God on the north bema pier at Hagia Sophia, Ohrid, from the eleventh century; and the mural icon of the enthroned Virgin of 1130 on one of the columns of the church of the Nativity in Bethlehem, which is Byzantine in form although Latin in patronage.[142] These examples show that Mary was depicted enthroned when she was presented independently as a devotional icon of mural scale. Such icons, however, began to become usual only in the second half of the twelfth century. Certainly this was the case on Cyprus, where two mural icons with the Virgin enthroned were installed in the last third of the twelfth century at St. Anthony, Kellia;[143] a third was painted in 1183 in the cell of St. Neophytos; a fourth was painted shortly thereafter in the refectory at his Enkleistra;[144] and a fifth, probably from the thirteenth century, occupies the south face of the northwest pier at the Panagia Angeloktiste, Kiti.[145] None of these is the strategically placed icon of the church's patron, as is the image at Asinou; for this one must wait for Lagoudera. None before Lagoudera, moreover, shows the Virgin with archangels.

The chronology of these examples makes it clear that the archangels can only have been a fourteenth-century feature; the throne, in turn, was a feature of the panel's role as a devotional icon. The attenuation of the Virgin makes it attractive to imagine that the initial figure on Asinou's south wall was not seated but standing.[146] Like the presence of an earlier figure of Mary here, this possibility cannot be proven, but it suggests a fruitful way of thinking about the image.

Among the most notable aspects of the fourteenth-century program is the way the central bay is set apart as a discrete capsule of space. This discreteness was determined by segmenting the naos with added responds and transverse arches. But it was enhanced by the painters in their treatment of the sanctoral cycle. The gentle animation of the figures unifies the circuit of saints; the figures of Peter and Paul turn eastward, separating the monastic saints of the western bay from the honor guard of warriors and patronal name-saints that ring the central space; and most significantly of all, the arches painted above the figures create an embracing armature, a kind of wrap-around templon that embraces the bay and enunciates its distinctive character as a space of petition in front of

---

"Political Meaning," fig. 2; Mouriki, "Τοιχογραφίες τοῦ Παρεκκλησίου τῆς Μονῆς Ἰωάννου," fig. 3. The enthroned Virgin at St. Stephen, Kastoria, is yet later, in the 13th century: see Pelekanides and Chatzidakis, *Kastoria*, 13, fig. 7; 19.

142. For Eğri taş Kilisesi see Jolivet-Lévy, *La Cappadoce médiévale*, figure on page 70. The icon at Ohrid is of debated date: Miljković-Pepek, "La fresque de la Vierge avec le Christ," 388–89, places it in the second quarter of the 11th century with the rest of the murals in the bema; Lazarev, *Storia*, 180 n. 90, places it in the 12th century, as does Grabar, "Deux notes sur l'histoire de l'iconostase," 410. On the Bethlehem panel, see Folda, *Art of the Crusaders*, 91–97, color pls. 1, 2; Kühnel, *Wall Painting in the Latin Kingdom of Jerusalem*, 15–22, pls. 3–6. A fourth example may be offered by the enthroned Virgin with archangels in the church of the Panagia ton Kastrianon, Kos, published as belonging to the early 12th-century phase of painting in the church, but perhaps added on a separate layer: see Papatheophanous-Tsoure, "Οι βυζαντινές τοιχογραφίες δυό μνημείων της Κώ," 357–58, fig. 1. I am endebted to Sophia Kalopissi-Verti for this information.

143. For the first of these, see Spanou, "Η τέχνη στη μητροπολιτική περιφέρεια Κιτίου," 27–28, fig. 6, where it is associated with the same hand as the paintings of 1160–80 at Perachorio. The second, which is probably somewhat later, is now removed from the wall and displayed in the museum of Kykkos Monastery: see Chotzakoglou, "Βυζαντινή αρχιτεκτονική και τέχνη," 2: fig. 342.

144. Mango and Hawkins, "Hermitage," figs. 107, 111.

145. Spanou, "Η τέχνη στη μητροπολιτική περιφέρεια Κιτίου," 36.

146. Not even on Mount Sinai—where Mary with the seated Child before her breast had special significance as the Virgin of the Bush—was the Child so inorganically suspended above her lap when she was seated: see the icon with the five Virgins, Soteriou and Soteriou, *Εἰκόνες*, 1:146–47, 2:125–28; Vassilaki, *Mother of God*, 144, fig. 87.

the sanctuary. This treatment of the bay heightens precisely the aspect of the twelfth-century program that had been most forward-looking: the clustering of intercessory icons of the Virgin before the bema. In 1105/6, when it had not yet become customary to close the view into the holy space of the bema, the devotional intensification of the area in front of the templon was not an issue. But as the templon became closed in, the images near it helped define and sanctify the space before it. In just this way, an image of the Virgin beside the south door in the initial program at Asinou may well have come, over time, to acquire a special role and character, amplified as the initial open templon was closed in the later thirteenth century,[147] and eventually articulated overtly in the fourteenth-century overpainting by the addition of the painted arches, the archangels, and the throne.

A final component of the sanctoral cycle is provided by the bust figures of saints in the soffits of the arches spanning the north and south walls. These, too, were overpainted in the fourteenth century. They represent four familiar clusters of martyr saints. On the north arch over St. Nicholas and the SS. Theodore rise medallion busts of four of the five MARTYRS OF SEBASTE, martyrs and miracle-workers celebrated on 13 December (Fig. 6.26): St. Mardarios (ὁ / ἅγι/ος / Μαρ/δά/ρι/ος), occupying the eastern end of the soffit, with a bright red cap on his short brown hair; St. Eugenios (ὁ / ἅγι/ος / Ευ/γέ/νι/ος), brown-haired with a white cross in his right hand; St. Auxentios (ὁ / ἅγι/ος / Αὐ/ξε(ν)/τιος), with long white hair and beard holding a white cross; and St. Eustratios (ὁ / ἅγι/ος / Εὐ/στρά/τι/ος), sallow with a white cross in his hand; Orestes, as noted below, is missing.[148] The martyrs of Sebaste are followed to the west by busts of the three MARTYRS OF 11 NOVEMBER (Fig. 6.27): Menas (ὁ / ἅγι/ος / Μι/ν(ᾶς)), Viktor (ὁ / ἅγι/ος / Βί/κτο/ρ), and Vikentios (ὁ / ἅγι/ος / Βι/κέν/τιος).[149] Finally, at the western end of the soffit, we meet St. Stephanites (ὁ / ἅγι/ος / Cτε/φα/νί/της), a figure otherwise unattested. Over the south wall, in turn, are busts of five of the ANARGYROI or "moneyless" saints, physician saints who healed without seeking recompense (Figs. 6.28, 6.29): St. Hermolaos (ὁ / ἅγι/ος / Ἑρ/μό/λα/ος), celebrated on 26 July, at the eastern end of the soffit; St. Panteleimon (ὁ / ἅγι/ος / Πᾶν/τε/λε/ήμ(ων)), celebrated on 27 July; St. Damian (ὁ / ἅγι/ος / Δα/μι/α/ν/ὸς); St. Cosmas (ὁ / ἅγι/ος / Κοσ/μ/ᾶς; see pp. 170–71 for feast dates of SS. Cosmas and Damian); and St. Thalelaios (ὁ / ἅγι/ος / Θα/λα/λε/ος, celebrated on 20 May).[150] They are followed by another cluster of three who share a saint's day and, in this

147. On the icons associated with Asinou, see pp. 28–29 and n. 86 above. The 12th-century icons associated with Asinou are epistyle icons; those of the 13th and 14th centuries are despotic icons.

148. The fifth member of the group, Orestes, is omitted. On these saints see especially the entry by N. P. Ševčenko in Nelson and Collins, *Holy Image, Hallowed Ground*, 174–77, no. 21; Mouriki, *Mosaics of Nea Moni*, 1:143–49; 2: pls. 61–65; Chatzidakis-Bacharas, *Les Peintures murales de Hosios Loukas*, 74–80, figs. 11–16; Weitzmann, "Illustrations to the Lives of the Five Martyrs."

149. On these figures see Nicolaïdès, "Étude iconographique," 131–32; Sinkević, *Church of Saint Panteleimon*, 72–73; Delehaye, *Synaxarium*, 212–23. Of the three, it is Menas who has drawn most attention, both because he conflates two saints, one associated with Egypt celebrated on 11 November and one associated with Constantinople celebrated on 10 December, and because of his attribute of a medallion with Christ, explained clearly by neither Vita. On Menas see Woodfin, "An Officer and a Gentleman"; Delehaye, "L'invention des reliques de Saint Menas"; Chatzidakis-Bacharas, *Les Peintures murales de Hosios Loukas*, 70–74. As to the disk, see Jerphanion, "Les caractéristiques et les attributs," 22 n. 4; he associates it with Menas of Egypt's preaching of Christ to idolaters, an association seconded by Xyngopoulos, *Τοιχογραφίες τοῦ Ἁγ. Νικολάου Ὀρφανοῦ*, 22. By contrast, Chatzidakis, "Particularités iconographiques," 92, links the disk with Christ's appearance in prison to Menas of Constantinople.

150. The first four are dressed as physicians and carry identical medical instruments; Thalelaios wears the tunic and chlamys of a martyr and carries a cross. Hermolaos, though often dressed as a physician, was a monk who converted St. Panteleimon and taught him spiritual healing: see Boyd, "Ex-Voto Therapy."

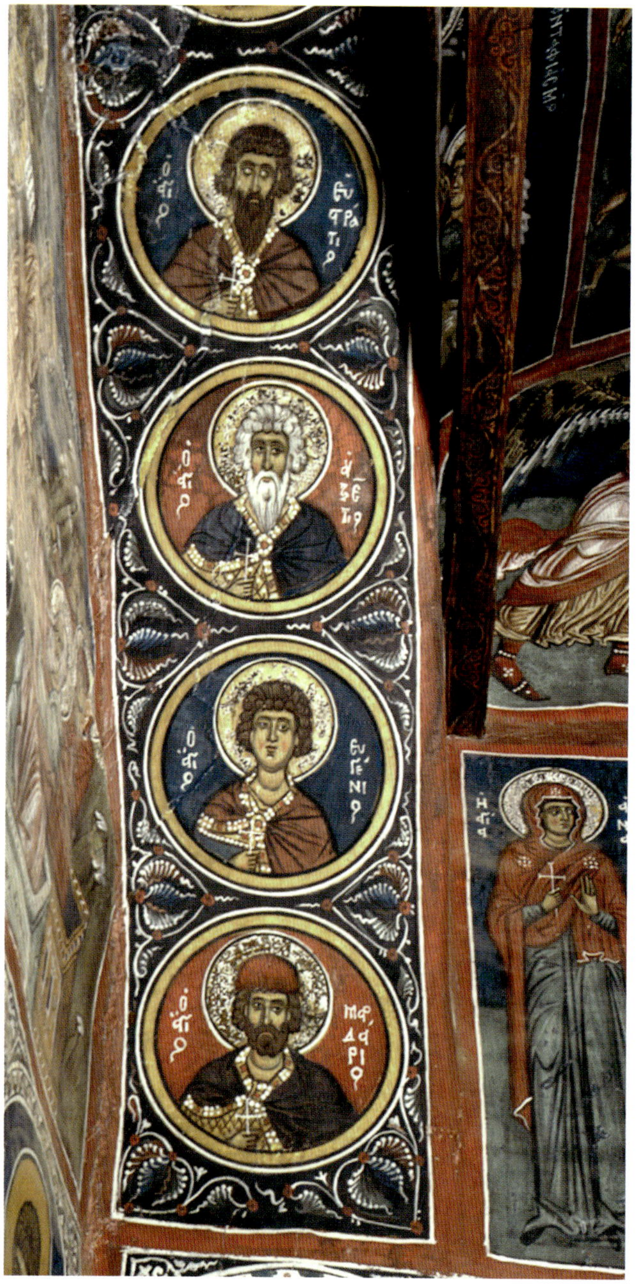

FIG. 6.26 Naos, central bay, soffit of north arch and north bema respond, looking east: Martyrs of Sebaste; St. Anna (photo courtesy of the Leventis Foundation and the Archaeological Research Unit, University of Cyprus, No. 006385)

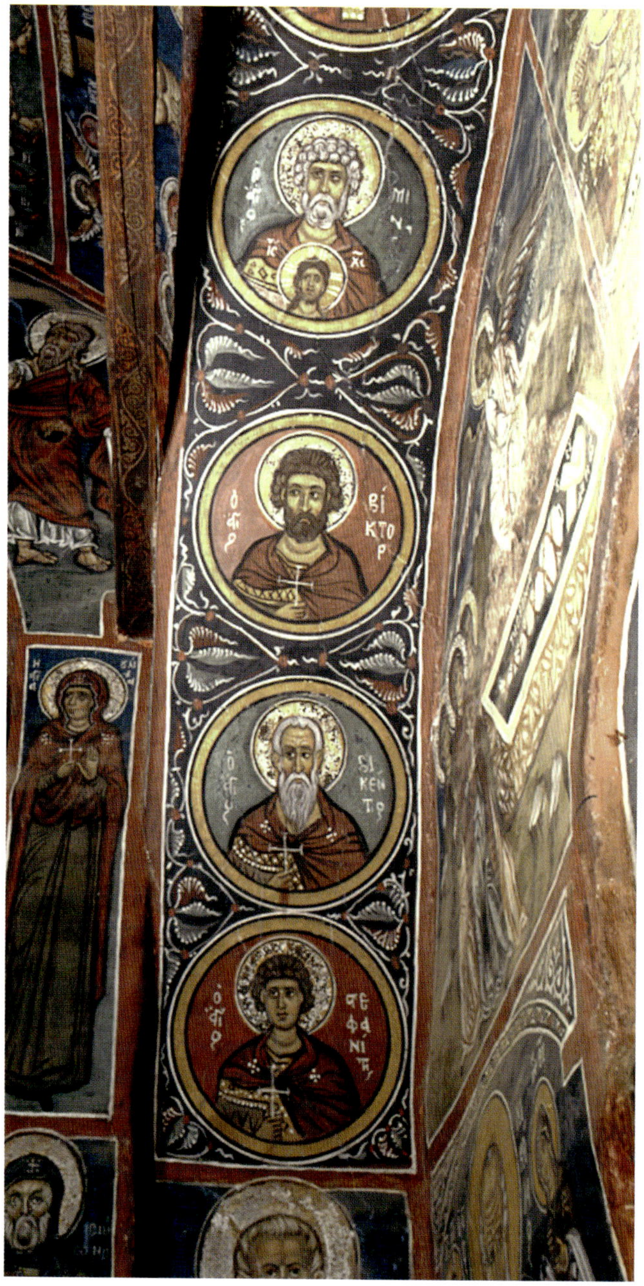

FIG. 6.27 Naos, central bay, north respond and soffit of north arch, looking west: St. Ioulitta; Martyrs of 11 November (photo courtesy of the Leventis Foundation and the Archaeological Research Unit, University of Cyprus, No. 006390)

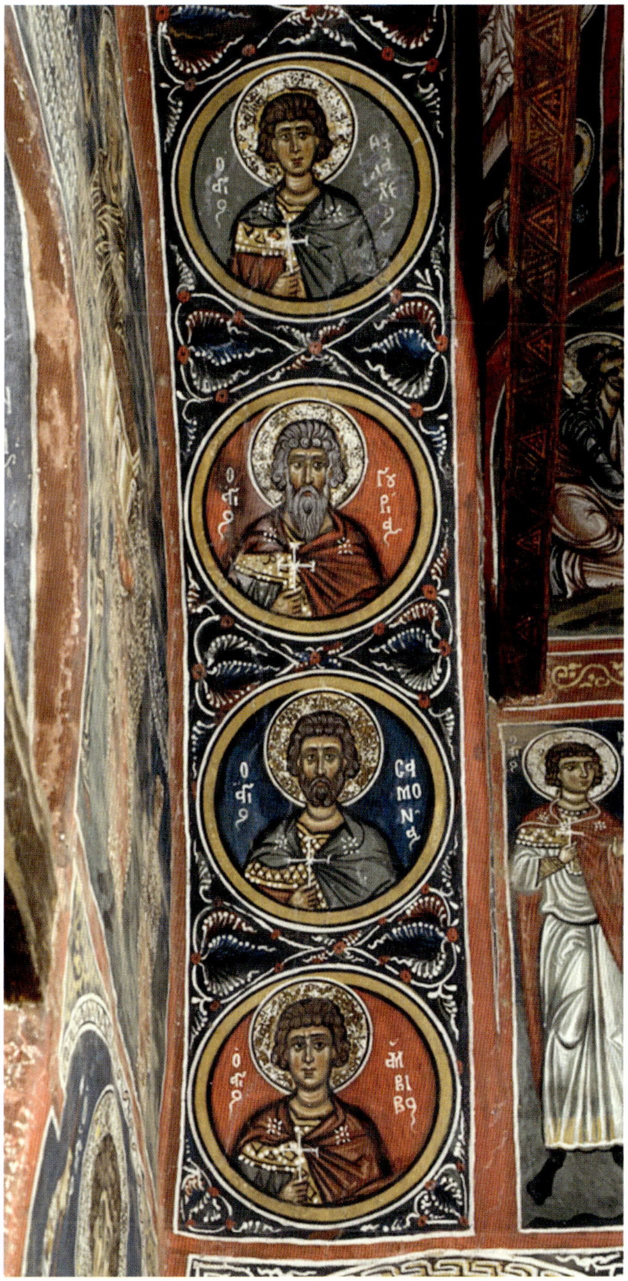

FIG. 6.28 Naos, central bay, south bema respond and soffit of south arch, looking west: Martyrs of Edessa; St. Kerykos (photo courtesy of the Leventis Foundation and the Archaeological Research Unit, University of Cyprus, No. 006389)

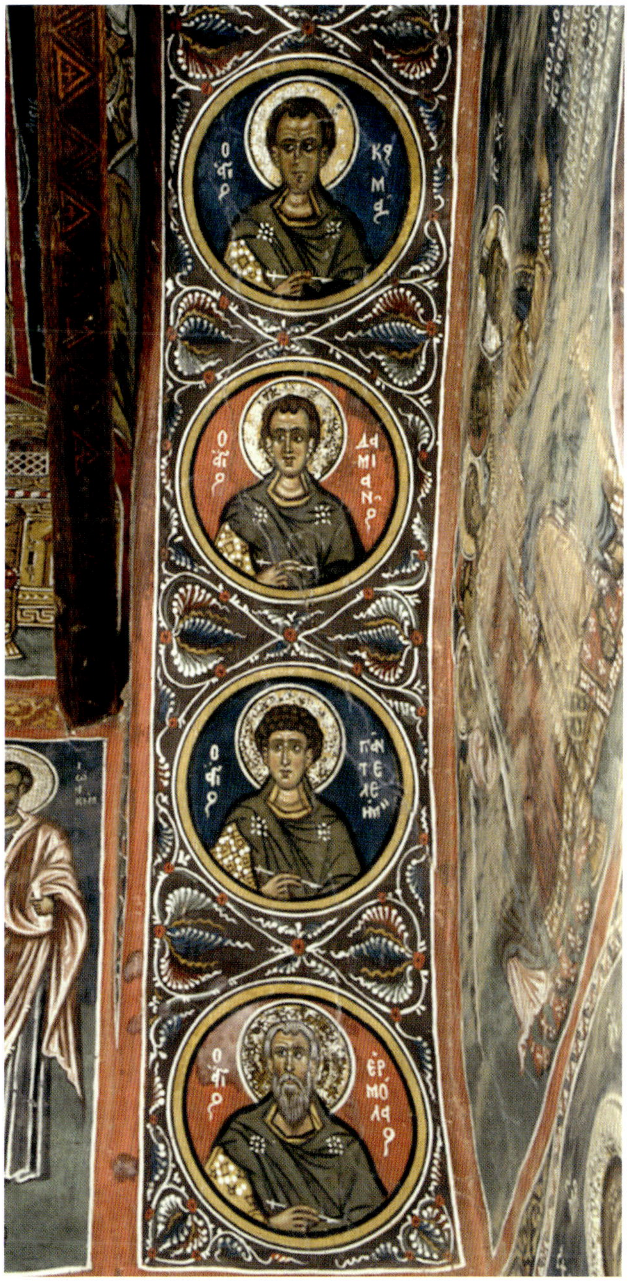

FIG. 6.29 Naos, central bay, soffit of south arch and south respond, looking east: St. Joachim; Anargyroi (photo courtesy of the Leventis Foundation and the Archaeological Research Unit, University of Cyprus, No. 006388)

case, a city of origin: the Martyrs of Edessa, Abibos (ὁ / ἅγι/ος / Ἄμ/βι/βος), Gourias (ὁ / ἅγι/ος / Γου/ρί/ας), and Samonas (ὁ / ἅγι/ος / Σα/μο/νᾶς), celebrated on 15 November.[151] The north and south arches, then, offer two clusters of five saints—the Anargyroi and the martyrs of Sebaste—and two clusters of three: the martyrs of Edessa and the martyrs of 11 November. All four groups were associated with healing miracles, either during their lives, as with the Anargyroi, or posthumously. Four further saints in the soffits of the window openings—John and Kyros on the south; Arethas and Artemios on the north (partially evident in Figs. 6.26–29)—were not overpainted and retain their twelfth-century forms.[152]

All four groups of saints in the arches appear frequently in middle Byzantine churches, and though none of the figures reveals a trace of the twelfth-century painting beneath him, they must repeat the saints used in the cycle of 1106. Two observations about them stand out: first, their widespread recurrence throughout the middle Byzantine world from the mid-eleventh century onward—one can practically call them "standard" saints—and second, their concentration on Cyprus at Asinou, Lagoudera, and, so far as one can tell, Perachorio—that is, in the most "standard" of the twelfth-century programs.[153] These examples reinforce the impression given by the standing saints: that, in its selection of protectors, the initial program at Asinou was more cosmopolitan than it was locally Cypriot.

Of the saints within these groups, a few assumed independent visibility as cult figures on Cyprus. This was true, above all, of the Anargyroi. SS. Cosmas and Damian, the most widely represented of all the Anargyroi, figure frequently in Cypriot panels and murals.[154] Panteleimon,

151. On these martyrs see usefully Nicolaïdès, "Étude iconographique," 131; Jolivet-Lévy, *Églises de Cappadoce*, 214, 225–26, 329. They are often juxtaposed with the Anargyroi or the Martyrs of Sebaste, as they are here. Thus in Karanlık and Elmalı kilise they are grouped in the western arches of the naos with the Martyrs of Sebaste (Restle, *Byzantine Wall Painting*, 2: plans 18, 22, fig. 230); at St. Nicholas Kasnitzes in Kastoria and the church of St. Strategos in Boularion, they face the Martyrs of Sebaste across the naos (Pelekanides and Chatzidakis, *Kastoria*, 52, plan; Drandakes, *Βυζαντινές τοιχογραφίες*, 430); and in the Christ church, Veroia, they join in one row with SS. Cosmas and Damian and the Sebaste five: Gounares, *Χριστός Βέροιας*, fig. 32.

152. John and Kyros were venerated as anargyroi but are otherwise unattested among the published programs on Cyprus; they are celebrated on 31 January and 28 June. On Artemios and Arethas see Walter, *Warrior Saints*, 191–99. Artemios, rare on Cyprus but portrayed also in the narthex of St. Nicholas of the Roof, was famous in pre-Iconoclastic centuries for his healing shrine at St. John Oxeia in Constantinople, specializing in genital ailments, but if not the functions, certainly the fame of the shrine had ceased by the 12th century, and Artemios was generally venerated as a warrior thereafter, as was Arethas of Najran, though he is far rarer and not paralleled on Cyprus. Why they are shown together is not clear, though their feast days are close, on 20 and 24 October respectively.

153. Though Cosmas, Damian, and Panteleimon, as noted below, are well attested, Hermolaos accompanies the Anargyroi only at Asinou and Lagoudera, and then again later in the 14th-century layer at Monagri and in the 15th century at the Palaia Enkleistra, Kouklia (Stylianou and Stylianou, *Painted Churches*, 133, 184, 244, 398). Thalelaios is seen elsewhere only in the 11th-century layer at St. Nicholas of the Roof (ibid., 55). Both the Martyrs of Edessa and the Martyrs of Sebaste appear on Cyprus only at Lagoudera (Nicolaïdès, "Étude iconographique," 128–29, 131). The Martyrs of 11 November appear only at Asinou and Lagoudera before the 16th century (Nicolaïdès, "Étude iconographique," 131–32; Stylianou and Stylianou, *Painted Churches*, 132, 182–83), though Vikentios appears at the Holy Trinity church at Koutsovendis (Mango, "Monastery of St. Chrysostom," 80, fig. 95) and Menas at Perachorio (Megaw and Hawkins, "Church of the Holy Apostles," 334, fig. 50), suggesting that the other members of the group were represented in these churches as well.

154. On the identity and Cypriot imagery of these saints, see above, pp. 170–71 along with notes 269–78; they are sometimes joined in Byzantine art with their mother, Theodote: see Drewer, "Saints and Their Families," 267, fig. 8 (Episkope).

in turn, is depicted on Cyprus in the twelfth-century apse of the church of the Holy Cross at Pelendri, wearing much the same physician's garb as here; he is also depicted in a full-length votive mural of the late twelfth or thirteenth century in St. Anthony, Kellia, where he is depicted in elegantly embroidered clothing.[155] Few Byzantine cycles were without Anargyroi, for the physician-healers were fundamental sources of comfort to the faithful.

St. Menas, too, was surely venerated in Cyprus: an icon in the Bishopric of Kition, often attributed to the tenth century but more likely belonging to the thirteenth, shows Menas holding the medallion of Christ and flanked by Viktor and Vikentios;[156] and he is prominently portrayed (though mislabeled as Viktor) in Trikomo holding a mirrorlike disk with the image of Christ.[157] In the "Nestorian" church in Famagusta he is portrayed as a white-haired warrior, an exceptionally beautiful late fourteenth-century icon shows Menas as a youthful equestrian, and legends of the saint on the island conjure a knightly image of him.[158] This said, the epithet Kallikedaros ("Beautiful-sounding") on the image of Menas in Perachorio,[159] an epithet associated with Constantinople,[160] makes it clear that Menas's presence in the twelfth-century church programs on Cyprus was due to his inclusion in a widely disseminated group of images that was cosmopolitan rather than provincial, and cannot be attributed to merely local predilection.

Yet despite all these instances of particular veneration, the saints in the medallions were more significant in the aggregate than individually, a host of heavenly healers—whether as actual physicians or more broadly as miracle workers—whose protection ringed the church and cloaked its worshippers, beginning with the donor. Their generic character seems to have become yet stronger in the fourteenth century, as indicated by the abrasion of individual types, seen in the martyrs of Sebaste (Fig. 6.26). The identifying features of these martyrs had already been codified in their earliest surviving images, from the late tenth century.[161] Mardarios's red hat remains in his image at Asinou, but Eustratios has lost the distinctive details of his costuming, and the fifth member of the group—Orestes—is not depicted at all. Some light may be cast on his omission by the figure of Stephanites, who follows the martyrs of

155. For Pelendri, see V. Karageorghis, *ARDAC* for 1986, fig. 15; for Kellia, see Karageorghis, *ARDAC* for 1980, fig. 20.

156. Spanou, "Η τέχνη στη μητροπολιτική περιφέρεια Κιτίου," 132, no. 2; Sophocleous, *Icons of Cyprus*, 76, no. 3, pl. 3 (as 10th-century); Carr, review of *Icons of Cyprus*, suggesting a 13th-century date. The presence of Menas's medallion makes a 10th-century date unlikely, though the way he holds it, in both hands, is striking.

157. Chotzakoglou, "Βυζαντινή αρχιτεκτονική και τέχνη," 1:606 n. 1055, 2: fig. 424.

158. For the Nestorian church, see Bacci, "Syrian, Palaiologan, and Gothic Murals," 214, fig. 5; for the icon, preserved in the Chrysaliniotissa church, Nicosia, see Papageorgiou, *Icons of Cyprus* [1992], 79, fig. 54. On the legends of St. Menas in Cyprus, see Papaskevopoulou, *Researches into the Traditions*, 115.

159. Megaw and Hawkins, "Church of the Holy Apostles," 334, fig. 50.

160. On this epithet, see Delehaye, "L'invention des reliques," 117.

161. They appear before 1000 in the Basil Menologion (*Menologio Basilio II*, p. 241) and in Kılıçlar kilise in Cappadocia (Jolivet-Lévy, *La Cappadoce médiévale*, pls. 62–64, with fine color pictures of the five in typical iconographic form), and then in Hosios Loukas (see Chatzidakis-Bacharas, *Les Peintures murales de Hosios Loukas*, 74–80), and in the Panagia ton Chalkeon of 1028: see Papadopoulos, *Die Wandmalereien des X. Jahrhunderts*, 36–37. Eustratios is sallow and dark-haired with a long, pointed beard, and often wears a cloak fastened with a cross-shaped clasp in front and a white string or handkerchief around his neck; Auxentios is white-haired; Eugenios is brown-haired and bearded; Mardarios is dark-bearded and wears a red hat, initially a beanie or pillbox but eventually—as in the Kariye Camii—a more pretentious fur-trimmed garment (contrast Mouriki, *Mosaics of Nea Moni*, 2: pl. 62 with Underwood, *Kariye Djami*, 2: pl. 142); and Orestes, who is omitted at Asinou, is in military dress, often with a cross around his neck and a javelin in his hand.

11 November (Fig. 6.27). Not only does he not belong to the group, he is also unprecedented in the litany of saints.[162] A person with a similar name is linked with the legends of 11 November. She is a woman named Stephanis, who witnessed the blinding of St. Viktor and is mentioned in the account of Viktor's martyrdom in the synaxarion.[163] It seems at least plausible that the fourteenth-century painter(s) accidentally put the youthful face intended for Orestes at the wrong end of the martyrs of 11 November and, searching to see who should go with the martyrs of 11 November, found the name Stephanis and adapted it.

Like the standing saints, the saints in medallions belong almost entirely to the twelfth-century program, and are notable for their widespread currency in Byzantine art. In this respect the naos contrasts sharply with the narthex, where many of the saints are associated especially with Cyprus. Such local preference is not seen in the twelfth-century program, either because the patron Nikephoros had more cosmopolitan interests, or because Cypriot identity was defined more strongly at this time by its membership in the empire.

The sanctoral cycle as a whole remains a twelfth-century program, but its repainting affected its interpretation. The twelfth-century program is notable in two respects. One is its cosmopolitan character, using up-to-date images (such as the Virgin Paraklesis on the bema respond), displaying saints who were venerated widely throughout the empire, and clustering them by their profession to create a kind of "honor guard of warriors" around the donor in the central bay. The other notable quality of the sanctoral program is its innovativeness, which is especially apparent in the concentration of iconic figures in the area in front of the bema. The intensification of devotional imagery in the space before the templon is a fundamental feature in the development of church programs during the century after 1105/6. Asinou anticipates this shift of devotional imagery in its cluster of major icons, especially of the Mother of God, in the central bay.

When one turns to the sanctoral cycle as a fourteenth-century work, however, two different features stand out in the imagery of the saints. The first is the introduction of elements that belong specifically to Cypriot tradition. Some are essentially programmatic. For example, the figure of John the Baptist—in conjunction with figures of the Virgin Paraklesis and Christ—takes the place that he had assumed in Kato Lefkara, Moutoullas, and the narthex of Asinou itself. And the image of Mary on the south wall acquired a throne and archangels, as pioneered at Lagoudera. But there are also shifts in cult attention, seen in the new image of Helena at the threshold to the bema, and in the addition of Eustathios, Tryphon, and Memnon as defenders against locusts. These modifications weave the sanctoral cycle into local traditions.

The second notable feature is the way the overpainting unifies the space of the central bay, integrating the figures through their gestures and the sequence of arches over their heads. The arches turn the figures into a circuit of individual, separately framed icons that are, at the same time, joined in a wrap-around templon of holy intercessors. This unification must, on the one hand, separate the saints of the central bay far more strongly than they had been in 1105/6 from those of the western bay, especially the Forty Martyrs of Sebaste, overemphasizing the sense of a distinction between lay and monastic saints (Fig. 6.15). On the other hand, such a concentration of saints gives fuller realization to that intensification of devotional imagery in the space before the templon which the twelfth-century program had anticipated with its cluster of iconic figures.

162. Thus Roueché, "Prehistory of the Cyprus Department of Antiquities," 160, quotes a letter to William Buckler from R. P. Hippolyte Delehaye responding to photographs of Asinou that the Bucklers had sent him: "Je suis étonné du nombre de nouveaux saints que vous rapportez de Chypre. ὁ ἅγιος Στεφανίτες m'est complètement inconnu. Il faudra faire une nouvelle édition de mes *Saints de Chypre*."

163. Delehaye, *Synaxarium*, 213.

The Crosses with Cryptograms

As in the narthex, so in the naos the portals were sealed with apotropaic crosses painted on their jambs (see above, pp. 190–92).[164] Three such crosses survive to greater or lesser extent, one on the east jamb of the south door and one on each jamb of the north door.

The cross on the east jamb of the south door stands on a rounded form representing the hill of Golgotha, and is wound with the crown of thorns (Fig. 6.30). It retains the letterforms that signal its formulas (Table 6.1).

Aside from the sequence of taus, which was used often in Cyprus but has never been satisfactorily interpreted, the only ambiguity lies in the fourth line, where the final letter could be either kappa or alpha. CA is unprecedented; ΞZCK, by contrast, is a widely used phrase and seems plausible in this case.[165] The association with Helena (line 6), which is widespread, recalls the figure of Helena on the north bema respond, suggesting that her presence on the jamb of the Holy Door evoked the cross and its apotropaic power. Scratched in the plaster in the upper margin of this cross is the record of a man's death; the year 1446 is still clearly seen: εγχρ(ο)νια ,ΑΥΜϚ' . . . εκυμιθι

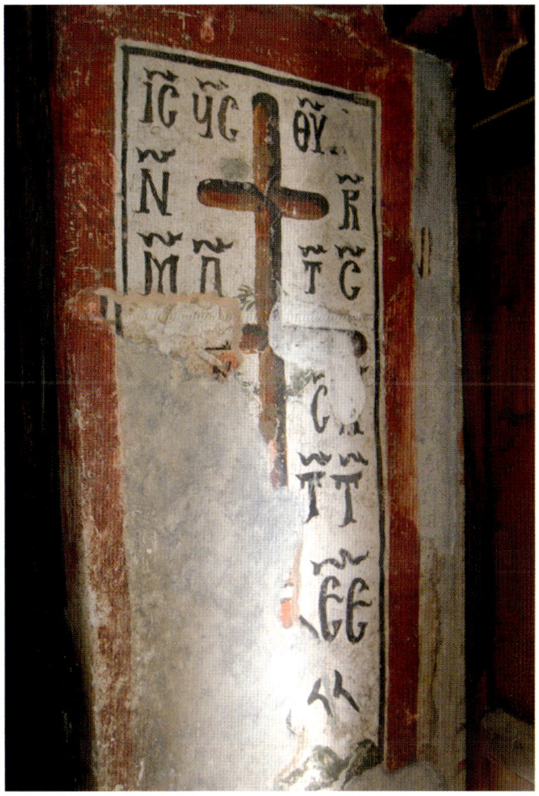

FIG. 6.30 Naos, cross on east jamb of south door (photo courtesy of A. Nicolaïdès)

TABLE 6.1 Transcription and translation of Fig. 6.30.

IC ΥC	ΘΥ [XC]	Ἰησοῦς Υἱὸς Θεοῦ [Χριστός]	Jesus, Son of God, Christ
N	K	νικᾷ	Conquers
M Π	T C	μαρτυρῶν πίστις τίμιος σταυρός	Martyrs' Faith, Holy Cross
[...]	C [A or K]	[ξύλον ζωῆς] σωτηρία κόσμου	[The Wood of Life], the Salvation of the World (?)
[T T]	T T	τ[...] τ[...] τ[...] τ[...]	
[E E]	E E	[Ἑλένης εὕρημα] ἐλέους ἔρεισμα or [Ἑλένη εὗρεν] ἐλέους ἔρεισμα or [Ἑλένη εὗρεν] εὕρημα ἐλέους	Helena's Discovery, the Staff of Mercy or Helena Found the Staff of Mercy or Helena Found the Discovery [that gives] Mercy

164. On the crosses, see in particular Walter, "IC XC NI KA"; Chatzoule, "Αμφίγραπτη εικόνα του Αγίου Νικολάου"; Babić, "Les croix," with earlier bibliography.
165. On this phrase, see Walter, "IC XC NI KA," 204, who notes that it is also used on the back of an 11th-century menologion icon at Mount Sinai, reproduced in Soteriou and Soteriou, *Εἰκόνες*, 1: pl.136–43, 2:123. Alpha usually appears in phrases including the word "beginning," as in ἀρχὴ πίστεως Μωσαϊκῆς σταυρός—see Zesiou, "Ἐπιγραφαὶ χριστιανικῶν χρόνων τῆς Ἑλλάδος," 132; Chatzoule, "Αμφίγραπτη εικόνα," 392—or, more occasionally, as "Ἀδάμ": see Chatzoule, "Αμφίγραπτη εικόνα," 392 no. 59: Ἀδὰμ πεπτωκὼς μετέστη σταυρῷ. Neither is compatible with the clear sigma here. At Lagoudera one encounters the phrase σταυρὸς ἀνάγει πρὸς πολέμου τροπαίον (the cross is raised as the tropaion of victory), but its CA sequence is at the beginning, not the end: see Nicolaïdès, "Panagia Arakiotissa à Lagoudéra" [1993], 132–34.

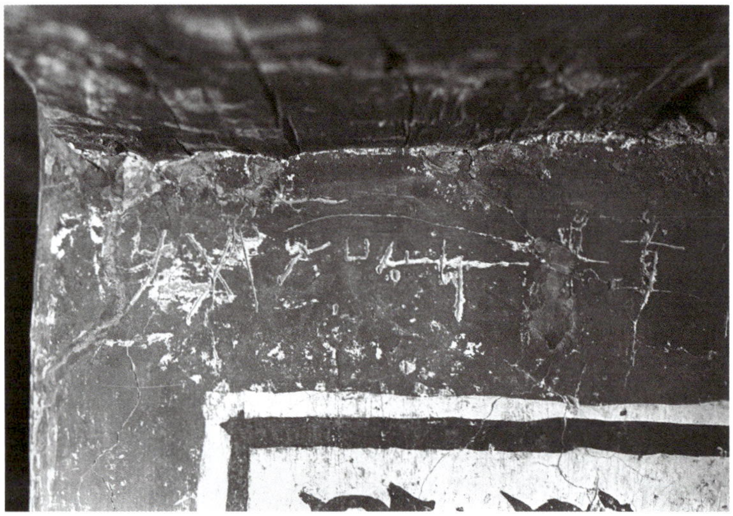

FIG. 6.31 Naos, cross on east jamb of south door: graffito incised in the upper border (photo courtesy of Dumbarton Oaks L.67.998 [IŠ])

TABLE 6.2 Transcription and translation of Fig. 6.32.

IC	XC	Ἰησοῦς Χριστός	Jesus Christ
ΥC	ΘΥ	Υἱὸς Θεοῦ	Son of God
N	K	νικᾷ	Conquers
Φ	[…]	φῶς [Χριστοῦ]	The Light [of Christ]
Φ Π	[…]	φαίνει πᾶσιν [ξύλον ζωῆς]	Appears to All [Wood of Life]
C K	E O	σωτηρία κόσμου ε[…] ο[…]	Salvation of the World […]
Θ T	H […]	θ[…] τ[…] η[…] […]	[…]
E E	E E	Ἑλένη εὗρεν ἐλέους ἔρεισμα or alternatives as in previous cross	Helena Found the Staff of Mercy

ω δουλ(ος) . . . (Fig. 6.31).[166] Like the year 1450 in the graffito on the east jamb of the north door discussed below, this year was significant in challenging the fifteenth-century date initially suggested

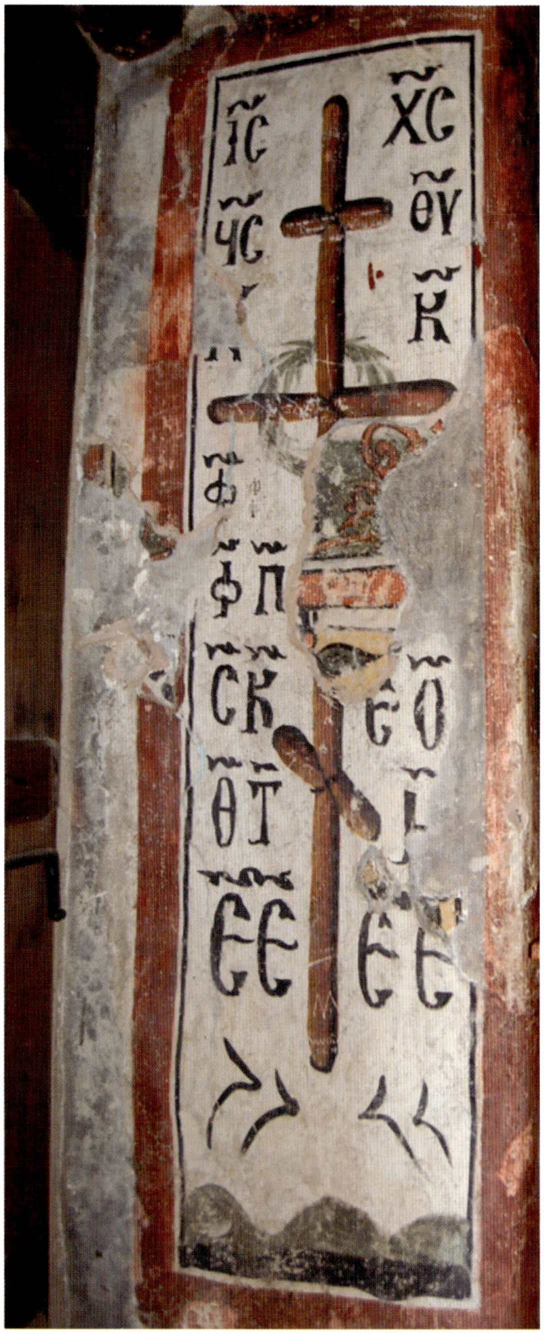

FIG. 6.32 Naos, cross on east jamb of north door (photo courtesy of A. Nicolaïdès)

for the frescoes of the central bay. The graffito is scratched into plaster of the fourteenth-century layer. A N in a pale red roundel survives from an earlier layer in the area of damage to the cross's left side. If this N belonged to the twelfth century, it

166. Winfield, *Asinou*, 4, 20. Ihor Ševčenko deciphered the graffiti on the two door jambs. I am indebted to him for transcribing them, and to Nancy Patterson Ševčenko for further help with them.

might indicate that a cross with the ancient formula IC XC NI KA originally stood at this place. There is no evidence that an apotropaic cross occupied the western jamb of this door in either the twelfth century or the fourteenth.

The second of the magic crosses, on the east jamb of the north door, also stands on a representation of the hill of Golgotha and has a crown of thorns woven around its central crux (Fig. 6.32). This cross, which has damage in its mid-section, allows a view of what was clearly the twelfth-century paint layer. A carpet of yellow lozenges and pink palmettes once occupied the lower half of the jamb; at the bottom of the upper half was a stretch of green ground giving way to a white ground above. Barely reaching into the white ground, the leafy end of a vine tendril coils from the center to the right frame and back again in a wide curve. Its point of origin is unclear, but it bears a striking resemblance to the tendrils that curl from the base of the cross when it is shown sprouting foliage as the Tree of Life, suggesting that a cross did stand here originally, though without the magic formulae that surround the fourteenth-century one. The letters visible on the fourteenth-century cross are shown in Table 6.2.

The Φ of the fourth line surely goes together with the ΦΠ of the fifth, to yield the often-used phrase φῶς Χριστοῦ φαίνει πᾶσιν, the only phrase on any of the crosses that has a parallel in the Byzantine liturgy.[167] The missing letters after ΦΠ may also belong with the first two in the next line as ΞZCK, though this leaves the EO unexplained. Scratched into the upper border of the cross is a graffito recording the death of a woman on 18 May 1450 (Fig. 6.33):

> \+ ἐκημ(η)θ(η) υ δουλ(η) τοῦ Θ(εο)ῦ λοιζε
> θηγατ(η)ρ του καστρὴς απο την λευ(κω?)σια
> τη(ν) ΙΗ μαίο ἐχρονια(ν) ΑΥΝ τοῦ Χ(ριστο)ῦ
> . . . εωνια η μνημ(η) ἀυτῆς

167. Vees, "Σύνταγμα ἐπιγραφικῶν μνημείων Μετεώρων," 578; Babić, "Les croix," 8.

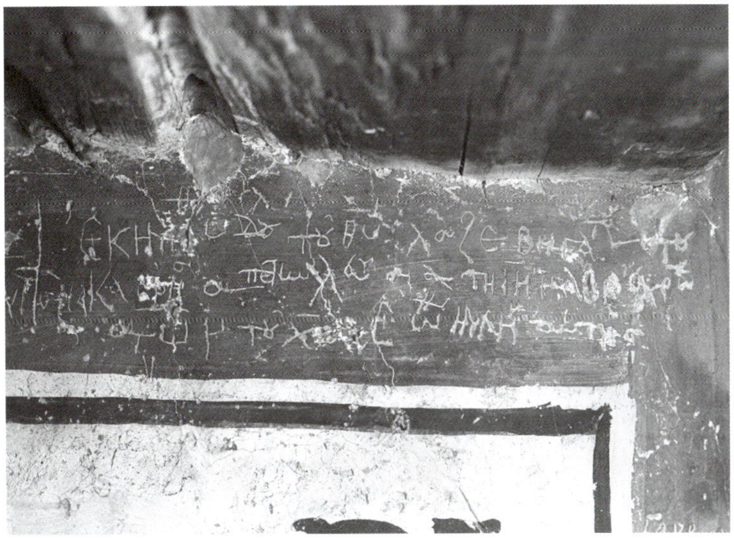

FIG. 6.33 Naos, cross on east jamb of north door: graffito incised in the upper border (photo courtesy of Dumbarton Oaks, L. 67)

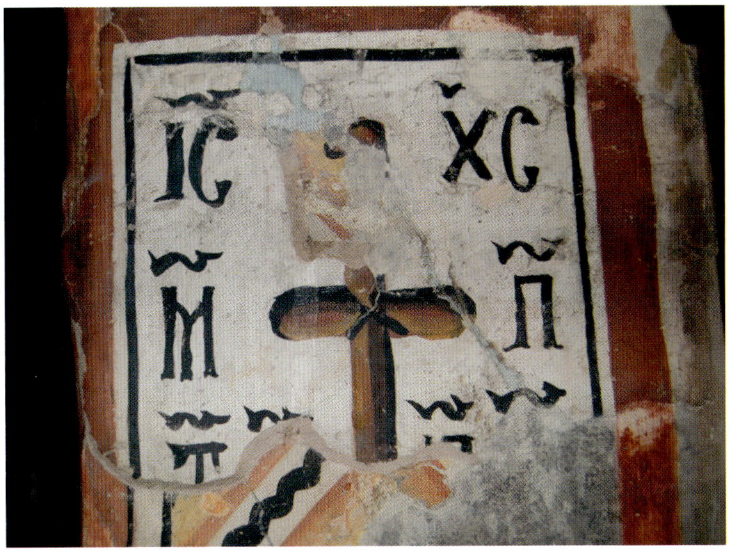

FIG. 6.34 Naos, cross on west jamb of north door (photo courtesy of A. Nicolaïdès)

TABLE 6.3 Transcription and translation of Fig. 6.34.

IC	XC	Ἰησοῦς Χριστός	Jesus Christ
M	Π	μαρτυρῶν πίστις	Martyrs' Faith
T [...]	Π [...]	τόπος [κρανίου] παράδεισος [γέγονε]	The Place [of the Skull has Become a] Paradise

= ἐκοιμήθη ἡ δούλη τοῦ Θεοῦ Λοίζα θυγάτηρ τοῦ Καστρῆς ἀπὸ τὴν Λευκωσίαν τὴν ΙΗʹ Μαίου ἐγχρονίαν ΑΥΝʹ τοῦ Χριστοῦ. Αἰώνια ἡ μνήμη αὐτῆς.

The servant of God Louisa the daughter of Kastres of Nicosia (?) died on May 18 in the year of Christ 1450. Everlasting be her memory.

Less survives of the cross that faces this one on the west jamb of the north door (Fig. 6.34). Its damage exposes what was clearly the jamb painting of 1105/6, with the familiar pattern of yellow lozenges and pink palmettes. There was no cross here originally. The remaining letters are shown in Table 6.3.

The final phrase is frequently used and has been associated by Glykeria Chatzoule with the beginning of a troparion.[168]

Like the imagery in the bay as a whole, the crosses echo the initial program, but were amplified to conform to fourteenth-century practice and to the preferences of the Cypriot locale.

The Vault and North Lunette

The South Side of the Vault

The cycle of saints in the central bay retains clear traces of its original imagery, exposed by the abrasion of the plaster on the lower walls. Thus a discussion of the saints inevitably becomes a discussion of their twelfth- as well as their fourteenth-century identities. No such glimpses of the earlier paintings exist on the vault, making the question of the relation of fourteenth- to twelfth-century imagery far more speculative. We know for sure only three things about the vault. First, we know, as Athanasios Papageorgiou points out (p. 58, above), that in the 1950s, when the wooden roof was removed for replacement, A. H. S. Megaw judged the existing vault to be the original one. This dispelled the belief that there might have been a dome and proved that the structure—though somewhat deformed—as clothed by the initial painter was still in place for the later painters. We also know, in the second place, that the western bay preserves scenes from 1105/6 that imply a more extensive cycle of the life of Christ. These scenes include the Raising of Lazarus, the Entry into Jerusalem, the Last Supper, and the Washing of the Feet (Figs. 6.35, 6.36)—in liturgical terms, the events of Holy Week from Lazarus Saturday to the reading of the Twelve Gospels on Holy Thursday. They imply the existence of scenes that both led up to and continued this segment of the story. Third, we know that originally there were scenes on at least some part of the vault. A small segment of original plaster survives behind the tie beam on the south wall at the base of the present scene of the Baptism. It is painted green and includes a small black boot. The boot is in profile, in a walking position, so it would have belonged to an active figure—one who was part of a scene. What scene it was is impossible to guess.

Beyond these facts, we know little. It may well be, as both David Winfield and Athanasios Papageorgiou suspect, that although the masonry of the vault survived the catastrophe(s) that prompted the structural repairs, the plaster with the murals did not, and that the fourteenth-century frescoes are the only layer of painting on the vault.[169] It would be probable under these circumstances that the fourteenth-century painters had never seen the imagery of 1105/6. The surviving scenes in the bema and in the western bay imposed a number of constraints upon them, however: the story of Christ had to be filled in; neither the Ascension nor the Pentecost was available as a subject to crown the central bay because these subjects already crowned the others; the number

168. Chatzoule, "Αμφίγραπτη εικόνα," 392 n. 57. Millet, Pargoire, and Petit, *Recueil des inscriptions*, 64, no. 212 also cite it.

169. See above, p. 63; letter to the author from David Winfield, 16 May 2007. In short, as Winfield emphasizes in his letter, overpainting in the naos may be limited to the figures of SS. Peter and Paul.

of feast scenes missing from Christ's early life was greater than from its end.

The very fact that the later painters heeded these constraints may be the strongest argument that at least some of the painting on the central vault remained. Nonetheless, the surface had been altered. Its curvature was flatter; the distance from transverse to transverse was probably somewhat narrower; and the diaphragm arches separated the central bay more sharply from those adjoining it. Under these circumstances it is unproductive to dwell on the original vault imagery. Though attentive to the ways in which the fourteenth-century forms and images were affected by the twelfth-century past, the discussion that follows will emphasize the vault cycle as a product of its own time. All too consistently it is treated as an inferior, provincial replica of the original frescoes. In fact, it is a cardinal witness to its own era.

Most striking in the vault is its organization as a uniform grid of scenes (Figs. 6.37, 6.42). In contrast to middle Byzantine modes of composition, which articulate the architectural forms, no central motif punctuates the apex of the vault here; no image delineates the integrity of the bay by stretching from one edge to the other of its surface; no scene breaks from its frame to flow organically into irregular areas of the architecture like spandrels. A gridlike alignment of rectangular scenes, on the other hand, does characterize the other fourteenth-century Gospel cycles on Cyprus—in the central vessel of the church of the Holy Cross in Pelendri,[170] and, in Famagusta, in the cathedral of St. George of the Greeks and in the Armenian church.[171] Asinou's grid of rectangular scenes falls into ready conformity with later medieval mural cycles, both on Cyprus and elsewhere.[172] Even in cases on Cyprus where a middle Byzantine cycle abandoned the "classic" scheme of one scene per surface, barrel vaults were usually divided vertically in tall, narrow scenes stretching from apex to base: witness the coupling of the Transfiguration and the Raising of Lazarus on the western vault at St. Nicholas of the Roof in Kakopetria[173] and the sequence of narrow scenes striating the barrel vault at Monagri.[174] The grid of horizontally aligned scenes at Asinou immediately looks late medieval.

170. Stylianou and Stylianou, *Painted Churches*, 223–32; Christoforaki, "Cyprus between Byzantium and the Levant."

171. On St. George of the Greeks, see Enlart, *Gothic Art*, 253–58; Papageorgiou, "Ἰδιάζουσαι βυζαντιναὶ τοιχογραφίαι," 201–12. On the date of the building see Vaivre and Plagnieux, *L'Art gothique en Chypre*, 286 (chapter by T. Soulard); on the date of its paintings, see Bacci, "Syrian, Palaiologan, and Gothic Murals," 207–20. On the Armenian church, see Vaivre and Plagnieux, *L'Art gothique*, 257–60, where P. Plagnieux and T. Soulard date the building to 1311–17; Enlart, *Gothic Art*, 286–88. Enlart dates the paintings to the 15th century; though the iconography of the Flagellation is paralleled only in the late 15th century in Cyprus, my impression of the style inclines me to a late 14th-century date.

172. In Cypriot cycles the scenes either flow with film-strip continuity in small quadrangles above a far larger register of standing saints, or they fill the surfaces of barrel vaults with picture grids of multiple scenes. The former, first encountered at Moutoullas, was well suited to the gabled medieval churches with their flat surfaces, and is well exemplified by the church of the Archangel Michael in Pedoulas of 1474 (Stylianou and Stylianou, *Painted Churches*, 331–43), the church of the Holy Cross of Agiasmati in Platanistassa and the church of St. Mamas in Louvaras, painted in 1494 and 1495 respectively by Philip Goul (ibid., 186–218; 246–55), and the Archangel-Theotokos church of 1514 and St. Sozomenos of much the same date in Galata (ibid., 90–97; 84–89). Key examples of the latter are the 14th-century murals at the church of the Holy Cross, Pelendri (ibid., 223–32), the 15th-century cycle in the vaults of St. Herakleidios at St. John Lampadistes, Kalopanayiotis (ibid., 298–304), and the cycle of ca. 1500 in the vaults of SS. Kerykos and Ioulitta, Letympou (ibid., 414–18). On these cycles see Christoforaki, "Η Τέχνη στην Κύπρο," with color plates 4–9; Emmanuel, "Monumental Painting in Cyprus," 245–51.

173. Stylianou and Stylianou, *Painted Churches*, fig. 19.

174. See Boyd, "Church of the Panagia Amasgou," fig. 19. One might counter that the grid system was in use at Trikomo, where four scenes are stacked on each face of the arches supporting the central dome in the naos. The arches here, however, are too narrow to be classed as barrel vaults.

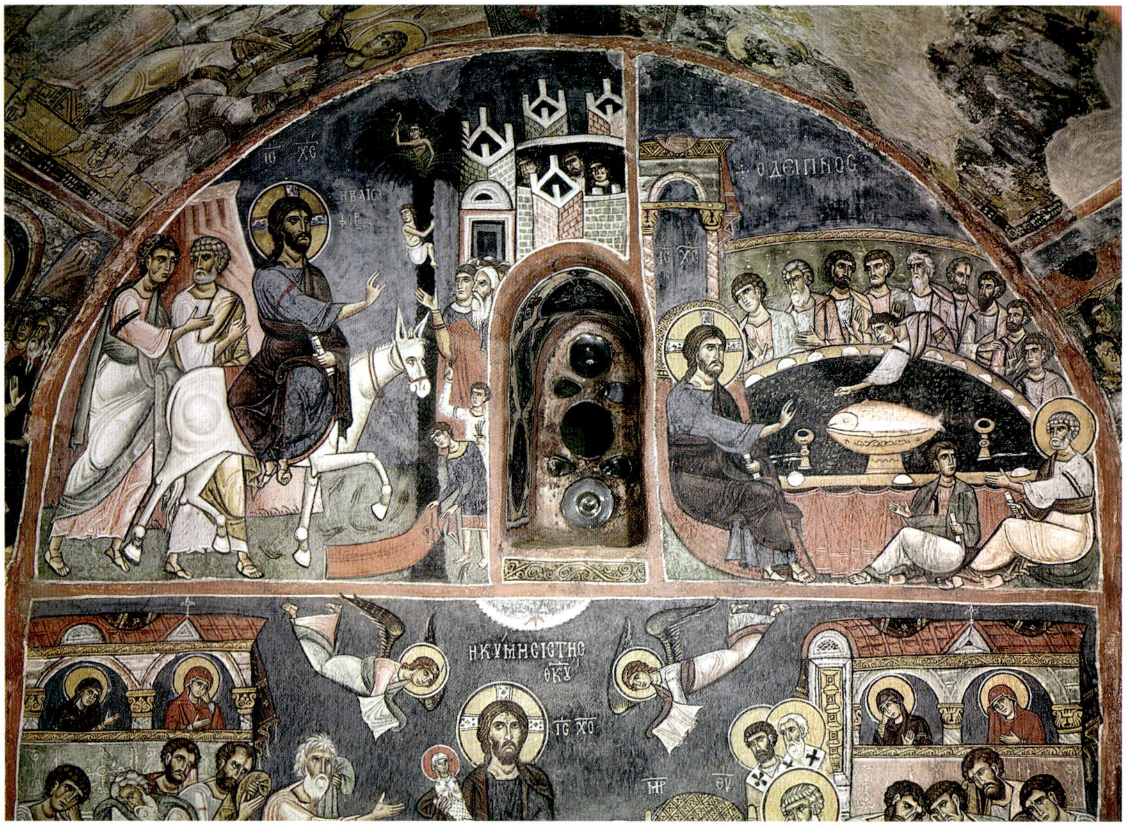

fig. 6.35

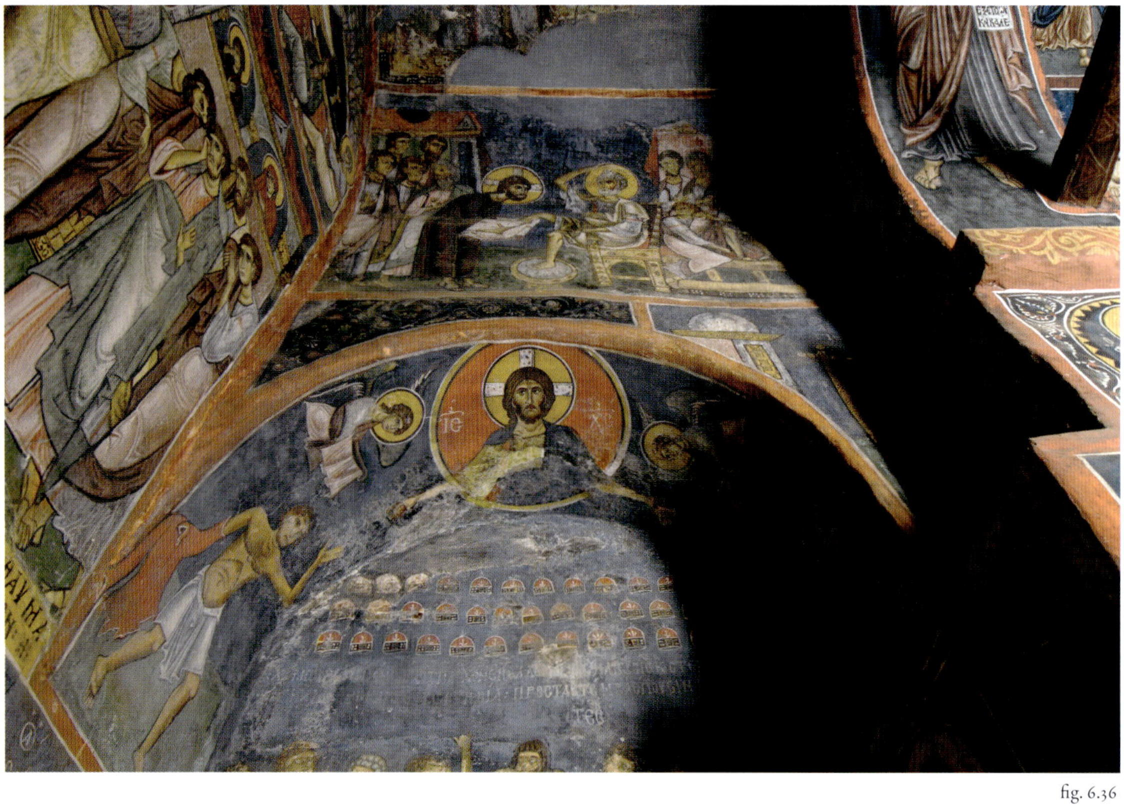

fig. 6.36

FIG. 6.35
Naos, west wall, lunette: Entry into Jerusalem, Last Supper. Below: Dormition (photo courtesy of Dumbarton Oaks, BF.T.As.J.6)

FIG. 6.36
West bay, north wall: Washing of the Feet, Forty Martyrs of Sebaste. Partially visible at left: Dormition (photo courtesy of G. L. Carr)

Some form of grid may have been used at Asinou in 1105/6, for an early twelfth-century precedent does exist on Cyprus: the western vault at Koutsovendis was laid out in a grid of eight rectangular scenes.[175] The Asinou Master knew Koutsovendis and drew on its solutions:[176] his west wall at Asinou resembles the south one at Koutsovendis, with multiple small scenes in the lunette above a single, huge icon on the wall below (Fig. 6.35). He may have drawn on the organization of Koutsovendis's vault, too. At Koutsovendis, though, the grid of scenes leaves ample space for a motif articulating the apex of the vault. The Asinou Master similarly punctuated the tops of his east and west vaults. He must have done the same in the central bay. The unarticulated grid at Asinou thus bespeaks a fourteenth-century sensibility.

Though often called narratives, the scenes in the south side of the vault are in fact all feast icons (Fig. 6.37). Following on the Annunciation on the bema arch, these images include the full sequence of major feasts preceding the Raising of Lazarus in the chronology of Christ's life: the Nativity, the Presentation, the Baptism, and the Transfiguration. All four are integral to the image of Christ's life as encapsulated in canonical middle Byzantine imagery; none is inconceivable in the cycle of 1105/6, and the cycle itself is probably inconceivable without at least some of them: all but the Transfiguration are frequent in Cyprus's middle Byzantine churches.[177] By contrast, no fourteenth-century cycle of Christ's early life other than that at Asinou survives on Cyprus,[178] though the Annunciation, the Nativity, and the Presentation were repainted in the late fourteenth century at St. Nicholas of the Roof.[179] Thus the four images at Asinou offer rare testimony to the history of these scenes.

The group opens with the NATIVITY (ἡ̃ν Χ(ριστο)ῦ / γέννησις; Fig. 6.38). A triangular mountain dominates the scene, its face opening in the

175. Mango, "Monastery of St. Chrysostom at Koutsovendis," 86–88, figs. 130–40. The Nativity of Christ, the Nativity of Mary, an indecipherable scene (the Presentation of Christ?), and the Presentation of Mary occupied the south side of the western barrel vault while the Entry into Jerusalem, the Dormition of Mary, and two lost scenes occupied the north side.
176. On the relation of the Asinou painter to the cycle at Koutsovendis, see Winfield, "Hagios Chrysostomos, Trikomo, Asinou," 285–91; Drossoyianni, "Some Observations on the Asinou Frescoes."
177. The Transfiguration is seen in the 11th century at St. Nicholas of the Roof, but not again until ca. 1200 at the church of Christ Antiphonetes, Kalogrea, and then in the 13th century in now nearly obliterated images at the Panagia Amasgou, Monagri (Boyd, "Church of the Panagia Amasgou," fig. 25), and the church of the Transfiguration at Sotera. Only in the 15th century does it become a regular component of Christological cycles (Stylianou and Stylianou, *Painted Churches*, index, s.v. Transfiguration). The Nativity, the Presentation, and the Baptism, by contrast, appear in almost all of the 12th-century cycles. Perachorio shows the Nativity, the Presentation, and the Baptism on its south wall; the south lunette at Kato Lefkara adds to these the Raising of Lazarus but not the Transfiguration (Papageorgiou, "Ἡ ἐκκλησία τοῦ Ἀρχαγγέλου," figure 40), and Lagoudera, which includes the Nativity, the Presentation, and the Baptism, offers no place for the Transfiguration.
178. Thus only the Passion cycles are legible in the two churches in Famagusta, though scenes of the Nativity and the Baptism were recorded by Enlart at the Armenian church (see note 171 above). At Pelendri the early life of Christ's mother, not Christ's own infancy, complements the cycle of Passion and post-Passion scenes (Stylianou and Stylianou, *Painted Churches*, 223–30). At St. Demetrianos, Dali, the decipherable scenes belong to the Passion (ibid., 426).
179. Stylianou and Stylianou, *Painted Churches*, 68–71, fig. 28.

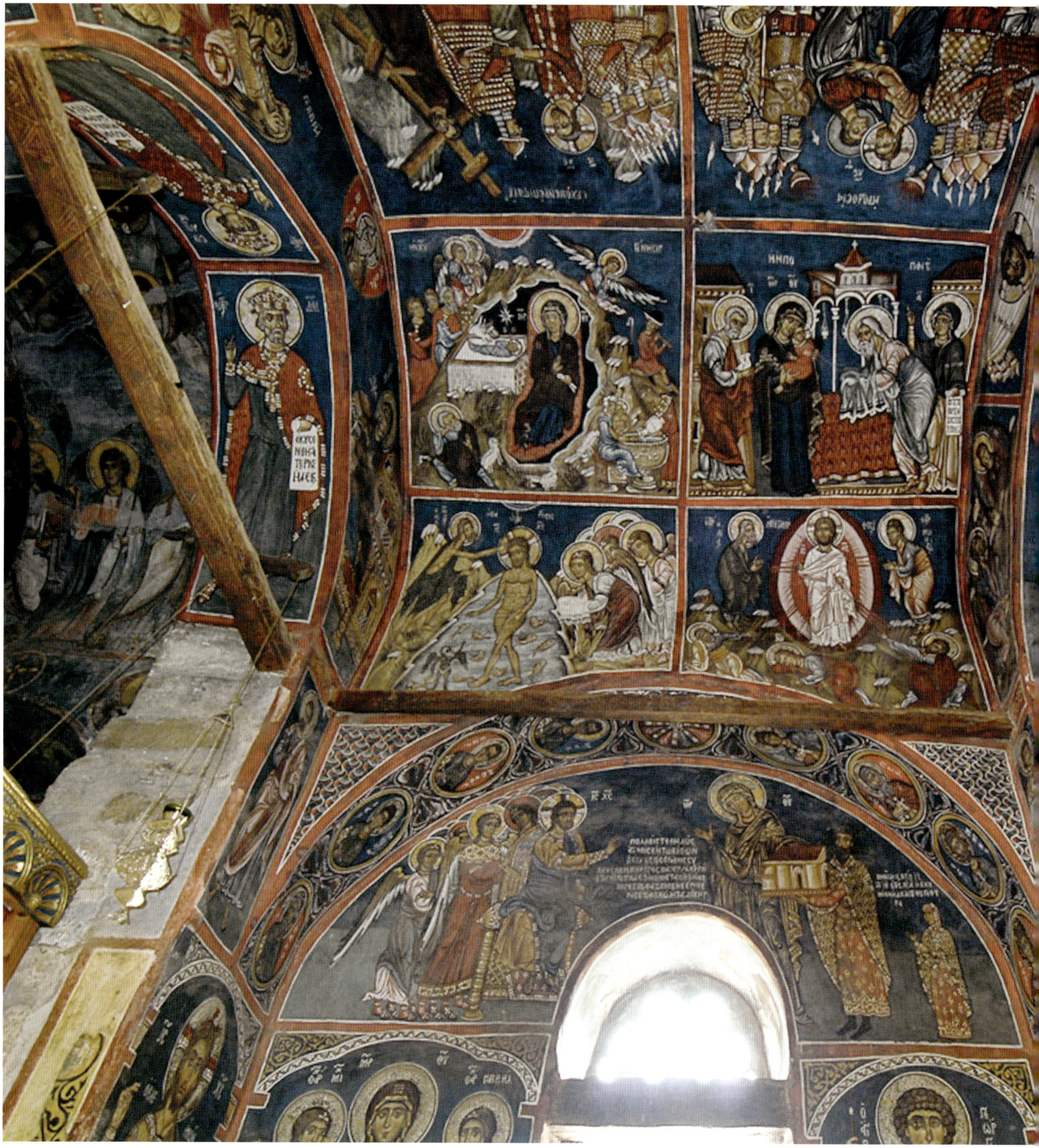

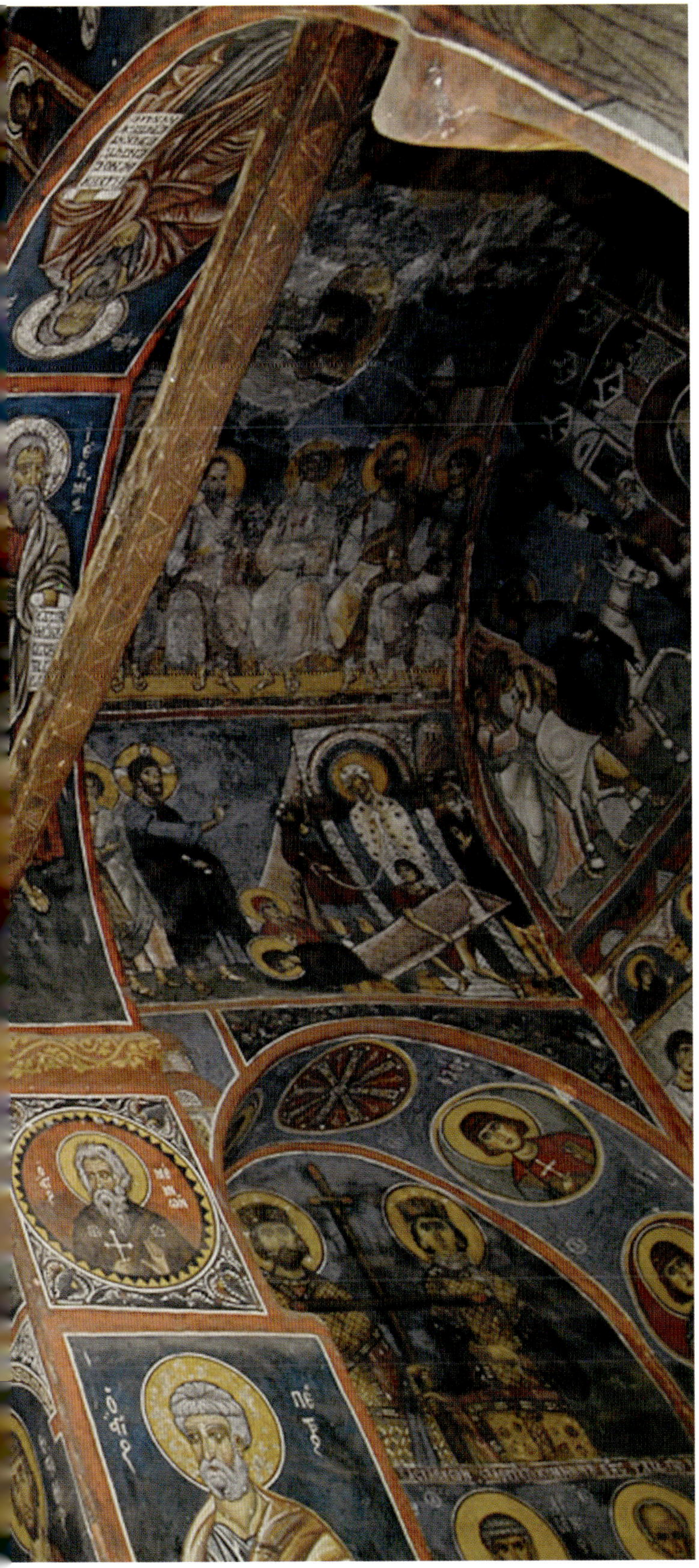

FIG. 6.37

Naos, central bay, south side of vault (photo courtesy of G. L. Carr)

cave containing a large, seated Mary (Μ(ήτ)ηρ / Θ(εο)ῦ), her child in a stone manger (Ι(ησοῦ)ς Χ(ριστό)ς), overlooked by the heads of ox and ass and the star of Bethlehem. Joseph and two small sheep turn toward Mary from the lower left; three more sheep and the scene of the bath occupy the lower right. A piping shepherd just above the bath turns to face an angel who emerges from behind the slope of the mountain; similarly, three magi and two angels emerge from behind the mountain above Joseph. An arc of heaven with a scalloped edge hangs from the top frame. The scene is linked to the Annunciation by the echoed gesture of Mary's raised hand, but it shares none of the Annunciation's assured panache. The brushwork is tentative and uneven; by comparison with the richly detailed Nativity at St. Nicholas of the Roof, moreover, the scene looks utterly conservative. Pensive Joseph, busy midwives, magi approaching on foot, piping shepherd, and heralding angels can all be traced in Byzantine imagery from the late tenth century onward.[180] Two features warrant particular attention. One is the clarity with which particular motifs can be paralleled in earlier paintings in Cyprus. Thus the composition is essentially the same as that of the Nativity at Lagoudera, with the triangular mountain, the figures emerging from behind its slopes, the midwife's classical-looking sleeveless clothing, and the weary pose of Mary sitting upright with her hand on her lap.[181] The angel admonishing a piping

180. See, for instance, the Nativity at Kılıçlar kilise in Restle, *Byzantine Wall Painting*, 2: fig. 265, though the shepherd stands here. The seated shepherd with his flute appears somewhat later, as at Karanlık kilise (ibid., 2: fig. 228) or Florence, Laurenziana, Plut. VI 23, 104v: Velmans, *Le Tétraévangile*, fig. 184.
181. On Lagoudera see Nicolaïdès, "Étude iconographique," 71–79, fig. 63; on Moutoullas see Mouriki, "Wall Paintings of the Church of the Panagia," 183–85,

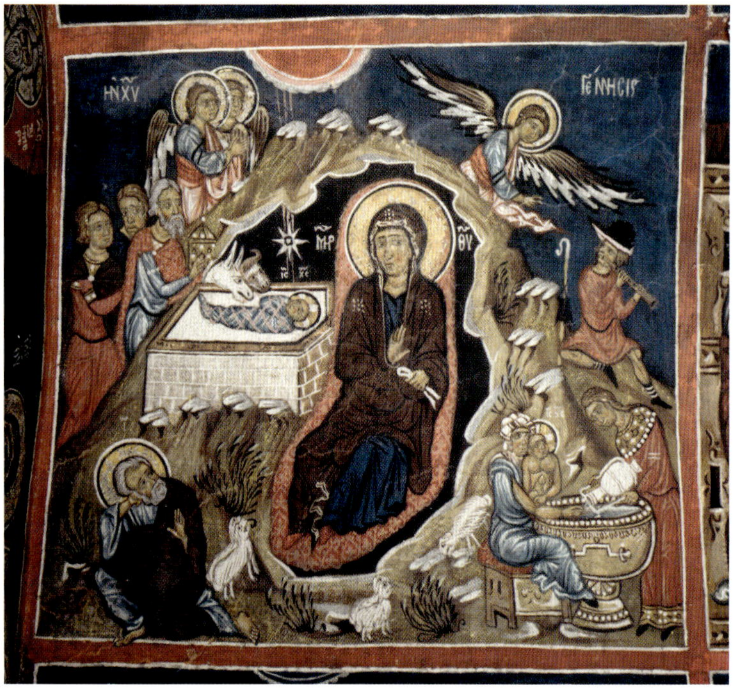

FIG. 6.38 Naos, central bay, south side of vault: Nativity (photo courtesy of the Leventis Foundation and the Archaeological Research Unit, University of Cyprus, No. 006306)

shepherd who turns up to face him is seen also at Perachorio;[182] the handkerchief in Mary's hand and the crouching posture of Joseph are both quoted from Moutoullas;[183] and the large, handled basin of the bath recalls the one at Monagri.[184] Thus the imagination of the painter seems to have been furnished by locally available models. The details have been simplified—the words of the angel's admonition are no longer written on the sky; the engaging still-life of the shepherd's staff, pouch, and satchel[185] has been reduced to an upright crook and wallet; and Joseph has lost the saddle on which he still sat at Moutoullas—but they reflect an important fact. The major Komnenian mural cycles, especially at Lagoudera, exercised a great force upon the painter(s) at Asinou. These cycles had become Cypriot classics. Many of their motifs can be traced back to earlier Byzantine painting, and it is not impossible that some were already available in 1105/6. But the dominant role in the Nativity is played by models from the late twelfth century.

The force of Cyprus's late Komnenian models is one feature that is important here; the other is the appearance of elements that are Palaiologan. Most visible is the treatment of the landscape. The dominating triangle of the mountain, though copied from Lagoudera, is far less perceptible here because its contour is no longer its defining feature. Instead, it is spangled with highlights and shadows that draw attention away from its contours and diminish its force as an abstract shape. The liberation of landscape from its role as a compartmentalizing envelope around the iconographic components of the scene, and its enlivenment with light, are features of Palaiologan painting that must have been stimulated at Asinou by contemporary Byzantine examples.

The same is true of individual iconographic motifs. This is shown by a closer comparison between the Nativity at Asinou and the late fourteenth-century example at St. Nicholas of the Roof. Both images share a similar core, with mother, manger, ox, ass, and star embraced by the womblike hollow of the cave, Joseph not brooding but raising his face

fig. 13. The type is seen also in Nereditsa, Kurbinovo, the Evangelistria at Geraki, St. Stylianos in Kastoria, and the Decorative Style manuscripts. On this pose see Tsigaridas, "La peinture à Kastoria," 317, figs. 9, 13; idem, *Οι τοιχογραφίες της Μονής Λατόμου*, 38–53, fig. 54A (Nereditsa); Georgitsoyanni, *Les peintures murales du vieux Catholicon*, 74. It is in the late 12th century, too, that her handkerchief appears in her idle hand: one sees it at Hosios David in Thessalonike and St. Stephen at Kastoria: Tsigaridas, *Οι τοιχογραφίες της Μονής Λατόμου*, 38, pl. 6.

182. Megaw and Hawkins, "Church of the Holy Apostles," 320, pl. 30. On the motif of the musician-shepherd see Kalopissi-Verti, *Die Kirche der Hagia Triada*, 87–91.

183. Mouriki, "Wall Paintings of the Church of the Panagia," fig. 13.

184. Boyd, "Church of the Panagia Amasgou, Monagri," color plate B and fig. 19.

185. As at Perachorio: Megaw and Hawkins, "Church of the Holy Apostles," fig. 32.

and hand in acclamation, and the infant in the midwife's lap.[186] The placement of the star inside the cave, though attested very sporadically in early and middle Byzantine art,[187] is seen consistently only in the late Byzantine period.[188] It seems to have belonged to a body of imagery that emerged in the mingled Italian and Byzantine context of the thirteenth century, and to have become established on Cyprus quite early, recurring regularly from the fourteenth century onward.[189] Similarly, the position of the Christ child in the lap of the midwife who bathes him, though not unprecedented,[190] becomes widespread only in the later thirteenth and fourteenth centuries, when one finds it not only at Asinou but throughout the Byzantine world.[191] The beaked hat of the piping shepherd is again a fourteenth-century addition. Headgear presumably intended to link shepherds with their counterparts in real life began to figure in Byzantine art in the eleventh century and soon appeared in Cyprus, as seen in the hooded cape of the shepherd in the Nativity at Trikomo.[192] Hoods are joined by caps somewhat later, as seen at Perachorio,[193] and the caps expand into broad-brimmed hats in late Byzantine painting.[194] The beaked hat seen here at Asinou, its earliest known occurrence in art, recurs in several later Cypriot paintings and may reflect a local garment.[195] Along with its strongly local inventory of models, then, the Nativity shows us a painter familiar with a number of current motifs and a grasp of fundamental shifts in the treatment of landscape. It tells us that the "naïve" colorism of the fourteenth-century paintings

186. Stylianou and Stylianou, *Painted Churches*, fig. 28.
187. It appears in the 6th-century box of Holy Land relics in the Vatican and then again around 1100 in Florence, Laurenziana, Plut. VI 23, 105r. See Weitzmann, "*Loca Sancta*," fig. 6; Velmans, *Le Tétraévangile*, fig. 185 and more clearly in Millet, *Recherches*, fig. 78.
188. Kalokyris, *Τὸ Ἄστρον τῆς Βηθλεέμ*, 67 passim. It makes its appearance in the mid-13th century in Cilicia and in the circle of Guido da Siena, recurs in Cyprus, and eventually becomes characteristic of post-Byzantine painting in Greece and the Balkans. For Cilician examples, see Der Nersessian, *Miniature Painting*, 2: fig. 378, Jerusalem, Library of the Armenian Patriarchate 2563, 21r (Queen Keran Gospels, 1272), and 2: color fig. 280, Jerusalem, Library of the Armenian Patriarchate 2568, 8v (Prince Vasak Gospels, 1268–84). For the circle of Guido da Siena, see Stubblebine, *Guido da Siena*, fig. 20, Guido da Siena, *Nativity* (Paris, Strolin Collection); and Millet, *Recherches*, fig. 45, Circle of Guido da Siena, *Nativity* (Siena, Accademia, no. 15).
189. It appears in the later 14th-century Nativity at St. Nicholas of the Roof (Stylianou and Stylianou, *Painted Churches*, fig. 28); in the late 15th century at the Archangel church in Pedoulas (ibid., fig. 198) and the Chryseleousa in Emba (V. Karageorghis, *ARDAC* for 1980, fig. 16); and in the 16th century at the Archangel-Theotokos church at Galata and the Savior church at Palaichori (ibid., fig. 149).
190. It is seen in the Cappella Palatina: see Grabar, *Byzantine Painting*, 130; see also Schiller, *Iconography of Christian Art*, 1: pl. 159. The infant Mary sits on the midwife's lap in the 12th-century scene of the Birth of the Virgin in the bema at Asinou itself. But characteristically the two nativity scenes are distinguished from one another, and do not repeat such motifs in the same monument.
191. It is seen in Paris. gr. 54 (Millet, *Recherches*, fig. 42), St. Nicholas Orphanos (Tsitouridou, *Ὁ ζωγραφικὸς διάκοσμος τοῦ Ἁγίου Νικολάου*, pl. 19), the Protaton on Mount Athos (Millet, *Monuments de l'Athos*, 10, 2), and at Mistra in both the Brontochion (Millet, *Monuments byzantins de Mistra*, pl. 95, 8), and the Peribleptos (ibid., pl. 124, 3). That this pose was more than an engaging piece of genre is illustrated emphatically by its use at Arilje, where the child lies across the midwife's lap in the posture of the Pietà: Millet, *La peinture du Moyen Âge*, 1: pl. 71, 3.
192. Stylianou and Stylianou, *Painted Churches*, fig. 297. A very similar hood appears in the 11th-century Athos, Panteleimonos 2, fol. 210r: see Pelekanides et al., *Treasures of Mount Athos*, 2: fig. 284.
193. Megaw and Hawkins, "Church of the Holy Apostles," fig. 30. An example from early in the 12th century is seen in the Skevophylakion Lectionary at the Great Lavra, Mount Athos, folio 114v: Pelekanides et al., *Οἱ θησαυροὶ τοῦ Ἁγίου Ὄρους*, fig. 7.
194. Good examples are in the Nativities of the Serbian churches: Millet, *La peinture du Moyen Âge*, 2: fig. 8, 1 (Sopoćani), fig. 53, 2 (Gradać); see also St. Nicholas Orphanos in Tsitouridou, *Ὁ ζωγραφικὸς διάκοσμος*, fig. 19, and Munich, Staatsbibliothek, slav. 4, 92v and 214r (the Serbian Psalter) in Strzygowski, *Die Miniaturen des Serbischen Psalters*, 2: pl. XXV (54) and LIV (131).
195. See Stylianou and Stylianou, *Painted Churches*, fig. 28 (St. Nicholas of the Roof), fig. 149 (Savior church, Palaichori).

need not imply naïve isolation from contemporary developments in the broader Byzantine world.

The PRESENTATION IN THE TEMPLE (ἡ ἡπο/παντῖ) follows the Nativity, the red of the Christ child's tunic echoing the rhythm of red rectangles in the Nativity and thus joining them visually (Figs. 6.37, 6.39). The Presentation has none of the Nativity's tentativeness. It is the most confidently painted of the scenes on the vault, with richly heaped drapery folds, robust volumes in the limbs and facial features, and a decorative play of color and ornament in the setting. Iconographically, on the other hand, the scene is totally traditional.[196] Mary (Μ(ήτ)ηρ Θ(εο)ῦ) and Symeon (C(υμεών)) face one another across the altar of the Holy of Holies. Mary holds the child; Joseph (Ι(ωσήφ)) follows her carrying two pigeons; and Anna (Α(ννα)) stands behind Symeon, bearing the scroll that had become customary by the mid-twelfth century.[197] It carries its usual message: τούτο το / βρέφ/ος οὐρα/νόν κ(αὶ) γ, that is, Τοῦτο τὸ βρέφος οὐρανὸν καὶ γῆν ἐστερέωσεν, "This is the child who established heaven and earth." The Presentation was a conservative image and—even after the emergence of the asymmetrical, Palaiologan version with Symeon facing all the other figures—the symmetrical, middle Byzantine formula was often preferred, as it was on Cyprus.[198] Even on Cyprus, however, Symeon holds the child from the thirteenth century onward, highlighting the conservatism of the version at Asinou.[199] Thus in emphatic contrast to the Nativity, the Presentation presents nothing that could not also be assigned to a painting of 1106. This is true even of the little cross on the dome of the Holy of Holies. Middle Byzantine paintings of the Presentation do not label the Holy of Holies with a cross. In the wake of the Crusades, however, images of the Temple became more assertive. With its many hanging lamps, the Temple here recalls the explicitly—possibly polemically—Christian images of the Temple on fourteenth-century pilgrimage glass from the Holy Land, which are topped with conspicuous crosses.[200] In fact, Holy Land history may have induced the fourteenth-century painter to claim the Temple explicitly with a cross.[201] Yet the cross itself was not an invention, for it is paralleled precisely in the little cross atop the dome in Asinou's Evangelist portrait of 1106 on the south wall of the naos. If the Nativity had taught us that a conservative iconographic matrix can nonetheless harbor fundamental later modifications, the Presentation alerts us that an

196. On the iconography of the Presentation, see Shorr, "Iconographic Development of the Presentation"; Schiller, *Iconography*, 1:91–92; Maguire, "Iconography of Symeon with the Christ Child"; Carr, "Presentation of an Icon"; Sinkević, "Changes in the Composition." Illustrating the conservatism of the scene at Asinou is the fact that virtually the same composition is seen already in 1028 at the Panagia ton Chalkeon: see Tsitouridou, *Church of the Panagia Chalkeon*, figs. 16–17.

197. Mouriki, "Icons," 385 n. 27 notes the famous icon of the Virgin surrounded by prophets at Mt. Sinai as perhaps the earliest surviving example of this motif; she dates the icon around 1130. The same text was used in both Kato Lefkara and Monagri: see Papageorgiou, "Η ἐκκλησία τοῦ Ἀρχαγγέλου," fig. 38, 3; Boyd, "Church of the Panagia Amasgou," fig. 23.

198. Certainly this was the case on Cyprus, where the Presentation is shown in this way in the later 14th century at St. Nicholas of the Roof and in the early 16th century at the Archangel-Theotokos church, Galata.

199. Mary still holds the child in Kato Lefkara (Papageorgiou, "Η ἐκκλησία τοῦ Ἀρχαγγέλου," fig. 38, 3), but in Xylotympou (Chotzakoglou, "Βυζαντινή αρχιτεκτονική και τέχνη," 1:627, 2: fig. 494) and Monagri (Boyd, "Church of the Panagia Amasgou," fig. 23) he is in Symeon's hands.

200. See in particular the enameled glass bottle from 13th-century Syria in the Furussiya Arts Foundation, Vaduz, Liechtenstein, beautifully reproduced in Carboni and Whitehouse, *Glass of the Sultans*, 242–45, no. 121, pl. on page 244.

201. The Dome of the Rock was believed to be the Temple, and pilgrims venerated it as the site of Christ's Presentation. Its Crusader conquerors conspicuously crowned it with a cross, which was equally conspicuously removed when the building reverted to Muslim control in 1187. On its removal, see Folda, *Crusader Art in the Holy Land*, 25, with further bibliography; on the Christian history of the Dome of the Rock, see Schein, "Between Mount Moriah and the Holy Sepulchre," 181–88.

iconographic eccentricity need not originate outside the twelfth-century program.

The Baptism (ἡ βά/πτισις) is below the Nativity (Figs. 6.37, 6.40).[202] Where Christ in the Presentation had carried over the horizontal rhythm of small red rectangles that ran across the Nativity, so the Christ of the Baptism creates a vertical continuity, his body aligned with the figure of his mother just above him, and the blue lines of the Jordan answering the blue bands of his own shroud-like swaddling in the manger beside her.[203] Christ (I(ησοῦ)ς / X(ριστό)ς) stands in a cone of water with ten fishes and an upright figure personifying the River Jordan; John (ο / ἅγι/ος / Ιω(άννης) / πρ(ο)δ(ρο)μ/ος) on the left gestures to Christ's head as a dove descends from an arc of Heaven and six angels approach from the right. The cape-like cascade of the Jordan creates an immediate impression of conservatism; Palaiologan versions of the scene draw the river back into a precipitous landscape that dramatizes the idea of Jesus's descent into the depths. The cross-legged stance of Jesus, the standing Jordan's lifting his face in response to Jesus's gesture of blessing, and the scant sling that clothes John the Baptist are also long-established conventions. Yet, as in the Nativity, the imagery points

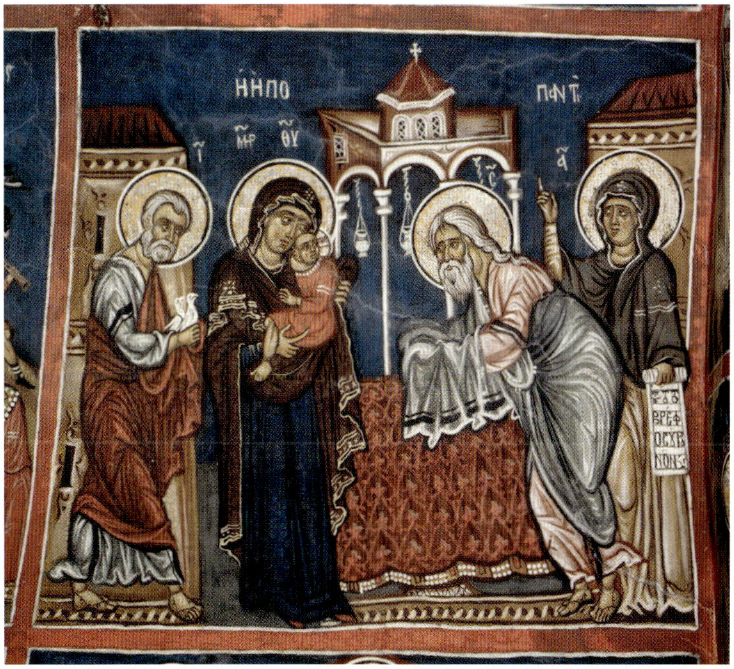

FIG. 6.39 Naos, central bay, south side of vault: Presentation of Christ in the Temple (photo courtesy of the Leventis Foundation and the Archaeological Research Unit, University of Cyprus, No. 006307)

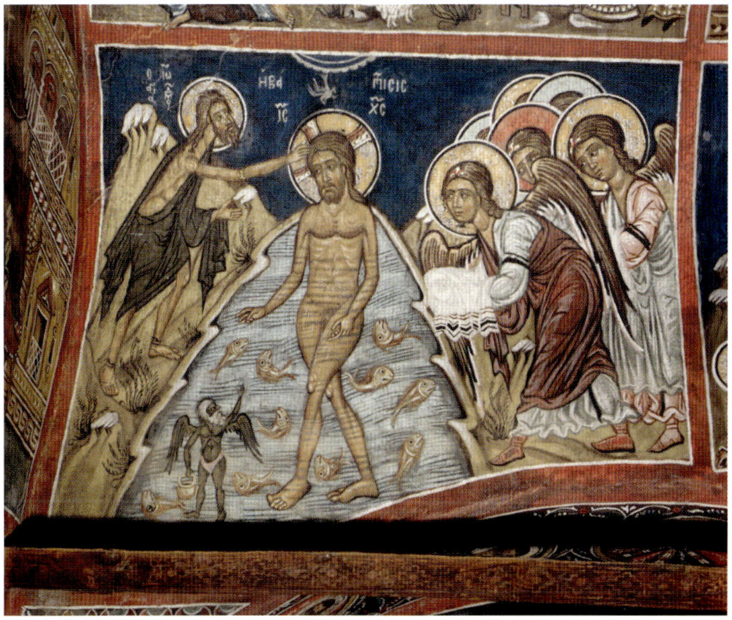

FIG. 6.40 Naos, central bay, south side of vault: Baptism (photo courtesy of the Leventis Foundation and the Archaeological Research Unit, University of Cyprus, No. 006308)

202. On the iconography of the Baptism see Millet, *Recherches*, 170–215; Schiller, *Iconography*, 1:134–37.

203. Such links are generally read as facilitating narrative continuity, but their intention may have been theological as well. Thus, as a second birth the Baptism was often linked with the Nativity. Theodore of Mopsuestia closes his catechetical sermon on Baptism saying, "[W]e have, by what we have said, wrapped you tightly in swaddling clothes, so you may grasp and remember firmly and unshakeably the birth that takes place": Theodore of Mopsuestia, *On the Lord's Prayer and on the Sacraments*, 69. The theme of light and being clothed with light that runs through the baptismal service, as in the troparion in tone 8 sung just after the chrismation in the Orthodox Baptismal liturgy, "[A] robe of divine light bestow upon me, O You that for vesture array Yourself with Light; and bestow many mercies, O Christ our God, who are plenteous in mercy," finds effective visualization in the Transfiguration, which follows the scene of the Baptism at Asinou.

to a more complex genealogy. The balletic twist of Christ's body and the bevy of angels on the riverbank behind him reflect a version of the Baptism formulated in the second quarter of the twelfth century and widely circulated in that century's second half: it is echoed in the Baptisms of the later twelfth century at Perachorio, Kato Lefkara, Lagoudera, Xylotympou, and Kalogrea on Cyprus,[204] and they are surely the examples that shaped the imagination of the fourteenth-century painter at Asinou. These are the same cycles that had so strongly affected the imagery of the Nativity. Here as elsewhere in the feast scenes, they emerge as particularly potent iconographic catalysts. The exuberant fish, in turn, become usual in mural painting only in the thirteenth century;[205] Monagri offers a good Cypriot example.[206] More intricate is the figure of Jordan himself. His dark skin and white hair are seen again at Kato Lefkara, Kalogrea, and Monagri,[207] reinforcing the importance of these churches as models. His spread wings, on the other hand, are new to Cyprus.

The dark-skinned Jordan has a fitful history and it is not clear if its various phases come together in a coherent story. The figure first appears in the late eleventh-century Column churches in Cappadocia, where a dark-skinned, youthful Jordan blows a trumpet in evocation of Psalm 28(29):3: "The voice of the Lord is upon the waters; the God of glory thunders."[208] His dark color must have been adopted to illustrate the concept of Jordan's waters as the watery depths. So long as this example remained unique, it was plausible to assume that the fourteenth-century figure in Asinou had been adopted from the program of 1105/6, which in turn reflected developments in Asia Minor. The figure did not remain isolated, though. A different form of dark-skinned Jordan, one with white hair and no horn, appeared in the early thirteenth century. This is found both on Cyprus, at Kato Lefkara and Monagri,[209] and in Lebanon in the bilateral Kaftoun icon.[210] The horn-blowing Jordan reappeared at this time in Cappadocia in the churches of Karşı kilise (1212) and the Archangel church, Çemil, but in these cases his dark skin color was abandoned.[211] The white-haired figure, being hornless, had no association with Psalm 28(29), but his tousled white hair and beard indicated a new dimension. These features associate him with Hades, long represented as dark.[212] The bond with Hades lends emphasis to his gesture with extended

204. See Megaw and Hawkins, "Church of the Holy Apostles," fig. 35; Papageorgiou, "Η ἐκκλησία τοῦ Ἀρχαγγέλου," fig. 39, 1; Chotzakoglou, "Βυζαντινή αρχιτεκτονική και τέχνη," 2: fig. 495 for Xylotympou; for Kalogrea, see Stylianou and Stylianou, *Painted Churches*, fig. 282. This version of the Baptism seems to emerge in the Kokkinobaphos manuscripts: see Stornajolo, *Miniature delle Omilie*, pl. 86.
205. See Jolivet-Lévy, "Nouvelle découverte en Cappadoce" (2002), 187; Belting, Mango, and Mouriki, *Mosaics and Frescoes of St. Mary Pammakaristos*, 66.
206. Boyd, "Church of the Panagia Amasgou," fig. 24.
207. See Papageorgiou, "Η ἐκκλησία τοῦ Ἀρχαγγέλου," fig. 39, 1; Boyd, "Church of the Panagia Amasgou," fig. 24. The figure of Jordan in the Baptism at Kalogrea is described as dark-skinned by Papageorgiou on 218, though the color reproduction in Stylianou and Stylianou, *Painted Churches*, figure 282, makes him look more ruddy than black.
208. His dark color at Karanlık kilise is clear in the color reproduction in Yenipınar and Şahin, *Paintings of the Dark Church*, 34; for Elmalı kilise see Restle, *Byzantine Wall Painting*, 2: fig. 174. The psalm passage is identified in Jolivet-Lévy, *La Cappadoce médiévale*, 202.
209. See note 207 above.
210. Immerzeel, "Holy Horsemen and Crusader Banners," pl. 24 with earlier bibliography, especially Hélou, "L'icône bilatérale de la Vierge."
211. For Karşı kilise see Jolivet-Lévy, "Images et espace cultuel," fig. 11. For Çemil, see Jerphanion, *Une nouvelle province de l'art*, 2:142; 3: fig. 157, 2.
212. The bond is made explicitly in Çemil, where paired paintings of the Baptism and Anastasis probably made in the 14th century give Jordan and Hades the same flying hair: see Jerphanion, *Une nouvelle province de l'art*, 3: fig. 157, 2. The link of blackness to Hades goes all the way back to the Khludov Psalter, where the illumination to Psalm 67(68):9, the second of two images labeled the "Anastasis of Adam," shows Hades as a sprawling, fat, old man with black skin: see Shchepkina, *Miniatiury Khludovskoĭ Psaltyri*, 63v. I thank Nancy Patterson Ševčenko for making me aware of this.

hand, which is adopted by the black Jordans at Kato Lefkara, Monagri, and Asinou: for, like Hades, with this gesture the figure acknowledges the life-granting power of the Christ who triumphs over him. Christ's life-granting power is visualized in the water, which teems with fish. The figure of Jordan at Asinou is very like the one at Kato Lefkara, with its hoary hair and loincloth. In both form and content, Kato Lefkara is a more plausible model than the horn blower in Cappadocia. But at Asinou the figure is winged.

Overtly demonic black figures with spread wings appear in thirteenth-century paintings of the Baptism from the eastern Mediterranean. The most dramatic are in Armenian manuscripts,[213] but there is also a Byzantine example in a Gospel book of the first half of the thirteenth century from Mytilene.[214] Slender, nude, wholly black, and hurrying away from Jesus, he is unmistakably demonic. But he also bears the gushing urn and is surely conceived as Jordan.[215] The figure at Asinou retains more clearly the features of Jordan. Thus he seems to be not simply a demon but a conflation of multiple ideas focused in Jordan. In this respect he bears closer kinship with yet a third cluster of Jordans, all winged and in some cases dark-skinned. These figures play a role in the Palaiologan art of early fourteenth-century Serbia and Macedonia.[216] The dark-skinned examples are in Veroia, in Kalliergis's Baptism of 1315 in the church of Christ and again a decade later in the murals of the Old Metropole.[217] As the winged Jordan had appeared in Cyprus in conjunction with the many exuberant fishes, so he appears in these examples in conjunction with a whole cohort of figures in and around the water. As such, he forms part of an expansive elaboration of the Baptism in Palaiologan art that presents the scene as a truly cosmic act of redemption embracing both humankind and nature.

The dark-skinned and winged Jordan is generally interpreted as the vanquished Devil, overwhelmed by the light and life of Christ.[218] The Devil was a participant in the Orthodox ritual of baptism,[219] and nowhere more visibly than in the events surrounding the blessing of the baptismal water, in which God's power is invoked to drive evil spirits from the water with the words, "may no dark demon lie hidden in the water."[220] Given the ubiquity of winged black nudes as devils in Byzantine art, the addition of wings would seem to assimilate the dusky old river god to the outright status of a dark demon, indeed the Devil himself. Nonetheless, the gesture of the white-haired Jordan in his school of lively fish accords better with the Jordans of Palaiologan Macedonia and Serbia than with the fleeing demon of the Mytilene Gospel

213. By far the most dramatic is the frantically fleeing demon in the Armenian Gospel book, Galata, Church of St. Gregory the Illuminator, MS 35, 19r, painted most probably in Cilicia in 1223: see Der Nersessian, *Miniature Painting*, 1:39, 2: fig. 121. In two instances it is transformed into a fish: see ibid., 2: color fig. 363, Jerusalem, Armenian Patriarchate 2568, 12v (Prince Vasak Gospels, 1268–84); and fig. 364, Erevan, Matenadaran 197, 20v, of 1289.
214. Boys Gymnasium, MS 9, 13v: Vocotopoulos, "L'évangile illustré de Mytilène," 380 and fig. 9.
215. A similar figure may have also appeared in the Gospel book Mount Athos, Iveron 5, of the third quarter of the 13th century, most probably from Constantinople. The figure in the water at Jesus's feet in the Baptism on folio 138r has been roughly slashed and erased, suggesting that it was seen as negative or harmful, and it seems to have been dark-skinned. See Pelekanides et al., *Treasures of Mount Athos*, 2: fig. 22.
216. Kono, "Personification of the Jordan and the Sea."
217. On the Old Metropole see Katsaros, "Η παράσταση της Βάπτισης," with earlier bibliography, especially Mouriki, "Revival Themes," 462. For the church of Christ, see Pelekanides, *Καλλιέργης*, fig. E′.
218. Kono, "Personification of the Jordan," 196, 212 passim.
219. Kelly, *The Devil at Baptism*, 163–69; Stewart, *Demons and the Devil*, 195–97. See also the sanctification of the waters on 6 January, which Kokosalakis, "Political Significance of Popular Religion," 48, speaks of as associated "with the purification of nature and the exorcism of dark and evil forces generally."
220. Whitaker, *Documents of the Baptismal Liturgy*, 80, translating the Barberini Euchologion. The text as given in Arranz, *L'Eucologio costantinopolitano*, 185–86: καὶ μὴ ὑποκρυβήτω τῷ ὕδατι τούτῳ δαιμόνιον. . . .

book.[221] They, too, acclaim Christ, appearing less as demons in the Christian sense than as demonic forces of nature that are not so much damned as tamed by the advent of Christ. Thus the wings of Asinou's Jordan may respond more to contemporary Byzantine conceptions of the Baptism than they refer to the demons of the thirteenth-century manuscripts. Seen in this way, the winged Jordan may reflect a genealogy not unlike that of the image of Moses at the Burning Bush on the transverse arch. In each, an iconographic motif that had circulated in the Crusader Levant—the Hades-like Jordan on the one hand, the burning bush on the other—was applied in the service of a religious conception current in Palaiologan Byzantium—the cosmic scope of redemption in the Baptism in one case, the veneration of Mary in her Old Testament prefigurations in the other. Such motifs show how layered the messages at Asinou were, for all the conservatism of their vocabulary.

The Transfiguration (ἡ μεταμόρ/φοσῖς) is the final scene on the south side of the vault (Figs. 6.37, 6.41). Like the Baptism, the Transfiguration saw a phase of energetic visual elaboration in the Palaiologan period that coincided with a heightened theological interest in its content.[222] The pervasive adoption of its dynamic new iconography, first seen in the late thirteenth-century Constantinopolitan Paris. gr. 54,[223] throws into stark relief the utter conservatism of the composition at Asinou. Christ (Ι(ησοῦ)ς / Χ(ριστό)ς) stands in a mandorla in a mountainous landscape, Elijah (ὁ πρ(ο)φ(ή)τ(η)ς / Η/λί/ας) standing to his right and Moses (ὁ πρ(ο)φ(ή)τ(η)ς / Μω/η/σῖς) to his left. John (Ιω(άννης)) lies prostrate at Christ's feet, with a kneeling Peter (Π(έτρος)) on the left and James (Ι(άκοβος)) on one knee on the right. The figures do not reflect the heightened emotional volatility of late twelfth-century versions of the scene,[224] much less the stunned and tumbling postures of the disciples in Palaiologan art. Only the light responds to modern conventions: Jesus's garment is now white, as it was so often in the Palaiologan period; his mandorla is painted in aggressively strong shades of red, its rays once glazed with a now-ruined reflective substance to make them shine; and the landscape is spangled with highlights. The showy mandorla contrasts with the conservative composition, which emerges as an awkward fourteenth-century pastiche.

The figure of Moses alerts us to look more carefully. Back-to-back with the Moses of the Burning Bush on the adjacent transverse arch, he links the two visions of God, veiled in the Old Testament and immediate in the New (Fig. 6.41). Possibly to underscore the connection, he lacks the tablets of the Law that he customarily carries in the Transfiguration, facing Christ with empty hands. Moreover, like his counterpart before the burning bush, he is grizzled and bearded. The bearded Moses is exceptional in Byzantine art and, until the fourteenth century, limited to images from Sinai.[225] It is to Sinai that the origin of Asinou's image of the burning bush has been assigned; Sinai, moreover, is associated with the scene of the Transfiguration, which adorned its apse and shaped its image as a pilgrimage site. The grizzled and bearded Sinaitic

221. These figures are inventoried in Kono, "Personifications," 196, and include the katholikon at Vatopedi of 1312 (Millet, *Monuments de l'Athos*, pl. 82, 1–2), an icon at the Peribleptos church in Ohrid of ca. 1314–20, the Christ church of 1315 and Old Metropole of the 1320s in Veroia (see note 217 above), the King's church in Studenica of 1313/14, St. George in Staro Nagoričino of 1316–18 (Millet, *La peinture du Moyen Âge*, 3: fig. 125, 5), St. Nicholas Orphanos in Thessalonike of 1310–20 (Tsitouridou, *Ο ζωγραφικὸς διάκοσμος*, fig. 22), and the katholikon at Chilandar of 1318–19 (Millet, *Monuments de l'Athos*, pl. 66, 1–2; pl. 67, 1; Underwood, "Some Problems in Programs and Iconography," figs. 9, 9a, 9b). On their relation to the other personifications, see esp. Jolivet-Lévy, "Nouvelle découverte en Cappadoce" (2002), 186.

222. On the Transfiguration, see Millet, *Recherches*, 216–31; Schiller, *Iconography*, 1:149–50; Weitzmann, "Metamorphosis Icon"; Nelson, "Text and Image," 34–42.

223. Paris. gr. 54, 213r: Lazarev, *Storia*, figure 393.

224. Nelson, "Text and Image," 34–42; Weitzmann, "Metamorphosis Icon," 415–21.

225. See note 67 above.

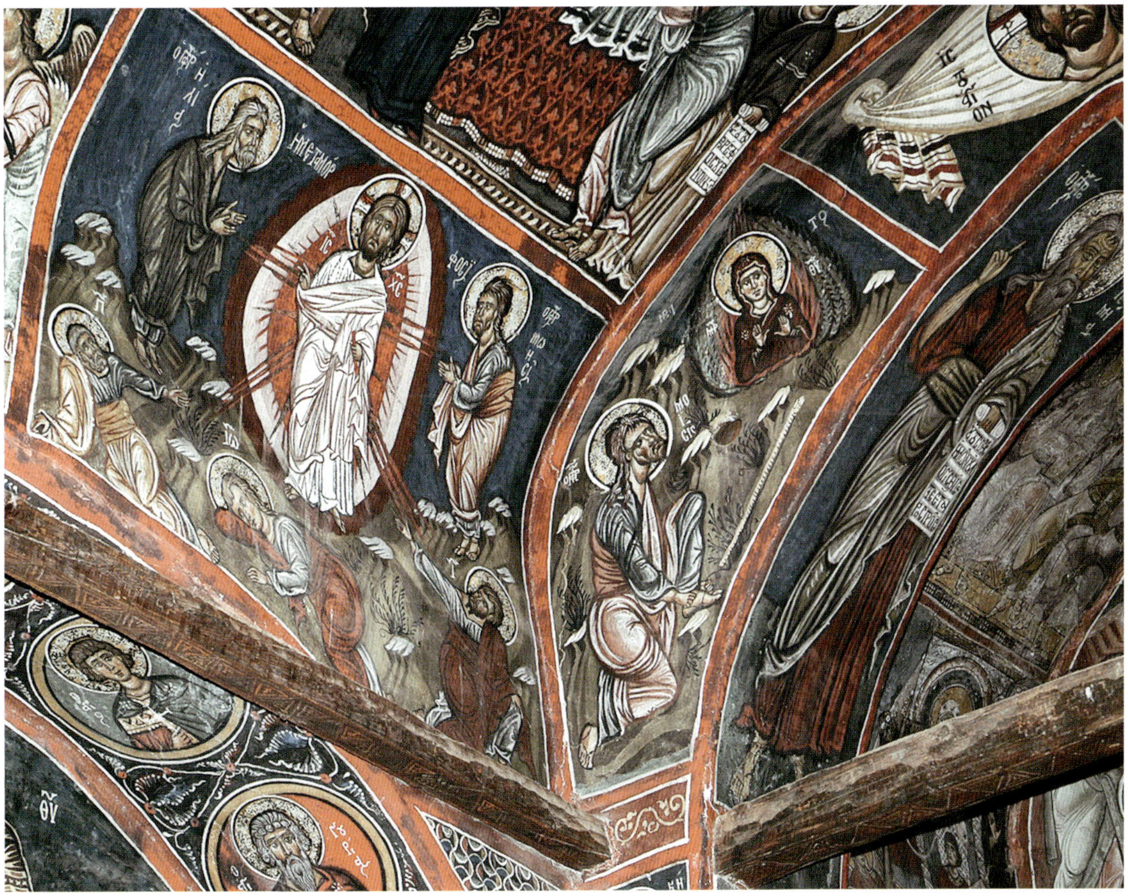

FIG. 6.41 Naos, central bay, south side of vault: Transfiguration and Burning Bush (photo courtesy of A.W. Carr)

Moses, linking two scenes associated with Sinai, shows a very deliberate shaping of both the program as a whole and the Transfiguration in particular. This parallel was not possible in the twelfth century, when the transverse arch did not yet exist and the image of the Burning Bush had not yet been formulated. It shows very clearly what the winged Jordan had implied—that the fourteenth-century painters used their time-worn compositions with deliberate and thoughtful nuance.

The four scenes on the south side of the vault form a coherent unit, intermeshed visually—and to some extent also intellectually—with one another by echoed shapes, colors, compositional axes, and motifs, like the waves of the Baptism that echo the swaddling bands of the Nativity. They belong together in the standard feast cycle, and lead logically to the Raising of Lazarus in the western bay. It is easy to assume that the same four scenes occupied the vault in 1105/6; certainly we know from the black boot below the Baptism that scenes were painted there, and we know from Koutsovendis that there could have been some form of grid composition. It is difficult, however, to draw any reliable conclusions about how such scenes must have looked. The middle Byzantine motifs employed in the vault have proved recurrently to be mid- or late twelfth-century ones, best paralleled in late twelfth-century churches in Cyprus itself. These churches have played a major role in modern art historians' conception of Byzantine art; Asinou's scenes make it clear that they played an equally powerful role in the visual imagination of medieval Cypriots, fundamentally shaping the way events of Jesus's life were expected to look. The intervention of this strong, local, late middle Byzantine phase of painting makes it difficult to see through the late twelfth-century conventions to elements of the scenes that might attest to the imagery used in 1106. We have seen in discussing the sanctoral cycle that Asinou's images of 1106 influenced later twelfth-century painters, and we cannot exclude the possibility that the iconography of the late twelfth-century churches of Cyprus was, to some fundamental degree, echoing canons established at Asinou itself. But if so, we cannot know in what ways that occurred.

If these existing scenes are evasive on the subject of the initial paintings, they are far more informative about the art of their own era. In this respect they are of special value, for fourteenth-century mural paintings of the birth and ministry of Christ are rare. Their recurrent reference to the imagery of the late middle Byzantine Cypriot cycles shows how deeply fourteenth-century art was rooted in local models. Cycles that might in the twelfth century have been valued as exoteric, reflecting Cyprus's bonds with Constantinople, are now embraced as integral to the local past. The reverence for local models, however, in no sense precludes an awareness of more cosmopolitan developments. A significant aspect of the scenes is their nuanced use of older images to construct contemporary messages. The sources of the older imagery are layered, including not only the Komnenian art on Cyprus but imagery from the mainland, like the Burning Bush and the Hades-like Jordan, imagery from the mingled Byzantine and Italian art of the thirteenth century, and the current art of Palaiologan Byzantium. The layered sources yield a kind of iconographic archaeology. When one turns to the scenes on the north side of the vault, the components of this layering emerge with greater clarity.

The North Side of the Vault and the Lunette

The north side of the vault continues the grid format, producing an impression of continuity with the south (Fig. 6.42). Yet fundamental contrasts between the two halves emerge in both composition and character. Where the scenes on the south side are all traditional feast scenes, those on the north are dominated by events of the Passion narrative. It is these northern scenes, and not the group as a whole, that warrant the label of "narrative." Compositionally, too, the scenes on the north are more loosely related to the architecture. Not only are the figures in the Crucifixion cut by the arc of the supporting arch, but the final episodes spill from the vault into the lunette below, turning the grid of four scenes into a larger group of six. These contrasts put one on guard, suggesting a shift in the conception of the program.

The scenes in the north side of the vault open with the Betrayal and Way to the Cross. The Betrayal (ἡ προδοσία; Figs. 6.42, 6.43) takes up the story of Christ where the west bay had left it, at the Washing of the Feet (Fig. 6.36). Stolid blocks of armed soldiers border the scene like bookends, framing the encounter between Jesus (Ι(ησοῦ)ς / Χ(ριστό)ς) and Judas (Ι(ούδας)). Christ strides eastward, his right arm extended toward the small knot of Peter and Malchus before him, as Judas lifts his arms in an embrace. Among the very earliest Passion scenes to enter Christian art,[226] the Betrayal had been largely excluded from the imagery of the naos in the middle Byzantine period by the compressed "classic" cycle of feast scenes, and it occurred—if at all—in the narthex until the expanded narratives of the Palaiologan period gave it a place once again inside the church.[227] Its

226. On the Betrayal, see Millet, *Recherches*, 326–86; Schiller, *Iconography*, 2:51–56; Mouriki, *Mosaics of Nea Moni*, 1:184–86. It already figured on early Christian sarcophagi and took a place—as the Crucifixion had not—in the earliest monumental Passion cycle that survives, at Sant'Apollinare Nuovo, Ravenna: see Deichmann, *Frühchristliche Bauten und Mosaiken*, fig. 187.

227. In Kılıçlar kilise of the 10th century, the scenes from the Passion cycle, including the Betrayal and Way to the Cross, already appeared in the western bay of the church as if in a narthex: see Restle, *Byzantine Wall Painting*, 2: figs. 271, 274. The Betrayal is seen in the narthex in the middle Byzantine churches of Nea Moni on Chios (Mouriki, *Mosaics of Nea Moni*, 1:184–85), Daphni (Diez and Demus, *Byzantine Mosaics*, figs. 96–98), Servia (Xyngopoulos, *Μνημεῖα τῶν Σερβίων*, fig. 11), Samari (Grigoriadou-Cabagnols, "Le décor peint," 179),

prominent appearance at Asinou thus suggests the intervention of a late Byzantine model. However, the Betrayal had always retained a place in monuments dedicated to the True Cross. Thus its inclusion in the naos program of the eleventh-century Column churches in Cappadocia has been related to the veneration of a cross relic in Çarıklı kilise, the earliest of the three,[228] and in Cyprus it reappears in the late twelfth-century naos cycle devoted to the Cross at the Enkleistra,[229] and again on the obverse of the early fourteenth-century silver Cross reliquary at Pano Lefkara.[230] More significantly for us, the Betrayal had appeared in the naos cycle of the Holy Trinity church in St. John Chrysostom, Koutsovendis.[231] Given the prominence of Koutsovendis and the fact that the Asinou painter knew it well, one cannot reject the possibility that the Betrayal was also adopted in the cycle of 1105/6.

If adopted from Koutsovendis, the scene was radically modernized in the fourteenth century. Especially notable is the full militarization of the group around Jesus.[232] Armored personnel were rare in Byzantine versions of the Betrayal before the twelfth century; then soldiers in arms began to infiltrate the posse around Jesus, and during the thirteenth century they often took it over entirely. This is more characteristic of Greece and Cyprus than of Serbia, where the Betrayals display deliberately diverse throngs of participants and onlookers.[233] Thus the militarization has been associated especially with areas of Crusader occupation, the hostile antagonists of Christ linked visually with the militant occupiers.[234] The soldiers at Asinou, with their stony profiles, illustrate this militarization forcefully. They wear generic Byzantine military garb, though,[235] so their militancy is hard to link in any polemical way with the Latins.

---

and St. Theodoros, Tsopakas, and the Holy Strategoi in the Mani: see Drandakes, *Βυζαντινές τοιχογραφίες*, 44, pl. 11; fig. 5 for St. Theodore; and 465, fig. 78 for the Holy Strategoi. The scene appears in the nave of both Monreale and San Marco in Venice—see Kitzinger, *I mosaici*, fasc. 4, fig. 94; and Demus, *Mosaics of Norman Sicily*, fig. 70; idem, *Mosaics of San Marco*, 1/2: color pl. 66—but these are truly huge churches that invited radically expanded cycles. In the Serbian churches of the early Palaiologan period, Petković, *La peinture serbe*, lists the Betrayal at the Virgin's church, Studenica (2:7), Žiča (2:10), Chilandar (2:19), Staro Nagoričino (2:25), Gračanica (2:33), Čučer (2:35), and Dečani (2:44). In Greece it is seen in the Christos church, Veroia (Gounares, *Χριστός Βέροιας*, fig. 30), and—among Greek cycles—with particular prominence in the tympanum of the south wall of the Transfiguration church, Pyrgi, in Euboia, where it faces the Anastasis: see Koumoussi's discussion of the scene in *Les peintures murales de la Transfiguration*, 78–80. I am indebted to Maria Panayotidi for my knowledge of this source.

228. The Betrayal appears in all three of the Column churches: see Restle, *Byzantine Wall Painting*, 2:181 (Elmalı), 2:207 (Çarıklı), 2:236 (Karanlık). On the connection with the True Cross, see Jolivet-Lévy, "Çarıklı Kilise," which associates the program at Çarıklı, and so perhaps at all of the three churches, with a relic of the "precious cross" represented in two of its paintings.

229. On the Enkleistra, see Mango and Hawkins, "Hermitage," 123–24 on Neophytos's relic of the True Cross and 140–60 on the iconography of the naos, where the cross was installed in a special reliquary cavity in the wall.

230. Papageorgiou, "Ο σταυρός των Λευκάρων," 2: fig. 133, 2.

231. Mango, "Monastery of St. Chrysostom," 83, figs. 103, 104.

232. Stylianou and Stylianou, "Militarization of the Betrayal."

233. Thus one can contrast the heavily militarized Betrayals in Cyprus and at Pyrgi and the church of the Soter Christos at Megara in Greece with the versions of the scene at the Peribleptos (St. Clement), Ohrid; St. Nicholas, Prilep; St. Niketas, Čučer; or St. George, Staro Nagoričino. For Pyrgi, see above, note 227; for Ohrid see Hamann-MacLean and Hallensleben, *Die Monumentalmalerei*, fig. 164; for Prilep see Millet, *La peinture du Moyen Âge,* 3: fig. 24, 3; for Čučer see ibid., 3: fig. 43, 3; for Staro Nagoričino see ibid., 3: fig. 85, 3–4.

234. In addition to the Stylianous, see Koumoussi, *Les peintures murales*, 78–80.

235. This is in marked contrast to the soldiers at Pyrgi, for instance, who wear unusual, surely contemporary, long coats of mail: see Koumoussi, *Les peintures murales*, 78–80, citing also the Betrayals at Oxylithos and St. Demetrios, Makrychori.

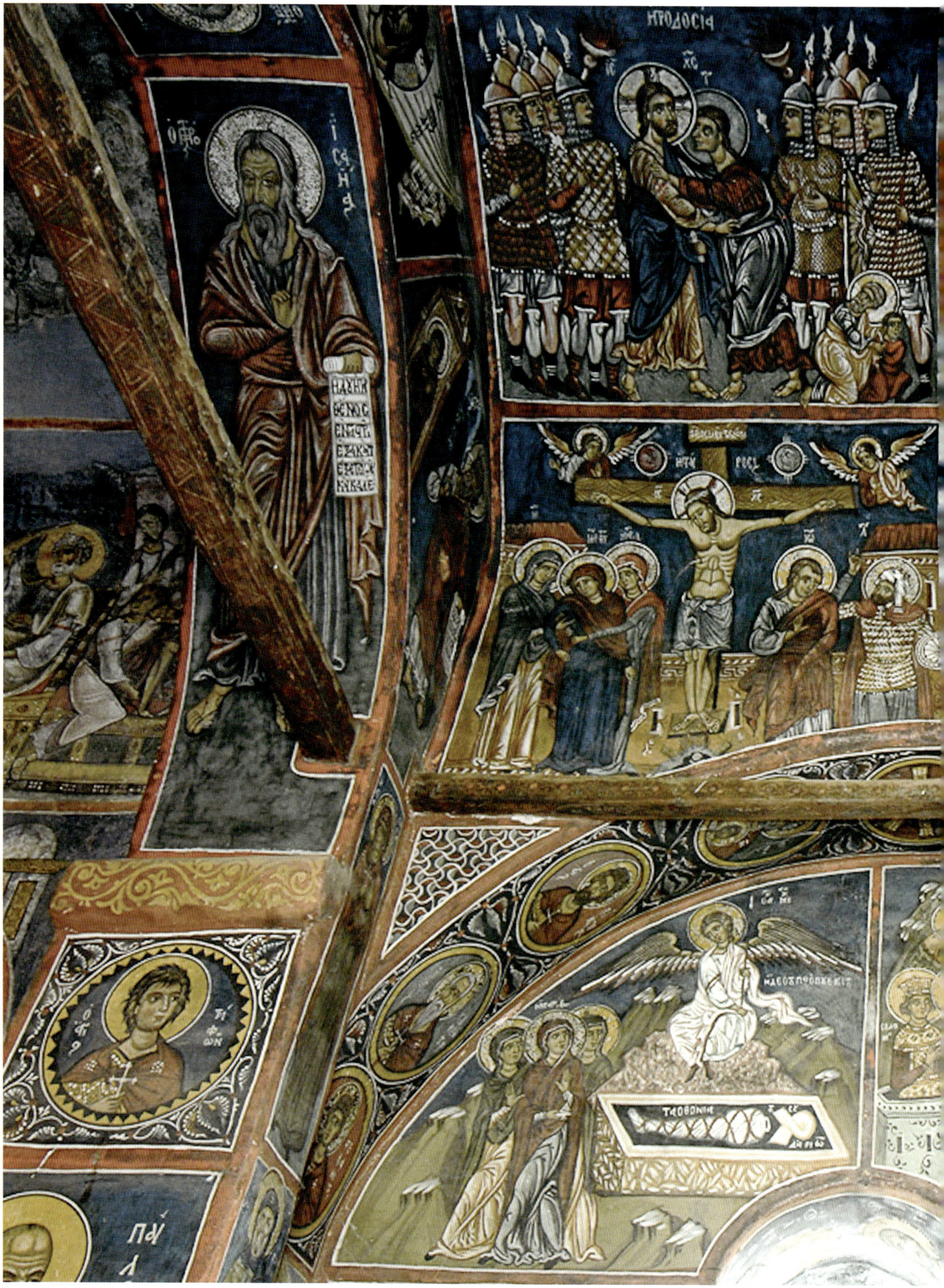

FIG. 6.42 Naos, central bay, north side of vault (photo courtesy of G. L. Carr)

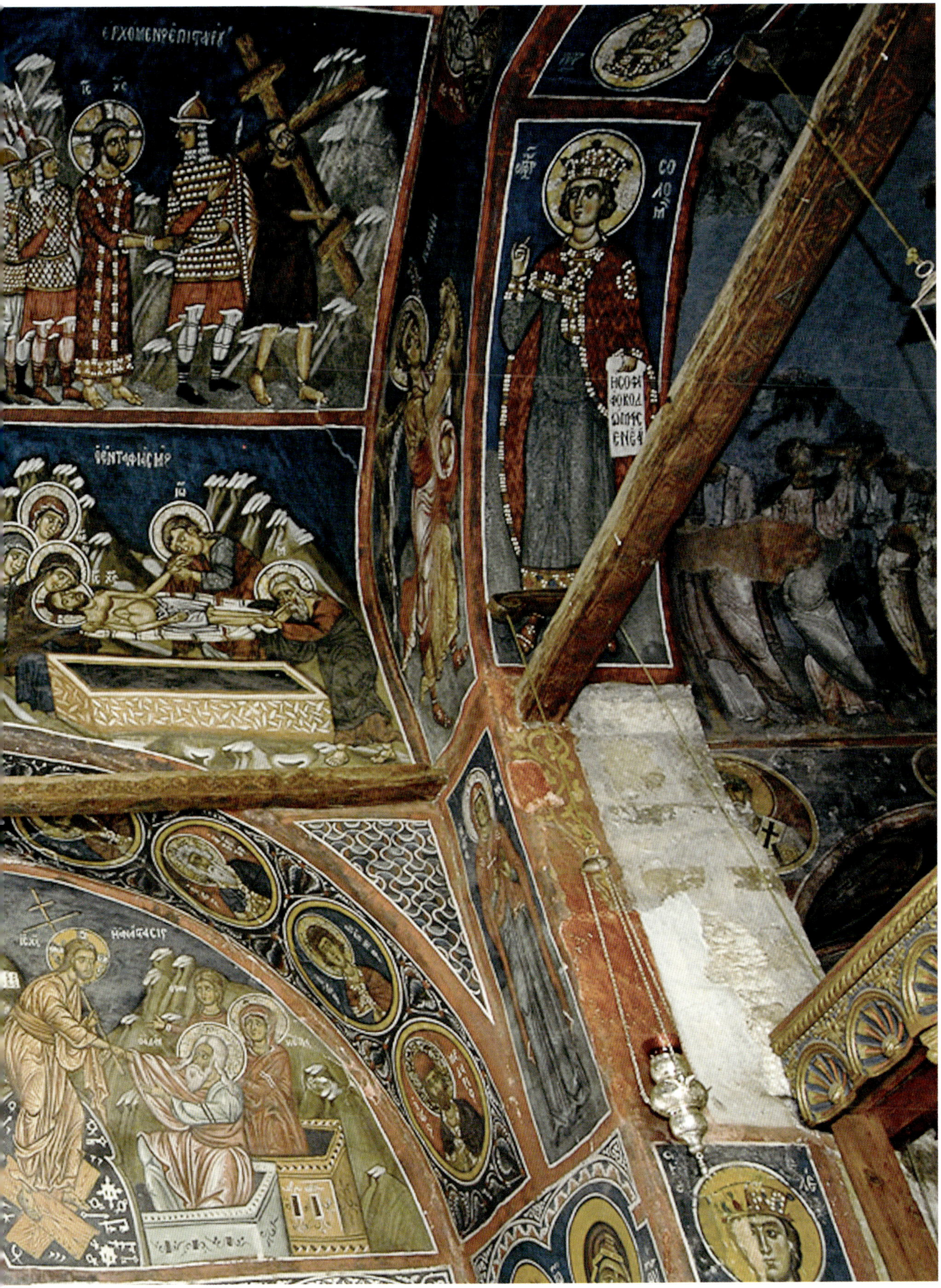

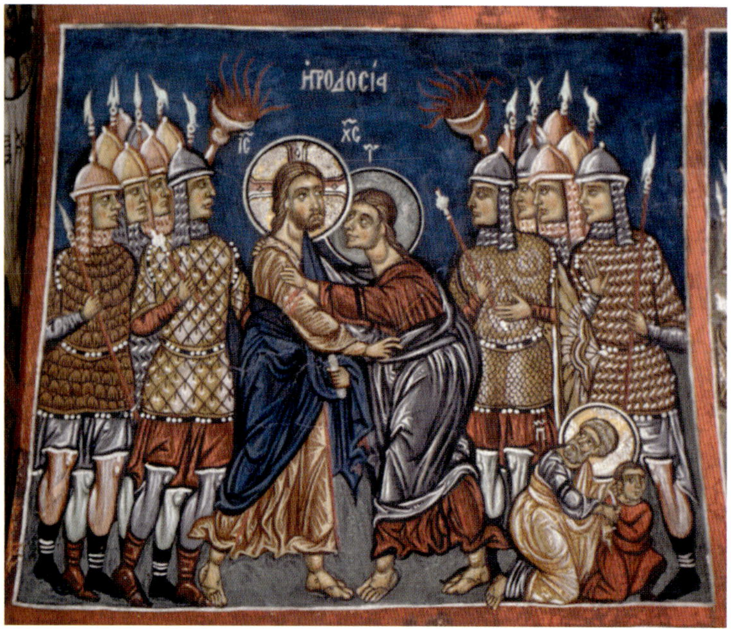

FIG. 6.43 Naos, central bay, north side of vault: Betrayal (photo courtesy of the Leventis Foundation and the Archaeological Research Unit, University of Cyprus, No. 006318)

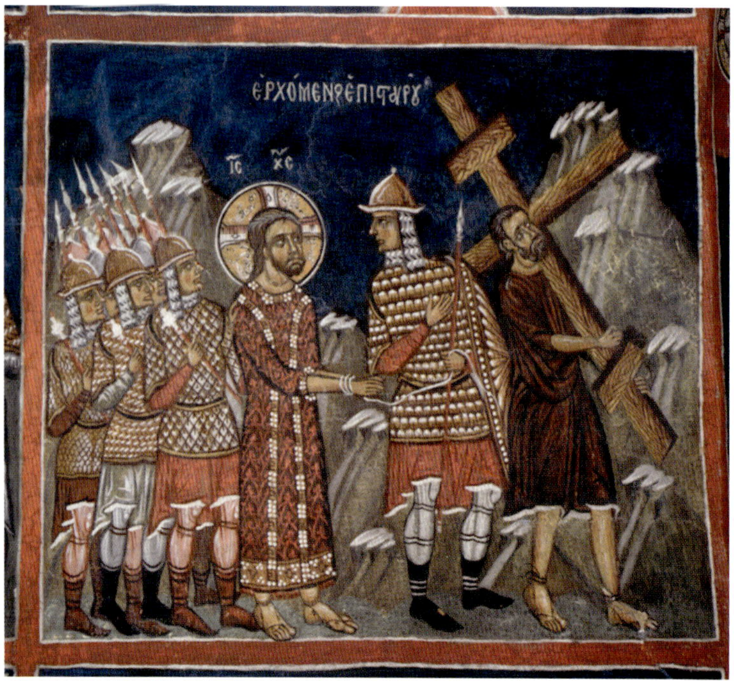

FIG. 6.44 Naos, central bay, north side of vault: Way to the Cross (photo courtesy of the Leventis Foundation and the Archaeological Research Unit, University of Cyprus, No. 006316)

More indicative of the scene's fourteenth-century refashioning may be its compositional efficiency, with the protagonists silhouetted against the bare ground and Christ reaching past Judas in the same direction as his stride to admonish Peter. The easy continuity of Jesus's forward gesture is best paralleled in the thirteenth century, in the Betrayal by Guido da Siena and in the churches of Euboia.[236] Similarly, the idea of framing the kiss against the bare ground, rather than in a churning ball of faces,[237] appears for the first time in the Enkleistra and the early thirteenth-century manuscript, Berlin, Staatsbibliothek, Graecus Quarto 66.[238] Thus it seems clear that, however rooted in early twelfth-century precedent the Betrayal might be, it has been rethought in fourteenth-century terms. The same composition is in fact repeated in the exactly contemporary Passion cycle at Pelendri.

The figure of Judas is especially interesting. His sycophantic profile is copied from the Judas of 1105/6 in the scene of the Last Supper on Asinou's west wall (Fig. 6.35). But his gray halo is an innovation. Judas was often shown unhaloed, but the negative halo is something else. Judas wears a gray halo in the Column churches,[239] but gray haloes

236. Stubblebine, *Guido da Siena*, fig. 25; Emmanuel, *Οἱ τοιχογραφίες τοῦ Ἁγ. Δημητρίου*, 64–67, fig. 15 for St. Demetrios in Makrychori, and fig. 45 for the Dormition church in Oxylithos.
237. Representative of the frontal type are the Betrayals in the Column churches and in San Marco, both cited in note 227 above. Representative of the type with Christ at the center of a churning ball of aggressors are the Betrayal at Monreale, also cited in note 227 above, and the miniature in the well-known Lectionary, Mount Athos, Dionysiou 587, folio 104v: see Pelekanides et al., *Treasures of Mount Athos*, 1: figs. 233–34.
238. For the Enkleistra, see Mango and Hawkins, "Hermitage," fig. 29; for Berlin Quarto 66, fol. 89r, see Carr, *Byzantine Illumination 1150–1250*, fiche 8D12. It recurs, then, in such Palaiologan works as St. Demetrios, Makrychori, of 1302 in Euboia: see Emmanuel, *Οἱ τοιχογραφίες τοῦ Ἁγ. Δημητρίου*, fig. 15; the Betrayal at Oxylithos is much the same: see ibid., fig. 45.
239. It is seen in both Karanlık and Çarıklı kilise, as seen well in the color reproduction in Yenipınar and Şahin, *Paintings of the Dark Church*, 83. I am indebted

appear on a number of figures there,[240] so gray was not distinctive to Judas. In Asinou, it is. This was not the case yet in the paintings of 1105/6, nor was it carried over into Pelendri. The same convention of the gray halo does appear, however, in the magnificent fourteenth-century Passion cycle in the south apse of the church of St. George of the Greeks in Famagusta. The gray halo had been used in 1281 in the superb fragmentary Betrayal from the church of the Virgin at Voulgarelion in Arta, and the motif may have reached Cyprus from Byzantium.[241] It was used in Trecento Italy, as well, however, and may have reached Cyprus from there.[242] The strongly Italianate architectural and ornamental motifs at St. George of the Greeks show how polyglot the art of the Lusignan cities was. The frescoes of St. George are too late to have inspired Asinou,[243] but they surely illustrate the kind of elite, cosmopolitan urban cycle from which a motif such as Judas's gray halo must have been adopted.

The Betrayal is followed by the WAY TO THE CROSS, labeled ἐρχόμενος ἐπι σταυροῦ (Figs. 6.42, 6.44).[244] Simon takes the lead, carrying a huge cross; a shield-bearing soldier follows him, pulling Christ (Ι(ησοῦ)ς / Χ(ριστό)ς) on a rope by his wrists, while the other soldiers take up the rear. Like the Betrayal, this scene was rare in middle Byzantine monumental cycles but retained a place in churches dedicated to the Cross, and it plays a pivotal role in the programs of both the Column churches and the Enkleistra.[245] The scene of the Way of the Cross became more widespread in thirteenth-century mural programs, reflecting their emphasis on the Passion, though at this point it joined with and was often displaced by the related scene of Christ at the foot of the already erected cross.[246] In Cyprus the scene retained a place in monumental cycles

to the Stylianous for pointing out the gray haloes in the Column churches, and heartily appreciate their complaint about the problems of working from black-and-white reproductions.

240. The disciples in the Last Supper, for instance, have alternating ocher and gray haloes, and in the Transfiguration the halo of Christ is gray. See the color reproductions of Karanlık kilise in Yenipınar and Şahin, *Paintings of the Dark Church*, 68–69 for the Last Supper and 89 for the Transfiguration.

241. Evans, *Byzantium, Faith and Power*, 86, no. 42; see also the Web site of the Byzantine Museum, Ioannina: http://hellas.teipir.gr/prefectures/greek/Ioanninon/Aksiotheata_Ioanninon/english_version/kastra-mouseia.htm

242. Schiller, *Iconography*, 2: fig. 105. I am indebted to Anne Derbes for drawing my attention to this. Later, in the 1430s, Fra Angelico would make the motif of Judas's anti-halo famous (ibid., 2: fig. 182).

243. Otten-Froux, "Un notaire vénitien à Famagouste," 42, 46, has published documents referring to the construction of the cathedral of St. George of the Greeks in the 1360s.

244. The scene has been studied extensively: Millet, *Recherches*, 362–79; Schiller, *Iconography*, 2:78–82; Wilk, "Die Darstellung der Kreuztragung Christi"; Katselake, "Ο Χριστός Ελκόμενος επί Σταυρού." It originated in early Christianity, was included at Sant'Apollinare Nuovo, and continued to be used in middle Byzantine manuscripts and icons though rarely in mural cycles, its frequency mounting with the growing interest in Passion imagery during the 12th century.

245. See Jolivet-Lévy, " Çarıklı Kilise," 310–11, on the way it guides the eye in Çarıklı and Karanlık; in the Enkleistra, it leads the eye around the corner to the wall where both the Crucifixion and the Cross relic itself were displayed: see Mango and Hawkins, "Hermitage," figs. 31, 32, 34.

246. An exemplary early instance of this second image is the great late 12th-century Cypriot icon in the Church of the Holy Cross, Pelendri; see Carr, "Thoughts on Seeing Christ Helkomenos." The jockeying of the two images is well illustrated by the churches of Kerkyra: see Chatzidakis and Bitha, *Ευρετήριο βυζαντινών τοιχογραφίων*, 32, pls. 10–11; 80, fig. 11; and 78, fig. 8 (St. Andrew, Perlengianika of the late 13th century); 252, pl. 1; and 255, pls. 7–8 (St. Nicholas, Noligates, of the 13th century). Both images were known as the "Helkomenos epi Stavrou" ([Christ] Drawn to the Cross), though the second image eventually preempted the title, and was later condensed to the powerful single-figure icon known from Cretan painting: see Foskolou, "Αναζητώντας την εικόνα του Ελκομένου." I am indebted to Sophia Kalopissi-Verti for alerting me to this article.

throughout the Middle Ages,[247] presumably because of the importance of the Cross relics on the island, and perhaps also because a segment of the rope, still venerated at Omodos Monastery today, may have been in Cyprus in the Middle Ages.[248] The Way to the Cross appeared in the naos at Koutsovendis and the narthex at the Apsinthiotissa in the early twelfth century and again in the Enkleistra at the end of the century;[249] it balances the Betrayal on the crossarms of the early fourteenth-century silver cross at Pano Lefkara;[250] and it figures in the fourteenth century not only at Asinou, but also in the church of the Holy Cross, Pelendri, and the Church of St. George of the Greeks in Famagusta. Of the four surviving fourteenth-century cycles on Cyprus, only that of the tiny Armenian church in Famagusta omits it. This steady recurrence, especially in the two early twelfth-century churches, makes it possible that the scene was included also in 1105/6 at Asinou. If so, however, it was wholly rethought in the fourteenth century: the man who leads Jesus, and the posse who follow him, are all armed soldiers;[251] Jesus's red garment is richly adorned with pearls;[252] and the cross carried by Simon is painted with a vigorous wood grain.[253] The sequence of figures, the garments, and the vigorously wood-grained cross all recur at the Church of St. George of the Greeks, Famagusta; by contrast, the version at Pelendri, though nearly identical in style to the one in Asinou, is quite different in composition. All three versions gain richness from Christ's robe, the armor, and the wood-grained cross. These fourteenth-century additions are what give the scene at Asinou its visual weight within the grid; the more modest version of the early twelfth century—if in fact used there—could not have had comparable force.

The CRUCIFIXION (ἡ σταύ/ροσις) occupies the next place, below the Betrayal (Figs. 6.42, 6.45). Over Christ's drooping head, with its crown of thorns, the title bar of the cross reads ὁ βασιλεῦ(ς) τις δόξις, "king of glory"; on its arms are his sigla, Ι(ησοῦ)ς / Χ(ριστό)ς. Below his right arm are three women, labeled in sequence from the left Μ(αρία),

247. Little is known of the cross relics on Cyprus before the Lusignan period, when they became very active, but the Abbot Daniel gives a vivid description of his visit to the relics on Stavrovouni in 1103, so they were already known at the time Koutsovendis and Asinou received their wall paintings: see Wilkinson, *Jerusalem Pilgrimage*, 125–26. See also Mango and Hawkins, "Hermitage," 124 n. 12 on early 12th-century evidence about Cyprus's relics of the cross.

248. Hackett, *History*, 454.

249. Mango, "Monastery of St. Chrysostom," 83, figs. 103, 104; Chotzakoglou, "Βυζαντινή αρχιτεκτονική και τέχνη," 2: fig. 442–43; Mango and Hawkins, "Hermitage," figs. 31, 32, 34. The paintings at the Apsinthiotissa no longer survive.

250. Papageorgiou, "Ο σταυρός των Λευκάρων," 2: fig. 133, 3.

251. On the militarization of scenes of the Passion, see notes 232 and 233 above.

252. As it is in St. Nicholas, Prilep, of 1298 (Millet, *La peinture du Moyen Âge*, 3: fig. 24, 3), and the church of the Panagia at Spilies, Euboia, of 1311 (Katselake, "Ο Χριστός Ελκόμενος επί Σταυρού," fig. 2).

253. The illusionistically painted wood grain, adopted widely on Cyprus after Asinou, was pervasive also in Trecento Italy, and it was probably from Italy that Cypriot painters learned how to achieve it. Perhaps most brilliantly employed by Pietro Lorenzetti in his Passion scenes in the Lower Church at Assisi, it is used as early as ca. 1300 by Pietro Cavallini in a Crucifixion at S. Domenico Maggiore, Naples, and then is found in many places. For Lorenzetti, see Carli, *La pittura Senese*, fig. 175 with the Crucifixion, fig. 178 with the Deposition; for Cavallini, see Castelnuovo, *La pittura in Italia*, 2:746. Other examples, all drawn from Castelnuovo, include a beautiful panel painting of the Deposition from the Cross by Pietro da Rimini of ca. 1320 (1: fig. 307), a fresco of the Crucifixion by an Emilian master of the first decade of the 14th century at Chiaravalle della Colomba near Piacenza (1: fig. 299), a Crucifixion of ca. 1355 by a Venetian painter, Vigo di Cadore, at St. Orsola (1: fig. 223), and a fresco of the Crucifixion by a Piedmontese master at Sant'Andrea, Savigliano (1: fig. 71). In the very late 14th century it is encountered occasionally also in Cretan painting: see Spatharakis, *Byzantine Wall Paintings of Crete*, fig. 249 with the Deposition at the church of the Panagia, Roustika, of 1391; idem, *Dated Byzantine Wall Paintings*, fig. 119 with the Lamentation at the church of St. John the Baptist, Kritsa, Merambellou, Lassithi, of 1389–90.

Μ(ήτ)ηρ Θ(εο)ῦ, and Μαρία. Under his left arm are John (Ιω(άννης)) and Longinus (Λ(ογγῖνος)). A half-length angel hovers at each end of the cross-arm, bracketing between them the sun and moon. The Crucifixion was surely a component of the initial cycle, and its *dramatis personae* remain very conventional. Its emphatic frontality is novel, however. Pressed to the picture plane, the figures are enlarged as much as possible, with the figures of John and Longinus even cut at knee level, as if in a close-up. Their immediacy is reinforced by the outward-facing turn of John and by the Mother of God; their gazes move out toward the viewer along the very diagonals that, in turn, draw the gaze of the viewer back inward toward Christ. Thus the central image claims attention, bringing the viewer's eye to a full stop. The words "king of glory" were first used in Cyprus only around 1200 and so are unlikely to copy an image of 1105/6.[254] The posture of Mary, supported not at the shoulders but around the waist, becomes frequent only in post-Byzantine art,[255] while John's outward gesture is unparalleled.[256] Assuredly used in the original cycle, then, the Crucifixion was equally surely rethought by the fourteenth-century painter(s).

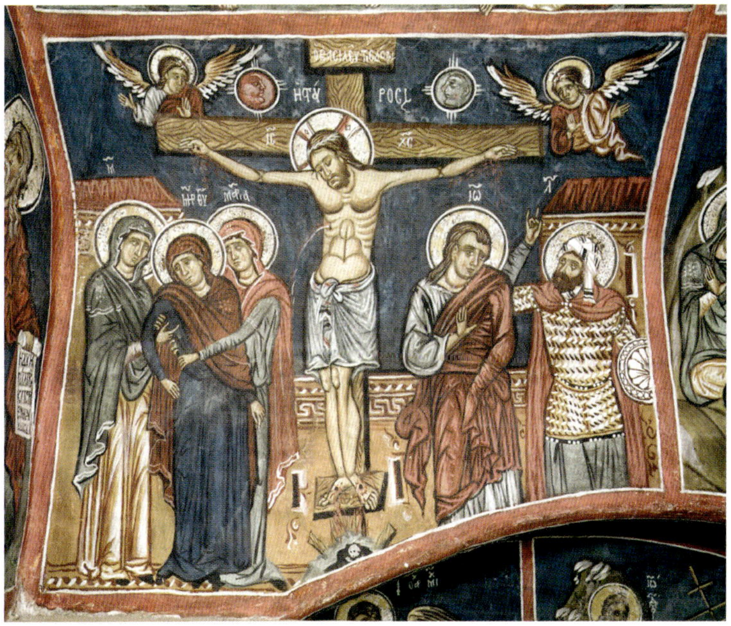

FIG. 6.45 Naos, central bay, north side of vault: Crucifixion (photo courtesy of the Leventis Foundation and the Archaeological Research Unit, University of Cyprus, No. 006317)

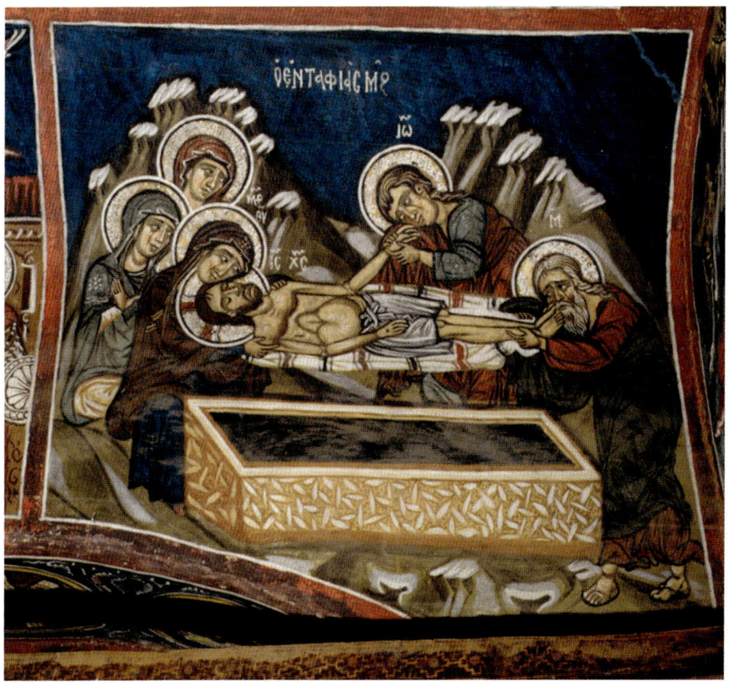

FIG. 6.46 Naos, central bay, north side of vault: Entombment (photo courtesy of the Leventis Foundation and the Archaeological Research Unit, University of Cyprus, No. 006344)

254. The formula is already found in early 11th-century Byzantine art, as in the beautiful triptych in the Cabinet des Médailles in Paris usually assigned to the 10th century: *Byzance: L'art byzantin dans les collections publiques françaises*, 236–37, no. 150. Kalavrezou-Maxeiner, "Eudokia Makrembolitissa and the Romanos Ivory," 324, dates it in the 11th century. In Cyprus the formula is seen in the naos at the Enkleistra and at Monagri; perhaps significantly, however, it does not figure in the two earlier images of the Crucifixion at the Enkleistra. Thus it may have become customary only around 1200. On the Enkleistra see Mango and Hawkins, "Hermitage," figs. 35 (naos), 89 (cell), and 106 (tomb); for Monagri see Boyd, "Church of the Panagia Amasgou," fig. 31.
255. As in the Crucifixion by Ioseph Houris (Papageorgiou, *Icons of Cyprus* [1992], pl. 132), or the 16th-century fresco at St. Andronikos, Kalopanayiotis (Stylianou and Stylianou, *Painted Churches*, figure 191).
256. John lowers his right hand from his face in the beautiful late 12th-century Crucifixion icon in Nicosia (Papageorgiou, *Icons of Cyprus* [1969], 27), but not in a gesture toward the viewer.

The episode that follows the Crucifixion is the most interesting in the cycle (Figs. 6.42, 6.46). It is labeled ὁ ἐνταφιάσμὅς or ENTOMBMENT, and shows the body of Jesus (Ι(ησοῦ)ς / Χ(ριστό)ς) hovering above an open stone sarcophagus. Mary (Μ(ήτ)ηρ Θ(εο)ῦ), attended by two women, cradles his head, while John (Ιω(άννης)) bends to raise Christ's left hand and a gray-bearded man, labeled "M," but surely Joseph of Arimathea, kisses his feet.

The name "Entaphiasmos" was adopted for any of a range of images evolved to fill the narrative gap between the removal of Christ's body from the cross and its placement in the tomb.[257] Middle Byzantine art characteristically focused on one of two: the lament over the body of Jesus, or its transport to the cave tomb. The former centered on the Mother of God; the latter initially excluded her, but soon evolved a synthesis of her lament and the walk to the tomb that culminated in the running lamentations of the late twelfth century.[258] Then, in the Palaiologan period, a different pair of scenes was favored, one showing the body exposed for shrouding on the stone of unction, and the other the fully shrouded mummy being carried by male mourners to the tomb, often followed by mourning women.[259] The change reflected the new prominence of the "red stone" of unction on which Jesus's body was supposed to have been prepared for burial. The stone had been installed in Constantinople by the emperor Manuel I Komnenos, and in the wake of its installation there it had begun to figure in art: Spatharakis signals its appearance already in the Georgian Gelati Gospels around 1170;[260] Millet associates it with the late twelfth-century figure of Christ in the sanctuary at Samari;[261] and, a half-century later, the scene of the lament on the stone began to acquire the new name of "Epitaphios Threnos."[262] In Crusader Jerusalem, too, the site of the preparation of the body was clothed in a special stone revetment.[263] These four "moments"—the lament, the running lament, the exposure on the stone of unction, and the transport—constitute the canonical history of the Entombment. But there was a fifth "moment" in the story, as well. This scene assumed brief but widespread prominence in the thirteenth century before being displaced by the lament at the stone of unction in Palaiologan art. It showed the body being

257. Characteristically signaled in modern parlance by the title "Threnos," the complex of scenes surrounding the lamentation of Jesus's body has been extensively discussed. See in particular Millet, *Recherches*, 489–516; Schiller, *Iconography*, 2:168–76; Weitzmann, "Origin of the Threnos"; M. Soteriou, "Ενταφιασμὸς—θρῆνος"; Hadermann-Misguich, *Kurbinovo*, 1:155–58. The title used here is applied to a range of compositions. Thus while the scene of Mary lamenting over Jesus's body at the base of the cross is called ὁ ἐνταφιασμός in both the Cathedral of the Transfiguration, Mirozhsky Monastery, Pskov, and the Gospel book in Parma, Biblioteca Palatina 5, 90v (Lazarev, *Storia*, figure 243), this title is applied at Asinou and in the Vatican steatite cited below in note 276 to the scene of the body over the sarcophagus, in Vatopedi to the lament over the stone of unction (Millet, *Recherches*, figure 561), and at Staro Nagoričino to the scene of Joseph of Arimathea and Nicodemus carrying the body to the cave tomb (Millet, *La peinture du Moyen Âge*, 3: figure 93, 2).

258. Seen at Kurbinovo (Hadermann-Misguich, *Kurbinovo*, 2: figure 75) and the church of the Anargyroi, Kastoria (ibid., figure 76). It was first intimated in images like the one in Vatican, gr. 1156, where the lamenting Mary sits in a "Knielauf" posture suggesting motion: Maguire, "Depiction of Sorrow," figure 38; M. Soteriou, "Ενταφιασμὸς—θρῆνος," figure 49, 2.

259. In Millet, *Monuments de l'Athos*, see the Protaton (figure 25), Chilandar (figure 73, 1), and Vatopedi (figure 93, 1 and 2); in idem, *La peinture du Moyen Âge*, vol. 3, see figs. 9, 3 and 26, 1 (Peribleptos, Ohrid); fig. 26, 1 (St. Nicholas, Prilep); and fig. 93, 2 (St. George, Staro Nagoričino). See also the Christ church, Veroia (Gounares, *Χριστός Βέροιας*, figure 34), St. Nicholas Orphanos (Tsitouridou, *Ο ζωγραφικὸς διάκοσμος*, figure 44), the Olympiotissa at Elasson (Constantinides, *Wall Paintings of the Panagia Olympiotissa*, 1: figure 126), and the churches in Mistra: see Millet, *Monuments byzantins de Mistra*, figure 88, 2 for the SS. Theodore; 122, 4 for the Peribleptos.

260. Spatharakis, "Influence of the Lithos," fig. 4.

261. Millet, *Recherches*, figure 536; Grigoriadou-Cabagnols, "Le décor peint," 182–84, figs. 4, 5.

262. As it does in Merenta: Coumbaraki-Pansélinou, *Saint-Pierre de Kalyvia-Kouvara*, figure 75.

263. Millet, *Recherches*, 498.

mourned before or while being placed in an open sarcophagus. Distinctive to this composition are the floating figure of Christ and the open sarcophagus placed prominently beneath it.[264]

The open sarcophagus was a staple of western European scenes of Christ's lamentation and burial throughout the Middle Ages.[265] In Byzantium, by contrast, the sarcophagus was rarely shown before the thirteenth century.[266] Three manuscripts of around the year 1200—Berlin Quarto 66, Harley 1810, and Mytilene 9—included an open sarcophagus in scenes of the holy women mourning Jesus's body.[267] And then, at mid-century, paintings in a range of media throughout the Mediterranean world portrayed the Mother of God lamenting her Son at a sarcophagus. In six of them Mary sits on or just over the sarcophagus, cradling in her lap the floating body of her son, stretched on its striped burial cloth. The best known of these are two Italian paintings—the Perugia polyptych by the St. Francis Master of ca. 1272,[268] and a mural at the church of the Holy Apostles in Venice[269]—that show her atop the closed tomb box. The other four monuments, of much the same date, modify this image by showing the box open, presenting it unequivocally as a sarcophagus. One of these is a Crusader icon at Mount Sinai;[270] the second is a wall painting at Merenta in Greece;[271] the third is a wall painting in the church of the Panagia at Myriokephala on Crete;[272] and the fourth—dated 1310—is the dramatic mural at the church of the Transfiguration in Pyrgi, Euboia.[273] Christ's body floats in all of them above the open tomb; at Sinai, Merenta, and Pyrgi the Mother of God still sits atop the sarcophagus, despite the fact that it is now open; in Crete she hovers in the landscape above it, and it is John the Evangelist who stands on the box. Asinou adopts a similar variant. Finally, three further images alter Mary's position more fundamentally, showing her not seated but bent over the body as it is lowered into the sarcophagus by mourning companions, among them the Magdalene, her hands thrown high in grief.[274]

264. Coumbaraki-Pansélinou, *Saint-Pierre de Kalyvia-Kouvara*, 145–46, discusses this image.

265. See the various images of the Entombment in western medieval art reproduced in Schiller, *Iconography*, 2: figs. 568, 570, 571, 573, 575–77.

266. The 10th-century Lectionary, St. Petersburg, Public Library, gr. 21, 7v, shows the holy women mourning beside a sarcophagus (Schiller, *Iconography*, 2: figure 565), a vignette repeated in the early 13th-century Gospel book, Berlin, Quarto 66, 96r, with the shrouded body visible inside (Carr, *Byzantine Illumination 1150–1250*, fiche 8E2; Hamann-MacLean, "Der Berliner Codex Graecus Quarto 66," figure 3; Maguire, "Depiction of Sorrow," figs. 18, 19, excellently juxtaposed with the scene in the St. Petersburg Lectionary). In the 11th-century frescoes in the crypt of Hosios Loukas, John and Joseph of Arimathea lower the body into a sarcophagus as Mary watches (Connor, *Art and Miracles*, fig. 68), and Florence, Biblioteca Laurenziana, Plut. VI 23, 201v shows Mary Magdalene on Easter morning before an empty sarcophagus (Velmans, *Le Tétraévangile*, pl. 64, fig. 299).

267. The scene of the holy women in Berlin, Quarto 66, is cited in the preceding note; London, British Library, Harley 1810, fol. 205v, includes the sarcophagus in the scene of Mary and John carrying the body to the tomb (Carr, *Byzantine Illumination, 1150–1250*, fiche 7A2), and Mytilene, Boys' Gymnasium, cod. 9, fol. 147v, includes it in the scene of the women on Easter morning (Vocotopoulos, "L'Évangile illustré de Mytilène," figure 237r).

268. Gordon, "Perugian Provenance." The image is well reproduced in Schiller, *Iconography*, 2: fig. 597.

269. Millet, *Recherches*, 508–9, fig. 555.

270. Weitzmann, "Thirteenth-Century Crusader Icons," fig. 12.

271. Coumbaraki-Pansélinou, *Saint-Pierre de Kalyvia-Kouvara*, pl. 75.

272. Spatharakis, *Byzantine Wall Paintings of Crete*, 145, fig. 194, color pl. 16b. Calling this scene unique ("Influence of the Lithos," 437), Spatharakis dates it to the very early 12th century, but I believe the schematic linearity of the forms rather suggests a date a century later.

273. This is reproduced in color in Liares, *Μεσαιωνικά μνημεία Εὐβοίας*, fig. IB′. What looks like a red stone of unction here in fact displays a long black rectangle below the floating body of Christ that can only be interpreted as the open mouth of the sarcophagus. Mary sits atop it.

274. The silver Cross reliquary at Pano Lefkara of the early 14th century shows a very similar Lamentation, though without the Magdalene. Here, however, it is difficult to tell whether the body lies on an exceptionally high stone of unction or in a sarcophagus. See Papageorgiou, "Ο σταυρός των Λευκάρων," 2: fig. 134, 5.

The Threnos at Pelendri, Asinou's close stylistic sibling, is the first of these images;[275] the second is a steatite in the Vatican attributed to the late thirteenth century (Fig. 6.48);[276] and the third is a panel from the circle of Guido da Siena.[277] It is with this last example that the image finds its customary art-historical niche: it became the canonical Italian Trecento image of the lament, with the clustered companions lowering the body into the open tomb. The composition had a briefer life in the Byzantine tradition, where the sarcophagus continued to figure in Palaiologan art but not in the lament.

The imagery of the sarcophagus outlined above took form in the thirteenth century, in the period most affected by the Crusader expansion. It surely became current in Byzantium as a result of contact with the West, and most probably at the site of the Passion itself, in Jerusalem. Three factors suggest this. First, during the twelfth century the sarcophagus-shaped tomb of Christ had become as real an aspect of Holy Land topography, for Christians of all creeds, as the stone of unction. Newly revetted by the kings of Jerusalem,[278] it had been given a golden lid by the Byzantine emperor Manuel Komnenos himself, as the Greek pilgrim John Phokas noted with pride.[279] The revetment had three holes in the side through which pilgrims could reach to touch the actual stone; it may be these holes that are indicated by the arches on the sarcophagus as it is portrayed in Berlin Quarto 66 and the steatite in the Vatican cited above (Fig. 6.48). Thus the attention drawn by the Crusades to the site of salvation came to center on a box-shaped tomb. It responded readily to Western expectation, but was at the same time endorsed by Byzantine imperial patronage and venerated by Greek pilgrims. A second index to Jerusalem is the concentration of early images of the sarcophagus in books with Holy Land associations. All three of the manuscripts cited—Berlin Quarto 66, Harley 1810, and Mytilene 9—belong to the Decorative Style group, for which an eastern Mediterranean origin has been proposed.[280] A third factor pointing to Jerusalem is the composition in the Georgian Gelati Gospels (ca. 1170) depicting the mourning Virgin seated with the body of her son.[281] Both she and Christ assume precisely the postures seen in the images just inventoried, with Mary's lament on the sarcophagus. Here, however, Mary sits on the flat stone of unction. This is the earliest clear image of the red stone that is known, and the composition may have been developed specifically to portray it. The Georgians had a particularly strong presence in Jerusalem, and would plausibly be in the vanguard of developments there in Passion iconography. It may well have been there that the image of Mary atop the stone was incubated and there, in turn, that the image was adapted from the stone to serve for the sarcophagus, as well.

275. The Entombment here is dramatic, with the male mourners lowering the shrouded body into the sarcophagus as the Mother of God bends to kiss it and the Magdalene throws both hands in the air. This composition was repeated a century later in 1474 in the Archangel church at Pedoulas (Stylianou and Stylianou, *Painted Churches*, 336). A similar composition appears also in St. George in Vasa: see V. Karageorghis, *ARDAC* for 1981, 16, fig. 12. With its bevy of extravagantly mourning women at one side, including the Magdalene with arms thrown high, the composition looks 15th-century, but it is difficult to judge it accurately from the published photograph.

276. Morello, *Splendori di Bisanzio*, 198–99, no. 80, where it is attributed to Venice and reproduced in color, but unfortunately in mirror-image; Kalavrezou-Maxeiner, *Byzantine Icons in Steatite*, 1:193–95; 2: pl. 118. The steatite's origin is not known, but its kinship to the scenes at Asinou suggests Cyprus. Steatite was carved in Cyprus from prehistoric times onward, and P. Hetherington, "Byzantine Reliquary at the Cathedral Museum," maintains his Cypriot attribution of the steatite diptych, now in Malta, with the arms of Hélion de Villeneuve, Grand Master of the Hospitallers (1319–46).

277. Millet, *Recherches,* 509, fig. 542.

278. Folda, *Art of the Crusaders in the Holy Land*, 82.

279. Wilkinson, *Jerusalem Pilgrimage*, 324, ¶14.18.

280. See Carr, *Byzantine Illumination*, 142–55; eadem, "Cyprus and the Decorative Style."

281. Fol. 85v: Spatharakis, "Influence of the Lithos," 437, fig. 4; Velmans, *La peinture murale byzantine*, fig. 100; Millet, *Recherches*, figure 533.

The twelve examples of the lament with the sarcophagus are striking for their geographical extent. They represent a broad cross-section of the Mediterranean, from Tuscany and the Veneto to southern Greece, Euboia, the islands, and the Holy Land itself. As such, they reflect a brief phase of iconographic homogeneity across the Mediterranean, in which shared motifs emerged in Italian and Orthodox art simultaneously, in a way that makes it impossible to assign them an origin in one culture or the other. They belong equally to both. A range of notable compositions can be associated with this brief but fertile phase of iconographic convergence.[282] Anne Derbes studied many of these;[283] the composition of the Doubting Thomas seen at Pelendri, analyzed by Ioanna Christoforaki, reflects the same paths of interchange.[284] This phase of iconographic community plays a significant role at Asinou, because not only the Entombment but also the star in the cave at the Nativity, the compact design of the Betrayal, and the Virgin of Mercy in the narthex (Fig. 5.1) all belong to it. The Entombment clarifies this layer, and with it the artistic history that lies behind the fourteenth-century murals at Asinou.

The Entombment is the first subject in Asinou's vault that cannot have been included in the program of 1105/6. On turning from the south to the north side of the vault, it had seemed that the scenes of the Betrayal and the Way to the Cross marked a definitive break from the liturgical formality of the feast scenes to a new narrative simplicity. But in fact it is still possible that the Betrayal and the Way to the Cross had appeared in the early twelfth-century program. The Entombment, by contrast, emerged only a century and a half after the original cycle was finished. The presence of the Entombment does not exclude the possibility that its place was initially occupied by the traditional lament of the Virgin over the body stretched on the ground, for this was popular in Cyprus and survives in three twelfth-century versions.[285] But the adoption of the Entombment had implications for the rest of the program: it demanded a new sequel.

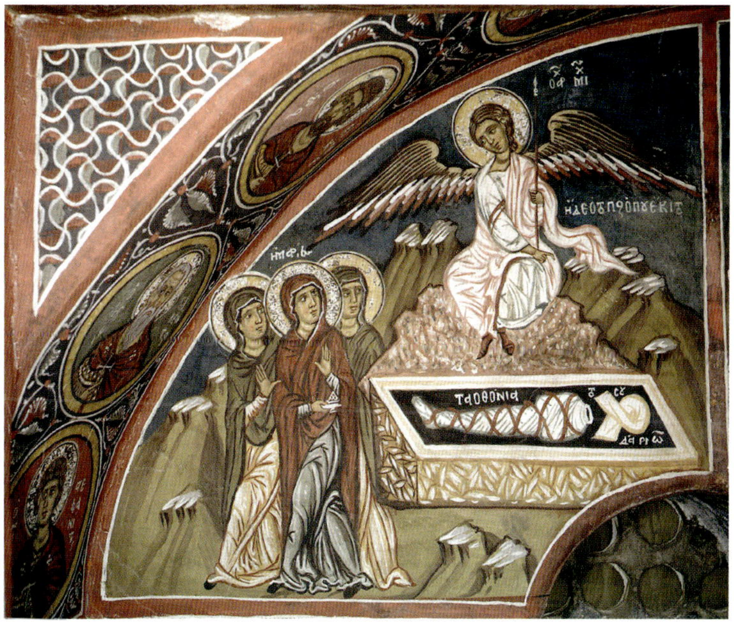

FIG. 6.47 Naos, central bay, north lunette: Women at the Tomb (photo courtesy of the Leventis Foundation and the Archaeological Research Unit, University of Cyprus, No. 006346)

282. An especially durable and widespread example is the composition of the Deposition from the Cross: see Millet, "L'art des Balkans et d'Italie." It is seen in the Francis Master's Perugia Polyptych (Millet, *Recherches*, figure 514; Gordon, "Perugian Provenance," figure 8), Guido da Siena's Palazzo Pubblica Madonna (Stubblebine, *Guido da Siena*, fig. 29), the Protaton (Millet, *Monuments de l'Athos*, pl. 27, 2), the reverse of the Cypriot icon of the Athanasiotissa (Papageorgiou, *Icons of Cyprus* [1992], fig. 49), and again in a Coptic panel of the 14th century published by Skalova, "Mourning with Indigo," fig. 2d.

283. Derbes, *Picturing the Passion in Late Medieval Italy*; eadem, "Siena and the Levant in the Later Dugento."

284. Christoforaki, "An Unsual Representation of the Incredulity."

285. See Mango and Hawkins, "Hermitage," 151 and fig. 120 for the scene from the ruined church at Koutsovendis, and fig. 36 for the remains of the Threnos at the Enkleistra. The scene at Kiti is unpublished.

The open sarcophagus that had given the Entombment its distinctive configuration appears again in the ensuing scene of the WOMEN AT THE EMPTY TOMB (Figs. 6.42, 6.47). Though untitled, it depicts the events of Easter morning. Three women, labeled ἡ Μαριε(ς), "the Maries," move in lockstep across a landscape that displays in its foreground the open sarcophagus, and, at its apex, the angel (ὁ ἀρχ(άγγελος) / Μιχ(αήλ)). The open sarcophagus now shows not the body but the empty burial wrappings, identified in accord with John 20:7 as τα οθόνια, "the shroud," and το / σου/δαριων "the sudarium."[286] Above the angel are words from Matthew 28:6: ἤδε ο τόπος ὁπου ἔκιτο, that is, ἴδετε τὸν τόπον ὅπου ἔκειτο, "See the place where he was laid." Having the angel speak in this way accords with the loquacity of Asinou's twelfth-century cycle, where Mary speaks across the bema opening to Jesus, Gabriel and the Virgin enact the Annunciation, the donor speaks to Mary, and the scenes speak by poetic inscriptions to the viewer. As such, it suggests that we have returned at this point to the imagery of 1106.

The scene of the Women at the Empty Tomb appeared widely in middle Byzantine art, including mural painting, and its composition throughout this period was stable, with the angel to one side on a boxlike block before the tomb, and two women approaching from the other side.[287] Then, in the late thirteenth and early fourteenth centuries, this formula gave way to a new, three-dimensional conception of the event in which three or even four women walk away from an open sarcophagus,[288] as if down a winding slope, while one or two angels sit atop its lid. The scene at Asinou, with its open sarcophagus and three walking women on the one hand, and its asymmetrical composition on the other, offers itself as a simple updating of a traditional middle Byzantine precursor of 1106.

Three factors suggest instead that the scene of the Women at the Empty Tomb was a new addition in the fourteenth century, to function in tandem with the scene of the Entombment. The theme itself, in the first place, was not the feast icon for Easter; this role was given to the Anastasis, and the great majority of middle Byzantine monumental cycles omitted it in favor of the Anastasis. In fact all the middle Byzantine cycles that we know on Cyprus omitted it. Thus the scene had no precedent there. The angel's words, reminiscent though they are of the "speaking" compositions of Komnenian art,[289] were quite as frequent in the fourteenth century; they appear on the Vatican steatite cited earlier (Fig. 6.48). The scene's twelfth-century roots, then, are tenuous. On the other hand, the version with the open sarcophagus was used consistently

286. On the words, see Mouriki, *Οἱ τοιχογραφίες τοῦ Σωτῆρα*, 25–28. The two textiles were often depicted in the upright cave tomb; only rarely, however, were they labeled. They are labeled at Kurbinovo: see Hadermann-Misguich, *Kurbinovo*, 1:159, 2: fig. 78, who calls the labels rare.

287. For the Column churches, see Restle, *Byzantine Wall Painting*, 2:211 (Çarıklı kilise); 2:239 (Karanlık kilise). These are reproduced in color in Yenipınar and Şahin, *Paintings of the Dark Church*, 86. The Cathedral of the Transfiguration, Mirozhsky Monastery, Pskov, offers a good mid-12th-century example: see Yamshchikov, *Pskov*, fig. 17. For an example from the late 12th century, see Kurbinovo in Hadermann-Misguich, *Kurbinovo*, 1:158–59; 2: fig. 78.

288. Three women are seen in the SS. Theodore, Mistra (Millet, *Monuments byzantins de Mistra*, fig. 8, 5); a number of the Serbian cycles including Prilep (Millet, *La peinture du Moyen Âge*, 3: fig. 26, 3), Staro Nagoričino (ibid., 3: fig. 85, 3), and Peć (Petković, *La peinture serbe*, 1: fig. 68a); and all of the Cypriot cycles, including the Church of St. George of the Greeks in Famagusta, St. Herakleidios at St. John Lampadistes in Kalopanayiotis, SS. Kerykos and Ioulitta in Letympou, and probably St. Catherine, Pyrga, though here there may be four. There are four at Vatopedi in Millet, *Monuments de l'Athos*, fig. 93, 2; and Gračanica: Petković, *La peinture serbe*, 1: fig. 44c. The issue of the identity of Mary of Bethany, and thus which and how many of the women came to the tomb, became especially aggravated in the Latin Kingdom of Jerusalem: Kedar, "Gerald of Nazareth," 55–57. As with the militarization of the soldiers around Christ in the Betrayal and the Way to the Cross, so here one wonders to what extent the motif still triggered a degree of partisan sensitivity.

289. On "speaking" images and their particular association with the 12th century see N. P. Ševčenko, "Close Encounters."

in the fourteenth- and fifteenth-century cycles on Cyprus: Pelendri, St. George of the Greeks, Pyrga, and St. Herakleidios all use it.[290]

Moreover—and this is the second point to consider here—those examples all use it in conjunction with the scene of the Entombment with an open sarcophagus. The form taken by the Entombment varies: Christ is mourned at Asinou as his body hovers outside the sarcophagus, at Pelendri as it is lowered into the sarcophagus, at Kalopanayiotis and Pyrga as it lies in the sarcophagus, and in Famagusta as it is carried to the sarcophagus. In each, however, there is a deliberate dialectic between the Entombment and Easter morning, as the open sarcophagus on the one hand receives the body, and on the other hand displays its absence. This is nowhere more evident than at St. George of the Greeks, where the south apse displays a grid of four scenes, with the Deposition above the Entombment, the Anastasis over Easter morning. Thus the descent/ascent of the adjacent Deposition and Anastasis is answered in turn by the dialectic of the tomb that receives and the tomb that yields the body of Christ below. Much the same grid is seen in the Vatican steatite, cited already several times (Fig. 6.48).[291] There, the Crucifixion flanks the Entombment above, with Easter morning and the Anastasis below. The two registers—of abasement above and exaltation below—are bound together by the open sarcophagus with its contrasting contents. Exactly the same matrix of four scenes is found at Asinou, extending beyond the grid of the vault into the lunette. The conformity of not just the iconography but also the selection and organization

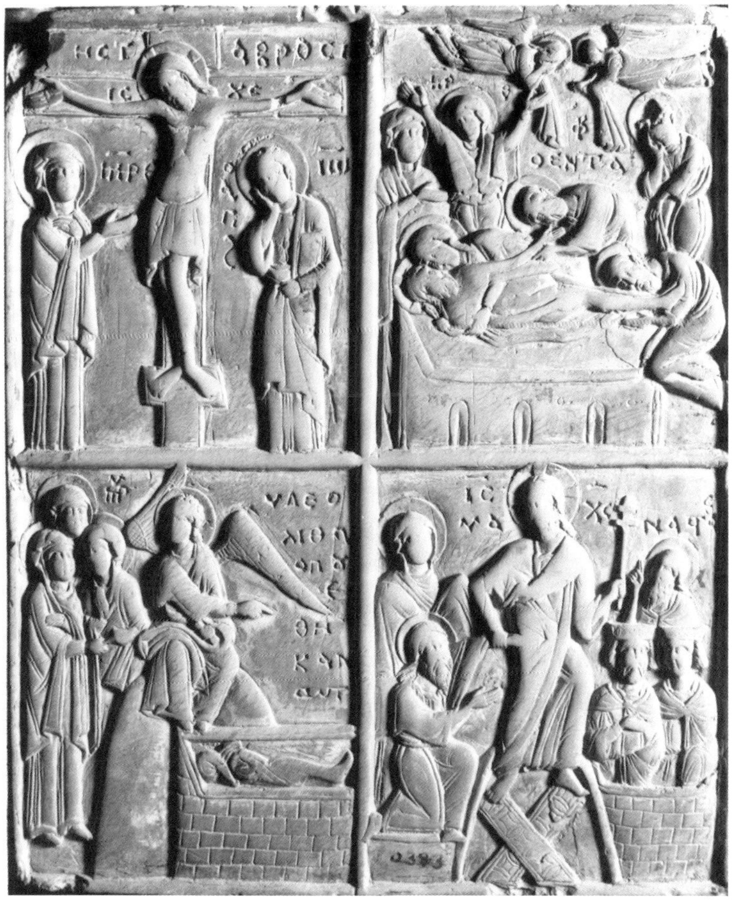

FIG. 6.48 Steatite with scenes of the Passion, late 13th century (photo courtesy of Vatican, Museo Sacro, No. 0393 [981])

290. The scenes at Pelendri are unpublished; of its post-Passion scenes, only the scene of Jesus appearing to the disciples at Galilee has been published: see V. Karageorghis, *ARDAC* for 1983, 19, figs. 11–12. The Entombment, described in note 275 above, is on the south side of the bema; Easter morning is on the eastern wall, along with Christ meeting his disciples at Galilee and the Palaiologan image of the *Noli me tangere* with Christ flanked by the two Maries. At the Church of St. George of the Greeks, the scene of the Entombment is balanced by one of Easter morning with two angels, one seated on the canted lid of the open sarcophagus and one on the hill behind: see Papageorgiou, "L'art byzantin de Chypre et l'art des Croisés," fig. 53, 3 and 4. At Pyrga, the sequence is idiosyncratic, with the women approaching a hole in the ground as an angel watches, and then a scene of the angel beside the sarcophagus and sleeping guards before it: see Emmanuel, "Monumental Painting in Cyprus," fig. 1. The motif of the grave as a hole in the ground is seen also in Mytilene, Boys' Gymnasium, cod. 9, 147v: see Vocotopoulos, "L'Évangile illustré de Mytilene," fig. 22. At St. Herakleidios, Jesus's enshrouded body in the sarcophagus dominates the lower portion of the Entombment. See illustration in Christoforaki, "Η τέχνη στη Κύπρο," fig. 16; while a similar sarcophagus, with the empty grave and burial cloths, dominates the lower portion of the Easter morning scene.

291. See above, note 276.

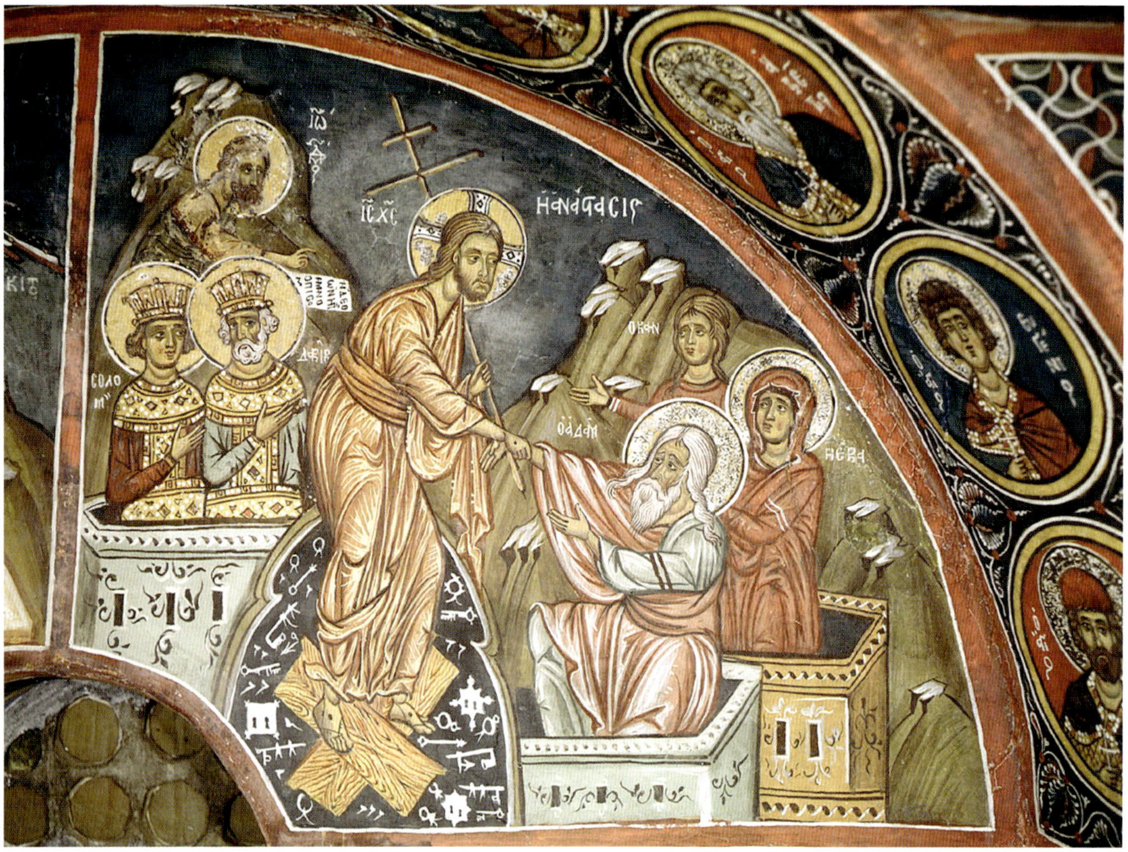

FIG. 6.49 Naos, central bay, north lunette: Anastasis (photo courtesy of the Leventis Foundation and the Archaeological Research Unit, University of Cyprus, No. 006342)

of the themes with the fourteenth-century examples makes it likely that the incorporation of the two episodes of the open sarcophagus was a fourteenth-century idea. This likelihood receives visual support from the fact that—in sharp contrast to the scenes above, the Betrayal and the Way to the Cross—these four respond to the images opposite them, the radiant angel of Easter morning wearing the same white clothing as the radiant Christ of the Transfiguration, and the abyss of Hades assuming the same triangular form as the river in the Baptism with its Hades-like personification of Jordan.[292] This kind of responsiveness seems to have characterized the fourteenth-century painter(s), as seen in the echoed gesture of Mary in the Annunciation and the Nativity, the play on the swaddling bands and waves of water in the Nativity and the Baptism, and the back-to-back alignment of Moses in the visions of the Transfiguration and the Burning Bush (Fig. 6.41). This reciprocation of imagery suggests that the fourteenth-century painter(s) introduced these scenes.

The third point at issue is the scenes' placement. To fit the full grid of four scenes into the space available, the painter was forced down into the lunette below the vault, giving it the same grid-like partition of scenes. Cypriot programs often packed the lunettes with multiple scenes;[293] the

292. The association of the Baptism and the Anastasis was long developed: see Kartsonis, *Anastasis: The Making of an Image*, 173–77.

293. The lunettes at Perachorio (Megaw and Hawkins, "Church of the Holy Apostles," figs. 30, 42) contain just one scene each, and they are beautifully coordinated

Asinou Master had done the same on the west wall. There, however, the subdivision of the lunette was counteracted by the monumental grandeur of the Dormition just below it (Figs. 2.25, 3.9). The donor portrait, which occupies the whole south lunette, gives the south wall a comparable monumentality (Fig. 6.37). It is tempting to believe that the north lunette, too, had a similar, monumental unity. The most likely candidate for this is the Anastasis, for it was not only a major feast but one that was emphasized at Asinou. Thus the poetic epigram on the north wall of the bema closes with a somewhat forced metaphor inviting the viewer to rejoice "seeing your resurrection (Anastasis)" (Fig. 3.2), as if invoking a scene of the Anastasis nearby and so tying the beginning of the painted cycle to its end; and a twelfth-century painting of the Anastasis just outside the north door (Fig. 2.18) seems to label it as the "Anastasis door." An Anastasis in the lunette would be in accord with these emphases. This presumes, however, that it occupied the full space, without the scene of Easter morning.

The scene of the ANASTASIS (Figs. 6.42, 6.49), labeled ἡ ἀνάστασις, shows Christ (Ι(ησοῦ)ς Χ(ριστό)ς) bending to the right to raise the protoparents Adam and Eve (ὁ Ἀδᾶμ and ἡ Ἐβα), while the prophets—John the Baptist (Ιω(άννης) / Πρ(ό)δ(ρο)μος), Solomon (Σολο/μ(ῶν)), and David (Δαβῖβ)—gather behind him.[294] This is the oldest of the types of the Anastasis, well attested in the eleventh century and plausibly composed around the window in the lunette in 1105/6. Even the inclusion of a child of Adam and Eve is possible in 1106, as a youth appears in the Anastasis at the Apsinthiotissa.[295] Only in later cases is this figure actually named.[296] The absence of a label in 1105/6 could help to explain his odd and surely erroneous identification as Cain (ο Καην) in the fourteenth-century painting. Only the scroll of the Baptist is clearly an addition to the traditional scene. First seen on Cyprus in 1183 in St. Neophytos's tomb in the Enkleistra and then repeated consistently in scenes of the Anastasis, the scroll bears a combination of words drawn from John 1:29–30: ήδε ο / ὼν ηπ'' / ημην ο / οπισο / μ, that is, ἴδε ὃν εἶπον ὑμῖν ὅτι ὀπίσω μου (ἔρχεται), "Behold the one of whom I said he comes after me."[297]

If plausible in 1105/6, however, the asymmetrical type of the Anastasis became widely popular once again in the Palaiologan period,[298] and is seen in fourteenth-century murals in both St. Nicholas of the Roof and Kato Lefkara.[299] Conceivable in 1105/6, the composition is yet more at home in the

with the architecture and with each other: Christ in the Dormition, literally displacing the window of the lunette to stand just over the north door, faces Christ of the Nativity, similarly aligned centrally over the south door. On the other hand, there are multiple scenes in the lunettes at both Koutsovendis (Mango, "Monastery of St. Chrysostom," figs. 9, 98, 103) and Kato Lefkara (Papageorgiou, "Ἡ ἐκκλησία τοῦ Ἀρχαγγέλου," fig. 40, showing the south lunette with scenes of the Nativity, the Presentation, the Baptism, and the Raising of Lazarus).

294. Kartsonis, *Anastasis*, 204, and figs. 63, 64, 67.

295. On the Apsinthiotissa, see Papageorgiou, *Christian Art*, 395–405. Kartsonis, *Anastasis*, 209–10, cites a son of Adam and Eve, surely Abel, also in Paris. gr. 74, fol. 64r, and the Skevophylakion Lectionary at the Laura on Mount Athos, now dated to much the same time as the initial Asinou program. For the Lectionary, see Pelekanides et al., *Οἱ θησαυροὶ τοῦ Ἁγίου Ὄρους*, fig. 6; and on its date, Anderson, *New York Cruciform Lectionary*, 98 n. 28. Abel's inclusion is often explained on the basis of a text assigned to the Cypriot St. Epiphanios: Kartsonis, *Anastasis*, 209–10; Der Nersessian, "Program and Iconography," 322.

296. The late 12th-century Abel in the Evangelistria in Geraki is among the earliest instances: see Moutsopoulos and Demetrokalles, *Γεράκι: Οἱ ἐκκλησίες τοῦ οἰκισμοῦ*, 130, fig. 200.

297. The text varies, often concluding with words to the effect that the one who comes will release humankind from the bonds of death: see Mango and Hawkins, "Hermitage of St. Neophytos," 185, and Nicolaïdès, "Étude iconographique," 91–92 with extensive bibliography on the phrase.

298. As pointed out by Mouriki, *Οἱ τοιχογραφίες τοῦ Σωτήρα*, 28–30.

299. The Anastasis at St. Nicholas of the Roof, though unpublished, is described in Stylianou and Stylianou, *Painted Churches*, 65. For Kato Lefkara, see Papageorgiou, "Ἡ ἐκκλησία τοῦ Ἀρχαγγέλου," fig. 46, 2.

fourteenth century. Thus it is hard to extract information from the Anastasis beyond the assertion that there was surely an image of the Anastasis in the twelfth-century program, and that without the intervention of the fourteenth-century group of four scenes bound together by the open sarcophagus, it is easy to imagine the Anastasis occupying the full lunette. The group of four functions as an intellectual unit, and it exacted as the price of its use the extension of the grid format into the lunette beneath the vault.

The Christological Scenes in Sum

Looking back on the images in the vault (Figs. 6.37, 6.42), three clusters of scenes emerge: the group of four feast icons from the early years of Jesus's life, the Betrayal and the Way to the Cross, and the final grid of four scenes focused on the open sarcophagus. On the basis of the conservatism not simply of the individual compositions but of the very themes selected for inclusion, the initial group seems to be based on the paintings of 1105/6. Surviving fourteenth-century programs on Cyprus are few, but they suggest a rather different mode of conceiving their cycles. Instead of tailoring a comprehensive (if selective) overview of Christ's life to fit like a glove around the available surfaces of the church, as had been the middle Byzantine habit, they spin narratives: the Passion narrative above all, but also the narrative of Christ's mother, which at Pelendri displaced the theophanies of Christ's infancy as the image of incarnation. The fourteenth-century painter(s) at Asinou acknowledged the emphasis on Mary in the incarnational imagery of the transverse arches. They did not, however, displace the feast scenes of Jesus's early life. The very fact of their inclusion gives the central vault a sense of belonging to the scenes in the west bay, and to the twelfth-century program that they still represent. The Betrayal and the Way to the Cross, in turn, are ambiguous. Best paralleled in the Passion narratives of the fourteenth century, their subjects had been included in early twelfth-century cycles on Cyprus, and so could have formed a part of the initial cycle. By contrast, the final group of four scenes—as a unit, at any rate—can be imagined only in the fourteenth century.

The three clusters of scenes run the gamut, then, from suggesting a twelfth-century origin at one extreme to a fourteenth-century one at the other. Their location may have played some role in their history. The structural damage was more severe on the north side of the church; thus the loss to the original paintings may also have been more severe there, inviting—even demanding—a more fundamental rethinking of the program on the north. Certainly the iconography of Christ's lamentation and burial had been elaborated significantly in both Byzantine and European art in the centuries since 1105/6, and this very plausibly colored the expectations held out for the fourteenth-century cycle. On the other hand, institutional memory may have demanded the retention of the older, more traditional theophanies from Christ's early life that were clustered on the south. What is not likely is that the fourteenth-century painter(s) simply copied the original scenes. The grid format, the deeply layered repertoire of iconographic motifs, and the visual links between scenes on the vault and scenes of undisputed fourteenth-century origin on the transverses all show this.

Perhaps least expected in the layered archaeology of Asinou's images, given the pervasive assessment of the murals as copies, is the role of contemporary Palaiologan themes and techniques—not just motifs like the radiance of the mandorla in the Transfiguration or the jeweled robe of Christ in the Way to the Cross, but compositional strategies like the light-spangled landscapes, and themes like that of the open sarcophagus in the grid of post-Passion scenes, or the cosmic imagery of the Baptism signaled in Jordan's wings. In the case of Jordan, an earlier image current in the eastern Mediterranean was adapted to a Palaiologan theme; in much the same way the Burning Bush had been adopted to produce a program of Marian prefigurations. Vault and transverse arches together reveal painters alert to Palaiologan ideas and adept at mobilizing older images in their service.

Among the earlier images thus adopted are motifs from visual traditions shared with the thirteenth-century mainland—like the grizzled Moses and Hades-like Jordan—and motifs incubated jointly in Byzantium, the Holy Land, and Italy, such as the open sarcophagus, Judas's anti-halo, and the heavily grained wood. These focus attention on Cyprus as a center of Mediterranean interchange, a brisk market of competing visual traditions in which the goods of converging cultures were exchanged and adopted.

By far the greatest share in this market, though, lay with the inherited traditions of Komnenian Cyprus. The thickest layer of themes and motifs comes from the later twelfth century. The programs of that period seem to have had as much a classic authority for the fourteenth-century painters at Asinou as they have for us today. It is hard to see through this very strong intervening layer to the period of Asinou's initial program. It is easy to believe, though, that before the final grid of post-Passion scenes was adopted, the north lunette displayed a single, large composition of the Anastasis. This idea of a single image in the north lunette responds to the present form of the south one, which is dominated by the single, large composition of the donor portrait (Fig. 6.50). We know the donor portrait, however, only as a fourteenth-century painting. It deserves scrutiny before too many judgments are based on it.

The Donor Portrait

Mary (Μ(ήτ)ηρ / Θ(εο)ῦ) dominates the donor portrait (Fig. 6.50). Her form is cut by the frame of the window, giving her a larger-than-life immediacy, akin to that of that John and Longinus in the Crucifixion scene. Behind her to the west are the patron Nikephoros, bearing in both hands a gabled church on which Mary rests her left hand, and the small figure of Gephyra with her identifying inscription (Fig. 6.51).[300] In front of Mary are Nikephoros's inscription asking for her protection on the final day (Fig. 3.7; p. 77–79) and the figure of the enthroned Christ (Ι(ησοῦ)ς Χ(ριστό)ς), who is surrounded by a host of angels and gestures affirmatively back to his mother.

That there was a donor portrait in the initial program at Asinou seems incontrovertible. The epigram transcribed on the present painting conforms to twelfth-century usage (see above, pp. 79–80); its dialogic form implies an accompanying image; and the figure of Nikephoros looks convincingly twelfth-century in style. His long-nosed face and his hairstyle echo Komnenian conventions; his chlamys-like costume resembles middle Byzantine courtly attire more closely than it does the caftans of Palaiologan Byzantium or the coats worn by Cypriot gentry in the fourteenth century;[301] and the church in his hands lacks its later narthex. To give the image of a donor such a prominent place is in full accord with middle Byzantine practice. The donors of Cappadocia, as Catherine Jolivet-Lévy points out, often displayed their images at the eastern end of the naos, close to the bema, where they could readily be addressed in the litanies performed

300. See above, pp. 18–19, 22, 53–54, and 77–80. The donor portrait has figured extensively in the literature: see in particular Buxton et al., "Church of Asinou," 342–43, 346–70; Stylianou and Stylianou, "Donors and Dedicatory Inscriptions," 97–99, fig. 1; Mango, "Chypre carrefour," 7 n. 14; Nicolaïdès, "Les *ktitores* dans la peinture"; Stylianou and Stylianou, *Painted Churches*, 114–17, fig. 57; Carr, "Palaiologan Funerary Icon," 602, where I assumed Gephyra was a child, given her small stature and the wreath on her head.

301. On the changing courtly and aristocratic garb of the 12th century, see Parani, *Reconstructing the Reality of Images*, 53–58. Fourteenth-century Cypriot garb is illustrated excellently by the 1317 portrait figure of Michael Katzouroumpos at Dali: see Stylianou and Stylianou, *Painted Churches*, 425–27, fig. 256; but see also pp. 115–30 above, for the donors in the narthex of Asinou itself. For the attire of the Constantinopolitan court around 1100, see the donor depicted on folio 1v of the mid-11th-century Athos, Dionysiou 61, or the emperor Alexios I Komnenos in Vatican gr. 666 in Spatharakis, *Portrait in Byzantine Illuminated Manuscripts*, figs. 77, 79. These images can be contrasted with the male figures in Oxford, Lincoln College, gr. 35 of the mid-14th century: ibid., figs. 145–51.

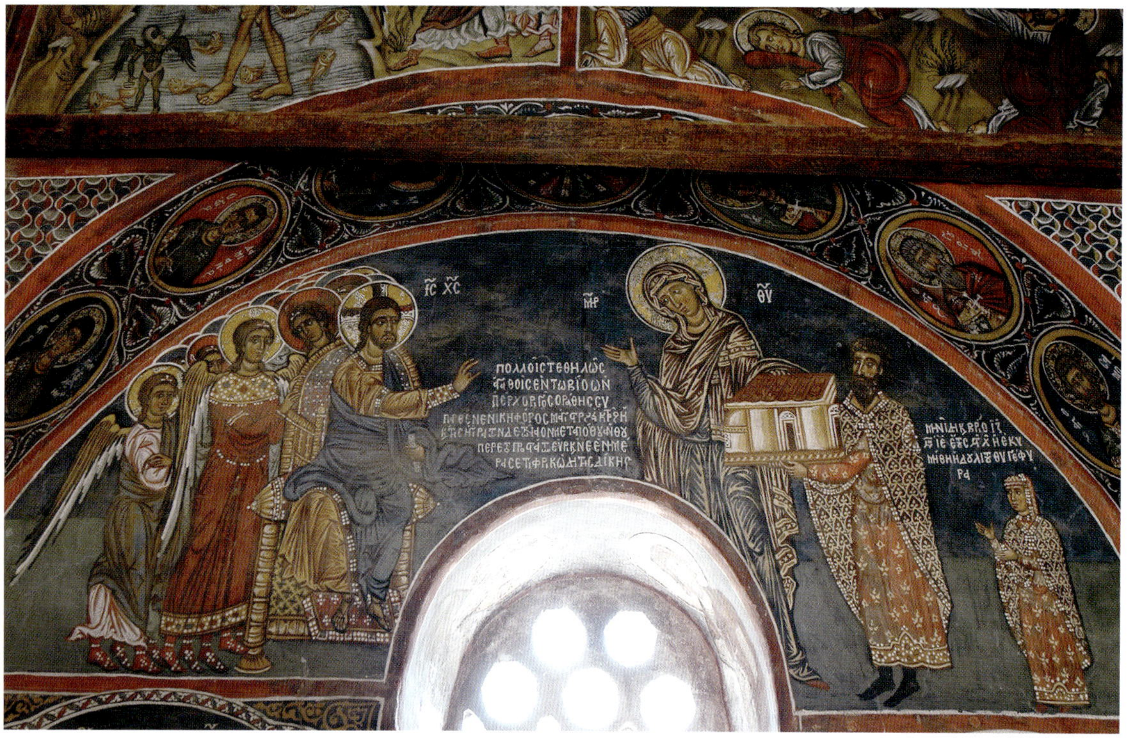

FIG. 6.50 Naos, central bay, south lunette: Donor portrait (photo courtesy of G. L. Carr)

there.[302] The same proximity was claimed by patrons on Cyprus: Eumathios Philokales placed his epigram—and possibly also his portrait—on the south bema pier of the church of the Holy Trinity at Koutsovendis;[303] the twelfth-century monk portrayed at St. Nicholas of the Roof stands by St. Nicholas's side in the monumental mural icon at the south end of the templon;[304] and later, in 1280 at the Panagia at Moutoullas, the patron John and his wife Irene installed their portraits inside the bema itself.[305] Like those at Koutsovendis and Kakopetria, the original portrait at Asinou must have occupied a place on the south side of the naos, as indicated by the Anargyroi over the lunette, for they were the favored guardians of patrons and their portraits.

Whether the image of Nikephoros originally occupied the south lunette, on the other hand, is harder to assess. Overdoors were favored sites for donor inscriptions in the twelfth century,[306] as illustrated on Cyprus by Leon Authentes' dedicatory inscription over the north door at Lagoudera and a fragmentary inscription on the south overdoor

302. Jolivet-Lévy, *La Cappadoce médiévale*, 55–90, esp. 79. On the portraits in Cappadocian churches see also the useful inventory given by Bernardini, "Les donateurs des églises de Cappadoce."
303. Mango, "Monastery of St. Chrysostom," 78–79, fig. 84.
304. Stylianou and Stylianou, *Painted Churches*, fig. 25.
305. Ibid., fig. 192. This practice is attested elsewhere. For Cappadocia, see Karanlık kilise, discussed below. For Greece, see Kalopissi-Verti, *Dedicatory Inscriptions and Donor Portraits*, 96–96, figs. 82–83 (a 13th-century monk in the Mavriotissa in Kastoria); 101, fig. 94 (a man in the sanctuary of St. Nicholas, Skaltsotianika, Kakomachi in the eastern Mani), and 101–2, figs. 95–97 (a couple in the apse of St. Kyriake, Marathos in Mesa Mani).
306. Thus in Kastoria both the churches of St. Nicholas Kasnitzes and the Anargyroi have inscriptions over their western doors: see Drakopoulou, *Η Πόλη της Καστορίας*, 41–42, 47.

in the Archangel church, Kato Lefkara.[307] The custom continued in the fourteenth century with the now incomplete donors' inscription over the western door of the central vessel at Pelendri.[308] Only with the portrait of Michael Katzouroumpos and his wife from 1317 at St. Demetrianos, Dali, however, does one find a painting of a donor above a door.[309] The portrait at Dali is strikingly like that at Asinou in conception and placement. But it belongs to the fourteenth century, not the early twelfth. A portrait over the door in 1105/6 would be exceptional. Far more in keeping with the evidence at Koutsovendis and the surviving portrait of the monk at St. Nicholas of the Roof would be a placement beside the standing image of the Mother of God postulated on the south wall, near the Christ on the south bema respond. Exceptional as a place over the door would be in the early twelfth century, however, it is also hard to imagine the circumstances that, after a gap of two and a half centuries, would favor a founder's promotion to a place as imposing as the south lunette. In the end, this may be the single best argument for assuming that the portrait occupied its present place from the very beginning.

The figure of Gephyra may reinforce this conclusion (Fig. 6.51). Gephyra's figure has perplexed scholars on almost every front, from her unusual name through the incompatibility of year (6608 = 1099) and indiction (15) in the date of her death to her diminutive size: no other portrait of a married couple in Cyprus depicts a wife in radically smaller scale than her spouse.[310] If her size is taken to imply that Gephyra was a child, then her mother should have been included in the image. Like Grivaud (pp. 53–54), I believe it is most plausible to read the indiction rather than the year as the accurate figure in Gephyra's mortuary inscription, placing her death in December of 1106: that is, a matter of months after the completion of the cycle of 1105/6. Too late to have been included in the original design, but too soon after its completion to have been left out, her figure was appended at the edge. Its small scale would thus be a record of nothing more than its tardy inclusion—she could have been the mother, daughter, sibling, or spouse of Nikephoros. But it would require that the portrait was always in this field, tucked into the descending arc of the lunette. How such a portrait might have originally looked, however, is far from obvious.

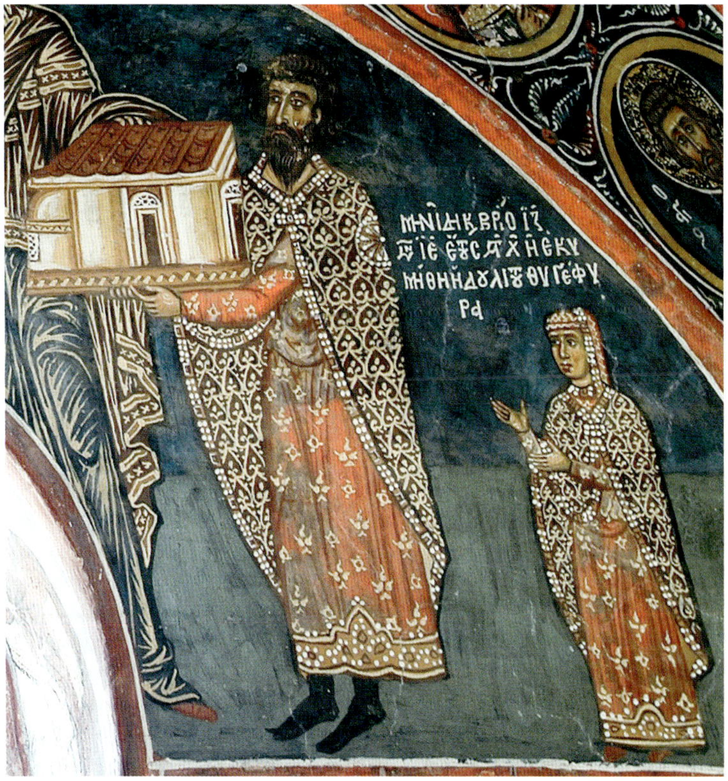

FIG. 6.51 Naos, central bay, south lunette. Donor portrait, detail: Mother of God, Nikephoros Ischyrios, and Gephyra (photo courtesy of G. L. Carr)

307. For Lagoudera see Nicolaïdès, "Étude iconographique," 4, fig. 2; for Kato Lefkara see Papageorgiou, "Ἡ ἐκκλησία τοῦ Ἀρχαγγέλου," 37, 1; reproduced also in Stylianou and Stylianou, *Painted Churches*, fig. 267.
308. Stylianou and Stylianou, *Painted Churches*, 223.
309. Ibid., fig. 256.
310. Not even a deceased wife or a second spouse is shown in smaller scale than her husband: see the icon of St. Mamas now in the Byzantine Museum, Nicosia, with portraits of a priest and his family, including his first and second wives and the children of each: Talbot Rice, *Icons of Cyprus*, no. 78; the portraits alone are reproduced in Marankou, *Η ζωή στην Κύπρο*, 27, figs. 10–11.

Portraits in which a devotee of Mary performs a poetic petition that is inscribed within the scene survive above all from the decades on either side of 1100, the period in which Asinou was first adorned. The finest examples are found in manuscripts,[311] but a monumental counterpart exists in the dedicatory mosaic of the admiral George of Antioch from 1146–47 in the Martorana in Palermo.[312] There the Mother of God addresses Christ in a scroll inscribed with a variant of the plea that she holds on the bema respond at Asinou, and he replies with an affirmative gesture from an arc of heaven above. Then, after about 1200 as Nancy Ševčenko points out, the interplay of word and image within the composition becomes infrequent, and portraits depend upon the image alone to carry their content.[313] The exceptions—the tomb portrait of the Russian prince Jaroslav Vsevelodović at Spas Nereditsa,[314] and the somewhat later thirteenth-century portrait of John, owner of a Gospel book, Athos, Iveron 5[315]—show the patron not with Mary but with Christ enthroned in judgment. Michael Katzouroumpos, too, addressed himself to Christ.

If the vogue for petitionary portraits with poetic epigrams coincides exactly with the first fresco campaign at Asinou, however, it is only Asinou's text that resembles them. The image at Asinou accords neither with these portraits nor with its own epigram. The text is a petition: Nikephoros asks for Mary's protection on the last day. The image, by contrast, is a presentation: Mary presents Nikephoros to the enthroned Christ surrounded by angels. The epigram he had addressed to her now hovers in the gap between Mary and her son: she has literally passed Nikephoros and his words on to Christ. Though Christ is implied in the reference to the last day, he is not the one addressed in the epigram. This contrasts with the twelfth-century images, in which the person speaking and the one spoken to were clearly indicated by the composition. At Asinou a displacement has occurred: a verbal interchange between Nikephoros and Mary has been set into a different picture, in which the interchange is between Mary and Christ.

Christ, especially Christ enthroned in judgment, plays a rather different role from his mother in donor portraits, with a rather different chronology. He appears perhaps for the first recorded time in a now-lost mosaic in the cathedral at Cefalù in which King Roger II was shown presenting the cathedral to Christ.[316] He is then encountered more consistently as one moves into the thirteenth century: in the funerary portrait of Jaroslav Vsevelodović at Spas Nereditsa; the funerary portraits of the Serbian kings; and the portrait of John, the owner of Athos, Iveron 5.[317] Unlike the petitionary portraits addressed to Mary, these portraits are distinguished by the act of presentation, in two senses. First, the patron recurrently carries the book or building being presented. The image confers upon the gift a juridical aura of legal confirmation.

311. See, above all, N. P. Ševčenko, "Close Encounters," 255–85, in particular the Lectionary, Jerusalem, Greek Orthodox Patriarchate, Megale Panagia 1, of 1061, in which the monk Basil crouches at the feet of a looming Mother of God with an invocation offering her the Lectionary volume itself and requesting in return her intercession with Christ for remission of his sins (ibid., 271–73, fig. 11), and the 12th-century Athos, Laura A 103, in which the petition of the aristocratic lay donor is voiced by the Virgin herself in a whole conversation with Christ not unlike that on the scroll of the Virgin Paraklesis (ibid., 266–67, fig. 7).

312. N. P. Ševčenko, "Close Encounters," 267–68, fig. 8, with earlier bibliography; on the date, see Kitzinger, *Mosaics of St. Mary's*, 262.

313. N. P. Ševčenko, "Close Encounters," 276.

314. Ibid., 275, with discussion of the date in either 1199 or ca. 1246; Velmans, "Le portrait dans l'art des Paléologues," 135; Lazarev, *Old Russian*, appendix fig. 57.

315. Folios 456v–457r. See N. P. Ševčenko, "Close Encounters," 273–75, fig. 13; Spatharakis, *The Portrait*, 85–86, figs. 53–54; Belting, *Das illuminierte Buch in der spätbyzantinischen Gesellschaft*, 36–37, 72.

316. Johnson, "Lost Royal Portraits of Gerace and Cefalù Cathedrals."

317. For Spas Nereditsa and Iveron 5, see above, notes 314 and 315. On the Serbian portraits and for their considerable bibliography, see Papamastorakes, "Επιτύμβιες παραστάσεις."

This official status is especially clear in the deliberately legal language of the inscriptions in the portrait of John in Iveron 5, as Hans Belting has shown,[318] but it was already present in the mosaic of Roger II, whose portrait attested to his gift.[319] Second, the portraits with Christ—except for the one at Nereditsa—display a distinctive composition that echoes court rituals of presentation, with Christ enthroned as a ruler in judgment and the petitioner led forward to be presented to him by a saintly patron, most often the Mother of God.[320] Early Christian donors had been shown in this way, but as Nancy Ševčenko points out,[321] this kind of courtly theatre is not known in middle Byzantine monumental painting. Only in the early thirteenth century does a comparable formula appear once again in churches, now for the portraits of donors buried in the church: affluent citizens like the deacon presented to Christ by St. Euphemia in the homonymous church in Constantinople,[322] and royal figures like the Serbian rulers, beginning with Stephan Nemanja, founder of the Nemanjid dynasty, at Studenica.[323]

The presentational content of Asinou's composition accords not with Nikephoros's epigram but with portraits of the thirteenth and fourteenth centuries organized around Christ. Other than a presumed original at Asinou, no such early twelfth-century courtly presentational portrait is known. The very church in Nikephoros's hands is anomalous. So seemingly timeless, such models cannot be found in the hands of nonroyal donors before the examples in Kastoria from the very end of the twelfth century.[324] They appear on Cyprus only with the portraits of 1280 at Moutoullas and 1317 at Dali.[325] In the disposition of the epigram, the introduction of the enthroned Christ, and the courtly choreography of presentation, the composition at

318. Belting, *Das illuminierte Buch*, 36–37 and 72 for Iveron 5; see also 77 for the similar interpretation of the multiple frontispiece of the Lincoln College Typikon.
319. By the 1220s it had been complemented by a sequence of four further images installed to confirm earlier privileges of the cathedral and to record the presentation of further new ones: see Johnson, "Lost Royal Portraits." On the use of mural images as legal documents, see Kalopissi-Verti, "Church Inscriptions as Documents," 79–80, where she points out that this practice seems to have grown in frequency in the Palaiologan period.
320. Its courtly origin is discussed by N. P. Ševčenko, "Close Encounters," 273–74.
321. Ibid., 273–77 and 283 n. 12.
322. For the tomb portrait in St. Euphemia, see Naumann and Belting, *Die Euphemia-Kirche*, 178–84, figs. 36–37.
323. On this kind of portrait and its fairly considerable bibliography, see Papamastorakes, "Επιτύμβιες παραστάσεις."

324. See Lipsmeyer, "Donor and His Church Model," 144–51 passim. Lipsmeyer assigns a significant role to Byzantium in the development of such models during the 10th and early 11th centuries, but the examples she assembles—the well-known mosaic of the emperors Constantine and Justinian over the south entrance to Hagia Sophia in Constantinople, and the Georgian and Armenian sculptures at Opiza, Aght'amar, Haghbat, Oshki, Ani, Doliskana, and Tbeti—all show royal patrons. Thus, as she says, they reflect the very highest rank of donors. The penetration of this elite motif to regional aristocrats and gentry seems to be a 12th-century development that is attested in surviving Byzantine monuments only two generations after the adornment of Asinou. It was more widely used in the West. In Sicily, as noted, Roger II (1130–54) was shown at Cefalù presenting a replica of the cathedral to the enthroned Christ (Johnson, "Lost Royal Portraits"). In Cappadocia the first example that Jolivet-Lévy cites (*La Cappadoce médiévale*, 86) is the image of Thamar at St. George, Belisırma, of 1283–95. Her Georgian origin may well be significant here. In Byzantium, the examples from the late 12th century at Kastoria thus assume particular importance. See Drakopoulou, *Η Πόλη της Καστοριάς*, 41–42, figs. 18–19 with the image of the magistros Nikephoros Kasnitzes in his church of St. Nicholas, from around 1170–90 in Kastoria, which is probably the first clear example. Ibid., 48–49, figs. 30–31 show the slightly later portraits in the church of the Anargyroi in Kastoria. Here the church, in the hands of Theodore Lemniotes in the north aisle, is a later addition; the monk Theodosios, also called ktetor and most likely Theodore himself in his monastic guise, was shown carrying a model of the church from the beginning.
325. Stylianou and Stylianou, *Painted Churches*, fig. 192 (Moutoullas) and fig. 256 (Dali).

Asinou draws upon formulas that are best known a century after 1105/6 and that differ from the intimate, petitionary content both of its epigram and of the early twelfth-century images composed around epigrams to Mary.

That the image at Asinou does bear the marks of a reconception is suggested by two purely internal anomalies. The first of these centers again upon the image of Christ. Enthroned though he is, Jesus shrinks in stature beneath Mary's towering gaze, his figure small and unstable with its bevy of surrounding angels. The gesticulative hem of his himation, apparently improvised to redress his diminution, only draws attention to the fact that the words that bridge him and Mary are not addressed to him. Had his figure been painted with its proper authority, it would have been at least isocephalic with that of Mary. The other anomaly is the figure of Gephyra. Crucial to the balance of the current composition, she seems integral to the scene. Yet her figure is a conundrum, too small in scale to represent the donor's wife, inappropriate as a daughter in the wife's absence. Her very costume, which replicates that of Nikephoros, is unparalleled in a culture of gender-specific clothing.[326] Her headdress, with its band over the crown leading down to pendant jewels, is very similar to those worn by the daughters of the Armenian king Levon III in the Queen Keran Gospels.[327] Her costume must reflect fourteenth-century conceptions of courtly attire; at the same time, it suggests that the fourteenth-century painter interpreted the little figure—whatever its original identity—as a child. It may be, as suggested above, that a figure awkwardly appended to the original composition has been regularized in the repainting; conversely, a remnant of a more coherent family portrait may have been salvaged in this one figure. But the figure as we see it now cannot replicate the initial composition. The initial image, in short, must have been different. Gephyra's garb, which elevates her to a princess as the Crusader kingdoms knew them, reveals quite graphically the romanticizing reconception of the courtly donors by a later, retrospective age.

It is hard to guess how the donor portrait of 1105/6, if not in the form of the present image, might have looked. Two considerations, however, are useful. First, the accurate form of the church in Nikephoros' hands, without the narthex, suggests that the little model was included in the portrait of 1105/6. Thus one can assume that the portrait did in some way participate in the presentational character of the later portraits with Christ. Second, the decades around 1100 offer several examples of flagrantly self-promotional portraits that, though not adopting the courtly choreography of the thirteenth-century presentational portraits, nonetheless do convey a comparable claim to privileged presence.[328] At Karanlık kilise from

326. While Ball, *Byzantine Dress*, 73 passim, often emphasizes that women and men wore the same basic garments in Byzantium, the chlamys was rarely a woman's garment, and (p. 51) courtly women do not look like their spouses when they are portrayed. Only deceased couples are shown uniformly attired: at least the Gothic funerary portraits of Cyprus depict male and female figures alike in an ankle- or floor-length garment with tight sleeves, fitted waist, wider hips, and full skirt with slits for pockets. See the funerary icon of Maria of 1356 in the Byzantine Museum, Nicosia; the two men—one named George—painted between SS. Peter and Paul at St. Theodosios, Akhelia; and the tomb slab of John Gavrilis, in Carr, "Palaiologan Funerary Icon," figs. 2, 7, and 9; Stylianou and Stylianou, *Painted Churches*, fig. 245. An excellent example is offered by the tomb slab of 1380 in the Limassol Castle showing Master Bonacours de Clarence and his daughter, Dame Catelin, both dressed in this type of garment: Imhaus, *Lacrimae Cypriae*, 1:149, no. F 278, pl. 126.

327. Der Nersessian, *Miniature Painting*, 2: fig. 641. This is folio 380r in Jerusalem, Library of the Armenian Patriarchate, MS 2563.

328. The issue of the presentational portrait in the middle Byzantine period has been the subject of considerable speculation. Thus, on the basis of surviving epigrams, Papamastorakes, "Επιτύμβιες παραστάσεις," 296, argues that compositions of courtly presentation must have already existed in the funerary portraits of early 12th-century Constantinople; and Bernardini, "Les donateurs," 120, proposes that the iconography of such

around 1100, for example, the patrons Nikephoros and Bassianos, accompanied by inscriptions opening with the word "deesis," kneel in the interstices of the Deesis adorning the apse; in essence they are being presented to Christ by the outstretched hands of the Virgin herself and the Prodromos.[329] In the opening diptych of Sinai manuscript gr. 172 of 1067, now detached as St. Petersburg, State Public Library, gr. 291, framed icons of Christ and his mother "come to life" to bless the donor couple, Theodore Gabras and Irene: Jesus places his hand on the head of Theodore, and Mary leads Irene firmly forward to meet her son.[330] And on Cyprus itself, Eumathios Philokales may have placed his portrait at Koutsovendis above his donor's epigram on the south bema pier, the customary place for Christ.[331] Nikephoros, then, would not have been alone if he had portrayed himself at Asinou in unusually large scale, claiming special, privileged access to holy figures.

The presentational character of the original composition, however it is imagined, raises the question of whether the portrait had a funerary function. Certainly the surviving examples of courtly, presentational portraits in monumental painting are predominantly funerary, beginning already with the earliest examples at St. Euphemia in Constantinople and the Virgin's church at Studenica. It is, moreover, to the funerary realm that Titos Papamastorakes looked in seeking precedents for the presentational portrait as early as 1100.[332] On the other hand, when the composition was used in manuscripts, as it was in the Gabras diptych or Iveron 5, it could not have carried a funerary connotation and it is not at all clear that Byzantium developed any portrait forms that were specific to funerary use.[333] At Asinou, the prominence of the Dormition, the inclusion of Gephyra's date of death, and the likely large scale of the original donor portrait all suggest that the building served a funerary function. To date, however, no archaeological evidence of burials confirms this, nor can the iconographic history of the presentational composition bind it unequivocally to a funerary use.

Imagining a differently composed donor portrait is challenging because the present fourteenth-century image functions so effectively. Accordingly, it is sensible to pause and ask what its functions were. The focal grandeur of the Mother of God, literally overlapping the architecture, establishes her centrality in the bay. In turn, the somewhat contrived introduction of Christ and the shift of the epigram heighten the juridical character of the image. The legalistic content latent in the courtly presentational composition may well have acquired an intensified significance in the fourteenth century when the portrait was reconceived. It is clear that the so-called compositions of legal witness, with a donor before the enthroned Christ, saw a particular currency in the Interregnum and early

scenes was significantly shaped by the patrons' social status, and that the now-lost Constantinopolitan portraits reflected courtly rituals in a way that was not often paralleled in peripheral sites, where presentational portraits still survive.

329. Yenipınar and Şahin, *Paintings of the Dark Church*, 62. The inscriptions make the donors participants in a ritual of petition in which they are at the same time presented to Christ, for they identify the figures' action as entreaty (deesis): δεησης του δουλου του Θ(εο)υ νηκηφορου πρ(εσβυτέρου), and δεησης του δουλου του Θ(εο)υ βας. . .ιου (the latter read variously as βασ(ηα)νιου or Βασ(ι)λ(ε)ιου: see Jolivet-Lévy, *Églises de Cappadoce*, 133).

330. Excellently reproduced in Cutler and Spieser, *Byzance médiévale*, pls. 258–59. See the vivid analysis of the image in N. P. Ševčenko, "Close Encounters," 275–76, fig. 14.

331. Mango, "Monastery of St. Chrysostom," 78–79, fig. 84.

332. Papamastorakes, "Επιτύμβιες παραστάσεις," 296.

333. This question hangs over all discussions of portraits in churches, as illustrated well in Jolivet-Lévy's discussion of the Cappadocian portraits: see *La Cappadoce médiévale*, 55–90. Her discussion on pages 78–79 of the standing figure with crossed hands shows clearly how uncertain it is that categories of specifically funerary imagery existed. This pose has been discussed as funerary by Carr, "Palaiologan Funerary Icon," 599–619; Stylianou and Stylianou, *Painted Churches*, 407; and Thierry, "Le portrait funéraire byzantin," 2: pl. 331.

Palaiologan periods, when issues of legal continuity may have been particularly strained. Such vulnerability surely persisted in areas like Cyprus. While we have no evidence that Asinou was threatened by its Latin overlords, Orthodox monasteries in other parts of Lusignan Cyprus were subject to the Latin fief-holders of the lands in which they lay.[334] Thus Asinou's monastic congregation may have found it singularly reassuring to assert with new emphasis the legitimacy of their institution's initial, autonomous dedication by reworking the donor portrait. No image in the central bay is so carefully or lovingly painted as this one. Nikephoros's memory may have been fed by the prominence of his initial portrait; its vivid reclamation, with its juridical elements visibly enhanced, may have been a focal motivation behind the full repainting of the bay.

The Central Bay in Sum

The aspect of Asinou that so engages its visitors—in the words of Harold Buxton, that one sees "the whole surface from dome to floor as a gallery of . . . paintings"[335]—is nowhere more forceful than in the central bay, which enfolds the viewer in an embracing cloak of color. Our analysis has separated this unity into discrete components. Yet its effectiveness as a whole is unequivocal, and so central to visitors' appreciation of the monument that it deserves to be acknowledged.

Assembling the messages of the central bay's chronologically and thematically diverse imagery depends on how it is approached. Paintings outside the north portal (Fig. 2.18) suggest that the monastic buildings lay in this direction, and therefore that this was the direction from which the church was most often approached by its own community. Thus entry was most typically on the short axis (Figs. 6.52, 6.53). Monks, like modern visitors, would have come into the central bay, surveying its circuit of saints and scenes as their first impression of the church. The centralized quality of this space is still expressed clearly in the actions of the church's Orthodox pilgrims, who make a circuit of the saints in the central bay before turning to admire the work of the Asinou Master in the west. As composed in the fourteenth century, the paintings seen from the north door function very differently from those seen from the south. Viewers entering from the north door enter through the Anastasis; the Passion is behind them, and what lies ahead is a panoply of theophanies (Fig. 6.52). Prominent among the saints, Helena, Ioulitta, Anna, and above all the Mother of God appear with their holy offspring in an affirmation of divine grace. The program offers the church as a site of theophany, congruent with the expectant imagery of Nikephoros, who stands as if already in the presence of God and his Mother.

The western door must have been the second-most common avenue of access to the building, given the importance of the fully adorned narthex (see intro. fig. 2). The view of the naos for those coming from the west was fundamentally reconfigured by the introduction of the transverse arches, which effectively both narrow and focus the visitor's attention through a series of diaphragmatic surfaces rising to pointed arches. These spaces are devoted to Mary, creating a coherent thematic axis that culminates in the apse. Passing the prophets Jeremiah and Isaiah, the viewer is riveted by the Annunciation; then, passing the acclamations of the prophet kings, the viewer's gaze comes to rest on the Virgin herself in the conch. Intellectually and visually coherent, the sequence pulls the eye from bay to bay, regardless of the discontinuities in style, era, organization, or narrative mode that separate them from one another. Only with the Annunciation is there a pause that alerts the viewer to stop, turn, and absorb the circuit of the central bay.

The south door, finally, was probably more often used as a mode of egress than of entrance.[336]

334. Schabel, "Religion," 200.

335. Buxton et al., "Church of Asinou," 328.

336. So, too, at Lagoudera; as David Winfield pointed out in conversation, the south portal there is adorned with St. Christopher. Because he is the patron of wayfarers, he therefore must adorn the portal as a gesture of farewell to those who leave.

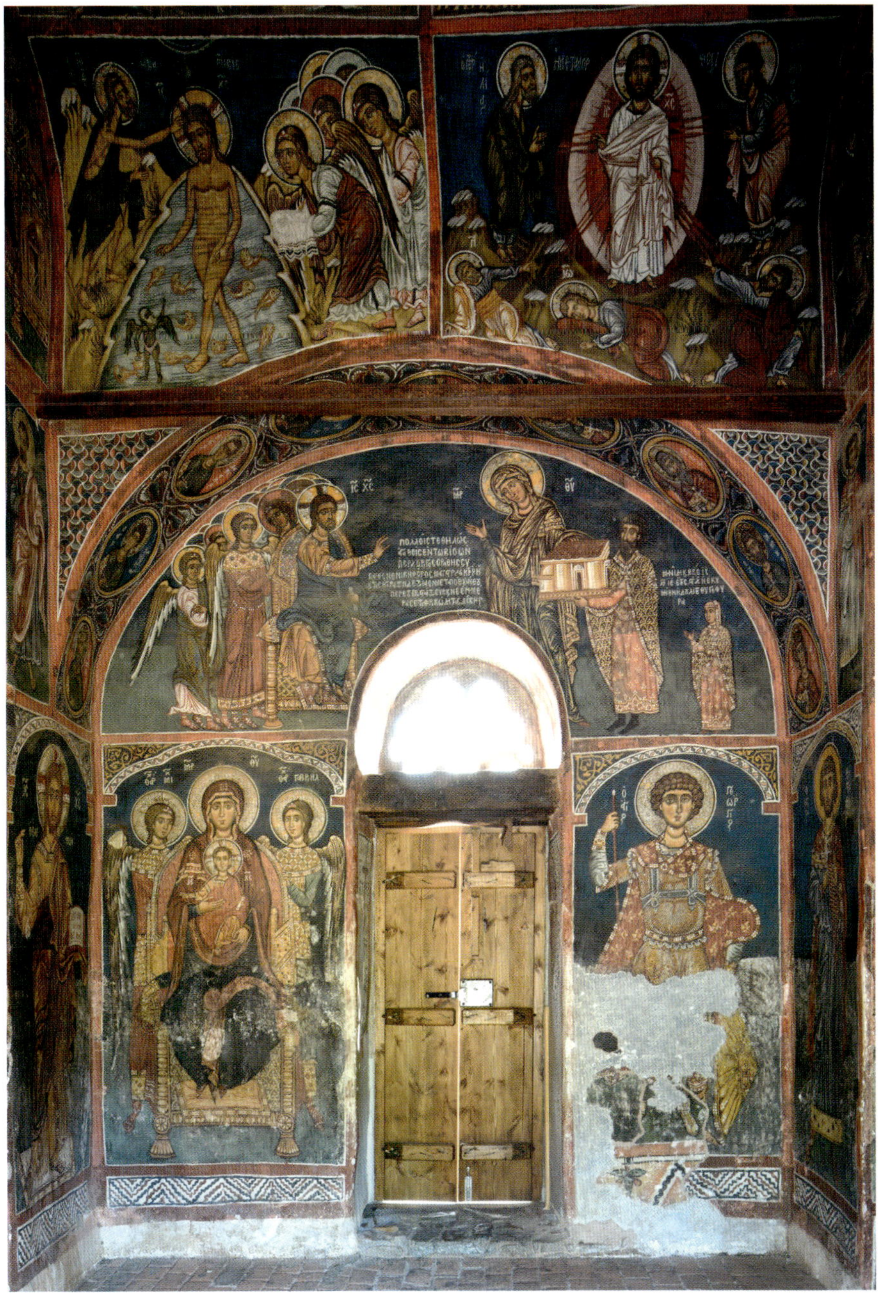

FIG. 6.52
Naos, central bay, south wall (photo courtesy of G. L. Carr)

It is ironic, then, that the south door is by far the most heavily used today. If people entering from the north do so through the Anastasis, with the Passion behind them and their face to the advent of God, those who enter through the south have the Passion before them (Fig. 6.53), while warriors—many rapt in the passion of Sebaste—dominate the sanctoral cycle. Form differs, too, as the cycle speaks without remission in the staccato sequence of gridlike scenes. No dominant icon draws this cycle to a close. Especially to the tourist and the historian, this vista offers the strongest possible contrast to the work of the Asinou Master. The result is almost inevitably a denigration of the paintings in the central bay. Much of the condescension with which they have been treated must be due to the circumstance of their being seen from the south door. In contrast to the gravity of the western bay,

FIG. 6.53
Naos, central bay, north wall (photo courtesy of G. L. Carr)

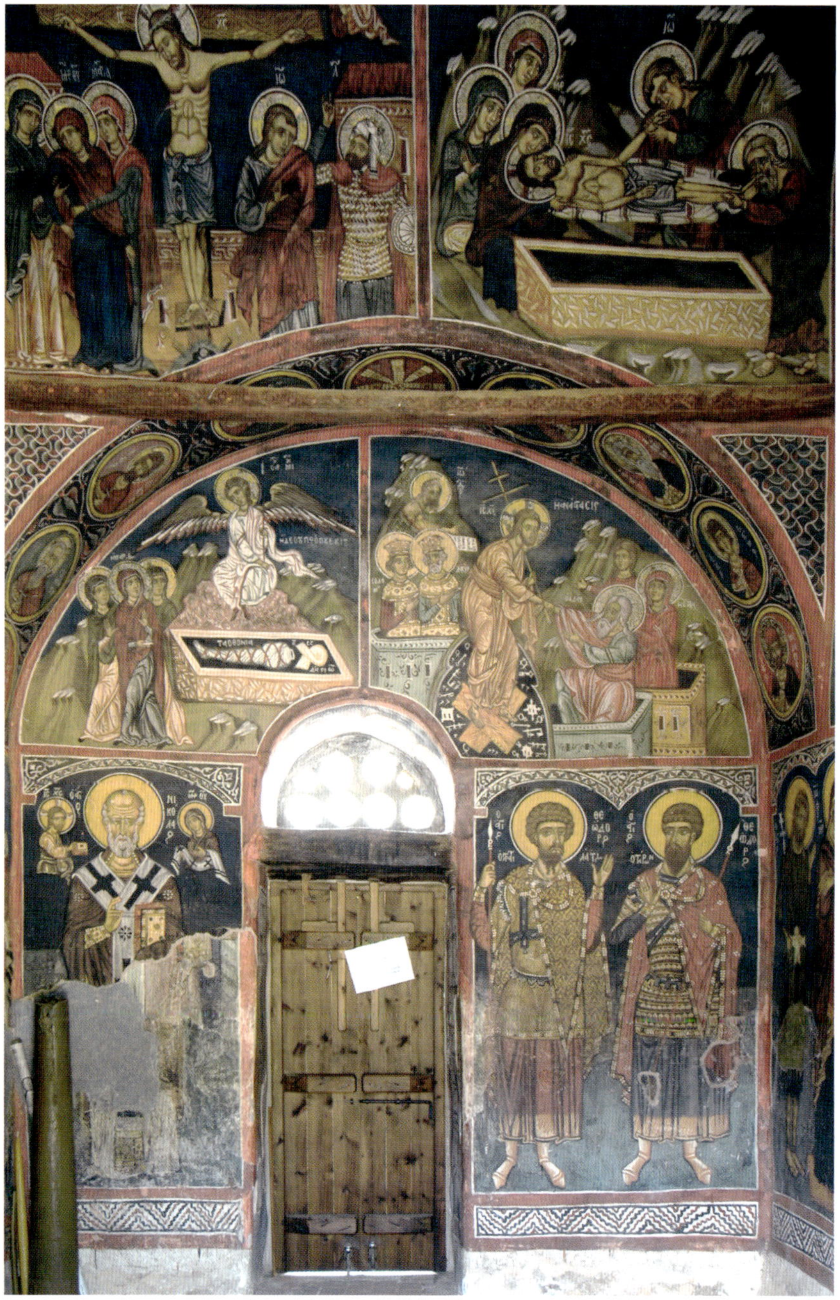

these scenes emerge as incoherent—garrulous and thematically disjointed. As such, they are dismissed as "local." The truth, as we have seen, may be just the opposite. If the central bay is incoherent, it is not because it is local, but because it is in fact radically diverse, joining a bedrock of regional but far from rustic middle Byzantine imagery with motifs drawn from the most radically cosmopolitan, Palaiologan, and pan-Mediterranean modernism. It is form and color that unite these paintings, clothing their diversity in a coherent carpet of style.

Ornament, Pastiglia, and Script

The purely visual aspects of the paintings in the central bay are able, as the iconography is not, to cast light upon the chronological relation of the naos to the narthex paintings of 1332/33. The graffiti from 1446 and 1450 in the door jambs made it clear that the paintings were earlier than the fifteenth-century date assigned them in early literature, but their relation to the paintings in the narthex remains ambiguous, David Winfield seeing them as contemporary with the narthex and the Stylianous placing them in the third quarter of the fourteenth century.[337] This question is most simply addressed in the patterns of the painted ornament and the raised gesso of the haloes.

All five patterns of painted ornament in the central bay are found also in the narthex. The decorative vocabulary in the two spaces is identical. They include: (1) the white panels painted with wavy lines of black and red that fill the dado of the central bay (Figs. 6.18, 6.22, 6.25); (2) the panel of crenellated lozenges in circles joined by a monochrome rinceau against an ocher ground, seen on the north face of the south bema respond next to Christ Eleemon (Figs. 6.25, 6.52); (3) the polychrome double axes that fill the spandrels on the north and south walls (Figs. 6.37, 6.42); (4) the floral motifs with white, heart-shaped linear patterns enclosing trefoils highlighted with white that fill in around the medallions of Saints Memnon and Tryphon and those of the saints in the soffits of the north and south arches (Figs. 6.23, 6.24, 6.26–29); and (5) the ocher tendril that runs above the portraits of Memnon and Tryphon (Fig. 6.42). Each of these is described and analyzed above by Sophia Kalopissi-Verti (pp. 192–93). Nothing shows more clearly the fact that the two programs are based on a common fund of artistic forms. This commonality is confirmed by the kinship in the letterforms of their inscriptions, reproduced in grids in the Appendix.

If the motifs are uniform, however, their execution is not. This is most evident in the polychromed double axes (Figs. 6.37, 6.42; 5.11, 5.15). Brightly and carefully painted in the narthex, they are more casually traced and less brightly colored in the naos. The floral motifs that fill in around medallions, too, are thinner in the naos (Figs. 6.23, 6.24; 5.11, 5.12). The crenellated lozenges, finally, are less smartly outlined, and the rinceau connecting them is heavier (Fig. 6.52; Fig. 5.29). The painter(s) of the naos seem to have quite deliberately undercut the fine draughtsmanship and clear local color that had given the paintings of the narthex their sense of quality. Such a shift may bespeak a number of variables—the abrasion of time, a clumsier hand, a more hurried work schedule, or a shift in aesthetic vision—but it clearly signals a discontinuity. Strong as the bond is between narthex and naos, their ornament indicates some break between them.

The patterned gesso of the haloes seems to confirm this distinction. No other Byzantine church has so much patterned gesso as Asinou does; and, so far as we know, certainly no other church adorned so many of its haloes—indeed, not just haloes but edges of furniture, too—with raised gesso. That this should have happened in Cyprus is not surprising. The technique of raised gesso—known as *pastiglia*—seems to have been known in Komnenian Constantinople, as suggested by the great mosaic icons from the Pammakaristos church;[338] it appears sporadically on panel-painted icons from the thirteenth and fourteenth centuries in both Greece and the Balkans,[339] and more occasionally on mural icons singled out for special votive or ex-voto significance.[340] Some fourteenth-century churches on

337. Winfield, *Asinou*, 5; Stylianou and Stylianou, *Painted Churches*, 123.

338. Mango et al., *Mosaics and Frescoes of St. Mary*, 10; G. Soteriou, "Η εἰκὼν τῆς Παμμακαρίστου." This antedates the Italian examples of pastiglia, which are from the 13th century.

339. See Kalopissi-Verti, "Διακοσμημένοι φωτοστέφανοι," 556, citing examples in Djurić, *Icônes de Yougoslavie*; see also the the icon of the Virgin enthroned with Archangels from St. Nicholas, Veroia (now Archaeological Museum, Inv. 88): see Vassilaki, *Mother of God*, 342–43, no. 33.

340. See the mural icon of the Mother of God Gorgoepikoos from the 13th century in St. Stephen, Kastoria (Pelekanides and Chatzidakis, *Kastoria*, fig. 7); the four churches of ca. 1300 in the Mani cited by Kalopissi-Verti, "Διακοσμημένοι φωτοστέφανοι," 556; and the example in Kera, Kritsas, Crete (ibid., 557).

Crete have quite a number of gessoed haloes.[341] But the technique survives nowhere more frequently than on the thirteenth- and fourteenth-century icons of Cyprus and Mount Sinai. Though pastiglia occurs less frequently in mural painting, it is seen on the murals of 1494 in the church of the Holy Cross of Agiasmati near Platanistassa,[342] and in the sixteenth century in the figures on the northwest respond at Asinou itself (Fig. 6.20). Thus the technique seems legitimately to have taken on a particularly sturdy life on Cyprus. It flourished in areas of Byzantium that were in contact with the West, but it embedded itself in Orthodox practice in these places, and there is no need to look for a Latin stimulus to its exceptionally extravagant employment at Asinou.

Pastiglia was a conspicuous sign of a patron's proud prosperity, but it is not entirely clear at Asinou what patrons these were. The pastiglia was applied not to the raw plaster of the wall but to the painted surface, and even there it was applied episodically—some prominent figures never received any. The frescoes would have presented a fully finished face had the patterned gesso never been applied. It was, in short, applied as an afterthought. It could have been added years, decades, or even centuries after the frescoes were finished—as it was to the figures of John and Kyros from 1105/6 in the south window. A feature of its application indicates, however, that the pastiglia was most likely produced at much the same time as the paintings. The gesso, as Ioanna Kakoulli shows (pp. 330–34, 344), was pressed into place either with flat wooden molds or with wooden rollers carved with the gridlike pattern of intersecting circles. Both the pattern and—as she emphasizes—the technique are the same in narthex and naos. Significantly, though, the molds differ. Their pattern is the same, but not their size. The intersecting segments measure very nearly exactly a centimeter from end to end in the narthex; while those in the naos measure 1.8 centimeters. Thus it seems likely that the narthex was gessoed after it was painted with one set of molds, and that the naos was then gessoed at a different moment, with much the same pattern but with a distinct set of molds. The shared technique indicates that narthex and naos were gessoed by people of the same tradition, but they were not undertaken in a single campaign. A gap of some kind intervened. To diagnose the character of that gap requires an examination of the paintings' style.

Style

The cardinal characteristic of the style in the central bay is its colorism: both contour lines and smoothly graduated surfaces recede, and forms take shape from the energy of the interacting areas of paint. This quality is clear already in the most general view of the ensemble, which is dominated less by shapes than by the glitter of highlights and bright colors—especially red—against the prevailing blue and brown of the scenes (Figs. 6.37, 6.42). The landscape settings, rather than being compartmentalized in broad, rhythmic shapes as in middle Byzantine painting, are spread in screens of small, sparkling units. Architecture is flattened to decorative coulisses; and space spreads in an ambiguous layer of flickering light and color. Figures speak more as colors than as clearly contoured shapes. The large forms of Jesus and Mary generally share the blue and brown tonality of the surface, creating pools of stability in the scenes, while the brighter tones and highlights play around them, glancing from the landscape and the other figures. The hues and highlights create an optical play of three-dimensional relief as bright tones twinkle in the foreground and heavier ones sink back, but the optical relief is neither tied to firmly closed and modeled contours nor meshed into a coherent spatial recession. Thus it does not stabilize the eye in a coherent three-dimensionality, but serves to keep the eye circulating within a thin, ambiguous spatial layer that spreads from highlight to highlight, scene to scene.

As Ioanna Kakoulli shows (see p. 320), the painter(s) operated with a remarkably limited

341. Kalopissi-Verti, "Διακοσμημένοι φωτοστέφανοι," 557, citing St. George in Vathenako and St. Fanourios in Valsamonero.

342. Argyrou and Myrianthefs, *Church of the Holy Cross*, figs. on pp. 32–39.

palette, building up their nuanced color repertoire by the optical interplay of a few unmixed hues variously juxtaposed. As hue is layered upon opaque hue, the scenes are truly "built," in the lapidary, architectural sense of the word as David Winfield has used it.[343] The forms produced in this way share certain recurrent conventions: faces are strongly modeled with rosy cheeks, long-lobed ears, and often an emphatic jowl; bodies are broad-hipped and small-footed and walk on tiptoe; garments have richly bundled folds and are decoratively enhanced with overlays of chrysographic highlights, star crosses, or spade-shaped patterns;[344] their borders are spangled wherever possible with pearls and gems, or if jewels are inappropriate—as in the robes of Mary or monastic saints—with rows of ocher x's; furniture is elaborate (Fig. 6.25); and architecture sports sawtooth and meander cornices and sometimes decorative latticework (Fig. 6.10).

Many of these mannerisms can be traced back to Cyprus's twelfth- and thirteenth-century murals and so echo in formal terms the allegiance to local precedent that has already been seen in the iconography. It is in the inflections with which these mannerisms are used, more than in the forms themselves, that the images reveal their fourteenth-century date. Other aspects suggest a bond with the eastern Levant. Thus, though the spangling of forms with pearls and patterns is also seen in fourteenth-century Cretan painting,[345] the colorful ornamentalism that enlivens both the architecture and the patterned fabrics at Asinou resembles more closely the paintings of the Cilician Armenian illuminator Sargis Pidsak, whose work is known from 1307 until 1352.[346] Finally, some elements, such as the landscape, seem persuasively Palaiologan. Similarly, the elaborately bunched and folded drapery in figures like John in the Crucifixion (Fig. 6.45), and the occasional band of drapery across the ankles in figures like the prophets in the Transfiguration (Fig. 6.41), seem to respond to the drapery patterns of Palaiologan art as reflected, for instance, in the Ascension at Pelendri;[347] but, above all, the colorism itself looks contemporary, in the sense that it moves attention from the contours into the body of the forms. Thus it echoes—though more simply—the way light pulls away from the edges to the center of the faces and forms in fourteenth-century icons.[348] In these respects one sees the painter(s) responding to contemporary currents in Byzantine painting.

The colorism of the paintings in the central bay distinguishes them from the paintings of 1332/33 in the narthex. As Sophia Kalopissi-Verti emphasizes (see above, pp. 121–22), the narthex paintings still reflect the fine linearism of the late thirteenth-century "maniera cypria." This is seen clearly in her comparison of Christ Eleemon in the narthex with

343. Winfield, "Middle and Later Byzantine Wall Painting Methods," 127–34.

344. The design of spades on the garments, though recalling patterns overpainted on Palaiologan fabrics in Constantinopolitan tomb portraits (Underwood, *Kariye Djami*, 3:535, 541, 547), is specifically paralleled to my knowledge only in the Schefer Maqamat from the so-called Baghdad School and may reflect Middle Eastern rather than Constantinopolitan techniques: see Ettinghausen, *Arab Painting*, 114: Paris, Bibliothèque nationale, arabe 5874, 26r.

345. As in the cycle of the life of Constantine in the church of SS. George and Constantine, Pyrgos Monophatsiou of 1314: Vassilaki, "Εικονογραφικοί κύκλοι από τη ζωή του Μεγάλου Κωνσταντίνου," figs. 22–23.

346. Der Nersessian, *Miniature Painting*, 1:142–53; 2: figs. 585–638, 650, 652. Among others, Sargis Pidsak illuminated a New Testament (Erevan, Matenadaran 242) that had been copied in 1318 in Cyprus (ibid., 1:144), and, though he probably never went to Cyprus, the ruling families of the two kingdoms were extensively intermarried and their clerics were in close contact (ibid., 1:134). A similar glitter of pale highlights and bright red against a dark ground is seen in a remarkable icon with the Nativity and the Crucifixion at Sinai that has been linked with both Cilicia and Cyprus: see Mouriki, "Icons," 120, fig. 71; Carr, "Icon-tact: Byzantium and the Art of Cilician Armenia," 98.

347. Stylianou and Stylianou, *Painted Churches*, fig. 129.

348. As, for example, in the superb figure of Christ now at Emba, see Papageorgiou, *Icons of Cyprus* (1969), 53; or the icon of Christ at the Archangel-Panagia church, Galata: *Ἱερὰ Μητρόπολις Μόρφου*, 276–77, no. 16.

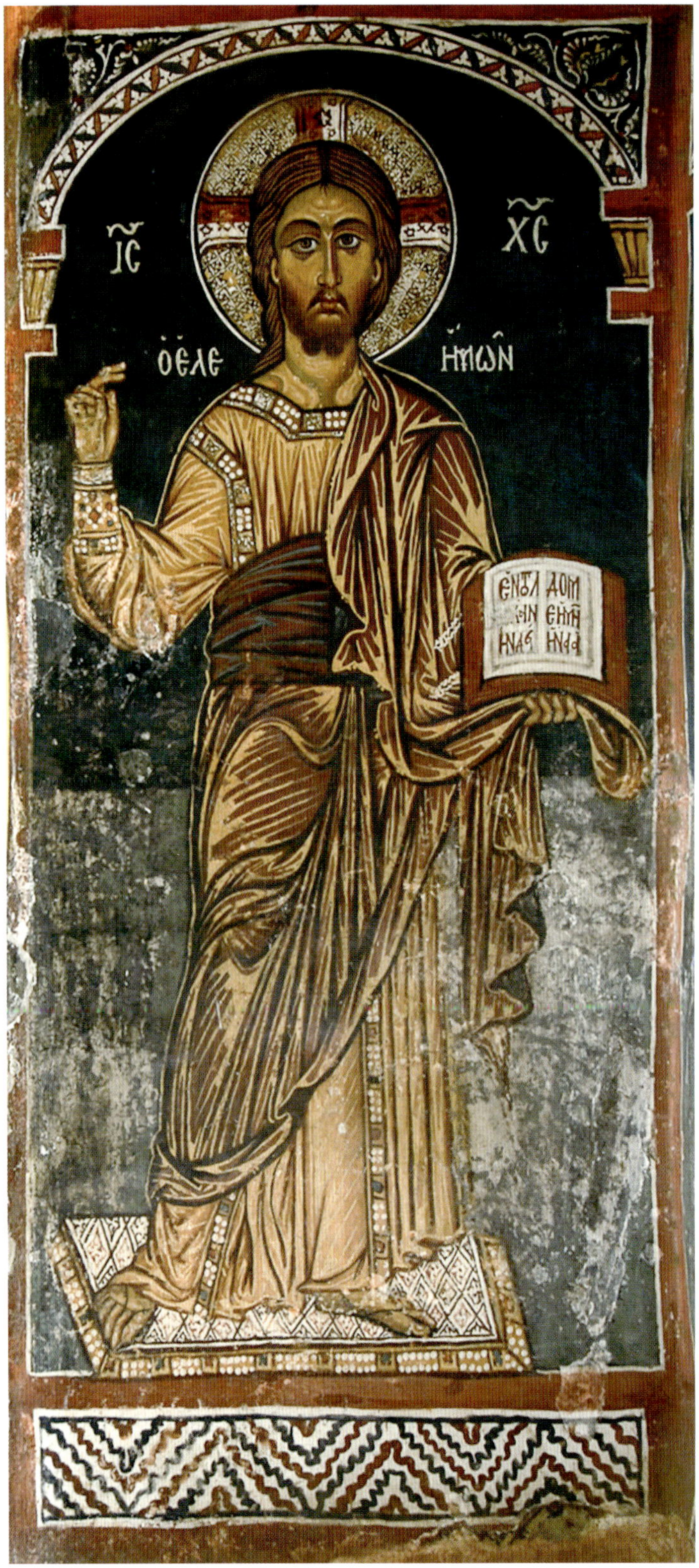

FIG. 6.54 Naos, south bema respond. Christ Eleemon (photo courtesy of G. L. Carr)

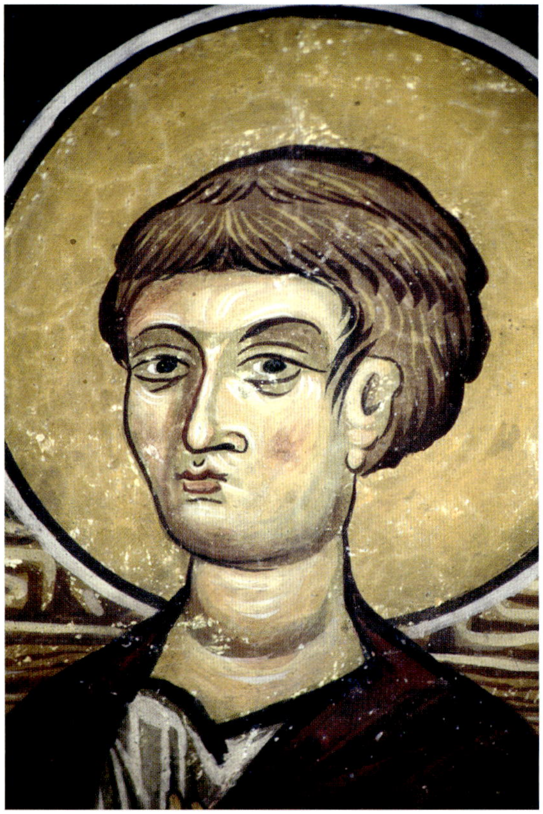

FIG. 6.55 Narthex, pendentive arch: Head of St. Thomas (photo courtesy of A. W. Carr)

the fresco of Christ from the church of the Panagia at Moutoullas from 1280 (Figs. 5.51, 5.60). In turn, a comparison of the figure of Christ Eleemon in the narthex with the Christ Eleemon on the bema respond gives a similarly clear picture of the relation between narthex and naos at Asinou (Figs. 6.54; 5.30, 5.51). The faces are similar enough in conception to have been drawn from a single template. But where the rendering of Christ's face in the narthex is smooth and linear, its surfaces only minimally modulated in either color or value and its features defined by their tight, cleanly drawn edges, the face in the naos is emphatically varied in both hue and value. Its lines play as fully into the coloristic definition of forms as into their linear rendering, and it recurrently draws attention away from the edges and into the volumes of the face—the mouth is perhaps the most striking example, but the deeply hollowed ears and brightly highlighted bulb of the nose are equally indicative. The contrast is reinforced by the himation: reticently modeled with a softly contrasting color, the himation in the narthex smoothes the body into a coherent support beneath the head; while in the naos it is modeled with pure optical force through an abrupt juxtaposition of light and dark that flashes over the whole surface. Rather than by any haptic continuity, the figure is integrated by a bright negative outline that surrounds it and separates it from its ground. Two points emerge from this comparison: the two programs draw on a remarkably similar repertoire of figure types, and they realize these types in contrasting ways. A number of comparisons can be drawn: between St. Sozomenos in the narthex and St. Paul in the naos (Figs. 5.30; 6.3); between St. Andrew in the pendentive of the narthex and St. Memnon in the naos (Figs. 5.17; 6.24); between the youthful St. Thomas in the narthex (Fig. 6.55) and St. Tryphon in the naos (Fig. 6.23). In these comparisons, the forms in the naos look later than those in the narthex.

That the naos paintings are in this respect more reflective of current, fourteenth-century developments is clear. Nor are they alone in this respect: the icon of the Mother of God from Moutoullas exhibits the same abandonment of line in favor of the play of hue and value that one sees in the faces of Mary in the naos at Asinou.[349] But two factors deserve further consideration. In the first place, as Sophia Kalopissi-Verti notes (see pp. 196–97), the forms in the narthex are not uniform but shift toward those of the naos. The contrasts are sharpest when forms from the naos are juxtaposed with figures from the vault of the narthex; they become more moderate when one turns to the figures in the lower register of the narthex. As one moves from the St. Thomas in the pendentive to the face of St. George Machairomenos in the lower register (Figs. 6.55, 6.56), the facial volumes change: no longer thin and subject to the deformations of willful contour lines, the face presents a firm, resistant ovoid whose form is established as much by the color-modeling as it is by the contour. In gathering its force away from the contour and into the body of the face, the St. George is more nearly akin to St. Tryphon in the naos (Fig. 6.23) than to the Thomas just above him. From St. George, in turn, one might move to the face of the Archangel Michael in the northern apse of the narthex (Fig. 6.57). Here the cool, porcelain continuity of surface evaporates in favor of color: the warmer ocher, the resulting heightening of color contrasts, and above all the stronger play of value contrasts now favor a reading of the face in terms of color and contrast rather than of line and surface.

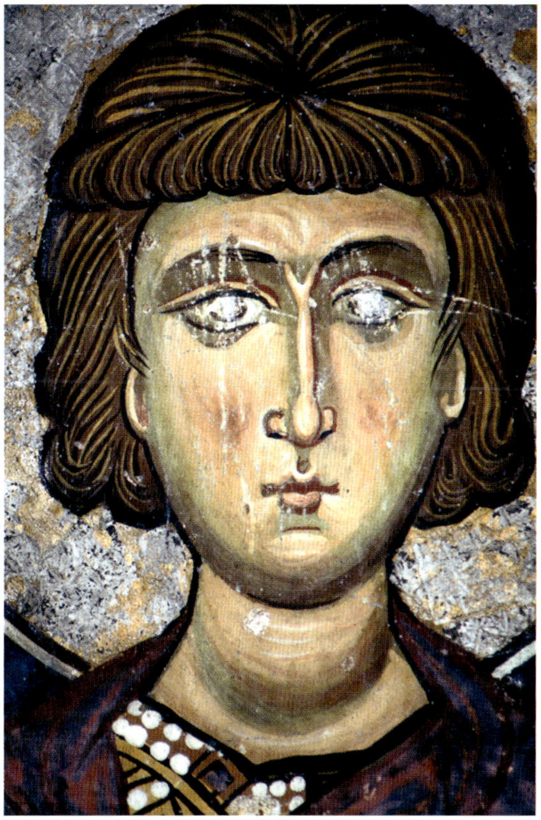

FIG. 6.56 Narthex, south apse: St. George Machairomenos (photo courtesy of A. W. Carr)

The play of value and color, in turn, is what characterizes the faces in the naos. A suggestive comparison is offered by the face of the enthroned Mother of God on the south wall, which, like that of Michael, is fully frontal (Figs. 6.57, 6.58). The face of Michael gives warmth and intensity to the surfaces but still relies on finely drafted lines

349. Papageorgiou, *Icons of Cyprus* (1969), fig. 29.

to define the features. In the face of Mary, lines broaden and blur. The laden strokes of red along the nose and nostrils, or of brown on the brows and in the eye sockets, no longer delineate the forms; instead, they offer relief within a system of color and value contrasts. There is, in fact, no contour line at all under the chin; the lower face is formed entirely by the shadowed effects of the green underpaint and brown wash. The Virgin's face stands to one side of the Michael as that of George Machairomenos does to the other (Figs. 6.56–58). They form an easy progression.

The forms in the narthex, then, are not uniform, but shift toward the colorism of the naos. They make this shift in what can easily be understood as the probable direction of the work, from top to bottom and from south to north.[350] The coloristic intensity seen in the face of St. Michael also characterizes the figures of Earth and Sea in the apse conch just above him (Fig. 5.29). These figures—with their round faces, loosely applied coloristic modeling, and sketchy locks of hair—are far closer to the St. Tryphon of the naos than they are to either St. George or St. Thomas in the narthex (Figs. 6.23, 6.55, 6.56). Much of what is called the contrast between naos and narthex, then, was already bridged in the narthex itself. No sharp gulf divides them. In short, the interval between the two need not be great.

This, however, leads to the second consideration. Chronology is only one aspect of the contrast between them. There is also—as intimated already in the discussion of ornament—a factor of quality. The paintings in the central bay are more loosely painted than are those in the narthex, abrading the purity of shape and line in which that manner had located its claims to excellence. There is also an issue of taste. The paintings in the naos introduce decorative highlights, spade-patterned fabrics, light-spangled architectural and landscape settings, and ornate furniture, reflecting a looser, more lavish sense of taste and exuberance quite alien to the narthex. Thus the two campaigns may not be the product of the same painter(s) moving from one scene to the other in unbroken continuity along lines of stylistic evolution. The shifts in taste and technique warn against using chronology alone to interpret the relation of naos and narthex. Rather than the slow, sequential evolution of a period style, the two may reflect the parallel work of different painters with different standards of taste.

The manner seen at Asinou was, in fact, practiced by different painters over a period of close to a century. Its repertoire of conventions recurs in no fewer than eight other mural cycles in Cyprus. They include the paintings of 1317 at St. Demetrianos in Dali;[351] the complex cycle in the central vessel and southern apse of the church of the Holy Cross at Pelendri;[352] the fragmentary figures on the east wall of the narthex at Lagoudera;[353] the prophets and saints in the western bay at Monagri;[354] certain individual figures in St. Marina, Pyrga;[355] and, with diminishing fidelity, the scenes in the cave of St. Sozomenos near Potamia[356] and scenes of the life of the Virgin and the martyrdom of St. Lawrence at St. Catherine, Pyrga.[357] These cycles are

350. Painters typically moved from top to bottom of their walls in order not to splash, scratch, or nick finished surfaces. But note Ioanna Kakoulli's observation, p. 343 below, that in the lunette and arch over the western doorway, "the upper *pontata* was painted after the bottom one."

351. Stylianou and Stylianou, *Painted Churches*, 425–27.

352. See Christoforaki, "Cyprus Between Byzantium and the Levant"; eadem, "Η τέχνη στην Κύπρο."

353. Winfield and Winfield, *Church of the Panaghia tou Arakos*, 68–69, 329–35 and 343; fig. 8, 300–303; Hein et al., *Cyprus*, fig. 57. These include on the south side a fragment of a Gospel scene showing Jesus seated on a hill and, below him, the standing figures of St. John of Damascus and St. Kosmas the Poet; and, on the north side, the fragment of a crowd of acclaiming apostles, and below it the torso of another monastic saint.

354. Boyd, "Church of the Panagia Amasgou," 323–27, figs. 54–63.

355. See pp. 201, 204 above.

356. Papageorgiou, "Λαξευτά ασκητήρια και μοναστήρια," 47–52; idem, *ARDAC* for 1990, 20, figs. 7–8.

357. Spanou, "Η τέχνη στη μητροπολιτική περιφέρεια Κιτίου," 49–51.

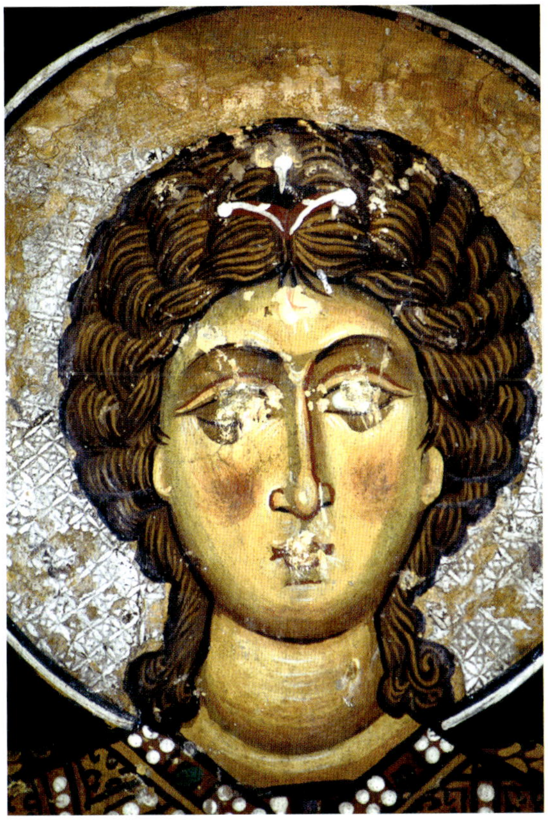

FIG. 6.57 Narthex, north apse: St. Michael the Archangel (photo courtesy of A. W. Carr)

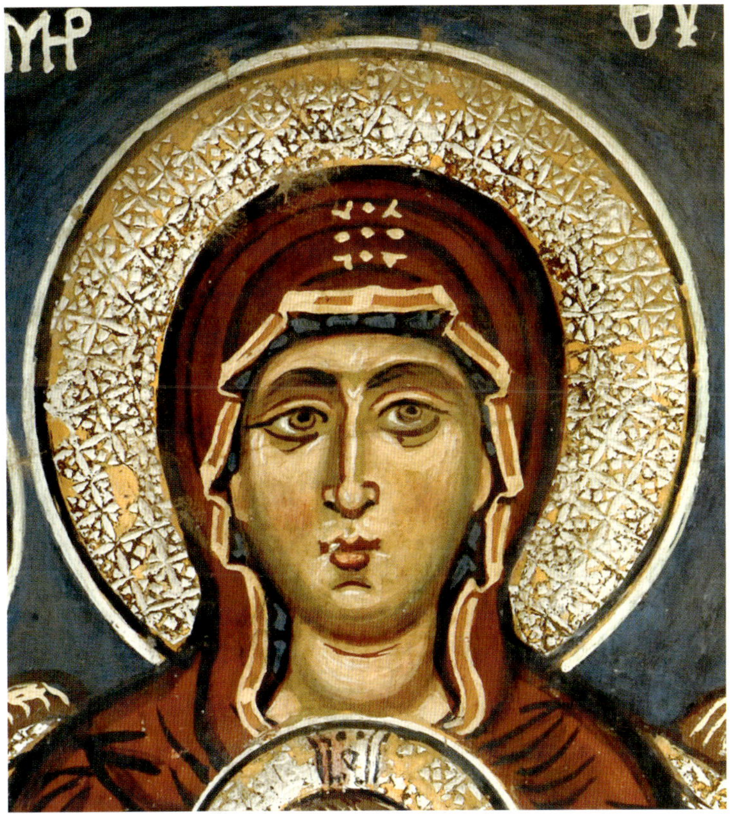

FIG. 6.58 Naos, central bay, south wall: Mother of God (photo courtesy of G. L. Carr)

loosely grouped as representatives of what is variously interpreted as a style, a workshop manner, or simply a particular mode of training.[358] Several of these cycles are dated: the donor portrait at Dali, as noted, bears the date of 1317; the Asinou narthex is dated by its inscription of 1332/33; Pelendri displays in its north vessel the armorial crest of Jean de Lusignan, brother to King Peter I, whose tenancy of Pelendri as a fief from at least 1353 until his murder in 1375 offers a likely span for the paintings there;[359] and the inscription over the door at Pyrga gives the year 1421.[360] Thus the group promises to be useful in pinpointing the date of Asinou's central bay.

358. As evidence of the organization of the painter's trade, these monuments would reward comparison with the early 12th-century cycles associated with the Asinou Master, for the two groups give interestingly different views into the way individuals, styles, and commissions interacted, presumably casting light on how painters worked within the different economic systems of the two eras.

359. Stylianou and Stylianou, *Painted Churches*, 224. On Jean de Lusignan's tenancy of Pelendri as a fief, see note 62 above.

360. The date has been challenged both by Spanou, "Η τέχνη στη μητροπολιτική περιφέρεια Κιτίου," 49–51, who favors a 14th-century date for some but not all of the frescoes, and by Wollensen, *Patrons and Painters on Cyprus*, who places them all around 1300. I believe the challenge is well taken, though I would favor a date in the reign not of Henry II but of Hugh IV, both because the images akin to Asinou seem to me to follow rather than to precede the murals of Asinou's narthex, and because of the connection that I perceive between the chapel and the relics of the True Cross that played such a powerful role in Hugh's reign: see Carr, "Holy Icons,"

The dated members—Dali, the narthex at Asinou, Pelendri, and Pyrga—reveal that the group is not especially obliging about lining up in a tidy stylistic progression. The paintings at Pelendri illuminate this admonition. The church of the Holy Cross at Pelendri is a cavernous, complicated space with a radically disjointed pictorial program painted by many different artists. Among them, the group in the central vessel interests us, as it includes familiar faces. One example, as Sophia Kalopissi-Verti shows (see p. 135), is the face of the apostle Peter on one of the piers in the central vessel. With his meticulously drafted cap of hair, his sunken profile, his heavily lined face, and his monochrome ocher robes, he is remarkably similar to the figure of Peter in the pendentive of the Asinou narthex. To a degree unparalleled in the Asinou naos, the figure at Pelendri invites interpretation as a work by one of the hands from the Asinou narthex, though the draftsmanship at Pelendri is drier, suggesting that it was later than that at Asinou. There is no hint of colorism in the form, however. The painter at Pelendri has maintained the values seen in the Asinou narthex. They are very different from those enunciated in the naos at Asinou. The two sites represent two distinct standards of value. They cannot be aligned in a graduated sequence of steps, as the idea of a stylistic evolution would have required.

There are also paintings at Pelendri that resemble those in the Asinou naos. These are the narratives of the life of the Virgin and of the Passion of Christ. They are the best known of Pelendri's paintings, and are often compared with the scenes at Asinou. A close look, however, suggests that they, too, are later than their Asinou counterparts. This emerges especially clearly from a juxtaposition of the Presentation of Christ in the Temple in Asinou with the Presentation of the Virgin to Joseph at Pelendri (Figs. 6.39, 6.59).The architectural setting at Pelendri has become congested, the drapery patterns have lost their definition and swirl over the surface instead of shaping the limbs, and the faces—though extremely painterly—are simplified to a scrawl of ocher squiggles over the brownish layer below. Only the face of the young Mother of God retains a play of color and, though it compares effectively with the face of St. Tryphon at Asinou (Fig. 6.23), it is far from displaying the deftly pooled puddles of color that form the face of Mary in the donor portrait there (Fig. 6.50). This painter, no less than the painter of St. Peter at Pelendri, seems to have moved onward from the manner at Asinou, but in his own way. Both manners seen at Asinou, then, are also seen at Pelendri. Both appear in what seem to be later stages. But at Pelendri they convey no sense that the painters have moved together in a uniform flow from linear to coloristic. The direction of stylistic change is episodic and depends on the taste of its particular practitioners. These practitioners—one related and possibly identical to the painter(s) seen in the Asinou narthex and the other related and possibly identical to the painter(s) of the Asinou naos—work together in one space but develop each in his own direction.

The evidence of Pelendri is crucial to an assessment of the relation of narthex and naos at Asinou. The work at the two sites cannot have been as much as a generation apart. If we believe that the painters who worked in the narthex pendentives at Asinou also worked at Pelendri, then the distance between these two monuments would be no more than a single painter's working lifetime. In turn, the distance between narthex and naos at Asinou would have to be less.

But the evidence of Pelendri is significant in another way. It challenges the faith in linear sequence. Not only do Asinou's two manners persist there without concessions to a shared sequential evolution; they also exist side by side in the same space. One might imagine them at Asinou, too, as belonging to contemporary campaigns overseen by painters of similar background but different taste—people who worked, as at Pelendri, in tandem.

The challenge Pelendri offers to any evolutionary interpretation of the various artistic manners in use in fourteenth-century Cyprus is reinforced by the paintings at Dali, which are simpler than either

---

315–20. The significant disjunctions in scale, iconography, and style among the images have yet to be understood adequately.

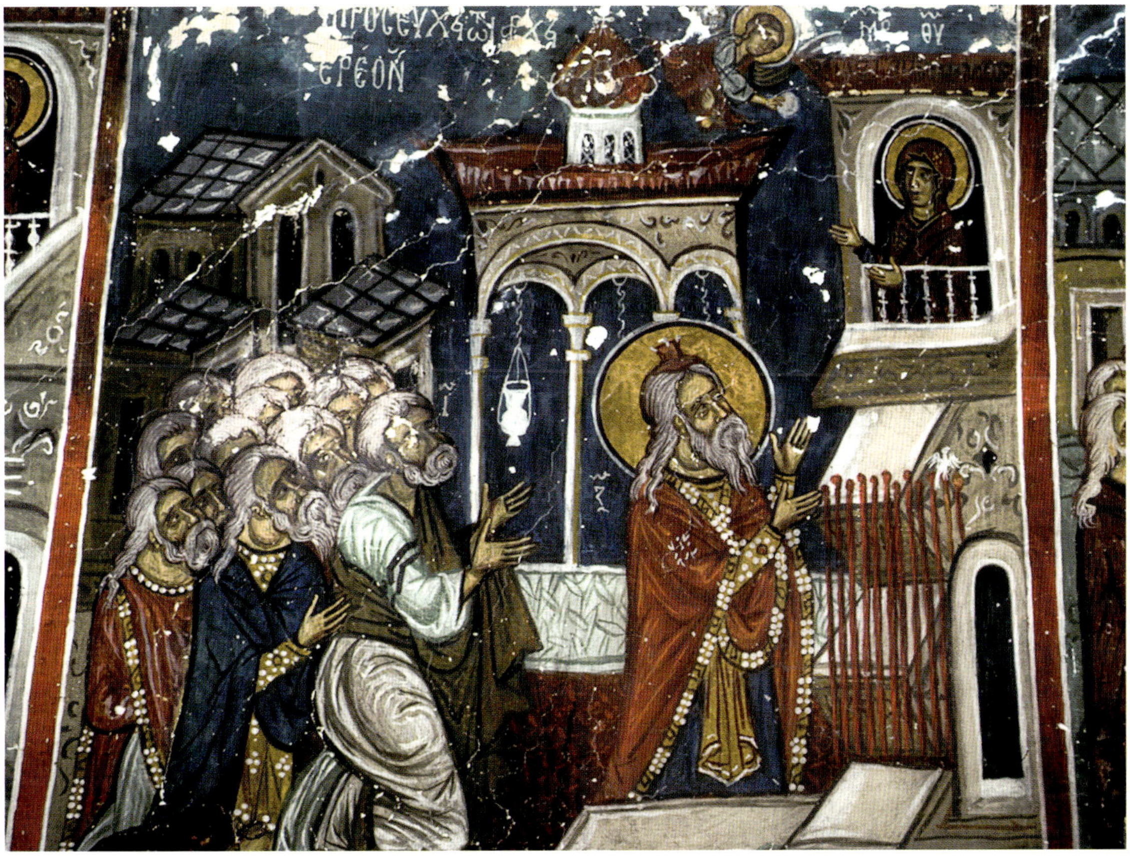

FIG. 6.59 Pelendri, church of the Holy Cross: Presentation of the Virgin in the Temple (photo courtesy of A. W. Carr)

campaign at Asinou but are not readily aligned with either one in an evolutionary sequence. This particularism makes it difficult to propose dates for the otherwise undated representatives of the group, like the central bay of the naos at Asinou. Stylistic testimony shows that the central bay of Asinou's naos is not far from the campaign of 1332/33 in the narthex, and that the two could be virtually contemporary. Two pieces of nonstylistic evidence speak in favor of attributing them to two campaigns separated by a span of years. One of these facts is the contrast in the pastiglia haloes; the other is the presence of the dedicatory inscription in the narthex (transcribed on p. 176). Its clear statement of termination suggests a campaign completed. Work in the naos would then have resumed as a new undertaking, plausibly under a new master and certainly with a new mode that is not merely more coloristic but also more exuberant in taste.

The naos at Asinou emerges from this deliberation as a work of the 1340s, close in date to the narthex but not coincident with it and quite surely complete by the middle of the century. Iconographically what had stood out about the paintings in the naos was their seamless integration of new and current ideas with deeply rooted conventions, conventions so strongly established in local usage that it was difficult to break through their mask of tradition to see if they could actually be tied to 1105/6 or not. Stylistically, in turn, the naos is even more striking in the way it accommodates the new, optical and volumetric tastes of the fourteenth century to the conventions of a powerfully rooted, local thirteenth-century manner. The product of this accommodation proves to be both singular and exuberant. It was not readily translated into the more meticulous medium of icon painting, and, in contrast to the manner seen in the narthex, it is barely attested in panel painting. In mural painting this manner remains particular, its warm color and ornamental vigor unparalleled even in the two monuments most closely akin to it, at Pelendri and in the narthex at Lagoudera. As such, the fourteenth-century painting offers an artistic statement that is at least as personal, as reflective of a given moment in the art history of its land, as the more famous murals by the Asinou Master that it covered over.

No less than for the master of 1105/6, one craves a name for the painter of the central bay. As both Sophia Kalopissi-Verti and David Winfield have pointed out, there is a painter of the fourteenth-century style whose name is known. This is the Deacon Leontios, who frescoed the now fragmentary east wall of the narthex at Lagoudera and left his name in an epigram over an image of the Mother of God Achrantos outside the north door (Fig. 5.61).[361] Leontios's forms do not share the linear clarity that distinguishes the narthex at Asinou; his execution is coloristic, though without the energetic warmth of the hues in the naos. Kalopissi-Verti associates his name with the narthex and Winfield with the narthex and naos alike. All painters have names, and it is stubborn to insist upon a particular name simply because it survives. Nonetheless, Leontios's colorism inclines me to align him with Asinou's naos, an alignment that receives unexpected reinforcement from his epigram. This quotes a heirmos of the seventh- or eighth-century hymnographer, Georgios Sikeliotes, that cites Habakkuk's prophecy of the incarnation to invoke the Mother of God:

> + Ἦχῳ εὐλάλῳ προδιαγνοὺς Ἀμβακοὺμ ἀραρότως ἐκ σοῦ, Παρθένε, Λόγου τὴν σάρκωσιν καὶ κόσμος λελύτρωται τῆς ἀρχεγόνου ἀρᾶς. Εὔχεσαι τῷ γράψαντι τὴν δέλτον ταύτην Λεοντ[ίου δια]κόνου. / Ἀμήν.
>
> With a clear sound Habakkuk firmly foretold the Incarnation of the Word through thee, O Virgin, and [so] the world has been delivered of its original curse. Pray for him who has written this tablet, Leontios the Deacon. Amen.[362]

The text, which is altogether in the spirit of the prefigurations used to visualize the theme of incarnation in the naos at Asinou, bespeaks a painter of some learning. Lagoudera's compositions, which Leontios knew, play persistently through those of the central bay in Asinou. These facts invite a link between Leontios and the program of the central bay of Asinou's naos. If they link him with the narthex, too, then we would have just what the modern viewer expects in an artist: a person whose work altered, often in unpredictable ways, over an evolving career.

361. Winfield and Winfield, *Church of the Panaghia tou Arakos*, 68–69, 329–35, 343; figs. 8, 300–303.

362. Ibid., 68.

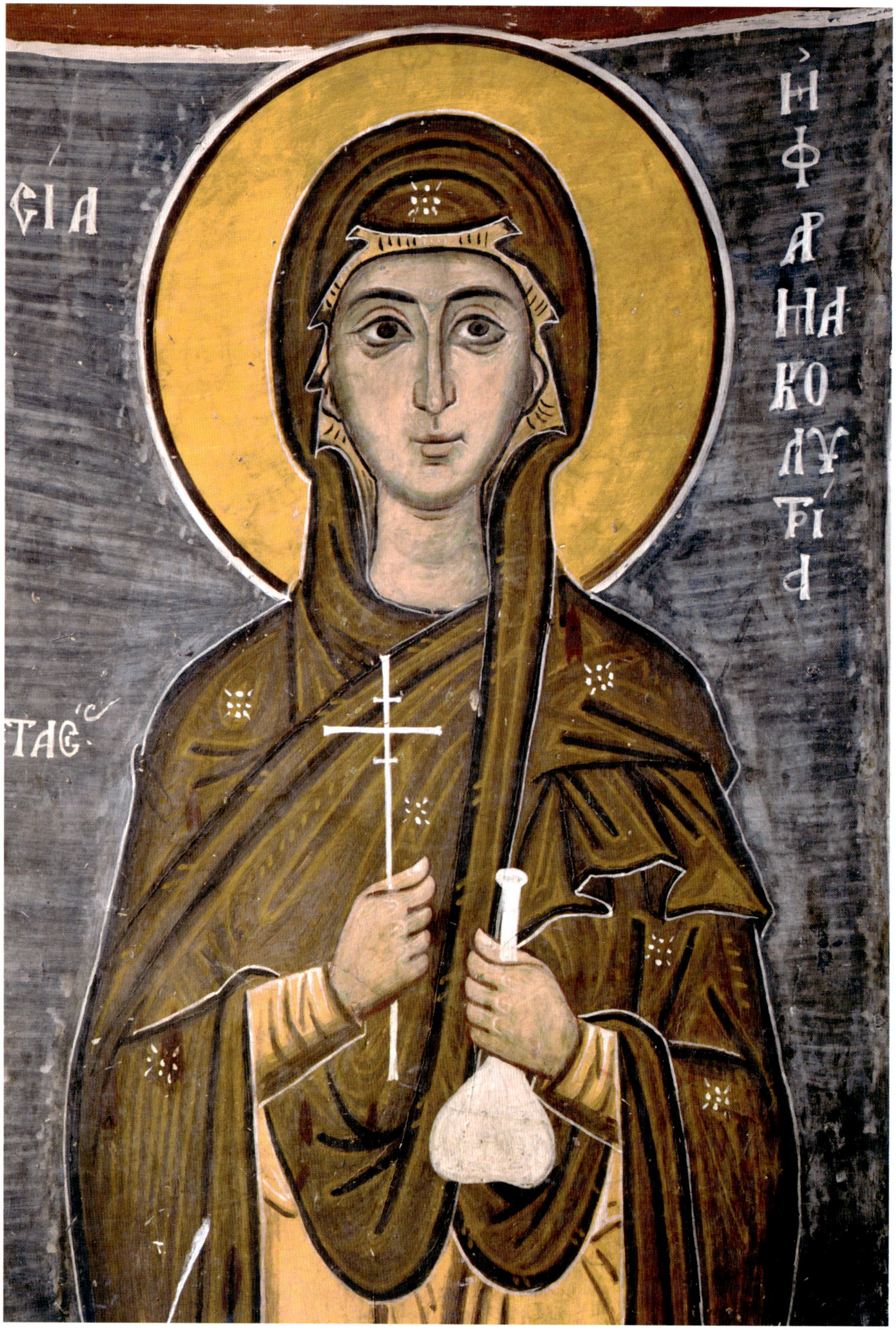

The church of Phanagia Phorbiotissa, narthex, south apse: St. Anastasia the Poison-curer, detail (photo courtesy of G. L. Carr)

The Murals of the Panagia Phorbiotissa

A Technical Examination

Ioanna Kakoulli,
Michael Schilling, and
Joy Mazurek

The technical study of western paintings is well developed. However, there has until very recently been surprisingly little such study of the vast corpus of surviving Byzantine wall paintings. Yet these paintings are particularly important, not only because they are distributed throughout the geographically extensive region that constituted the eastern survival of the Roman Empire, but also because they represent a virtually uninterrupted tradition from late antiquity into the eighteenth century. Despite this continuity, they display a diversity of expression depending on region. Is this continuity and diversity also reflected in the technological tradition? Available studies, both published and unpublished, suggest that there may have been technological diversity, but they are not sufficiently conclusive.

An early comprehensive study of the techniques of Byzantine mural painting was published by David Winfield in 1968. Although of considerable value, this study was based on in situ observation and the primary literature, without the benefit of sampling or technical analysis. In the late 1990s interest began to grow in the technical study of icons and wall paintings (witness the excellent CD-ROM produced by the Benaki Museum in Athens[1] and the establishment in 1996 of the Diagnostic Centre for the Research and Study of Byzantine Hagiography at Ormylia, in northern Greece), reaching unprecedented levels in the last decade. Examples include the study of the pigments and plasters of the wall paintings at Tokalı kilise in Cappadocia;[2] the study of the thirteenth-century wall paintings in the Protaton church at Mount Athos, attributed to Manuel Panselinos, one of the most celebrated painters (*hagiographoi*) of the Byzantine period;[3] the study of the 1557 painting program at Dousiko in Meteora, Greece, signed by George, the famous painter of the Cretan School;[4] the

1. Benaki Museum, *Conservation of Icons.*
2. P. Schwartzbaum, "Appendix 1" in Epstein, *Tokalı Kilise*, 52–59.
3. Daniilia et al., "Protaton Church, Mount Athos."
4. Chiavari et al., "Analytical Pyrolysis."

study of wall paintings at the church of Antiphonitis in Cyprus;[5] the study of the fourteenth-century St. Euthymius wall paintings in the Cathedral of Thessaloniki;[6] studies of wall paintings at Monagri and Askas; and the study of the twelfth-century wall paintings in the rock-cut Enkleistra of St. Neophytos in Paphos.[7]

Clearly, technical studies can contribute to our understanding of the Byzantine painting tradition, and the research published here aims to provide a comprehensive examination of the materials and techniques of the painted programs in the church of Asinou in their historical and artistic context. An important aim of this study is to indicate ways in which technical findings can be used to enhance our understanding of artists' working methods and our ability to "date" their works—in the case of Asinou, the paintings of uncertain date between ca. 1100 and 1600. Particular issues to be addressed include: (1) What are the techniques and painting materials used for the various iconographical programs? (2) Do techniques and imagery relate to one another? Are certain pigments and media characteristic of or unique to a particular program or period? (3) On what bases can we group paintings of uncertain date with other securely dated and classified paintings? (4) How do the Byzantine painting techniques identified at Asinou relate to the broader context of Byzantine and western medieval painting traditions?

The study was based on a comprehensive technical analysis of the paintings, involving the following procedures: noninvasive in situ examination, scientific examination and analysis of microsamples in the laboratory, collection of comparative data through the study of Byzantine and medieval treatises on painting, gathering of information from modern technical studies, and collection of analytical data on other Byzantine and medieval paintings.

The in situ examination was based on careful visual observation and employed special lighting and photographic methods for recording and documenting the paintings. This examination revealed important features and allowed the development of hypotheses concerning the techniques and materials involved. Scientific methods of analysis carried out on microsamples from representative areas of the painting were then used to test these hypotheses. The materials were examined and analyzed for: physical and chemical characterization of the constituent materials and structure of the plasters; identification of pigments and study of their microstructure and manufacture (if synthesized) as well as their application method; identification of the gilding methods and coatings; identification of the binding media employed.

Methodology of Technical Study

Noninvasive In Situ Examination and Recording

Techniques were chosen to minimize the number of required samples. These included raking-light (using focused oblique illumination), false-color infrared,[8] and ultraviolet-induced visible fluorescence photography.[9]

5. Daniilia and Minopoulou, "Discolouration"; and Daniilia et al., "Christ Antiphonitis."

6. Sotiropoulou et al., "Degradation Issues."

7. *Monagri and Askas*: Howard, "Church of Archangel Michael"; Kakoulli, "Philaretos' Akra Tapeinosis"; Frieden, "Ioannis Prodhromos, Askas." *Paphos*: Fischer and Kakoulli, "In Situ Reflectance" and eidem, "Innovative Approach."

8. False-color infrared photography involves a technique that can capture a narrow region of the near infrared from the electromagnetic spectrum that is recomposed, together with the red and green components of the visible RGB image of the identical subject, to form a trichromatic false color image. Because the color of the resulting image represents intensities outside the visible region and therefore differs from a true-color image (an image that appears normal to the human eye), this type of imaging is called false-color infrared.

9. In ultraviolet-induced visible fluorescence photography, black lights (which emit in the ultraviolet region with $\lambda^{\text{exc. max.}} = 365$nm) are used to illuminate an object, while a barrier filter in front of the camera or detector cuts off residual reflected ultraviolet and infrared light so that the resulting image represents only the fluorescence in the visible region.

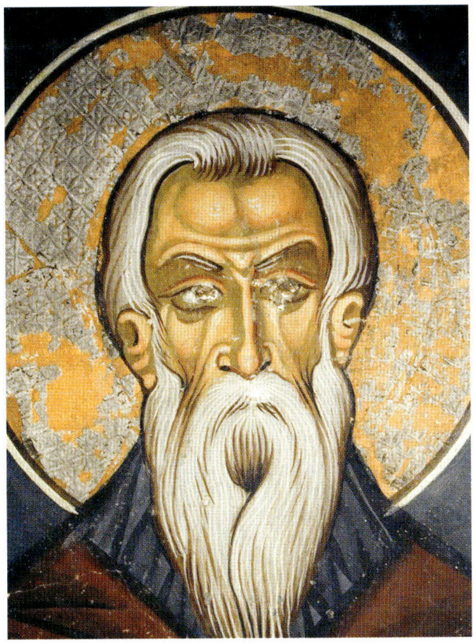

fig. 7.1a

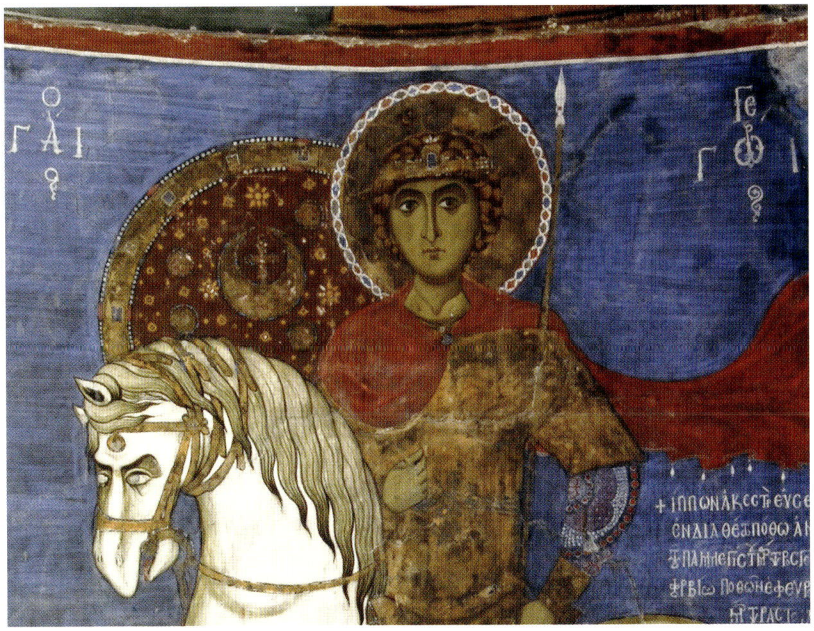

fig. 7.2a

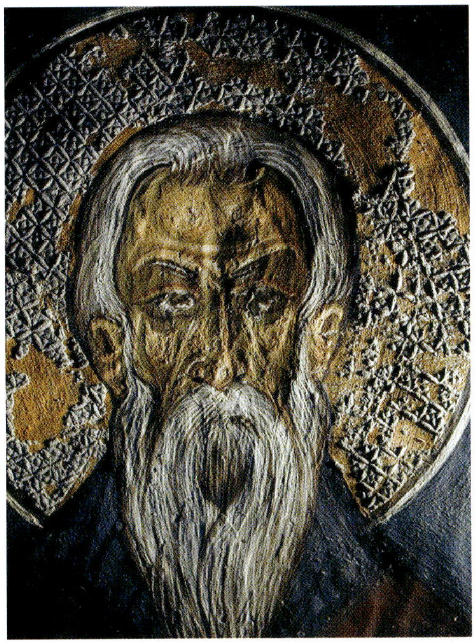

fig. 7.1b

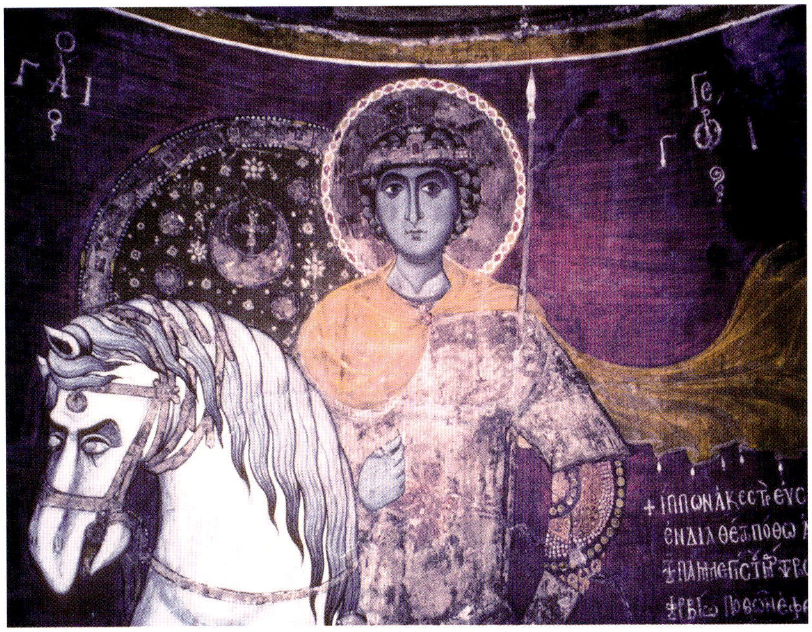

fig. 7.2b

Fig. 7.1 Diffuse (a) and raking-light (b) photographs of St. Sozomenos in the narthex (1332/33 painting program). The image photographed with raking light (b) reveals the tooling of the plaster in the center of the saint's face and the strong surface texture created by the paint brushstrokes, and it enhances the stucco relief in the halo (photos courtesy of Conservation of Wall Painting Department [CWPD], Courtauld Institute of Art).

Fig. 7.2 Diffuse light (a) and false-color infrared (FCI; b) photographs of the figure of St. George in the narthex (late twelfth century). The FCI image (b) displays pseudo-colors characteristic of the chemical composition of the pigments; hence the red mantle of the saint, which was painted in cinnabar, appears lemon yellow in FCI; while the blue background, painted in ultramarine blue, appears fuchsia (photos courtesy of CWPD, Courtauld Institute of Art).

Raking-light photography revealed topographical details such as incisions, irregularities of the paint layer, brush strokes, and paint flakes (Fig. 7.1). Ultraviolet-induced visible fluorescence imaging assisted in the detection and—sometimes—the identification of materials based on their characteristic fluorescent properties, while false-color infrared photography aided in the mapping of areas of the painting altered by previous conservation interventions and by environmental factors, areas not easily distinguishable with the naked eye.[10] In addition, false-color infrared photography provided information regarding the composition of pigments, based on the specific "false" color rendition of each individual pigment (Fig. 7.2).

Sampling

Sampling was unavoidable for the study of the paintings at Asinou. Since sampling is an invasive process, samples were taken only from areas for which crucial information was required to answer specific questions related either to the materials and technique of the painting or to its subsequent conservation. To avoid damaging the painting, samples were taken from edges of losses or cracks. The average sample size obtained for microanalysis was approximately 0.5–1.0 mm in diameter (nearly the size of a sand grain); wherever possible, each sample contained the whole stratigraphy of the painting, but where this was not possible, two or more successive samples were taken.

During this research, in total eighty-three paint samples, including eleven plaster samples, were taken from the various painting programs and were analyzed (see Appendix 1 for locations). Sampling was carried out during two consecutive campaigns, with the permission of the Department of Antiquities of Cyprus and the Bishopric of Morphou.

For the preparation of the microsamples, the use of a binocular microscope was invaluable, since their size made them very difficult to handle. While under magnification (between 10× and 30×), most samples were cut in half. Each half was then treated in various ways, depending on the analytical technique required to answer specific questions. In general, half the sample was mounted in resin and polished to reveal the paint-layer stratigraphy, while the rest was used for other analytical techniques and for the preparation of dispersion samples.[11] In exceptional cases, where samples were large enough (approximately 3–5 mm in diameter), thin sections were prepared.[12]

Laboratory Microanalysis

The heterogeneous nature and small size of the samples imposed many restrictions on the analyses, which involved the use of both nondestructive (in which the sample is retrievable and reusable) and destructive methods (requiring the consumption of the sample to yield results). Different analytical techniques were employed for the study of microsamples. As much information as possible was gathered through nondestructive means before techniques were used that would alter or destroy the sample. Known materials were tested in various concentrations to establish the sensitivity and limitations of the instrumentation and methods used for the analyses.

10. Fischer and Kakoulli, "Multispectral and Hyperspectral Imaging."

11. For the preparation of dispersion samples, a few particles from individual paint layers were separated under the binocular microscope and placed on a glass slide. These particles were placed in a drop of thermoplastic resin (Meltmount) with a refractive index of 1.662, after been heated at a temperature around 50° C. A cover slip was pressed gently over the dispersed particles with a pencil eraser to eliminate the formation of air bubbles and assist in the homogenous dispersion of the particles in the resin (to allow their mineralogical characterization). Upon cooling at room temperature the resin solidifies with the pigment particles well dispersed within the resin. Dispersion samples are examined using transmitted light on a polarized light microscope for the characterization and identification of the pigment particles.

12. Thin sections were prepared only for the plaster analysis. Samples of this size involved cylindrical sections of plaster taken from areas of existing paint losses, using a variable speed microdrill and diamond-coated hollow bits of 3 and 5 mm diameter.

The primary optical and analytical techniques used were polarized light microscopy (PLM), scanning electron microscopy (SEM) with energy-dispersive x-ray spectroscopy (EDS), Fourier transform infrared (FTIR) spectroscopy, and gas chromatography–mass spectrometry (GC-MS). For the resultant inorganic and organic analyses, see Appendices 2, 3, and 5. Microchemical tests were also carried out on selected particles (see Appendix 2).

Results

The complex stratigraphy of overlapping programs of wall paintings in the church of Asinou has intrigued art historians because it provides a microcosm of major developments in Byzantine wall painting from the twelfth to the seventeenth centuries.

Painting Techniques

Two techniques—fresco and secco—were identified in all painting programs of the church. These techniques are discussed in Appendix 4. The base colors, in a flat tonality, seem to have been applied in fresco (i.e., fresh plaster), while the modeling and highlights were added later, in secco (dry plaster), using an organic binding medium or lime (calcium hydroxide). Blue pigments of the background and gilding were also applied in secco using organic binding media and mordants.

Although this mixed technique (involving a combination of fresco and secco) is found in all painted programs ranging from the twelfth to the seventeenth century, small differences—such as the plaster's consistency and application, special features of the setting-out techniques, and the manner of painting—assisted in the differentiation of the programs and the classification and attribution of the paintings of uncertain date.

Plasters

Composition

The preliminary in situ investigation, combined with the microscopic examination of thin sections, suggested the presence of single plaster layers in all programs of painting studied. These plasters were lime based and were rich in organic fibers. The latter help reduce shrinkage and increase the flexural strength of the plaster. Two different types of fibers were identified: a thick type with the morphological characteristics of chaff; and a finer type, probably flax tow or hemp.[13] The varying use of these fibers created differences in the plaster's texture. Variations in the color and texture of the plaster layers also were influenced by the presence of inert inorganic aggregates (in minor quantities) such as chalk, ferric oxide particles, sandstone fragments, muscovite, quartz, and micrite. The presence or absence of certain aggregates and their combination, together with chaff, flax tow, or hemp, assisted in classifying certain paintings of uncertain date.

Comparing the plaster of the paintings at Asinou with other Byzantine paintings in Cyprus, it seems that the addition of fibers was a very common practice. Fiber-rich lime plaster was also found in Philaretos's eighteenth-century paintings at Monagri. The plaster, applied in a single layer 0.5–1.5 cm thick directly over the stone support, included chaff and flax tow.[14] Likewise, at Askas, the plaster was applied either in a single or a double layer.[15] The most common filler identified in Byzantine wall paintings has been chaff. Only in a few cases was the lime mixed with flax tow to form a smooth layer.[16]

13. Dionysios of Fourna describes a method for preparing plaster, the first using refined lime and fine chaff as the first layer, with a second and final layer consisting of lime and flax tow. Although Dionysios was writing in the first half of the eighteenth century, his manuscript, which draws from ancient and then-current sources, describes a longstanding Byzantine painting tradition. Dionysios of Fourna, *Hermeneia*, 6, 13.

14. Howard, "Church of Archangel Michael"; Kakoulli, "Philaretos."

15. Frieden, "Askas," 19.

16. For an example without flax tow: Lime plaster with chaff, quartz, and albite (a silicate with stoichiometry $NaAlSi_3O_8$) was also identified in the thirteenth-century Protaton paintings at Mount Athos: Daniilia et al., "Protaton," 105–7.

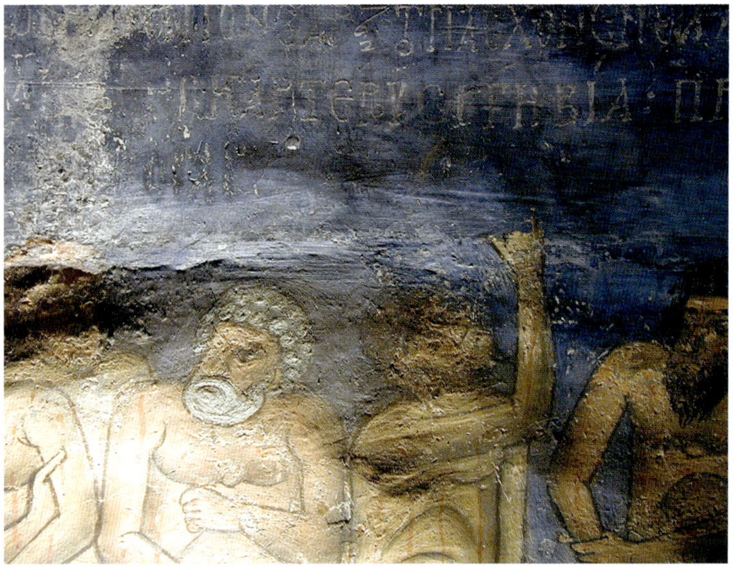

Fig. 7.3 Raking-light photograph of a detail from the scene of the Forty Martyrs (1105/6) on the north wall of the naos. This image illustrates a horizontal plaster join, corresponding to the height of a scaffolding lift and known as a *pontata* (photo courtesy of CWPD, Courtauld Institute of Art).

Application

Plaster joins (seams between sections of plaster applied at different times) were identified during the preliminary investigation on two different phases of painting: the 1105/6 program in the naos and the 1332/33 program in the narthex. These plaster joins are either run horizontally between *pontate* (large, rectangular sections of plaster corresponding to the height of the scaffolding lifts) as, for example, in the scene with the representation of the Forty Martyrs in the naos (Fig. 7.3); or they define *giornate* (plaster applied in patches, corresponding to the work that an artist can complete on fresh plaster in a given day). The *giornate*, which follow the outlines of the smaller scenes, can be seen in the dome of the narthex. Plaster joins in general do not necessarily indicate a fresco technique; large *pontate* might just as easily feature in secco paintings. By contrast, the use of *giornate* would certainly imply the use of fresco technique at least for the application of the base

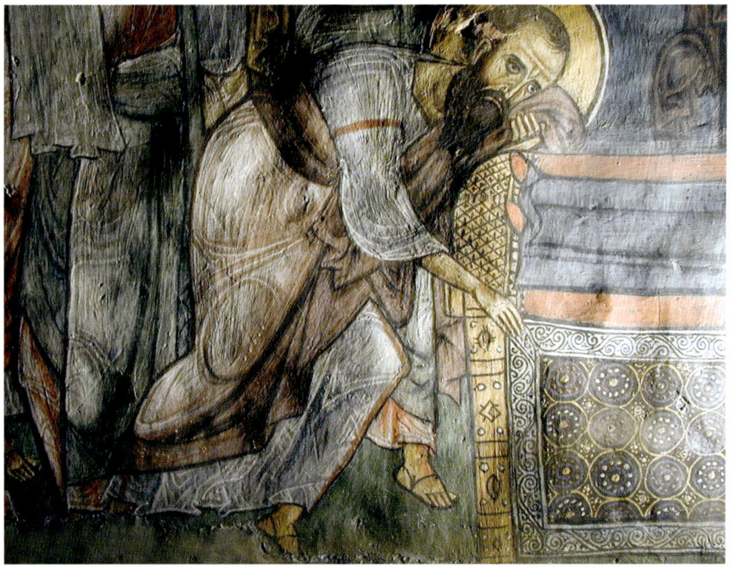

Fig. 7.4 Detail from the Dormition scene (1105/6) on the west wall of the naos, photographed in raking light. The image shows the strong surface texture in the painted figure and the undulating surface of the plaster (photo courtesy of CWPD, Courtauld Institute of Art).

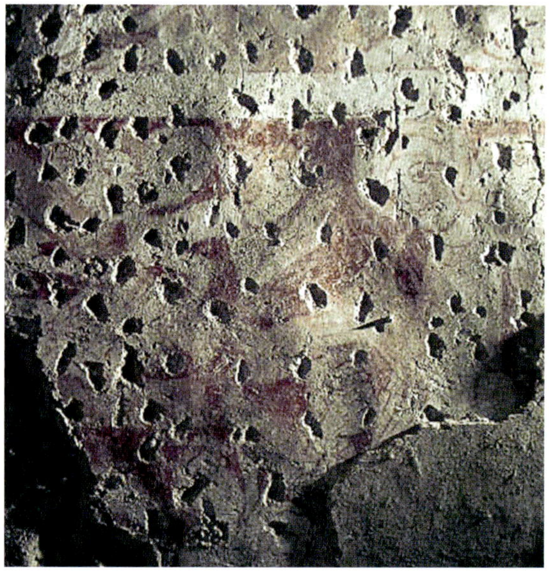

Fig. 7.5 Detail of the Romanesque painting in the church of St. Mary the Virgin, Houghton-on-the-Hill, near Norfolk, England, photographed in raking light. The image shows a keyed, undulating plaster (photo courtesy of CWPD, Courtauld Institute of Art).

Fig. 7.6 Detail of St. Paul from the Dormition scene (1105/6) on the west wall of the naos, photographed in raking light. The image shows the characteristic preparatory drawing using dilute brown paint to outline the figures. The preparatory drawing can be better observed in the area outlining the fingers (photo courtesy of CWPD, Courtauld Institute of Art).

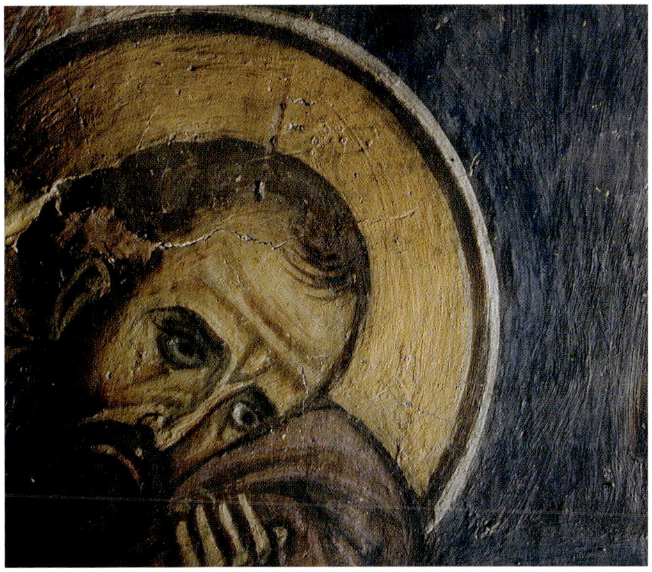

colors. The application of plasters for individual painting programs at Asinou is discussed below. Examples of plaster joins suggesting a fresco application were identified in other Byzantine paintings in Cyprus (at Monagri and Askas),[17] as well as in the Protaton paintings at Mount Athos.[18]

The texture and appearance of the plaster layers at Asinou vary considerably, influenced by the nature and size of the aggregates, the thickness of the plaster, and the tools used for its application. For example, the plaster of the 1105/6 program has a very characteristic undulating texture (Fig. 7.4), quite similar to contemporary medieval paintings in western Europe; an example is found at the church of St. Mary the Virgin, Houghton-on-the-Hill, near Norfolk, England (Fig. 7.5).[19] The later paintings in the Asinou church have very smooth, flat plaster surfaces; extensive fourteenth-century examples can be seen in the in the narthex.

Preparatory Drawing and Setting-out Techniques

Most of the paintings in the church at Asinou were sketched on the plaster using diluted black or brown paint (Fig. 7.6). Evidence of freehand incised preparatory drawing was observed in only four painting programs: the Anastasia painting in the narthex (late thirteenth century; Fig. 7.7); the older layer of painting depicting SS. Peter and Paul on the westernmost piers in the naos (possibly late thirteenth century; p. 213); the Pantokrator in the dome of the narthex

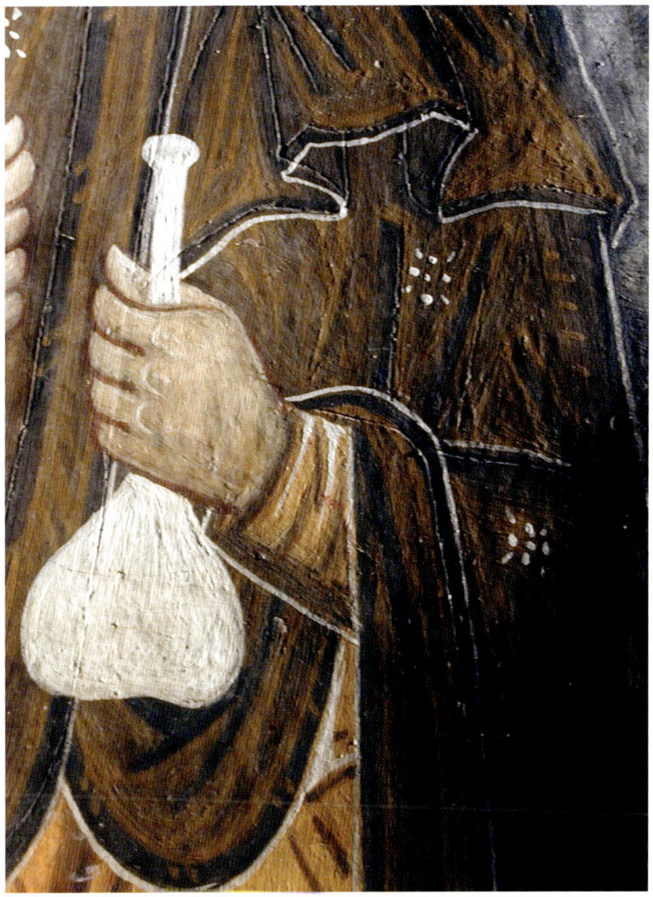

Fig. 7.7 Raking-light photograph of a detail from the late thirteenth-century painting of St. Anastasia in the narthex, showing the incised preparatory drawing (photo courtesy of CWPD, Courtauld Institute of Art).

17. Howard, "Church of Archangel Michael"; Frieden, "Askas," 8–19.
18. Daniilia et al., "Protaton," 105–7.
19. Kakoulli and Cather, "Houghton-on-the-Hill."

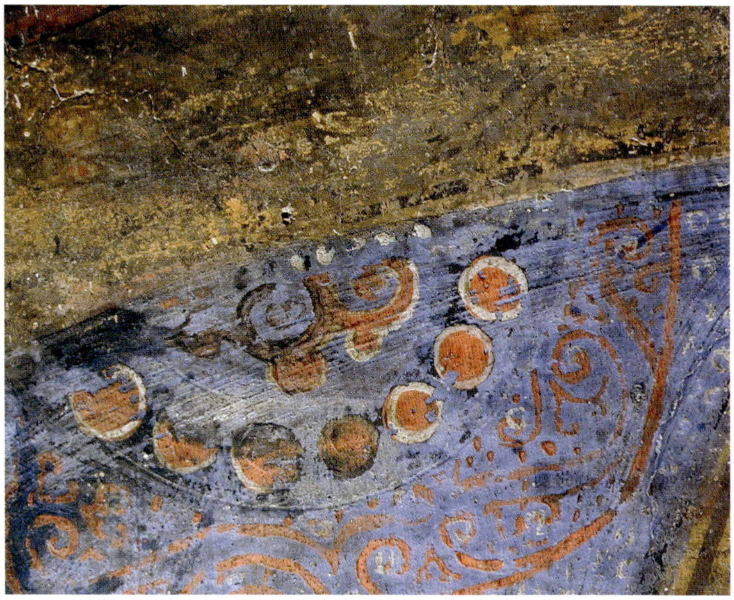

Fig. 7.8 Photograph of the painting of St. George in the narthex. This photograph, taken under raking light, shows incisions made by using a compass to outline the circular motifs on the garments. The center of the circle is visible as a hole in the plaster, made by the point of the compass (photo courtesy of CWPD, Courtauld Institute of Art).

(fourteenth century; p. 197); and the Pantanassa painting in the conch of the apse in the bema (possibly late thirteenth century; p. 215).[20] Compass incisions were also recorded, for example, to outline the circular motifs on the garments of St. George in the narthex (possibly last quarter of the twelfth century; Fig. 7.8). Evidence that halos were incised using a compass was also seen, for example, in the sixteenth-century paintings in the church.

Incised preparatory drawing has also been identified in the paintings at Protaton, Mt. Athos, primarily for outlining the garments of the figures. A few *pentimenti* (corrections of the preparatory drawing by the painter) were also visible in that painting program.[21] Dionysios of Fourna describes the use of incised preparatory drawing, particularly to inscribe halos. He also mentions the use of yellow ocher to outline the figures; at Asinou, diluted black or brown paint was used.

Pigments and Methods of Application

The following pigments, both natural and artificial, were identified: lapis lazuli, consisting mainly of lazurite $[(Na,Ca)_{7\text{-}8}(Al,Si)_{12}(O,S)_{24}[(SO_4), Cl_2,(OH)_2]$, diopside, and pyrite minerals;[22] azurite $[2CuCO_3.Cu(OH)_2]$; green earth, mainly celadonite mineral $[K(Mg,Fe^{2+})(Fe^{3+},Al)Si_4O_{10}(OH)_2]$; hematite-rich red ocher $[\text{-}Fe_2O_3]$; amorphous red ocher $[Fe_2O_3.nH_2O]$; cinnabar [HgS]; red lead or minium $[Pb_3O_4]$; yellow ocher or limonite $[FeO.OH.nH_2O]$; goethite-rich yellow ocher $[\alpha\text{-}FeO(OH)]$; jarosite $[KFe_3(SO_4)_2(OH)_6]$; natural sienna (a form of limonite); massicot or litharge (both PbO); lime white or bianco di San Giovanni $[CaCO_3$ and $Ca(OH)_2]$; and carbon black [C].

The pigments used were either pure, mixed with white or black for tonal adjustments, or mixed with each other to obtain different hues. An example of the last is the combination of cinnabar with lapis lazuli to form a purple, as found in the garments of the St. George in the narthex. In other cases, pigments were layered to enhance their color, as for example the blue pigments applied over a black intermediate paint layer. The use of lime white in the mixtures also affected the opacity and texture of the paint layers. The mixing and layering of pigments, in some cases, influenced the attribution of the paintings to specific programs (see below).

The pigments identified in the different painting programs are presented in Table 7.1.[23]

20. Winfield, "Wall Painting Methods," plates 11, 14–17.
21. Daniilia et al., "Protaton," 94.

22. Plesters, "Ultramarine Blue"; Gaetani et al., "Egyptian Blue"; Klein and Hurlbut, *Manual of Mineralogy*; Kakoulli and Michaelides, "Tomb Paintings."
23. For a very similar palette of colors see the thirteenth-century paintings of Panselinos at Protaton, which included lime white, carbon black [C], limonite, red ocher, caput mortuum, green earth (celadonite), azurite, cinnabar, and minium. The last two were used only occasionally for the red highlights. The pigments used were either pure or in simple combinations: Daniilia et al., "Protaton," 108–9.

Table 7.1. Occurrence of pigments

	1105/6 paintings in naos and bema	1105/6 and 14c: Phorbiotissa in narthex	late 12c: St. George in narthex	late 13c: Pantanassa in bema	late 13c: SS. Peter & Paul in naos	late 13c: St. Anastasia Pharmakolytria in narthex	1332/3 paintings in narthex	14c paintings in naos	16c paintings in naos
lapis lazuli	•		•						
azurite		[a]•		•			•	•	•
green earth	•		•	•	•		•	•	•
hematite-rich red ocher	•	•				•	•	•	
amorphous red ocher	•		•	•	•	•	•	•	•
cinnabar	•	•	•	•		•	•	•	•
red lead	•		•					•	•
yellow ocher (limonite)	•	•	•	•		•	•	•	•
goethite-rich yellow ocher		•			•	•	•		•
jarosite	•		•	•		•	•	•	
natural/raw sienna							•		
massicot or litharge							•		
lime white	•	•	•	•	•	•	•	•	•
carbon/charcoal black	•	•	•	•		•	•	•	•

[a] Azurite found in 14th-c. additions to the painting, not the original 1105/6 composition.

Blue Pigments

Two blue pigments were identified: lapis lazuli and azurite.

Lapis Lazuli (Natural Ultramarine)

Lapis lazuli or natural ultramarine blue was an extraordinarily expensive pigment, and its use at Asinou indicates a lavish commission. It is prepared from the semiprecious stone lapis lazuli, composed mainly of lazurite, a feldspathoid silicate mineral $[(Na,Ca)_{7-8}(Al,Si)_{12}(O,S)_{24}[(SO_4),Cl_2,(OH)_2]]$. Asinou represents one of the earliest examples in western European and Byzantine wall painting where lapis lazuli was used as a pigment, though it was available in antiquity and can be found in Chinese and central Asian paintings as early as the sixth century and in Byzantine illuminated manuscripts from the seventh century on.[24] At Asinou, lapis lazuli was identified in the 1105/6 program in the naos and bema and in the painting of St. George in the narthex (late twelfth century) using PLM and SEM-EDS.[25]

Microscopically, lapis lazuli has a very characteristic appearance in its translucent particles with conchoidal fracture and squared corners (Fig. 7.9). These blue particles are isotropic with a refractive index lower than 1.662.[26] SEM-EDS analysis indicated the presence of sodium, aluminum, silicon, oxygen, sulfur, and chlorine, all characteristic of lazurite. Cubic particles yielding the elements iron and sulfur were identified as pyrite, often found as the accessory mineral of lazurite.

Because of its low refractive index, lapis lazuli is much brighter when applied in tempera rather than in oil (see below, Binding Media). The quality of the lapis lazuli blue and the binding media used for its application seem to have contributed to the difference in chromatic appearance between

24. Howard, "Blue in the Lewes Group."
25. Gettens and Stout, *Painting Materials*, 166.
26. For the examination of the blue particles using PLM, a dispersion sample was prepared by dispersing a few blue particles in Meltmount (a thermoplastic resin) with refractive index 1.662.

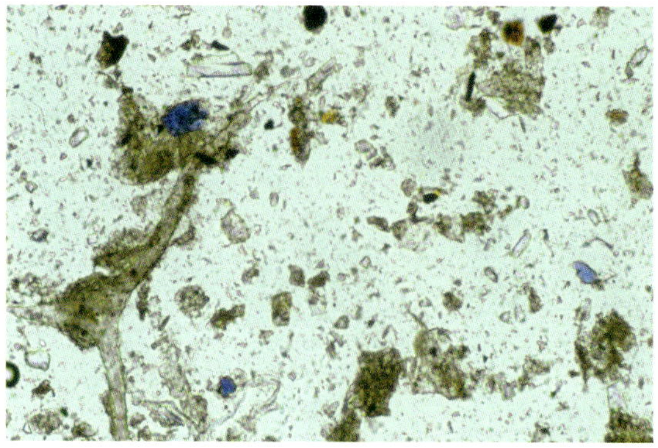

Fig. 7.9 Photomicrograph of sample 23 (acc. no. 2889), photographed in plane-polarized light, showing translucent blue particles with conchoidal fracture and squared corners, characteristic features of lapis lazuli particles (photo courtesy of Ioanna Kakoulli, 2001).

the blue backgrounds in the paintings of the 1105/6 program and in the St. George (see Figs. 7.1a and 7.1b). In the former, the blue was applied with linseed oil, while in the latter it was applied using egg, resulting in an enhanced blue color.

The method of extracting a good blue pigment from the raw lapis lazuli stone is well described in the *Craftsman's Handbook* (written in the early fifteenth century) by Cennino d'Andrea Cennini, a painter influenced by Giotto. Cennini suggests that the mineral be kneaded in a weak solution of lye with a paste or dough of wax, pine resin, gum mastic, and linseed oil.[27] The dough retains the impurities of silica, pyrite, calcite, and so on, while the blue particles of lapis lazuli settle out in the alkaline solution. According to Gettens and Stout, the first extraction gives the best color. Each subsequent extraction gives a color less pure, until a grey blue known as "ultramarine ash" is obtained.[28]

Azurite

Azurite is a natural blue pigment derived from the mineral azurite, a basic copper carbonate, by

27. Cennini, *Il libro dell' arte*, 36–39.
28. Gettens and Stout, *Painting Materials*, 166.

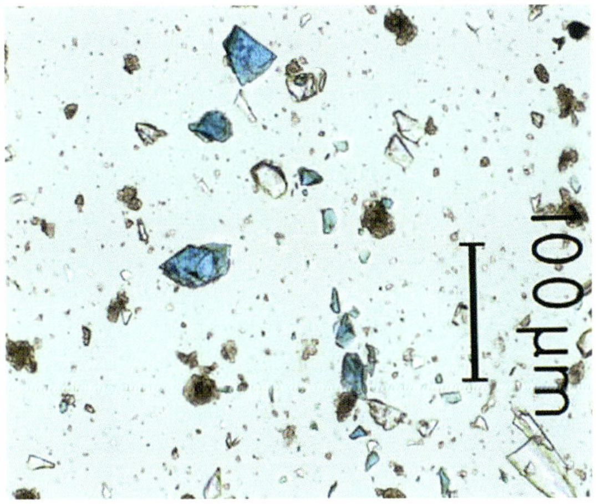

Fig. 7.10 Photomicrograph of azurite particles in plane-polarized light, displaying the characteristic large bluish-purple crystals with well-defined contours and relief pleochroism (photo courtesy of Ioanna Kakoulli, 2001).

grinding, washing, levigation, and flotation.[29] It is crystalline and highly refracting and birefracting. As with lapis lazuli, azurite performs better when applied in tempera; in oil it appears muddy and dark. But the coarseness of its particles made azurite difficult to apply in tempera, so sizing, which bette holds it in place, was often used instead.[30] Sizing degrades easily under humid conditions, however, and therefore blues applied with it have often perished.

Azurite appears for the first time at Asinou in the paintings of the late thirteenth century, in accordance with roughly contemporary evidence from both Byzantium and western Europe of its adoption as a substitute for costly natural ultramarine.[31]

In the church of Asinou, azurite was applied either pure over a smooth black layer for the background,[32] or in mixtures with black or white to achieve tonal variations. In all cases, it was applied using linseed oil rather than sizing, contrary to recommendations in the ancient treatises.

In the samples from Asinou, the use of azurite was attested by its characteristic large bluish-purple crystals with well-defined contours and relief pleochroism (Fig. 7.10). Under crossed polars, the blue particles displayed distinct birefringence and vivid interference colors. The presence of copper—the main constituent element of azurite—was further confirmed by SEM-EDS analysis.

Green Pigment

Green Earth (Celadonite)

Green earth, composed mainly of the mineral celadonite, was consistently used in all painting phases at Asinou. It has been identified in all paintings sampled, with the exception of the Pharmakolytria and the Phorbiotissa paintings in the narthex (of which the green paint was not sampled for analysis). Green earths vary in composition, but they always include one or both of the micaceous minerals celadonite and glauconite. Of the different methods available to identify these minerals—most commonly SEM-EDS, FTIR, x-ray diffraction (XRD), and Mössbauer spectroscopy—this study used SEM-EDS and FTIR supplemented by PLM and microchemical tests.

Under transmitted light (plane- and cross-polarized), microscopic examination of dispersion samples from Asinou enabled a general characterization of the green pigment particles: the properties displayed were characteristic of micaceous green-earth pigments (Fig. 7.11). The presence of a green earth pigment (most likely celadonite mineral) was further confirmed with the identification of ferric and ferrous ions through microchemical spot tests. Optically, however, celadonite can be confused not only with glauconite but also with other micaceous minerals, and the small size of the pigment particles (0.5–5 μm) further restricts their identification by PLM. At high magnifications

29. Ibid., 95; Thompson, *Techniques*, 131–32.
30. Thompson, *Techniques*, 133.
31. Raft, "Blue Colour," 4.
32. It seems to have been common practice in ancient and Byzantine painting that when the upper paint layer was limited in coverage (for example, where a blue pigment was used), black was chosen for the background, since, by absorbing light, it would accentuate the color of the upper layer. Kakoulli, "Technical Literature," 65.

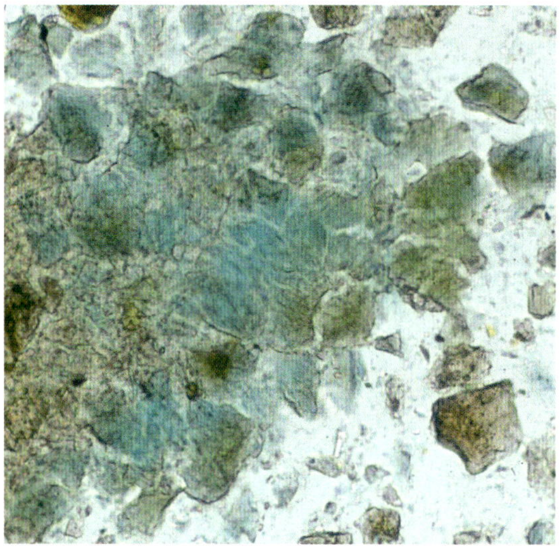

fig. 7.11

Fig. 7.11 Photomicrograph of a green pigment (sample 24, acc. no. 2890), photographed in plane-polarized light, displaying the characteristic bluish-green color and fibrous texture typical of micaceous green-earth pigments (photo courtesy of Ioanna Kakoulli, 2001).

Fig. 7.12 FTIR spectra of celadonite from Cyprus (lower blue spectrum) and from Verona, two important sites in antiquity for the mining of the mineral (spectra courtesy of Ioanna Kakoulli, 2001).

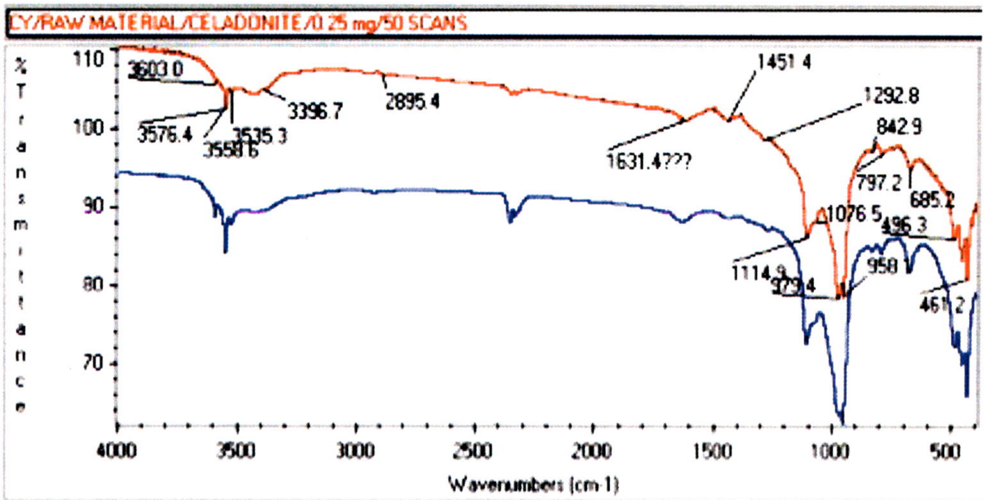

fig. 7.12

using the SEM, celadonite could be identified more securely, showing well-defined variable particle shapes, platy habits, and lamellar forms.[33]

The identification of the green-earth samples as celadonite was further confirmed using FTIR spectroscopy.[34] Van der Marel and Beutelspacher give the absorption peaks characteristic for the distinction between the two principal minerals, celadonite and glauconite.[35] Owing to its very good crystal order, celadonite produces very sharp FTIR spectra with characteristic absorbencies, thus allowing its identification.

Two sources for fine-quality green earth are well known in the Mediterranean—Cyprus and Verona—and both characteristically contain celadonite. During this study, samples from the natural sources were taken from both sites and were analyzed using FTIR. The characteristic absorption bands were very sharp and similar; these are presented in Table 7.2 and Fig. 7.12.

All micaceous green paint samples from Asinou analyzed by FTIR were prepared in high dilution in

33. Delamare, "Terres vertes," 348–50.
34. Farmer, "Infrared Spectra."
35. Van der Marel and Beutelspacher, *Clay Minerals*, 120.

Table 7.2. FTIR characteristic absorption bands (wavenumbers in cm^{-1}) of celadonite from Cyprus and Verona

Cyprus													
3603	3576	3559	3535	1631	1115	1077	979	958	843	797	685	496	461
Verona													
3603		3559	3534	1641	1114	1076	976	959	839	801	682	494	459

a potassium bromide matrix, thus displaying the silicate absorption band near 1000 cm^{-1}.[36] The samples were all ground to a fine powder using a grinding mill, since the particle size seems to influence the shift of the absorption bands;[37] 0.2 mg of the ground powdered pigment was mixed with 180 mg of potassium bromide (KBr) and compressed into a pellet under vacuum. The spectra obtained had absorbencies in the same regions as the standard samples analyzed from Cyprus and Verona.

Red Pigments

Three different red pigments were identified in the paintings at Asinou: hematite-rich red ocher and amorphous red ocher, cinnabar, and red lead.

Hematite-Rich Red Ocher and Amorphous Red Ocher

Two different forms of red ocher were identified in the paintings at Asinou. A hematite (iron oxide) rich-red ocher and a less-pure pigment contained oxyhydroxide phases. Hematite is a pure form of anhydrous ferric oxide that provides the red color of the pigment generically called red ocher. The crystal order of anhydrous ferric oxide provides distinguishing properties, allowing firm identification using PLM supplemented with elemental analysis using SEM-EDS and microchemical tests.

Hematite was readily identifiable microscopically, while the hydroxide phases varied both in composition and particle size according to the source. Hematite displayed hexagonal, almost tabular crystals, and a birefringence masked by the pigment's strong body coloration, showing only an intense red color. The less pure forms, however, could not be easily characterized and further chemical analyses were needed. Microscopically, the oxyhydroxide pigment particles displayed subrounded habit and a dark red-brown color. Particles were isotropic when viewed under crossed polars.

Cinnabar

Cinnabar derives from the main ore of metallic mercury, containing approximately 86.2% mercury and 13.8% sulfur.[38] It was considered an expensive pigment when these murals were painted, and seems to have been employed in the decoration of only the most important and richest sites or commissions. It has been found consistently in all painting programs at Asinou, with the exception of the painting of SS. Peter and Paul. Its absence from this particular painting (only part of which survives) does not imply, however, that cinnabar was deliberately excluded from that specific painted program, believed to belong to the late thirteenth century.

In this study, cinnabar was first identified using PLM. The particles of cinnabar showed very distinctive features: hexagonal fractured crystals with an intense red color and perfect cleavage.[39] When viewed under crossed polars, the crystals, though birefringent, displayed only an intense red color. In general, optical means alone are insufficient for distinguishing cinnabar, a naturally occurring mineral, from vermilion, a synthetic pigment with the

36. Russell, "Infrared Methods," 295–99. High dilution, as opposed to high concentration, in the KBr matrix will give a broad band of absorption that will mask the defined peak identified. If a different type of FTIR was used, sample preparation would be different.
37. Ibid.

38. Klein and Hurlbut, *Manual of Mineralogy*, 362.
39. Gettens et al., "Vermilion and Cinnabar," 50.

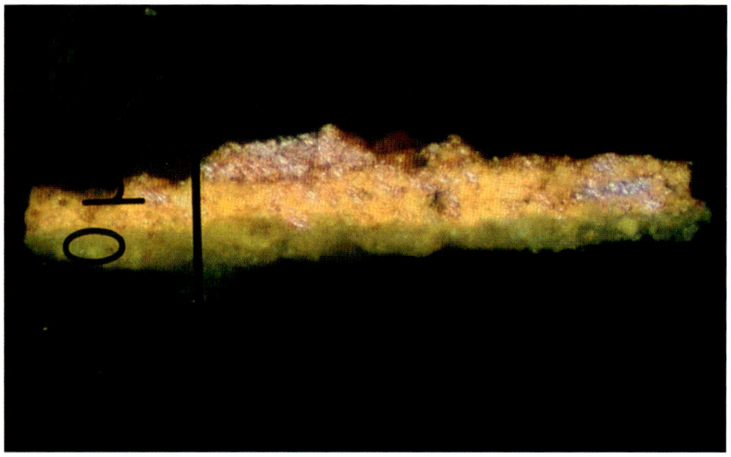

a

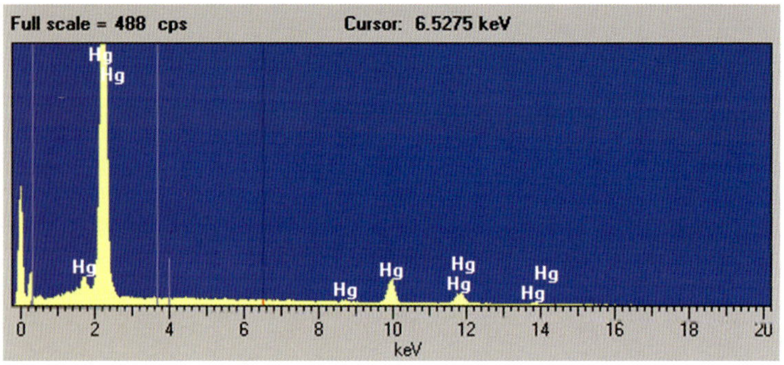

b

Fig. 7.13 Photomicrograph of a cross-section of sample 7 (acc. no. 2873) showing a multi-layered paint sample consisting of three distinct layers. From bottom up, (a) a yellow ocher layer, red lead mixed with cinnabar, and cinnabar and (b) the EDS spectrum of mercury (Hg) in the red particles in the top layer, confirming the presence of cinnabar (mercuric sulfide) (photo and spectrum courtesy of Ioanna Kakoulli, 2001)

same chemical composition. The dry (sublimation) method of making vermilion may yield crystals similar enough to those of cinnabar to be confused with them. Such confusion would be likely if a chemically pure sample were found; while purity is to be expected in manufactured vermilion, very pure cinnabar also exists in nature. At Asinou, however, impurities and associated minerals found in the pigment suggested a natural source, and thus an identification of the pigment as cinnabar.

SEM-EDS analysis was the principal method used for the exact characterization of the pigment. EDS analysis identified the x-ray photons characteristic of mercury and sulfur (the two elements that compose cinnabar). The characteristic x-rays for sulfur, namely the Kα (2.31 keV) and Kβ (2.46 keV), are found very close to the Mα (2.195 keV) x-ray photon emission for mercury, which renders the labeling of the peaks difficult. For the identification of cinnabar it was therefore important to search for the Lα (9.987 keV) and Lβ (11.823 keV) x-ray photons characteristic for mercury, emitted at higher energies (Fig. 7.13). In those cases where SEM-EDS analysis was not available, a microchemical test for sulfide was carried out on a few dispersed particles under the binocular microscope.[40]

Red Lead

Red lead had been used since antiquity, but the name "minium" was applied to the pigment in the Middle Ages. It was used extensively in Persian and Byzantine manuscripts.

Red lead is an orange-red mineral, a tetroxide of lead (Pb_3O_4 or, for analytical purposes, $PbO_2.2PbO$) produced artificially since antiquity by heating litharge (PbO) or white lead ($2PbCO_3.Pb(OH)_2$) to around 480°C for a few hours. If the temperature goes too high the pigment will revert to litharge. If the raw material is white lead, the final product will have less free litharge. The pigment has a very intense scarlet color, fine texture, and good hiding power.

In the samples analyzed, red lead was identified using PLM and SEM-EDS. Its particles have a high refractive index, with moderate birefringence and interference colors that range from orange-red to green. Microchemical tests indicated the presence of lead ions. Further confirmation was obtained by SEM-EDS (Fig. 7.14).[41]

Yellow Pigments

At Asinou, four different yellow pigments were identified: limonite, goethite-rich yellow ocher, jarosite,

40. Plesters, "Cross-sections," 143.

41. The emission of the characteristic x-rays at high energies Lα1 = 10.55 keV and Lβ1 = 12.61 keV indicated the presence of lead.

raw sienna, and massicot or litharge. The last was identified only in a single case, while goethite and jarosite were abundantly found as associated minerals in many samples (see Table 7.1). Limonite contains in various amounts the different earth minerals described below, primarily goethite and jarosite, and therefore will not be discussed individually.

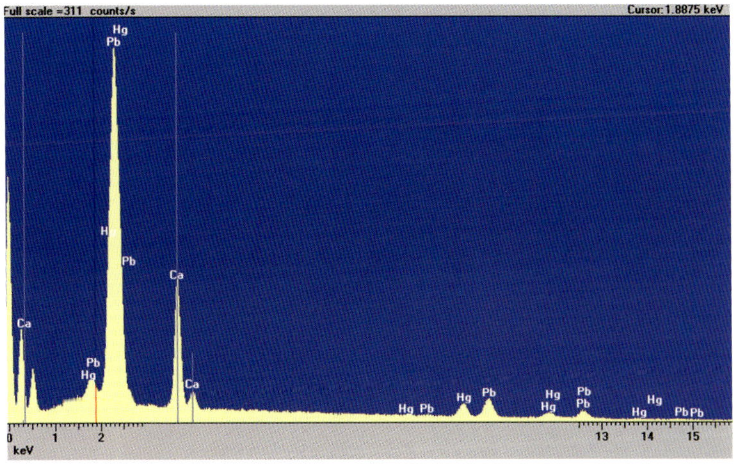

Fig. 7.14 Detail of fig. 7.13b, EDS spectrum of the orange-red particles from sample 7 (acc. no. 2873), showing photon emissions characteristic of lead (Pb) and mercury (Hg), confirming the presence of red lead in addition to cinnabar (spectrum courtesy of Ioanna Kakoulli, 2001).

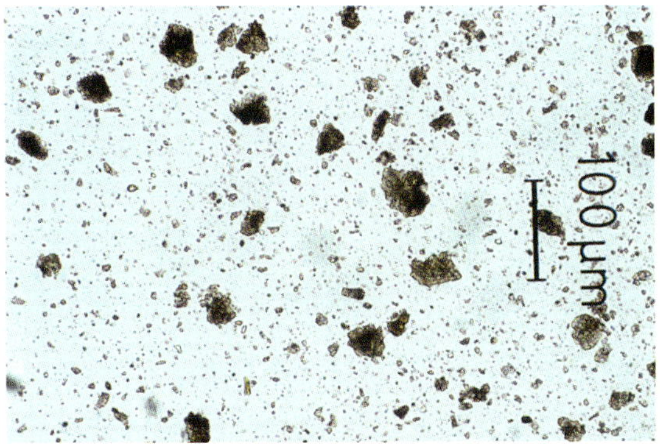

Fig. 7.15 Photomicrograph of yellow pigment particles photographed in plane-polarized light, displaying a yellowish brown color, rounded habit, spherulitic texture, and perfect cleavage, characteristic features of goethite mineral (photo courtesy of Ioanna Kakoulli, 2001).

Goethite

Goethite derives from the weathering of iron-bearing minerals such as siderite and pyrite. It is therefore found in the oxidizing zones (called gossans) of these ore bodies. Goethite was identified microscopically by its characteristic optical properties;[42] in plane-polarized light, the particles displayed a yellowish brown color, rounded habit, spherulitic texture, and perfect cleavage. In most samples, the particles were isotropic when observed under crossed polars (Fig. 7.15).

Analysis of polished paint cross-sections was carried out using PLM and SEM-EDS. The particles of goethite displayed a fibrous texture and rounded habit, confirming the presence of the mineral goethite. The high-resolution images of the SEM were capable of showing such details of the microstructure, while EDS provided information about the elemental composition.

Where sufficient quantities of a sample were available, FTIR analysis was also carried out. Although the spectrum of goethite obtained was weak, IR absorbencies were recorded at 3140–3100, 900–880, 673, 461, and 428 cm^{-1}.[43]

Jarosite

The presence of jarosite in the paintings at Asinou was attested by its mineralogical and elemental composition. Microscopically, the particles of this pigment display a translucent yellow color with tabular and angular crystal habit. When observed under crossed polars they are strongly birefringent with distinct extinction. SEM-EDS analysis pointed to the presence of iron, potassium, and sulfur, three constituent elements of jarosite (Fig. 7.16).

FTIR was used to further confirm the presence of jarosite, which displays strong FTIR absorbance. Van der Marel and Beutelspacher's example of jarosite gave a clear spectrum with the characteristic wave numbers presented in Table 7.3.

42. Deer et al., *Rock-Forming Minerals*, 579.
43. Van der Marel and Beutelspacher, *Clay Minerals*, 192.

Table 7.3. FTIR characteristic absorption bands (wave numbers in cm^{-1}) for jarosite

Jarosite															
3380	**3350**	3280	2310	2070	1980	**1185**	**1091**	**1019**	1007	668	**635**	581	**512**	**480**	449

The wave numbers in bold correspond to intense peaks of the mineral.

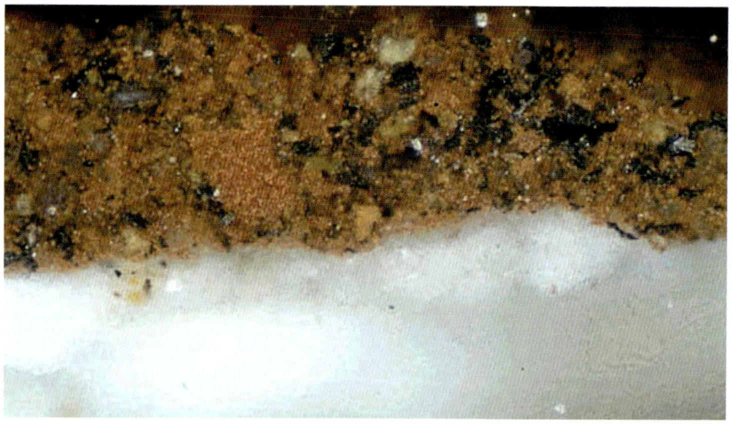

a

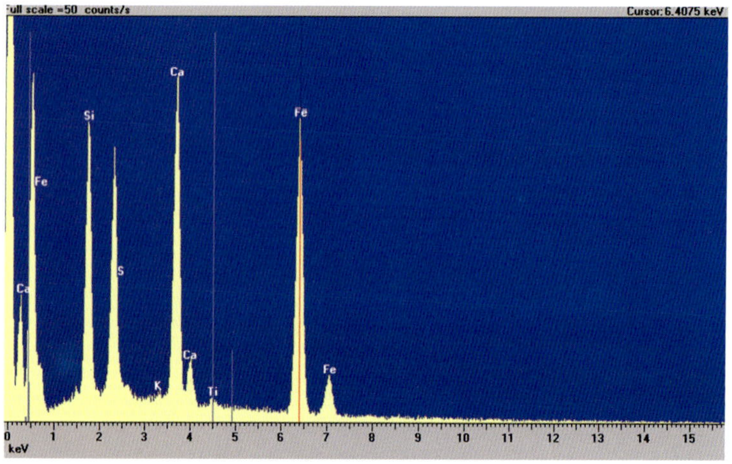

b

Figs. 7.16 Photomicrograph (a) and spectrum (b) of a reddish-brown painted layer (sample 9, acc. no. 2875). The particles of this pigment are tabular with an angular crystal habit. SEM-EDS analysis of the particles yielded the presence of iron (Fe), potassium (K), and sulfur (S), indicating the presence of jarosite (photo and spectrum courtesy of Ioanna Kakoulli, 2001).

Jarosite is found as a secondary mineral in the gossans of ore bodies, usually in association with goethite and quartz. Because it differs considerably from goethite, it can easily be distinguished.

Raw Sienna

In color, raw sienna is very similar to goethite. It gets its name from Siena, the Tuscan city where one of the best grades of this color can be found. Raw sienna is a hydrated ferric oxide (like goethite) associated with alumina and silica, but with slightly warmer tone than goethite and more transparent. Good quality sienna also consists of at least 50% ferric oxide/hematite (Fe_2O_3). Manganese dioxide (MnO_2) is also present but only as a trace element (0.6–1.5%).[44]

Raw sienna was identified by its characteristic microscopic properties, displaying a mixture of particles, some transparent and colorless, others with a slight yellow and brownish coloration. The latter particles are moderately birefringent and have a yellow body color when observed under crossed polars. Some of the particles are isotropic. SEM-EDS analysis confirmed the presence of iron, silicon, aluminum, and manganese (characteristic elements of the associated minerals of the pigment).

Massicot or Litharge

Massicot and litharge are both yellow monoxide of lead (PbO) and are naturally occurring minerals. Massicot can be obtained by heating white lead (basic lead carbonate) at 300°C, decomposing it into carbon dioxide, water, and the yellow powder of PbO. Litharge is formed by the direct oxidation of molten lead, is more orange in

44. Gettens and Stout, *Painting Materials*, 156.

color than massicot, and is not normally found as a pigment.[45]

Massicot or litharge was identified only in the 1332/33 paintings in the narthex. The pigment was identified by means of PLM and SEM-EDS. Under the PLM and the SEM, the particles appeared small and amorphous, while the EDS spectrum indicated the characteristic x-ray photon emissions of elements at high energies typical for lead.

White Pigment

Lime White

Lime white was found in several forms: as chalk, as calcite, and as the microcrystalline calcite known as "bianco di San Giovanni." The last material is of exceptional value in the fresco technique because it includes a high proportion of calcium hydroxide and therefore can function as both a pigment and a binder.[46]

Black Pigment

Charcoal Black

Charcoal (carbon) black derives from the partial burning of wood in kilns. The final product is not carbon alone but contains various impurities. It is a very stable pigment, unaffected by moisture or light.

Most of the samples examined showed the characteristic features of an opaque pigment. It appears with a black, lustrous color and with a few brownish flakes. The particles appear opaque with an elongated, splintery habit.[47]

Binding Media

Since research on identifying binding media in Byzantine wall paintings is a rather recent endeavor, the results from the analysis of samples from the paintings at Asinou are of primary significance.

The use of more sensitive and accurate techniques such as GC-MS allows for an unprecedentedly precise characterization of binding media. From the analysis of the samples, it can be suggested that linseed oil was extensively used for the paintings of 1105/6 at Asinou (see Appendix 5). It was identified as the medium used for the application of the blue pigment on the background and for the modeling of the garments, although traces of egg were also identified in the garments. Similarly, linseed oil was identified in the paintings dating from the fourteenth century in the naos. It was used for the application of azurite on the background, for painting the blue garments of the Virgin, and in the gilding (see below).

Of the paintings sampled, only the St. George in the narthex shows a more "traditional" Byzantine painting technique.[48] To make the background, the blue pigment—lapis lazuli—was applied using egg over a black intermediate layer, while some type of oil (linseed or walnut oil) was used for the pigments that have siccative properties (that is, pigments that contribute to the drying of the oil film), such as cinnabar and red lead. As with the fourteenth-century paintings, traces of oil (linseed or walnut) were also identified in samples taken from the gilded areas (see below).[49]

The surprising identification of the abundant use of linseed oil at Asinou requires a revision of our understanding of the Byzantine tradition of painting. It was always believed that egg was the primary binding medium used in Byzantine painting, although in the *Hermeneia* by Dionysios of Fourna the type of media used for the "upper" paint layers in wall paintings remains vague.

Recent analyses of the thirteenth-century wall paintings by Panselinos at Protaton indicated the use of an egg-based tempera,[50] whereas animal glue was identified in the sixteenth-century paintings at Dousiko, Meteora, Greece.[51]

Both pigments and binding media are important parameters affecting the appearance of a paint

45. Ibid., 129.
46. Denninger, "Bianco di San Giovanni."
47. Gettens and Stout, *Painting Materials*, 104.

48. The term "traditional" refers to a painting technique that follows closely the methods and materials of painting as described in the *Hermeneia* by Dionysios of Fourna.
49. Thompson mentions the use of "oil glazes" where oil has been used, often with tempera painting: Thompson, *Techniques*, 66.
50. Daniilia et al., "Protaton," 108.
51. Chiavari et al., "Analytical Pyrolysis," 1148–50.

layer; its color depends on the pigment, because the binding medium in which the pigment is dispersed is colorless. However, the nature of the binding medium is responsible for the transparency of the paint layer, the optical properties of which are determined primarily by the binding medium's refractive index. When a pigment is mixed with a binding medium, the degree of chemical and physical compatibility of the two phases in the suspension renders each pigment more suitable in a specific medium. The latter should also have the property of film-forming, so that upon drying it can create a stable, coherent film that adheres well to the support, and that has good mechanical and optical properties.

The appearance of a paint layer is also determined by the nature and particle size of the pigment. In general, the finer the pigment particles, the greater the diffusion or scattering of light and hence the opacity of the paint layer. In addition, this hiding power (or opacity) of the pigment is influenced by the tonality of its color, its concentration in the medium, and the difference between its refractive index and that of the medium. Depending on the hiding power of a given paint layer, as determined by the properties of the pigment and the binding medium used, medieval artists were able to create transparent paint layers and also to enhance the color qualities of pigments. As we have seen, the radiance of the lapis lazuli was visibly affected by the use of different binding media in the 1105/6 paintings and in the St. George.

Raised Halos

Samples taken from the raised gilded halos found in the fourteenth-century paintings in the naos and the 1332/33 paintings in the narthex at Asinou displayed similar technical features: the halos were first raised using lime plaster and were subsequently painted yellow. Over the yellow, a layer of plaster of paris was thickly applied and modeled, probably using a mold made of wood, stone, or metal. This relief stucco addition was gilded using tin leaf applied with linseed oil and likely glazed using a yellowish dark oil or resin (probably copal, as indicated from the analysis; Fig. 7.17). A similar

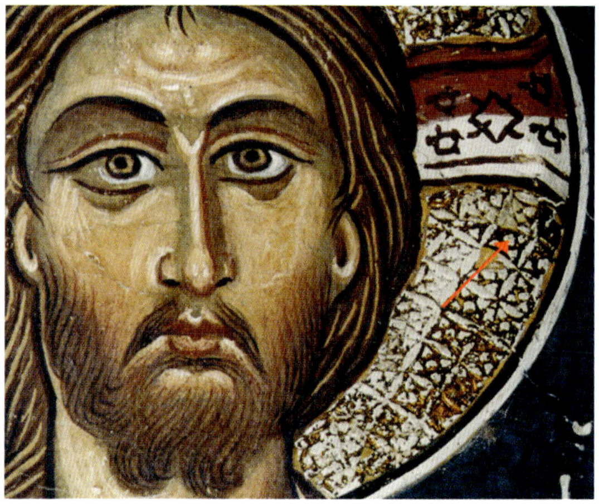

a

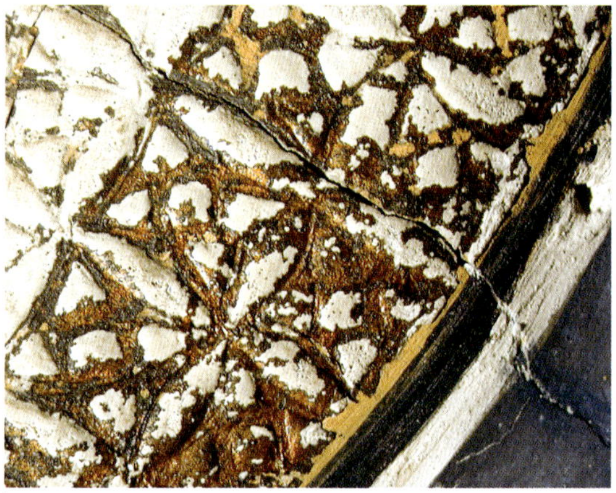

b

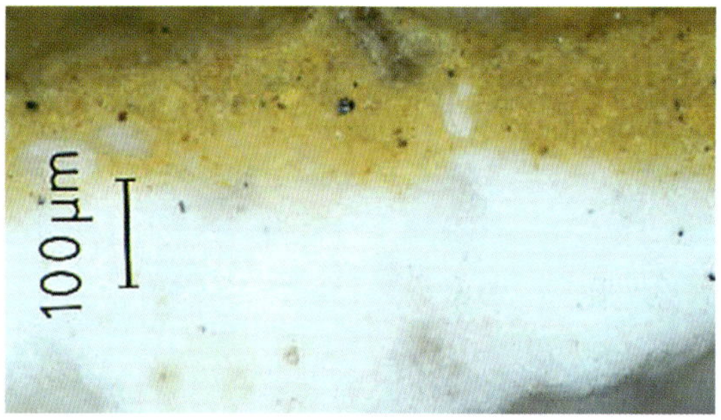

c

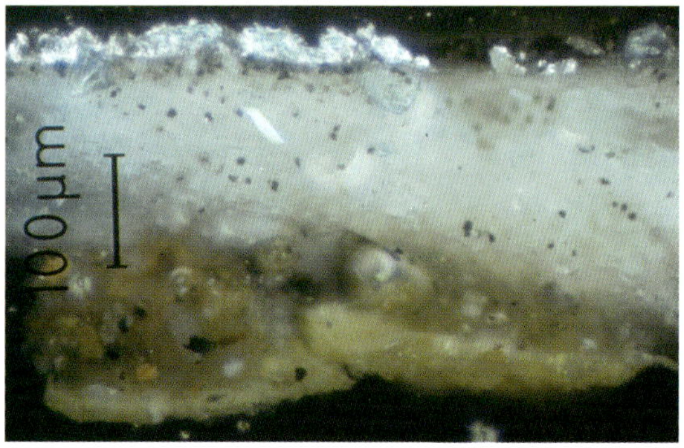

d

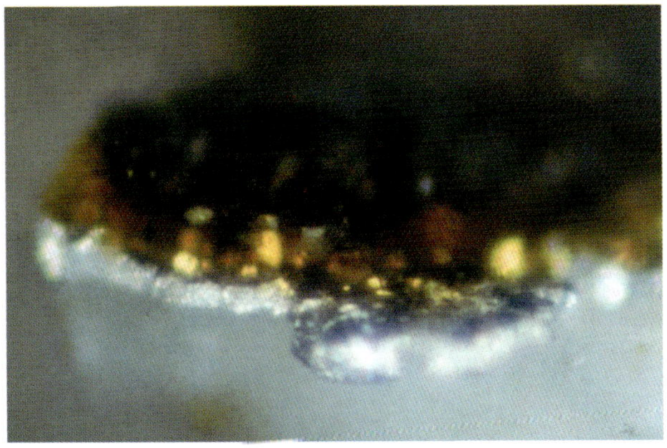

e

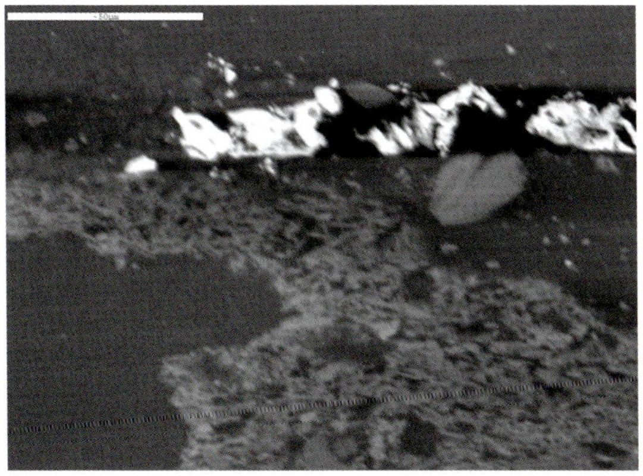

f

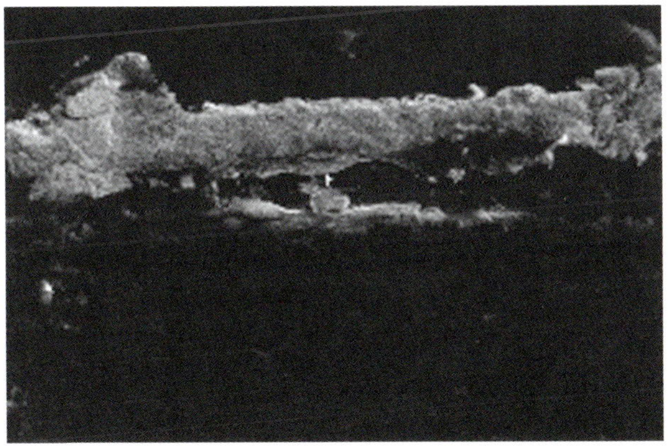

g

h

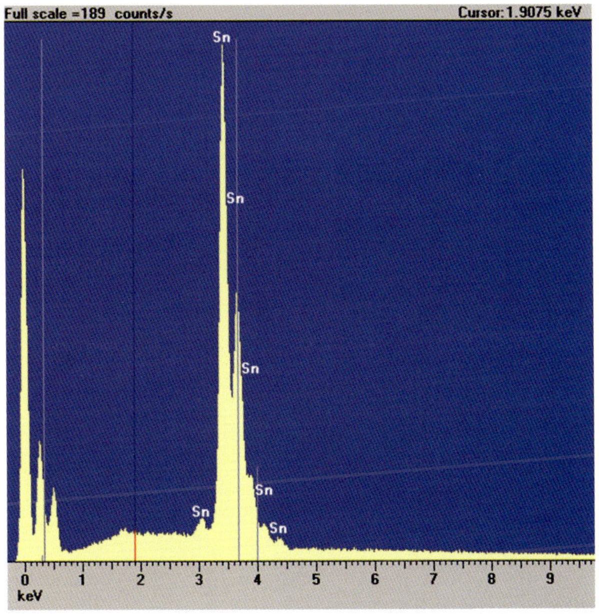

i

Fig. 7.17

Photographs illustrating the location, stratigraphy, and composition of sample 11 (acc. no. 2877), taken from the halo of Christ in the fourteenth-century program in the naos. Figs. a and b show the location of the sample (indicated by an arrow). Figs. c–f illustrate the sample's stratigraphy (in consecutive images), typical for raised halos in the fourteenth-century paintings at Asinou, from the bottom up: in c, part of a lime-based plaster used to raise the halo overlaid by a yellow ocher intermediate paint layer; in d the ocher layer again but richer in binding medium, a white layer of plaster of paris probably shaped in a mold, a thin layer of organic binder (identified as linseed oil) used as the mordant for the gilding, and a layer of tin leaf; and in e, the tin leaf again, with a final yellowish dark oil or resin glaze (probably copal, as indicated by the analysis) to give the gold color. Fig. f shows a magnified image of d in backscattered electrons (BSE) with the tin foil appearing bright white owing to compositional contrast; fig. g is also a BSE image of a detail of the "gilding" in the same sample with the corresponding distribution map of tin (Sn) (fig. h). Fig. i shows the EDS spectrum with the characteristic photon emissions of tin (Sn) (spectrum and photos courtesy of Ioanna Kakoulli, 2000 and 2001).

technique for gilding was also identified in the much later sixteenth-century paintings in the naos. The fact that the sixteenth-century paintings overlay the twelfth-century program might suggest that the former partly covers the earlier paintings.

Gilding

Because very little evidence exists in the technical literature on gilding techniques for Byzantine wall paintings, information concerning gilding practices derives from the primary literature and treatises. However, results from the analysis of the painting samples from Asinou (ranging between the twelfth and the seventeenth centuries) have provided significant data that enrich our knowledge of gilding practices and techniques of the Byzantine and post-Byzantine periods. The gilding materials identified are listed in Table 7.4.

Table 7.4. Materials used in gilding identified in the various programs at Asinou

	1105/6 paintings in naos and bema	1105/6 and 14c: Phorbiotissa in narthex	late 12c: St. George in narthex	late 13c: Pantanassa in bema	late 13c: SS. Peter & Paul in naos	late 13c: St. Anastasia Pharmakolytria in narthex	1332/3 paintings in narthex	14c paintings in naos	16c paintings in naos
gold and silver leaf	•		•						
tin leaf							•	•	•
plaster of paris							•	•	•

Metal Leaves

At Asinou, different metal-alloy foils applied as thin leaves were used for the decoration of the halos. The analysis of samples taken from the 1105/6 program in the bema indicated the presence of an alloy of gold and silver (60:40 ratio; Fig. 7.18). The absence of copper (often found alloyed with gold) in the alloy and the ratio between the two metals suggests that it is probably electrum, a natural alloy. This was applied directly over an intermediate, yellow ocher layer. The gilding technique identified in the painting of St. George in the narthex uses metal leaves of an alloy of gold and silver with a higher concentration of silver (55:45 ratio) applied over a yellow ocher layer. Between the yellow ocher layer and the metal leaf there is a thick layer of mordant, while in the 1105/6 program the mordant was applied very thinly.

In the samples taken from the fourteenth-century paintings in the naos (Fig. 7.17) and the 1332/33 paintings in the narthex, the metal leaf was identified as tin, glazed to imitate gold (Fig. 7.19). Tin foil was very commonly used in the Middle

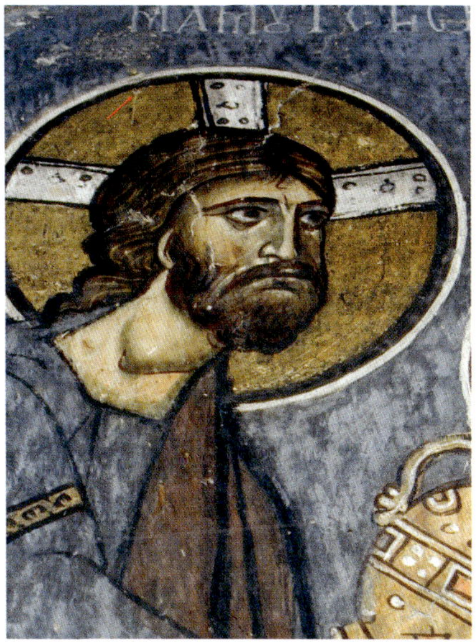

a

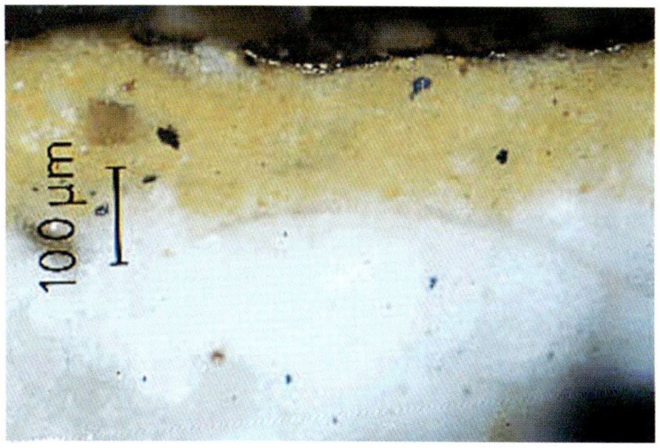

b

Fig. 7.18 Photographs illustrating the location, stratigraphy, and composition of sample 65 (acc. no. 2971), taken from the halo of Christ in the bema (1105/6). Fig. a shows the location of the sample (illustrated with an arrow); b shows the stratigraphy of the sample, from bottom up: the plaster layer, a yellow ocher layer, a thin layer of an organic binder (mordant) and the gilding (metal foil). Fig. c shows the secondary and back-scattered electron images of the sample in b, and x-ray distribution maps of the characteristic elements in the area analyzed, indicating the presence of a metal alloy of gold (Au) and silver (Ag) used for the gilding and the presence of a yellow ocher in the yellow layer (d), the EDS spectrum of the metal leaf with the characteristic photon emissions of Au and Ag (spectrum and photos courtesy of Ioanna Kakoulli, 2000 and 2001).

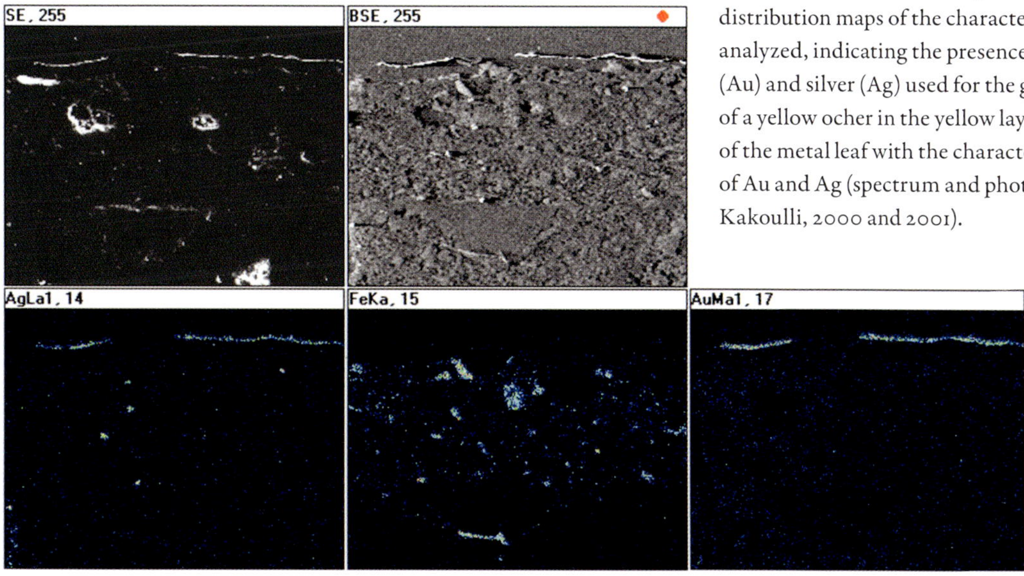

c

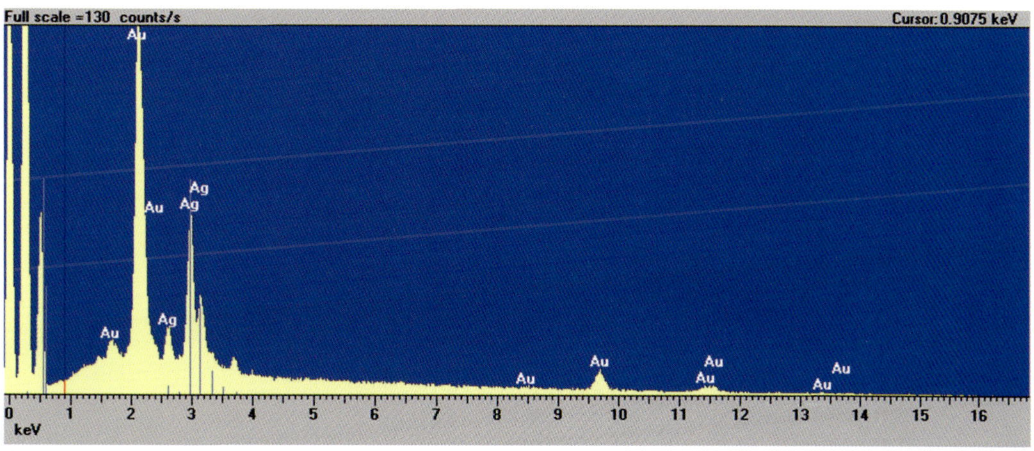

d

Ages either to imitate silver or, when lacquered yellow, to imitate gold.[52] The gold-imitating glaze for tin was known as "auripetrum." In his book *On Divers Arts,* Theophilus describes the preparation and glazing of the leaves to look like gold by beating the tin leaf on an anvil and coating it with glair and saffron yellow.[53]

The application of the tin leaf, however, needs further investigation; the presence of stucco relief decoration using a mold and the thickness of the tin foil could also suggest the use of the "tin relief" method found in northern Europe during the Middle Ages.[54]

Mordants

Samples from gilding, either on flat surfaces or over stucco relief decoration, were taken from the various paintings at Asinou. Based on the results from the samples analyzed, the technique indicated the use of mordant gilding employing linseed oil, although walnut oil was not ruled out for the gilding of the painting of St. George (see Appendix 5).

The use of siccative oil as the mordant for gilding on a panel or wall painting was a common practice in the medieval years.[55] A siccative oil mordant was also identified using pyrolysis and gas chromatography combined with mass spectrometry (Py-GC/MS) in two samples containing gold leaves from the paintings at Dousiko at Meteora, Greece.[56] Traces of shellac and gum Arabic were also identified in the Dousiko samples.

Discussion

Relation of Technical Study to Painting Programs of Uncertain Date

A number of art historical questions make it difficult to "date" the various painting programs. In characterizing the materials and the application methods used in paintings, scientific analysis may aid in their technological differentiation by identifying similarities and differences. The most significant art historical questions raised were:

- Do the paintings of the Virgin Phorbiotissa (over the western door to the naos, originally on the building's exterior but now within the narthex) and the remaining exterior fragments of the north wall belong to the original decoration of the church (dated to 1105/6)?
- Is the painting of St. George in the narthex coeval with the 1105/6 program in the naos and the bema, although their styles differ considerably?
- Does the Anastasia painting in the narthex belong to the same painted phase as the Pantanassa painting in the conch of the apse? What is their relation to the paintings of SS. Peter and Paul shown beneath the fourteenth-century homonymous paintings of the westernmost supporting pillars in the naos?
- Do the paintings dating from the fourteenth century in the naos correspond to the same painted phase as the paintings dated to 1332/33 in the narthex?

The Painting of the Panagia Phorbiotissa in the Narthex and the Remaining Exterior Fragments of the North Wall

The in situ examination and the results from the microanalysis of samples suggest that the painting of the Panagia Phorbiotissa, as well as the

52. Gettens and Stout, *Painting Materials*, 160; Thompson, *Techniques*, 66, 180.
53. Theophilus, *On Divers Arts*, 31–32.
54. Nadolny, "Gilded Relief Decoration"; Nadolny, "Relief Backgrounds"; personal communication with J. Nadolny, February 2002.
55. Thompson describes how oil was applied thickly (sometimes mixed with some pigment) over the surface to be gilded and left to dry. When it was almost dry, but still somewhat sticky, the gold leaf was laid on. The oil varnish was sometimes applied very thinly so the gold leaf would be flat on the surface, while in other cases it was applied very thickly, so the gilded surface was significantly raised: Thompson, *Techniques*, 227.
56. Chiavari et al., "Analytical Pyrolysis," 1150.

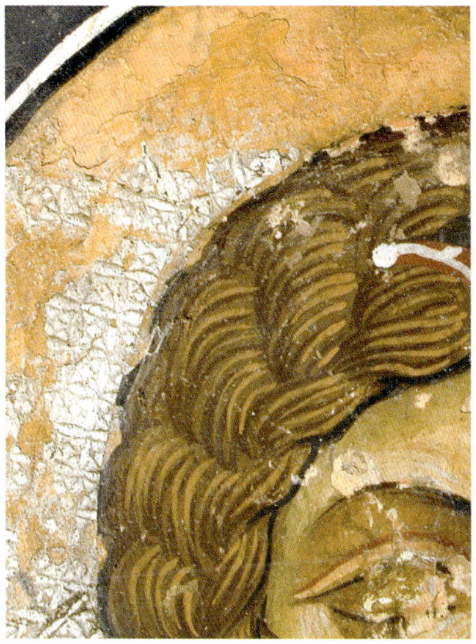

a

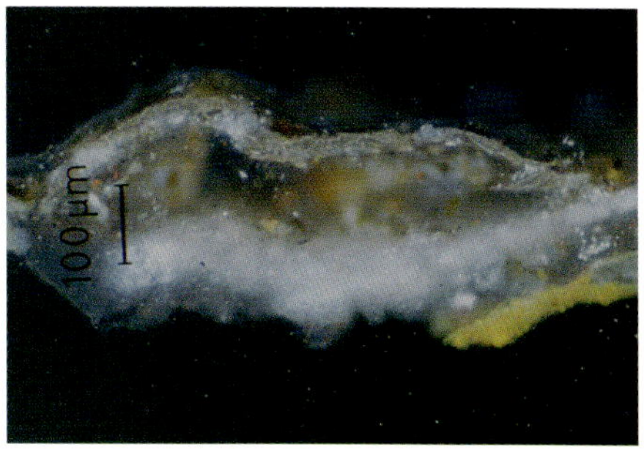

b

Fig. 7.19

Photographs illustrating the location, stratigraphy, and composition of sample 46 (acc. no. 2934), taken from the halo of Archangel Michael in the narthex (1332/33 painting program). Fig. a shows the location of the sample (illustrated with an arrow); b shows the stratigraphy of the sample, from bottom up: a yellow ocher layer (applied over a lime-based plaster layer, not visible here), a plaster of paris layer used to raise the halo (create the relief), a translucent layer of organic origin used as the mordant, the tin foil, and a yellow glaze to imitate the color of gold. Fig. c shows a secondary and a backscattered electron image of the stratigraphic sample seen in b and spatially resolved x-ray maps of the elements silicon, sulfur, and tin. Fig. d shows a spectrum of the tin foil yielding the characteristic photon emission of the element (spectrum and photos courtesy of Ioanna Kakoulli, 2000 and 2001).

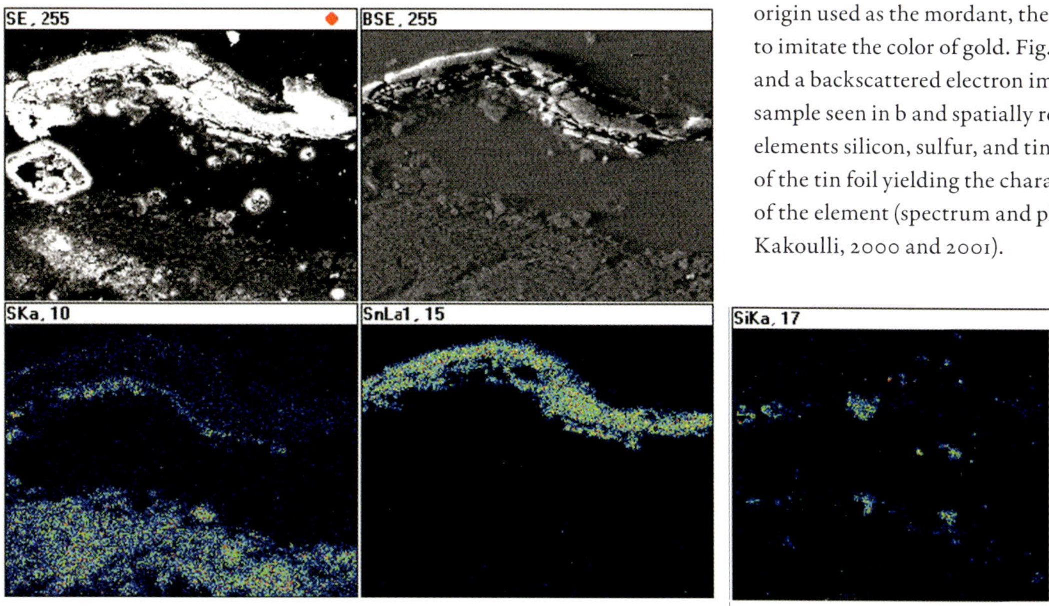

c

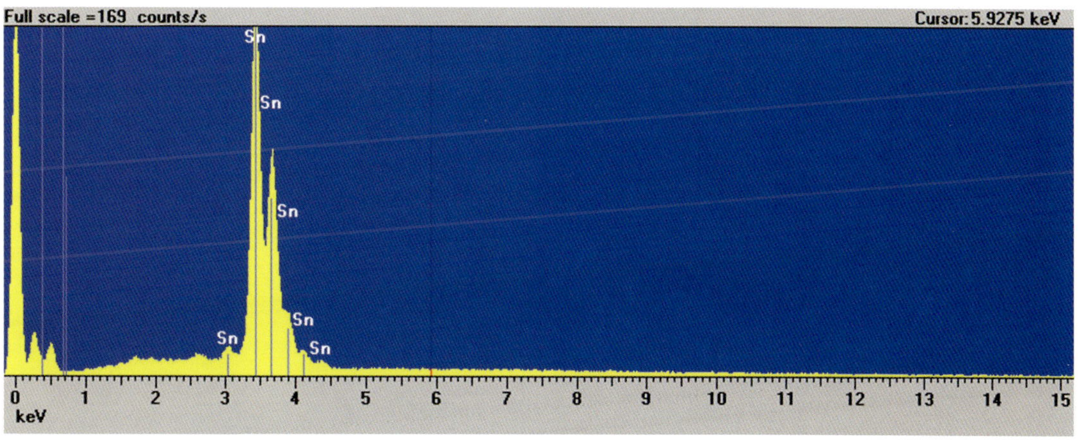

d

fragmentary paintings on the exterior of the north wall, belong to the original 1105/6 program (Fig. 7.20). Although the Panagia Phorbiotissa has undergone extensive repainting, probably in the fourteenth century, it retains technological features characteristic of the 1105/6 phase.

Plaster

Examination of a plaster sample from the Panagia Phorbiotissa indicated the presence of a lime matrix with dispersed thin fibers (probably flax tow or hemp), sandstone aggregates, ferric oxide particles, muscovite, and micrite. This is identical to the plaster layer sampled from two areas of the 1105/6 program in the naos and the bema (Fig. 7.21). In raking light, all the original plaster, including that of the Panagia Phorbiotissa and on the exterior, shows the same randomly oriented striations indicative of the tool used, the method of application, and the leveling.

Setting-Out Techniques

The Phorbiotissa painting shows a painterly drawing in dark color with a fine, light-color outline, the latter probably a later addition. The dated 1105/6 program shows similar setting-out techniques, using primarily fine, brown lines, with black used only to enhance certain features.

Paint Layers

Only a few samples were taken from the Phorbiotissa painting in the lunette. The blue background—although very similar to the fourteenth-century paintings, in that azurite was applied over charcoal black—preserves in some

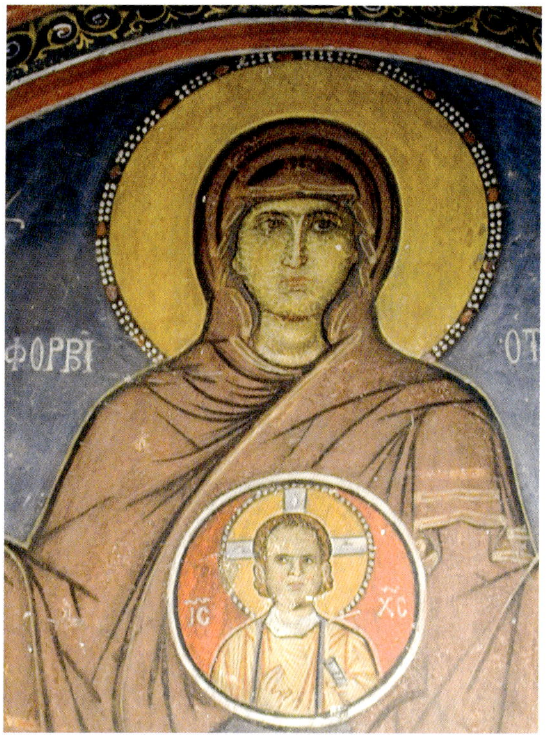

a

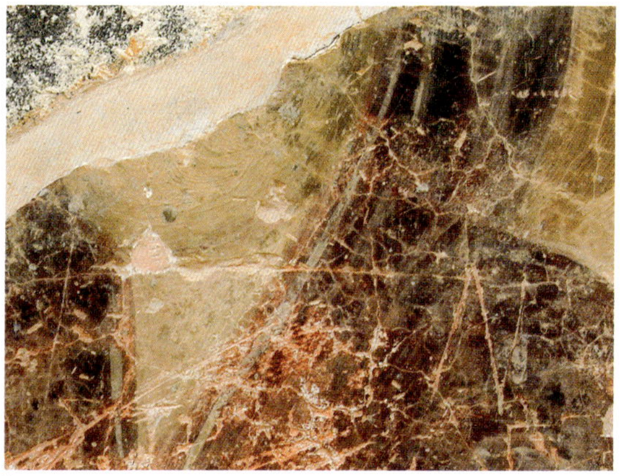

b

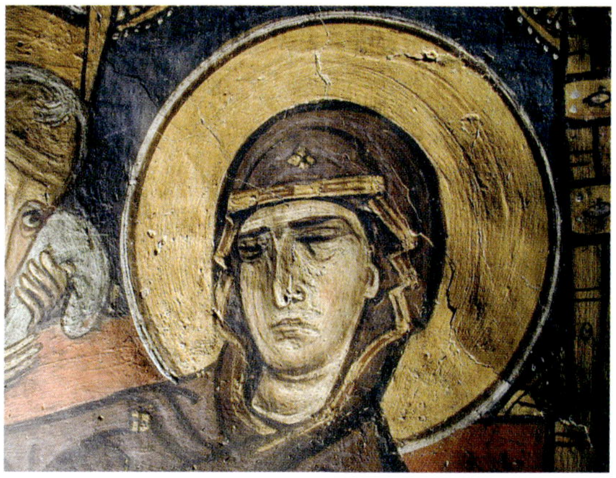

c

Fig. 7.20
Photographs of the Virgin Phorbiotissa (a), the fragmentary painting of the Virgin on the exterior of the north wall (b), and the Virgin from the Dormition scene of 1105/6 in the naos (c). Technological features resulting from similar pigments and composition of the paint, mainly that used for the flesh tone, suggest that these paintings are contemporary to one another (photos courtesy of Ioanna Kakoulli, 2000).

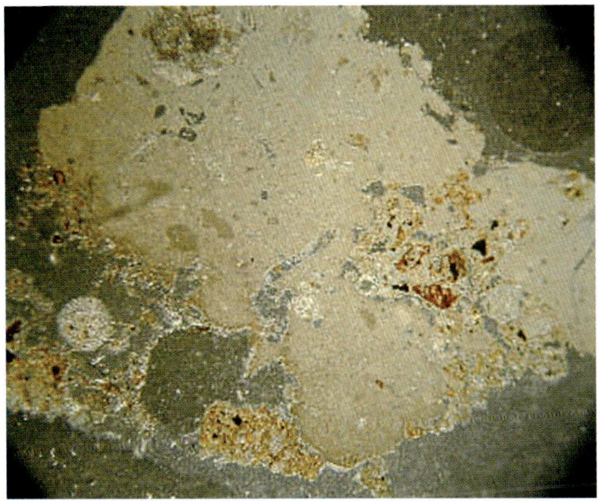

a

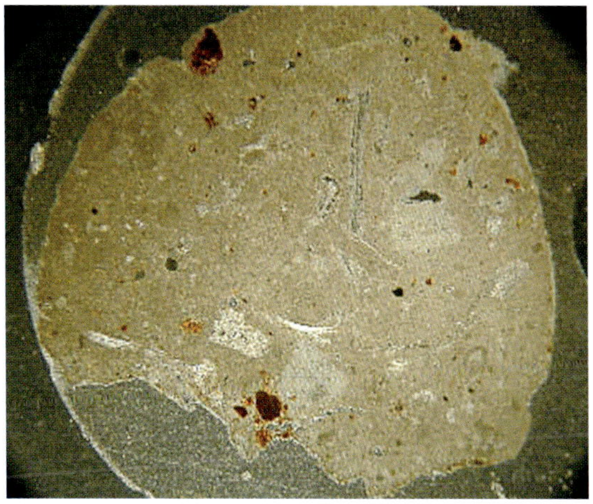

b

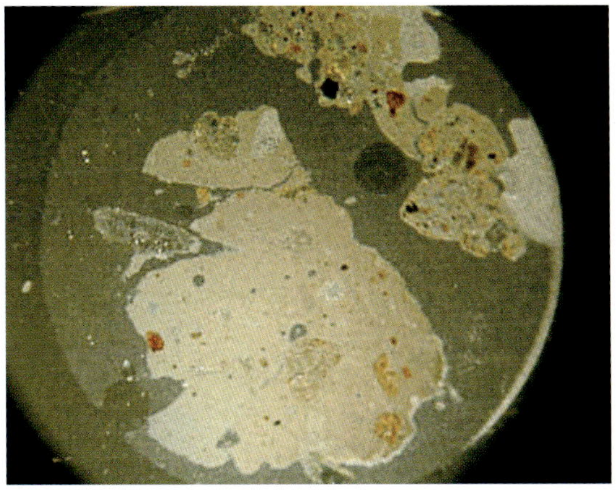

c

Fig. 7.21
Thin sections in plane-polarized light from different plaster layers. Fig. a shows sample P10 (acc. no. 2965), taken from the plaster used for the Virgin Phorbiotissa painting. It indicates the presence of a lime matrix with dispersed thin fibers (probably flax tow or hemp), sandstone aggregates, ferric oxide particles, muscovite, and micrite. Figs. b and c show two thin sections photographed in plane-polarized light from two distinct areas of the plaster from the 1105/6 program in the naos (b; sample P11, acc. no. 2966) and the bema (c; sample P9, acc. no. 2964). All three samples show very close affinity (photos courtesy of Ioanna Kakoulli, 2001).

areas traces of lapis lazuli, indicating the presence of an earlier layer corresponding to the 1105/6 program. The flesh tone used in all the paintings from the 1105/6 phase is made of a single layer of yellow applied over the plaster (Figs. 7.22–23). By contrast, the other paintings have a different flesh tone, similar to the *verdaccio* described by Cennino Cennini (Fig. 7.24).[57]

Binding Media

An analysis of the binding media used in the 1105/6 paintings indicated the presence of linseed oil for the application of lapis lazuli. Although medium analysis was not carried out on the Phorbiotissa or the exterior painting, they both display extensive craquelure, the characteristic typology of cracks associated with the drying of oil.

The Painting of St. George in the Narthex

Plaster

Examination of a thin section taken from the plaster layer of the St. George scene from the narthex shows short and abundant chaff fibers mixed with flax tow, chalk, micrite, red ocher, quartz, and fragments of sandstone (Fig. 7.25). The fibers can easily be seen in the paint layer, since they have surfaced, probably from the smoothing of the plaster.

The plaster is carefully smoothed and leveled and is approximately 1 cm thick. Identical plaster appears on the geometrical decoration immediately beneath the St. George, thus confirming the

57. Cennini, *Il libro dell'arte*, 45–46.

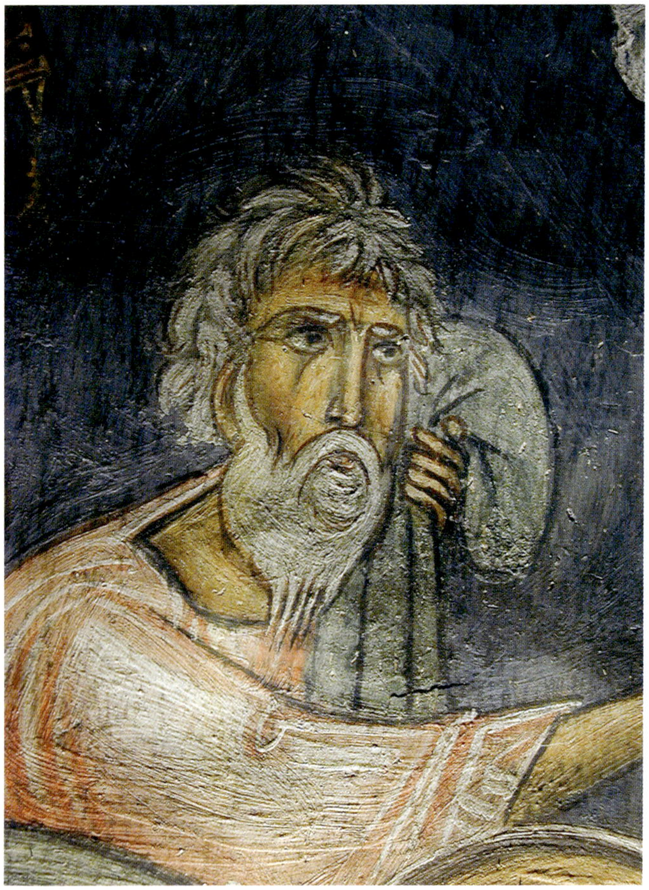

fig. 7.22a

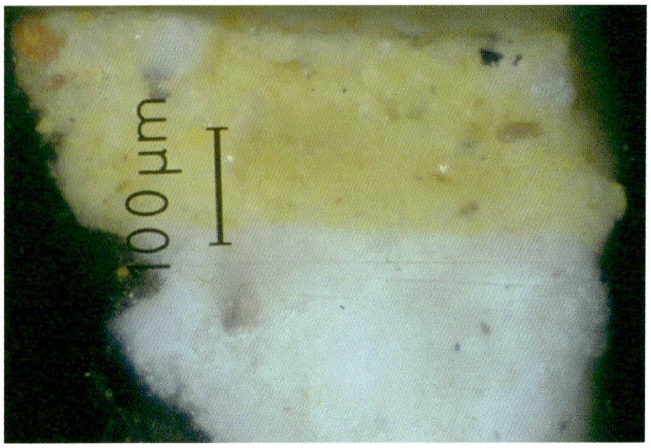

fig. 7.22b

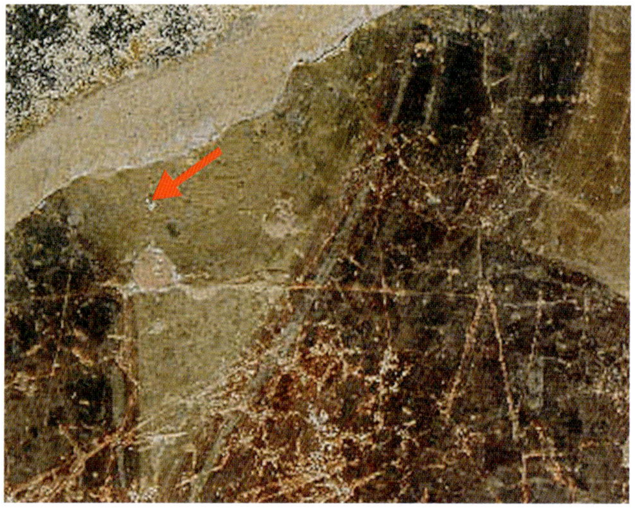

fig. 7.23a

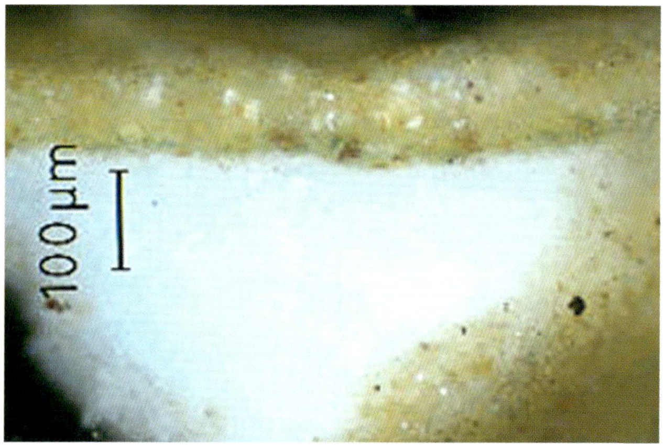

fig. 7.23b

Fig. 7.22
Detail of the standing figure behind St. Paul in the Dormition scene of the 1105/6 program in the naos (a), photographed in raking light, showing the location of sample 22 (acc. no. 2888). The sample, taken from the flesh color, shows a simple stratigraphy (b) consisting of a plaster layer and a pale yellow ocher paint layer (photos courtesy of Ioanna Kakoulli, 2000 and 2001).

Fig. 7.23
Detail of the Virgin depicted on the exterior north wall of the church, with a red arrow (a) showing the location of sample 39 (acc. no. 2927). The sample, a polished cross-section (b), shows a simple stratigraphy similar to that in Fig. 7.22b (photos courtesy of Ioanna Kakoulli, 2000 and 2001).

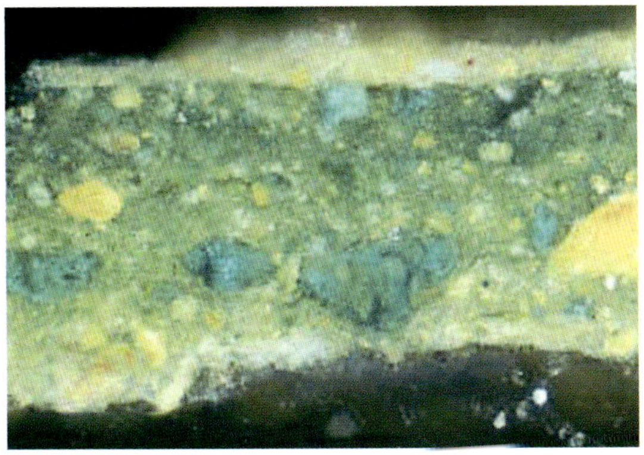

fig. 7.24

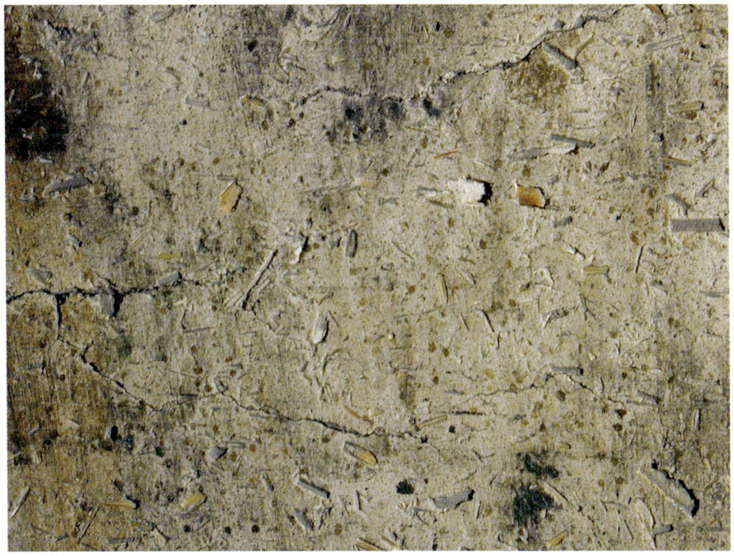

fig. 7.25a

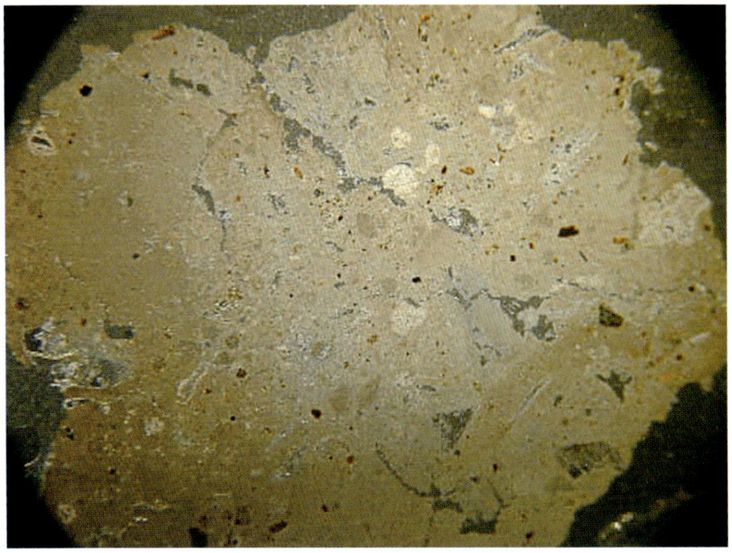

fig. 7.25b

Fig. 7.24
Photomicrograph of a polished cross-section (sample 8, acc. no. 2874) from the flesh color of St. George in the narthex (late twelfth century). The sample consists of a paint layer rich in green earth and yellow ocher applied over a plaster layer, which is not visible in this photograph (photo courtesy of Ioanna Kakoulli, 2001).

Fig. 7.25
Close-up photograph of the plaster layer in the painting of St. George in the narthex (a) and photomicrograph of a thin section taken from this plaster layer, photographed in plane-polarized light (b). The thin section shows chaff fibers mixed with flax tow, chalk, micrite, red ocher, quartz, and fragments of sandstone (photos courtesy of Ioanna Kakoulli, 2000 and 2001).

continuation of the same painting phase, the first painting program after the closing of the south doorway leading to the narthex.

Setting-Out Techniques

In setting out the program, painterly and incised techniques were used to outline the composition. For the decorative rounded motifs there is extensive evidence of compass use, while freehand incisions are visible on the outlines of garments and in the figure of St. George. Within the church there are only a few examples of incised preparatory drawing, such as the painting of Anastasia in the narthex, the first program of paintings on the westernmost pillars in the naos, and the sixteenth-century paintings in the naos. Because the type of incision differs considerably from one program to another, each type of preparatory incised drawing can indicate a different painted phase. For example, the incisions visible in the painting of St. George are rather smooth and shallow, almost invisible to the naked eye (Fig. 7.8). In contrast, the incisions in the paintings of Anastasia in the narthex, the Pantanassa in the bema, and those of SS. Peter and Paul in the naos, are very sharp and primarily vertical (Fig. 7.7).

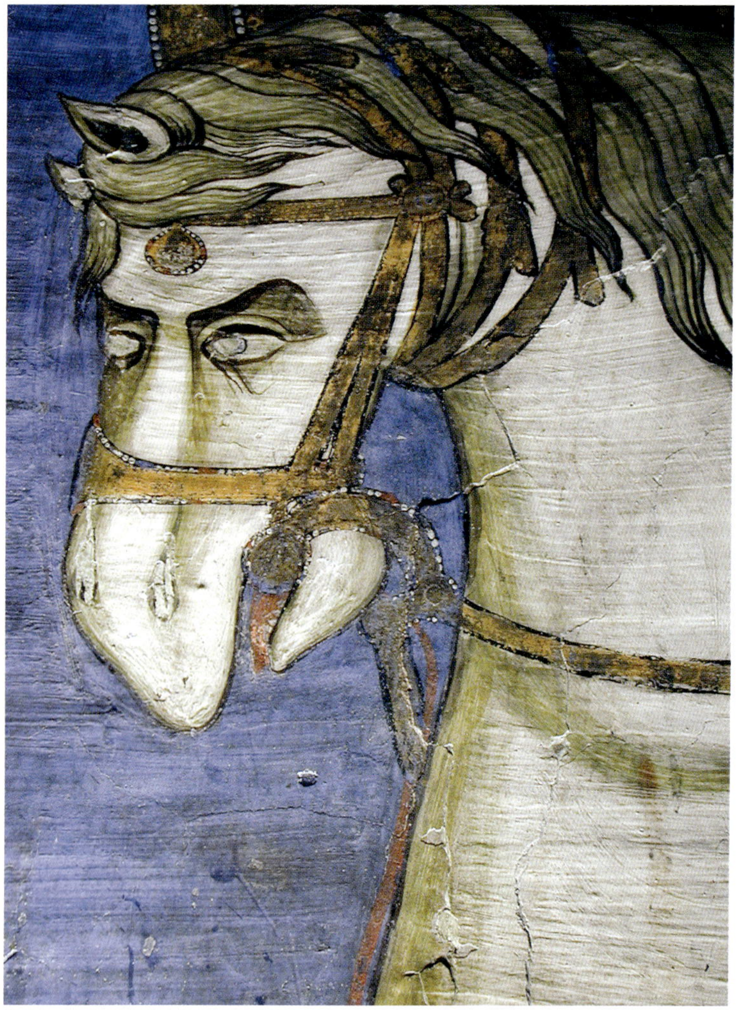

fig. 7.26

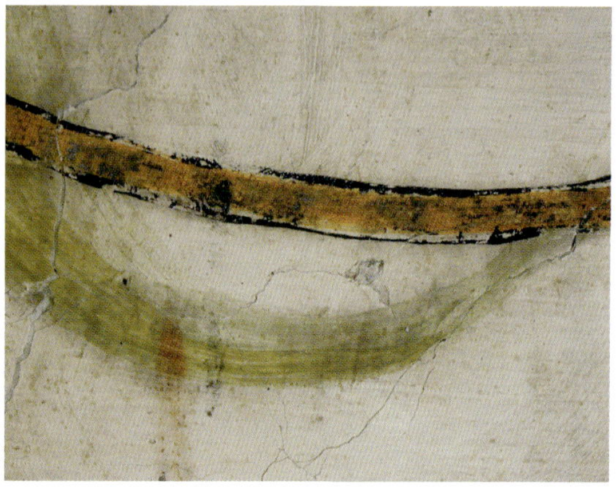

fig. 7.27

Fig. 7.26
Detail of the horse from the painting of St. George in the narthex (late twelfth century), showing a highly stylized painting technique (photo courtesy of CWPD, Courtauld Institute of Art).

Fig. 7.27
Detail of the neck of the horse from the painting of St. George in the narthex, showing horizontal brushstrokes for the application of the base colors, with final touches laid down in random directions (photo courtesy of CWPD, Courtauld Institute of Art).

Paint Layer

The highly stylized painting of St. George is unique in the church (Fig. 7.26). However, the painting has lost much of its modeling, applied as indicated by the analysis with the *secco* technique, and therefore much information concerning the technical aspect of style has disappeared. From the surviving painting, it can be observed that the preliminary or base colors were applied primarily using horizontal brushstrokes with final touches in random directions. Evidence can be seen on the area of the horse's neck and in the background near the shield and the horse's head (Fig. 7.27).

Gilding

The gilding materials and the method of applying the gold leaves on the surface of the painting in the St. George's program in the narthex is similar to the treatment for gilding in the 1105/6 program and distinctively different from the later fourteenth-century painted programs, suggesting a chronology for St. George closer to the 1105/6 paintings rather than later. The gold leaves made of an electrum of silver and gold (simply as in the 1105/6 paintings) were cut into squares and applied over a yellow intermediate paint layer using a mordant. Results from organic analysis indicated the use of either linseed or walnut oil (see Appendix 5). Traces of a modern consolidant present on the surface of the metal leaf restricted the identification of any original surface coating.

The Paintings of St. Anastasia Pharmakolytria in the Narthex, the Pantanassa on the Conch of the Apse in the Bema, and SS. Peter and Paul in the Naos

There appear to be close stylistic and epigraphic kinships among the paintings of Anastasia in the narthex, the Pantanassa in the conch of the apse in the bema, and SS. Peter and Paul from the first program on the westernmost pillars in the naos (Figs. 7.28a and 7.28b, along with 6.2 and 6.3; see also above, pp. 215–17). The technical study of these paintings, however, has revealed differences in technique that cast doubt on the correspondence between the paintings of SS. Peter and Paul, on the one hand, and the Anastasia and the Pantanassa paintings in the narthex and the bema on the other.

Judging from in situ examination and the results from the study of the samples, the paintings of Anastasia and the Pantanassa seem to belong to the same painted phase, while the paintings of SS. Peter and Paul, although similar in style and setting-out techniques, seem to belong to another based on differences in their execution.

Plaster

The thin section sample taken for analysis from the Anastasia painting has a pinkish color and consists of a lime-based plaster with thick pieces of chaff, flax tow or hemp, quartz, ferric oxide particles, and micrite. The sample taken from the figure of St. Paul is yellower; it contains much less quartz and ferric oxide, and it lacks the thick chaff pieces. However, in both cases the plaster is very smooth and compact.

Setting-Out Techniques

All the paintings discussed in this section show sharp incisions that were used as the preparatory guidelines for the painting. Painterly drawing in fine brown paint was also used. Uniquely in the Anastasia painting, the garments of both the saint and her devotee are finely outlined in white.

Paint Layer

The paintings of Anastasia and the Pantanassa have a very similar technical style of painting. Observations using raking light show a characteristic direction of the brushstrokes, particularly in the halos and the background; the brushstrokes come to a very visible and definitive conclusion, ending in a splash of paint where the brush tip would have been removed from the painting surface (Figs. 7.28c–f). Such a technique is not visible in the paintings of SS. Peter and Paul.

The pigments and pigment admixtures used in the Anastasia and Pantanassa paintings are very similar: the yellows consist of limonite and jarosite diluted with lime white, while the dark brown is a mixture of limonite, hematite-rich red ocher, and charcoal black. The green pigment was identified in all cases as the naturally occurring mineral celadonite, but in the background of the painting of St. Peter in the naos, that pigment was diluted with lime white and applied over a reddish ground; in the other cases it was used in pure form over a charcoal black intermediate layer.

The Fourteenth-Century Paintings in the Narthex and the Naos

Art historical reservations about the exact dating of the fourteenth-century program in the naos led to a comprehensive study of the painting samples. Technical comparisons were made with the dated 1332/33 paintings in the narthex; despite the several similarities in technique and materials, there are some differences that make it possible to question an attribution of the naos paintings to that date. These differences could be explained by the passage of a span of years between the execution of the two programs, or they could simply be attributable to the different techniques of two distinct but contemporary teams of painters at work in the church.

Plaster

There are small differences in the plasters used for the decoration of the two fourteenth-century

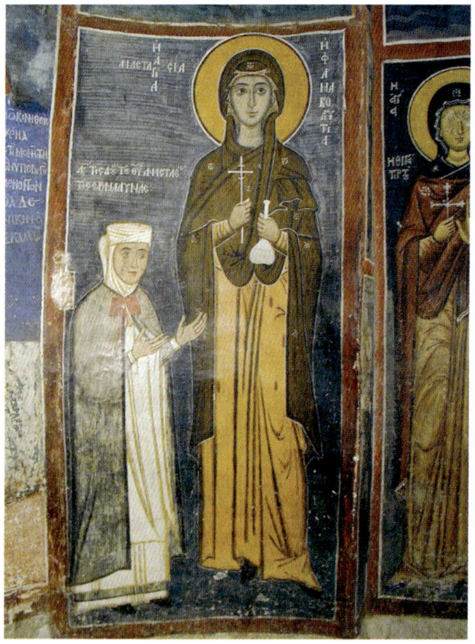

a

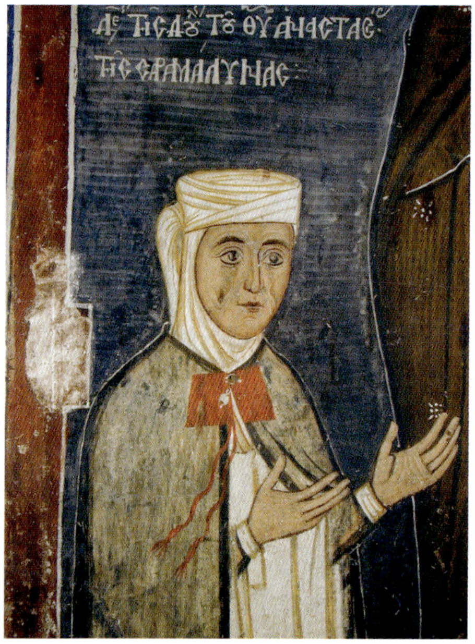

b

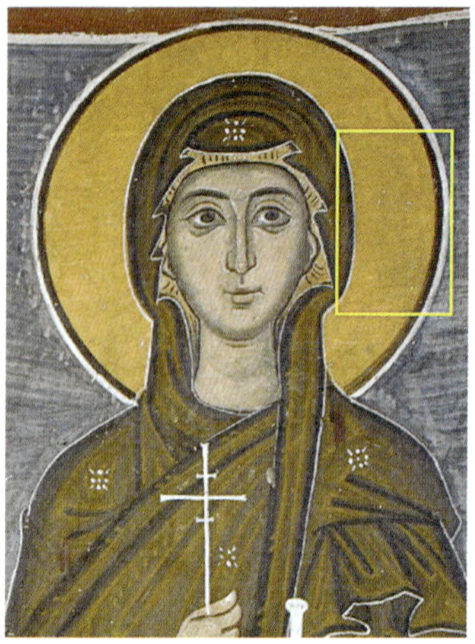

c

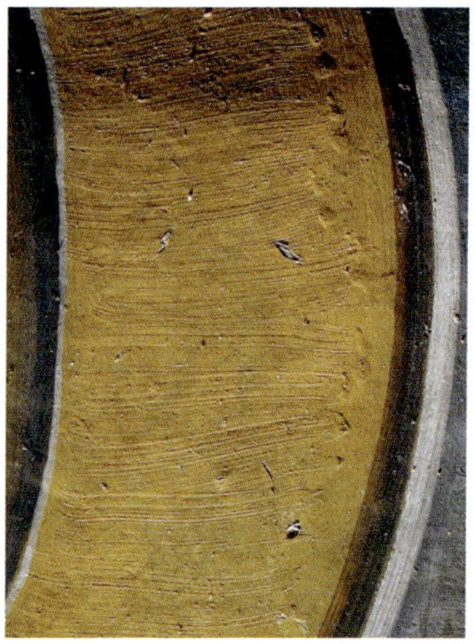

d

Fig. 7.28
The paintings of Anastasia in the narthex (a–d) and the Pantanassa in the bema (e–f) share similar stylistic and technical features, such as the painterly technique of the backgrounds and halos (photos courtesy of CWPD, Courtauld Institute of Art).

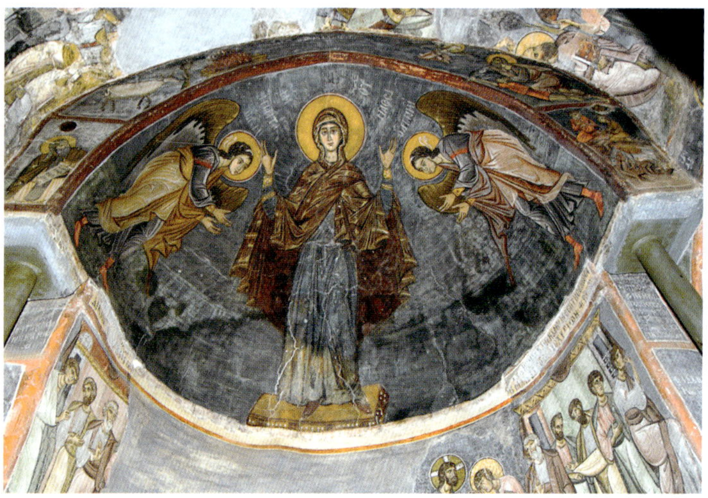

e

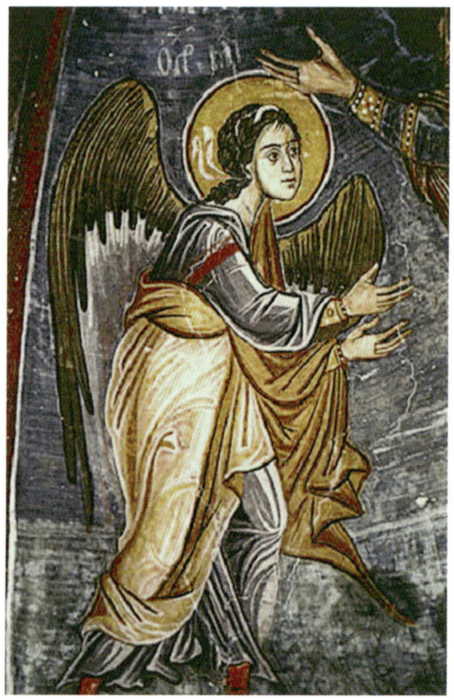

f

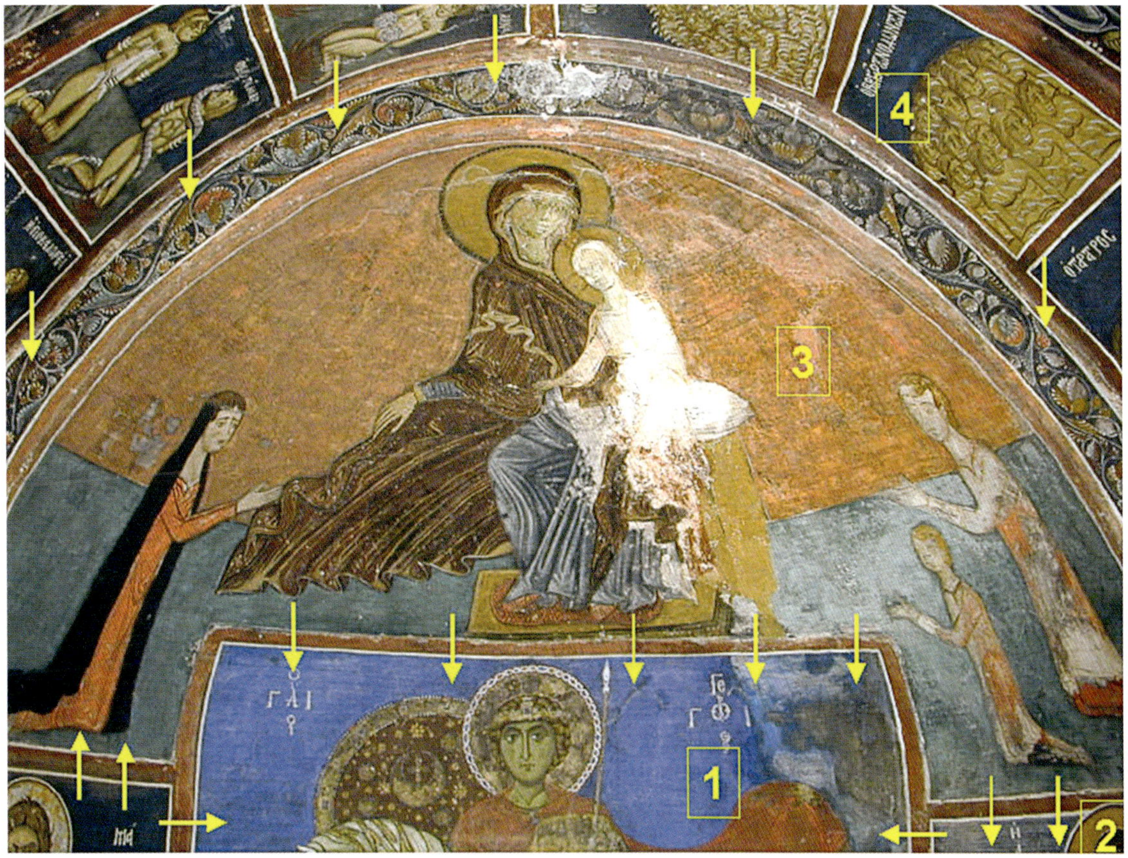

Fig. 7.29 View of the south apse in the narthex, illustrating how plaster joins can be used to help date paintings. Arrows indicate a join between two sections of plaster; the arrow points from the later to the earlier section. Numbers show the relative chronology of the sections (photo courtesy of G. L. Carr).

painting programs. The sample taken from the narthex consists of flat and cylindrical fibers, probably chaff and hemp, chalk aggregates, micrite, dispersed particles of ferric oxide, and quartz. The plaster from the fourteenth-century painting in the naos, however, consists of chaff and probably flax tow or hemp, chalk, quartz, and micrite. There is no evidence that cylindrical fibers were present in the other paintings.

The painting in the narthex made use of *pontate* and *giornate*, especially in the central area of the dome, while in the naos there is no clear evidence of such plaster joins. One of the *pontate* in the narthex, for example, includes the whole lunette and arch over the western doorway (Fig. 7.29). As in the 1105/6 program, the upper *pontata* on each vertical wall was painted after the bottom one; however, the vault and pendentives were probably painted first.

Setting-Out Techniques

The preparatory drawing of the paintings in the narthex was made with brown and black paint outlining for both the figures and the objects. This is in many respects similar to the fourteenth-century paintings in the naos.

Paint Layer

In the narthex, the background was painted in vertical brushstrokes, with final brushstrokes following the pattern of the composition. In some paintings, primarily in the southern part of the narthex, there is a darker green wavy pattern in the green background. The paintings on the north side do not show this detail. However, other technical features, such as the relief stucco decoration, do show close parallels. As a whole, the paint-layer techniques here are in many respects similar to those found in the fourteenth-century naos paintings.

Gilding and Raised Halos

In the narthex the raised halos seem initially to have been built up simultaneously with the plastering. Raised halos can be seen on the east wall and north apse of the narthex in the figures of the archangel Michael and St. Sozomenos. The relief decoration was then added later, using plaster of paris. Judging from the regular pattern and visible joins of the relief stucco sections, it seems that the decoration of the raised halos was executed with a wooden pattern used as a mold. It is uncertain, however, whether the plaster of paris was modeled in situ or whether the relief decoration was prepared elsewhere and then glued on. Evidence of a shiny material near the hair of selected figures with such raised halos might suggest the latter technique, although Dionysios of Fourna describes in his treatise a method of making raised halos in situ, which finds parallels in the fourteenth-century paintings at Asinou.[58] Raised halos can be seen on the east wall of the narthex and on the north apse, on the figures of Archangel Michael and St. Sozomenos (Figs. 7.1, 7.19a; see also pp. 205, 167).

Identical relief-gilded stucco decoration is also found in the fourteenth-century paintings in the naos (Fig. 7.17). Examples of such applications with clear technical features can be observed on the figure of St. George depicted on the south wall of the naos (Fig. 6.22), to the west of the southern door. In both programs, a pseudogilding technique was applied, using glazed tin leaf to imitate gold (see above, Gilding). Analysis indicated the presence of linseed oil and probably copal oil as the final coating over the tin leaf (see Appendix 5).The identification of the latter, however, is not conclusive.

58. Dionysios mentions a technique of making raised halos, which finds parallels in the method used in the fourteenth-century paintings at Asinou. Dionysios of Fourna, *Hermeneia*, 15.

Conclusions and Further Research

The lack of both contemporary Byzantine treatises and complete and systematic modern technical studies renders any conclusions about the Byzantine wall painting tradition open to doubt. Nonetheless, the church at Asinou yields evidence that is not only informative but also, in some cases, unparalleled, and so enhances our understanding. In two areas especially, Asinou's paintings are exceptionally informative. One is in the binding media, the other in the use of tin for the gilding. Though less exceptional, its pigments, too, expand our knowledge and provide a sample of the Byzantine palette used for painting from the twelfth to the fourteenth century. In addition, the technical study of the paintings in the church of Panagia Phorbiotissa at Asinou has assisted in the classification and attribution of painting phases of uncertain date.

Throughout the church a common painting technique was identified in the plastering of the walls, the selection of painting materials, and their application. A mixed technique of fresco and secco was employed: the base pigments were applied in fresco, whereas superimposed pigments, mixed with lime or an organic binding medium, were applied in secco. Of particular interest was the presence of siccative oils. Although oil has been identified as the binding medium in some icons and was used extensively in medieval wall paintings in western Europe, this was the first time that linseed and possibly walnut oil were identified on twelfth-century Byzantine murals.

Egg tempera was another binding medium identified in the wall paintings. The application of certain pigments with a specific binding medium (oil or egg) seems not to have been circumstantial. The physical and chemical compatibility of certain pigments with specific binding media affects both the properties and the appearance of the paint film. This is evident in the aesthetic appearance of the blue backgrounds in the paintings of 1105/6 in the naos, which are dull and grey, and that of St. George in the narthex, which has a vivid violet-blue hue. The former was identified as lapis lazuli applied in oil, while the latter is lapis lazuli applied in egg tempera. In both cases, the lapis lazuli particles have the same size, shape, and color, thus suggesting a good quality pigment and not an inferior one, often referred to as ultramarine ash.

A common palette of pigments was identified throughout the painting programs with the only apparent variation being the use of azurite instead of lapis lazuli from the end of the thirteenth century on. Gilding materials and methods also presented a chronological variation; the earliest paintings show mordant gilding on flat surfaces using thin metal foils of gold and silver electrum. The paintings after the fourteenth century, however, have replaced the foils of natural alloy with glazed tin foils.

The possible use of "tin relief" technique for gilding in the fourteenth-century and later paintings is an important discovery that emerged from the analysis. This technique, though common in western Europe, was never before identified in Byzantine wall paintings.[59] Its presence in the fourteenth-century paintings at Asinou suggests western influences or a local development that reflect the sociopolitical environment in Cyprus then.

Scientific investigations using a multiscale and multianalytical approach have proved critical for the study of the paintings at Asinou. New discoveries regarding the technological characteristics of the various painting programs have assisted in the interpretation of art historical questions and, in some cases, have led to the attribution of certain paintings to specific phases. Conversely, there are still unanswered questions that require further investigation, such as the dating and attribution of the paintings visible under the 1332/33 program in the narthex, although data suggest a date close to the 1332/33 phase, and the evidence of an earlier painting beneath the dedicatory inscription of the fourteenth century in the naos.

59. Nadolny, "Gilded Relief Decoration."

Chapter Seven
Appendix 1
Sample Locations

Sample no.	Acc. no.[A]	Location and type of sample	Figures
GILDING AND PAINT SAMPLES			
1	2867	Narthex. St. George. Gilding from the vest of St. George.	
2	2868	Narthex. St. George. White paint from the horse of St. George.	
3	2869	Narthex. St. George. Green paint from the background.	
4	2870	Narthex. St. George. Dark reddish or brown paint from the wavy background.	
5	2871	Narthex. St. George. Blue paint from the background.	
6	2872	Narthex. St. George. Purple paint from motif decorating the saddle of the horse.	
7	2873	Narthex. St. George. Red paint from the mantle of St. George.	7.12–14
8	2874	Narthex. St. George. Flesh paint from the hand.	7.24
9	2875	Narthex. St. George. Brown paint from the shield of St. George.	7.16
10	2876	Narthex. St. George. Light green paint from tail of horse.	
11	2877	Naos. South wall. Virgin and Child. Raised halo of Christ. Gilding.	7.17
12	2878	Naos. South wall. Virgin and Child. Raised halo of Archangel Gabriel. Lower gilding layers.	
13	2879	Naos. East wall. Christ Eleemon. Flesh paint from Christ's neck.	
14	2880	Naos. East wall. Christ Eleemon. Green paint from belt.	
15	2881	Naos. East wall. Christ Eleemon. Blue paint from background.	
16	2882	Naos. South wall. St. George. Yellow paint from cloak.	
17	2883	Naos. South wall. Virgin and Child. Green paint from lower background.	
18	2884	Naos. East wall. North side. Virgin. Blue paint from dress.	
19	2885	Naos. North wall. St. Theodore. Red paint from mantle.	
20	2886	Naos. East wall. South side. Christ. Yellow paint from sleeve.	
21	2887	Naos. South wall. 1st program. Orange paint from shoe of St. George.	

SAMPLE LOCATIONS *continued*

Sample no.	Acc. no.[A]	Location and type of sample	Figures
GILDING AND PAINT SAMPLES			
22	2888	Naos. West wall. Dormition. Flesh paint from standing figure behind St. Paul.	7.22
23	2889	Naos. West wall. Dormition. Blue paint from background.	7.9
24	2890	Naos. West wall. Dormition. Green paint from lower background.	7.11
25	2891	Naos. West wall. Dormition. Red paint from decoration of Virgin's bed.	
26	2892	Naos. West wall. Dormition. Yellow paint from Virgin's sleeve.	
27	2893	Naos. West wall. Dormition. Pink paint from St. Paul's garments.	
28	2894	Naos. West wall. Dormition. Bluish grey paint from St. Paul's garments.	
29	2895	Naos. West wall. Dormition. Green paint from the clothes of the second figure from left.	
30	2896	Naos. West wall. Dormition. Yellow paint from the halo of St. John.	
31	2897	Naos. South wall. SS. Helena and Constantine. Blue paint from background.	
32	2898	Naos. South wall. SS. Helena and Constantine. Flesh paint from Helena's hand.	
33	2899	Naos. South wall. SS. Helena and Constantine. Green paint from background.	
34	2900	Naos. South wall. SS. Helena and Constantine. Blue paint from Helena's garments.	
35	2901	Naos. South wall. SS. Helena and Constantine. Olive green paint from Constantine's garments.	
36	2902	Naos. South wall. SS. Helena and Constantine. Yellow paint from Helena's halo.	
37	2903	Naos. South wall. Western recess. West face. Red paint from St. Floros's garments.	
38	2904	Naos. West wall. Dormition. Blue paint from decorative elements on Virgin's bed.	
39	2927	Exterior. North wall. Flesh paint from Virgin's hand.	7.23
40	2928	Exterior. North wall. Plum red paint from Virgin's garments.	
41	2929	Narthex. South apse. Eastern part. Lower decorative program with circles. Yellow paint.	
42	2930	Narthex. South apse. Eastern part. 1st program. Yellow paint.	
43	2931	Naos. Northwest respond. South face. 1st program. Flesh paint from foot of standing figure.	
44	2932	Naos. Southwest respond. North face. 1st program. Green background.	
45	2933	Narthex. North apse. Archangel Michael. Reddish-purple paint from sleeve.	
46	2934	Narthex. North apse. Archangel Michael. Gilding from halo.	7.19

SAMPLE LOCATIONS *continued*

Sample no.	Acc. no.[A]	Location and type of sample	Figures
GILDING AND PAINT SAMPLES			
47	2935	Narthex. East wall. Virgin Eleousa. Bluish-green paint from sleeve.	
48	2936a	Narthex. East wall. Christ Eleemon. Yellow paint from raised halo.	
49	2936b	Narthex. East wall. Christ Eleemon. Flesh paint from Christ's neck.	
50	2937	Narthex. Arch over doorway to the naos. St. John. Blue paint from background.	
51	2938	Narthex. North apse. St. Cosmas. Green paint from garments.	
52	2939	Narthex. North apse. St. Marina. Red paint from garments.	
53	2940	Narthex. Arch over doorway to the naos. St. John. Green paint from background.	
54	2941	Narthex. East wall. Virgin Eleousa. Brown paint from garments.	
55	2942	Narthex. North apse. 1st program beneath Archangel Michael. Yellow paint from decoration.	
56	2943	Narthex. Anastasia. Red from donor's bow.	
57	2944	Narthex. Anastasia. Flesh paint from donor's hand.	
58	2945	Narthex. Anastasia. Yellow paint from Anastasia's garments.	
59	2946	Narthex. Anastasia. Brown paint from Anastasia's garments.	
60	2947	Exterior. North wall. Pinkish paint from garments.	
61	2967	Narthex. Lunette. Virgin Phorbiotissa. Blue paint from background.	
62	2968	Narthex. Lunette. Virgin Phorbiotissa. Flesh paint from Virgin's hand.	
63	2969	Narthex. Lunette. Virgin Phorbiotissa. Brown paint from Virgin's garments.	
64	2970	Narthex. Lunette. Virgin Phorbiotissa. Red paint from Christ's medallion.	
65	2971	Bema. Apse. Communion. Gilding from Christ's halo.	7.18
66	2972	Bema. Conch of apse. Blue paint from Virgin's dress.	
67	2973	Bema. Conch of apse. Green paint from background.	
68	2974	Bema. Conch of apse. Brown paint from Virgin's shoe.	
69	2975	Naos. Northwest respond. St. Nikephoros. Blue paint from background.	
70	2976	Naos. Northwest respond. St. Symeon Stylites. Flesh paint from hand.	
71	2977	Naos. Northwest respond. St. Onouphrios. Gilding from halo.	
72	2978	Naos. Northwest respond. St. Nikephoros. Red paint from book.	
PLASTER SAMPLES			
P1	2948	Narthex. North face. Intrados of arch. East side. Plaster sample.	
P2	2949	Naos. North pillar. South Face. Dado. 1st program. Plaster sample.	
P3	2950	Naos. North jamb of west door. Plaster sample.	

SAMPLE LOCATIONS *continued*

Sample no.	Acc. no.[a]	Location and type of sample	Figures
PLASTER SAMPLES			
P4	2951	Narthex. East wall. South side of door. Dado. 1st program. Plaster sample.	
P5	2952	Narthex. South apse. Dado. Below St. George. Plaster sample.	
P6	2953	Narthex. South apse. St. George's program. Plaster sample.	
P7	2954	Narthex. South apse. Anastasia. Plaster sample.	
P8	2955	Narthex. North apse. East from door. 1st program beneath Archangel Michael. Plaster sample.	
P9	2964	Bema. East wall. Dado. Beneath niche. Right lower corner. Plaster sample.	
P10	2965	Narthex. Tympanum. Virgin Phorbiotissa. Plaster sample.	
P11	2966	Naos. South wall. Virgin and Child. Plaster sample.	

[a] Accession numbers for Courtauld Institute of Art.

Chapter Seven
Appendix 2
Inorganic Analysis

Identification of Pigments

Paint samples were first examined with a Kyowa Optical RFB-7 binocular microscope at magnifications between 10× and 45×. This examination of the unmounted microsamples is important for characterization of the surface (pitting, dirt, coatings, etc.) and for preliminary characterization of the pigments present, either unmixed or combined, within the various layers. Information concerning the physical properties of the particles (shape, color, etc.) and surface characteristics were recorded, together with data on the presence of surface salts, alteration products, microbiological growth, etc. Binocular microscopic examination also assisted in the interpretation of the analytical results.

Cross-sections, thin sections, and dispersion samples were initially examined using a Leica Leitz DMRD polarized microscope, providing fundamental information on the stratigraphy of the samples. The cross-sections were then carbon-coated and examined using a Jeol JSM-35CF SEM equipped with a backscattered electron detector at 15–25 keV. Energy-dispersive analysis was carried out with an Oxford Link Pentafet spectrometer with an ATW2 window for the detection of light elements using Link Isis software. Another SEM, used at the Ancient Monuments Laboratory at English Heritage, is an LEO Stereoscan S440 SEM, which was also equipped with a backscattered detector and an Oxford Instruments EDS detector with an ATW (atmosphere thin window) detector allowing it to detect light elements down to atomic number five (boron). During analysis of the samples, the energy of electrons used was 20 keV and therefore L-series and sometimes M-series x-rays were used to detect heavy elements.

Dispersions were examined primarily in transmitted light, both plane-polarized and with crossed polars.

Samples in powder form were analyzed using FTIR spectroscopy (a Nicolet Magna-IR 550). Spectra were recorded in percent transmission (%T) over the range of 4000 to 400 cm^{-1}. Infrared spectroscopy is a nondestructive technique providing structural and molecular information which can assist in the identification of both inorganic and organic materials. In this study, FTIR was used primarily for the identification of inorganic pigments and plaster constituents. Data was acquired using either diffuse reflectance or infrared transmission powder; the latter was extensively used in this study.

Microchemical tests provided complementary analysis. These tests employ specific reagents that assist in identifying the materials present.[1] They were performed directly on individual particles isolated under the microscope. These tests are destructive, therefore only a few particles were used. The microchemical tests used in this study could detect carbonate, ferric, lead, and sulfide ions.

1 Plesters, "Cross-sections."

Carbonates (such as calcium carbonate)

For the identification of carbonates, a drop of dilute hydrochloric acid (HCl) is added to a few particles of the unknown material placed on a glass slide. Effervescence—the release of carbon dioxide—indicated the presence of carbonates.

Ferric oxides (such as ochers)

The test for ferric ions, characteristic of all iron pigments, uses HCl and potassium ferrocyanide ($K_4[Fe(CN)_6].3H_2O$). A few grains of the pigment are combined with concentrated HCl and left to dry under an infrared lamp. The samples are then cooled and a drop of dilute HCl added, immediately followed by a drop of $K_4[Fe(CN)_6].3H_2O$. Blue staining of particles and solution suggests the presence of ferric ions.

Lead ions (found in white and red lead pigments)

This test uses HCl and potassium iodine (KI). A drop of the dilute HCl is added either to pigment particles or to a cross section. In the presence of lead white (basic lead carbonate $2PbCO_3.Pb[OH]_2$), there is a slow effervescence from the breakdown of the carbonates. Red lead discolors to white in the presence of HCl (probably due to the formation of lead chloride). Analysis is confirmed by adding KI, which turns lead-containing pigments deep yellow.

Sulfide (such as ultramarine, cinnabar)

A drop of sodium azide-iodine reagent is added to the powdered pigment. The reaction was observed through the microscope. A careful check was made for any gas release. In this case, the "effervescence" results from the escape of nitrogen gas in the solution.

The reaction occurs only in the presence of sulfur, which catalyzes the reaction between the nitrogen and the iodine:

$$2NaN_3 + I_2 \xrightarrow{S^{2-}} 2NaI + 3N_2\uparrow$$

$$\textit{sodium azide} + \textit{iodine} \xrightarrow{\textit{sulfide}} \textit{sodium iodide} + \textit{nitrogen gas}$$

This reaction occurs in the presence of pigments containing sulfur, such as cinnabar, ultramarine blue, realgar, orpiment, cadmium yellow, and cadmium red.

Identification of Plasters

Plaster samples were first examined using binocular microscopy to allow selection and separation of particles, which were then prepared as pellets and analyzed using FTIR. Larger samples were prepared as thin sections and examined using PLM to determine the stratigraphy and the type and morphology of aggregates and fibers.

Chapter Seven
Appendix 3
Organic Analysis

Identification of coatings and binding media

Samples of the paint and coating layers were removed for identification of organic binding media and other substances. Gas chromatography with mass spectrometry (GC-MS) was used to identify the organic binding media through procedures for the analysis of oils, fats, and proteins. Fourier-transform infrared spectroscopy (FTIR) was performed in order to identify materials in the coatings.

The GC-MS technique can be used to identify organic binding media, such as proteins, oils, waxes, resins, and plant gums, in addition to many types of paint additives. The samples must be treated with reactive chemicals prior to analysis, and each type of medium may require a specific pretreatment procedure. Procedures were developed at the Getty Conservation Institute (GCI) for the identification of the common organic binding media.[1] Moreover, for plant gums, proteins, and oils it is possible to measure the amount of medium present in the sample. Proteinaceous binding media were identified by comparing the amino acid composition of

1 The sample was weighed on an ultramicrobalance and transferred to a 0.1ml conical reaction vial, and norleucine internal standard was added. Then, 50µl of 6.0N hydrochloric acid was added and the vial capped with a Mininert valve. Air was removed from the vial by thrice alternating between vacuum for 20 seconds and nitrogen purge for 5 seconds. The vial was heated at 105°C for 24 hours. The sample was centrifuged after cooling, and the contents evaporated to total dryness under a stream of nitrogen while heating to 60°C. The vial was rinsed with 40µl of high-purity water, centrifuged, and evaporated as before. The rinsing process was repeated using 200-proof ethanol to thoroughly dry the contents prior to silylation.

Next, the silylating mixture was added to the vial and the Mininert valve was replaced. The solvent for silylation was silylation-grade pyridine, and the reagent was 99% MTBSTFA with 1% TBDMCS (Pierce Chemical). The silylating mixture was composed of 30% MTBSTFA/TBDMCS and 70% pyridine solution (v/v). For typical paint samples, 1µl of reagent was used per 2µg of sample. The vial was warmed at 60°C for 30 minutes on a hot plate, then heated in an oven at 105°C for 5 hours. After cooling, this was centrifuged and 1µl injected into GC-MS.

Quantitative analysis of the TBDMS derivatives was performed on a Hewlett Packard 5972 gas chromatograph/mass spectrometer. A DB-5MS capillary column was used for the separation (30m × 0.25mm × 0.25µm). Helium carrier gas was set to a linear velocity of 45cm/sec. The splitless injector was set to 260°C with a 60 sec purge-off time. The MS transfer line was set to 280°C. The GC oven temperature program was: 80°C for 1 minute, then ramped to 320°C at 20°C/minute, followed by a 3-minute isothermal period. A solvent delay of 4 minutes was used. The mass spectrometer was used in selected ion monitoring mode. A mixture of amino acids, fatty acids, and glycerol was used for calibration.

The use of MTBSTFA is described in Šimek et al., "Capillary Gas Chromatography." A manuscript that describes the complete GC-MS analysis procedure is currently in preparation.

the sample to that of standard reference materials.[2] Similarly, oils and fats present in the samples were identified by comparison to reference materials.[3]

The FTIR technique has a number of advantages over GC-MS. FTIR can be used directly on a paint sample without requiring aggressive chemical pretreatment. Because samples may be recovered for subsequent analysis by other methods, it is termed a nondestructive technique. Furthermore, it can identify pigments and other nonvolatile species (such as acrylic media) that cannot be detected by GC-MS. However, it can detect components present only in concentrations above 5–10% by weight, although many substances are well below that level in commercial paints. Herant Khanjian, GCI assistant scientist, tested the samples. A representative sample particle was placed on a barium fluoride (BaF_2) window, flattened by a stainless steel roller, and analyzed by a transmitted infrared beam with an aperture of approximately 100 × 100 microns, using a 15× objective. Each spectrum was the sum of 200 scans at a resolution of 4 cm^{-1}. Based on the results from the initial analysis of bulk material, extraction was made by placing a microdroplet of solvent on the sample, and analysis was performed on the resultant extracted dry solvent ring. Infrared spectra of the samples contain bands that correspond to the paint components. To identify materials in a paint sample, the infrared spectrum may be matched to spectra for reference materials using a computer algorithm. Of course, other components may be present in the samples at concentrations below the 5% detection limit.[4]

2. In order to identify the protein, the amino acid composition of the sample was compared to the compositions of standard casein, glue, and egg by correlation coefficients and other mathematical procedures. Data interpretation is discussed in detail in Schilling and Khanjian, "Amino Acids."

3. Data interpretation follows the methods described in Mills, "Fatty Acid Composition," and in Mills and White, "Organic Mass Spectrometry." Because glycerol is present as the backbone of all triglycerides, glycerol was analyzed quantitatively in order to estimate the oil and fat content of the samples (% glycerol × 10 = oil content).

4. For more details see Derrick, "Infrared Microspectroscopy."

Chapter Seven
Appendix 4
Wall-Painting Techniques

Fresco Technique

Fresco ("fresh" in Italian) technique refers to any painting executed on a moist, lime-rich plaster layer. The pigments are applied with water and are fixed by the formation of a carbonate lattice during the setting of the lime (calcium hydroxide). Lime is one of the oldest and most favored binders for plasters. It was used as early as the Neolithic period in the form of lime wash and throughout the centuries it has been used as a plaster by admixture with various inert aggregates,[1] such as fragments of rocks and minerals. The Greeks and later the Romans explored the use of mildly reactive hydraulic materials to produce a stronger plaster, known as *opus signinum*. Hydraulic fillers can be natural (volcanic or diatomaceous earth) or artificial (crushed bricks and other refractory materials).

The extensive use of lime can be related to the abundance of limestone throughout the Mediterranean. The use of lime-based plasters and the existence of lime kilns in archaeological sites prove that ancient civilizations were familiar with the technology of lime.

Lime is made by calcining limestone, which consists essentially of calcium carbonate. The limestone is heated to high temperatures (700–900° C) to obtain quick lime (CaO).

1. Torraca, *Porous Building Materials*, 67.

$$CaCO_3 \xrightarrow{700\text{–}900^\circ C} CaO + CO_2$$

$$\text{calcium carbonate} \longrightarrow \text{calcium oxide} + \text{carbon dioxide}$$

$$\text{limestone} \longrightarrow \text{quick lime}$$

Slaking of lime is the next step, which involves the reaction of quicklime with water to produce calcium hydroxide ($Ca[OH]_2$), or slaked lime.

$$CaO + H_2O \longrightarrow Ca(OH)_2$$

$$\text{calcium oxide} \longrightarrow \text{calcium hydroxide}$$

$$\text{quick lime} + \text{water} \longrightarrow \text{slaked lime}$$

The setting of lime is based on a chemical reaction between the calcium hydroxide and the carbon dioxide (CO_2) of the atmosphere.

$$Ca(OH)_2 + CO_2 \longrightarrow CaCO_3 + H_2O\uparrow$$

$$\text{calcium hydroxide (slaked lime)} + \text{carbon dioxide} \longrightarrow \text{carbonated lime} + \text{water}$$

During this chemical reaction there is a loss of water, causing contraction and cracking. Hence, when used as a plaster, lime is always mixed with an inorganic (inert or hydraulic) aggregate (also termed charge or filler), with or without the addition of organic additives. Organic materials may be used as additives to provide plasticity to the plaster, and these typically include chaff, fibres, animal hair, blood, and urine.

Owing to the high alkalinity of the lime, only a small number of pigments are compatible with the fresco technique. Those available in the ancient world included Egyptian blue, ultramarine blue, green earth, yellow ocher (ferric hydroxide), red ocher (ferric oxide), calcium carbonate white, China clay, ivory black, bone and carbon black, and manganese dioxide (pyrolusite). However, other mineral pigments such as cinnabar, azurite, malachite, and red and white lead are often found on wall paintings in fresco technique. These have normally degraded over the course of time, and their alteration may generally be related to their incompatibility with the technique.

In a fresco application, painters often apply the plaster patch by patch, each patch representing the area of painting that could be completed before the plaster dried out. These small sections of plaster are usually called *giornate* (singular *giornata*, "day"). The horizontal plaster sections, known as *pontate* (singular *pontata*, meaning story of scaffolding), were normally used for areas with geometrical decoration. Although this terminology was introduced with the study of Renaissance paintings, *giornate* can be found in Roman paintings, examples of which are well preserved in Pompeii.[2]

Secco Technique

Secco ("dry" in Italian) technique involves no chemical reaction for the fixation of the pigments. As suggested by the etymology of the word, secco painting involves the use of dry plaster or whitewash, onto which the pigments are fixed by using an additional organic binding medium. This technique is therefore not restricted to lime plasters. They can also involve clay, gypsum, or calcium carbonate as the principal plaster binders. In many cases the painting is executed directly on the support (rock-cut surface, stone blocks).

2. Mora et al., *Conservation of Wall Paintings*, plates 54–56.

Chapter Seven
Appendix 5
Synoptic Organic Analysis Report

Sample 1 (acc. no. 2867)
coating over metal leaf
Reason for sampling: identify coating
Results from FTIR analysis: The spectrum showed bands from poly(vinyl acetate), calcium oxalate monohydrate, and chalk.
Conclusions: Poly(vinyl acetate) originates from a restoration. The origin of the chalk and oxalate is unclear.

ground
Reason for sampling: identify binding medium in gilding ground
Results from GC-MS analysis:
Protein data: 0.3% protein, 0.987 correlation coefficient of amino acid composition to egg yolk plus a trace of animal glue.
Oil data: 2.7% oil content, A/P 3.4, P/S 2.43
Conclusions: The oil content of the sample is much higher than the protein content. The fatty acid data are consistent with linseed oil with traces of egg fats, although walnut oil cannot be ruled out entirely. One possible explanation for the findings is that egg and glue originate from ground, and oil is present in the overlying yellow paint layer.

Sample 4 (acc. no. 2870)
coating over red paint
Reason for sampling: identify coating
Results from FTIR analysis: The spectrum showed bands from poly(vinyl acetate), calcite chalk, and iron oxide ocher.
Conclusions: Poly(vinyl acetate) must originate from a restoration, whereas chalk and ocher may be present in the underlying red paint.

Sample 5 (acc. no. 2871)
blue paint
Reason for sampling: identify binding medium
Results from GC-MS analysis:
Protein data: 0.7% protein, 0.953 correlation coefficient of amino acid composition to egg yolk plus a trace of glue.
Oil data: 1.7% oil content, A/P 0.34, P/S 2.42
Conclusions: The protein and oil results are consistent with egg.

Sample 7 (acc. no. 2873)
red paint with some yellow
Reason for sampling: identify binding medium
Results from GC-MS analysis:
Protein data: 1.7% protein, but no high correlation coefficient of amino acid composition to common proteinaceous media.
Oil data: 8.7% oil content, A/P 1.58, P/S 2.19
Conclusions: The oil results are consistent with linseed oil (although walnut oil cannot be ruled out entirely), plus contamination by proteinaceous or non-proteinaceous materials.

Sample 11 (acc. no. 2877; Fig. 7.17)
colored substrate for gilding (also contained bits of white ground)
Reason for sampling: identify binding medium. Medium thought to be animal glue
Results from GC-MS analysis:
Protein data: 6.3% protein, 0.994 correlation coefficient of amino acid composition to egg yolk.
Oil data: 3.2% oil content, high content of oleic acid, A/P 0.43, P/S 1.99; fatty acid composition is consistent with fats from egg, mixed with linseed oil.
Conclusions: Binding medium in bole layer identified as linseed oil. Egg may originate from white ground layer. Evidence for animal glue was not found.

white ground under gilding (also contained bits of colored substrate for gilding)
Reason for sampling: identify binding medium. Medium thought to be animal glue
Results from GC-MS analysis:
Protein data: 3.9% protein, 0.979 correlation coefficient of amino acid composition to egg yolk.
Oil data: 1.6% oil content, high content of oleic acid, A/P 0.69, P/S 1.87; fatty acid composition is consistent with fats from egg, possibly with linseed oil.
Conclusions: Binding medium in ground layer identified as egg. Linseed oil may originate from colored substrate. Evidence for animal glue was not found.

coating with orange and colorless areas
Reason for sampling: identify coating over tin foil. Shellac was traditionally used.
Results from FTIR analysis: On an orange area of the coating, the spectrum showed bands from Acryloid B-72 and copal oil medium, whereas on a clear area of the coating only Acryloid B-72 was evident.
Conclusions: Acryloid B-72 originates from a restoration; oil or resin substances may originate from the original coating. Evidence for shellac was not detected by FTIR.

Sample 15 (acc. no. 2881)
blue paint
Reason for sampling: identify binding medium
Results from GC-MS analysis:
Protein data: 0.3% protein, >0.9 correlation coefficient of amino acid composition to non-proteinaceous contaminants.
Oil data: 3.3% oil content, azelaic to palmitic acid ratio (A/P) 0.76, palmitic to stearic acid ratio (P/S) 1.76
Conclusions: Binding medium in blue paint identified as linseed oil.

Sample 18 (acc. no. 2884)
blue paint with some white and brown
Reason for sampling: identify binding medium
Results from GC-MS analysis:
Protein data: 0.6% protein, >0.9 correlation coefficient of amino acid composition to non-proteinaceous contaminants.
Oil data: 3.6% oil content, A/P 1.74, P/S 1.86
Conclusions: The oil results are consistent with linseed oil. Although the protein analysis results are inconclusive, they are not totally unexpected. Experience has shown that, over time, objects may become contaminated with proteinaceous and non-proteinaceous materials, such as human epidermis, certain natural resins, insect debris, and many other materials.

Sample 23 (acc. no. 2889; Fig. 7.9)
blue paint
Reason for sampling: identify binding medium
Results from GC-MS analysis:
Protein data: 0.4% protein, >0.9 correlation coefficient of amino acid composition to non-proteinaceous contaminants.
Oil data: 2.4% oil content, A/P 0.68, P/S 1.78
Conclusions: The binding medium was identified as linseed oil with non-proteinaceous contaminants.

Sample 28 (acc. no. 2894)
blue paint
Reason for sampling: identify binding medium
Results from GC-MS analysis:
Protein test: 0.8% protein, 0.960 correlation coefficient of amino acid composition to egg yolk plus a trace of glue.
Oil data: 7.3% oil content, A/P 1.52, P/S 1.39
Conclusions: The binding medium in blue paint was identified as linseed oil. Egg may originate from traces of the underlying white ground layer.

Sample 31 (acc. no. 2897)
blue paint
Reason for sampling: identify binding medium
Results from GC-MS analysis:
Protein data: 0.3% protein, >0.9 correlation coefficient of amino acid composition to non-proteinaceous contaminants.
Oil data: 5.2% oil content, A/P 0.43, P/S 2.01
Conclusions: The binding medium was identified as linseed oil with non-proteinaceous contaminants.

Sample 34 (acc. no. 2900)
blue and green paint over brown
Reason for sampling: identify binding medium in blue and green paint
Results from GC-MS analysis: There was a problem with test, and the sample was completely consumed.
Conclusions: No analytical results were obtained.

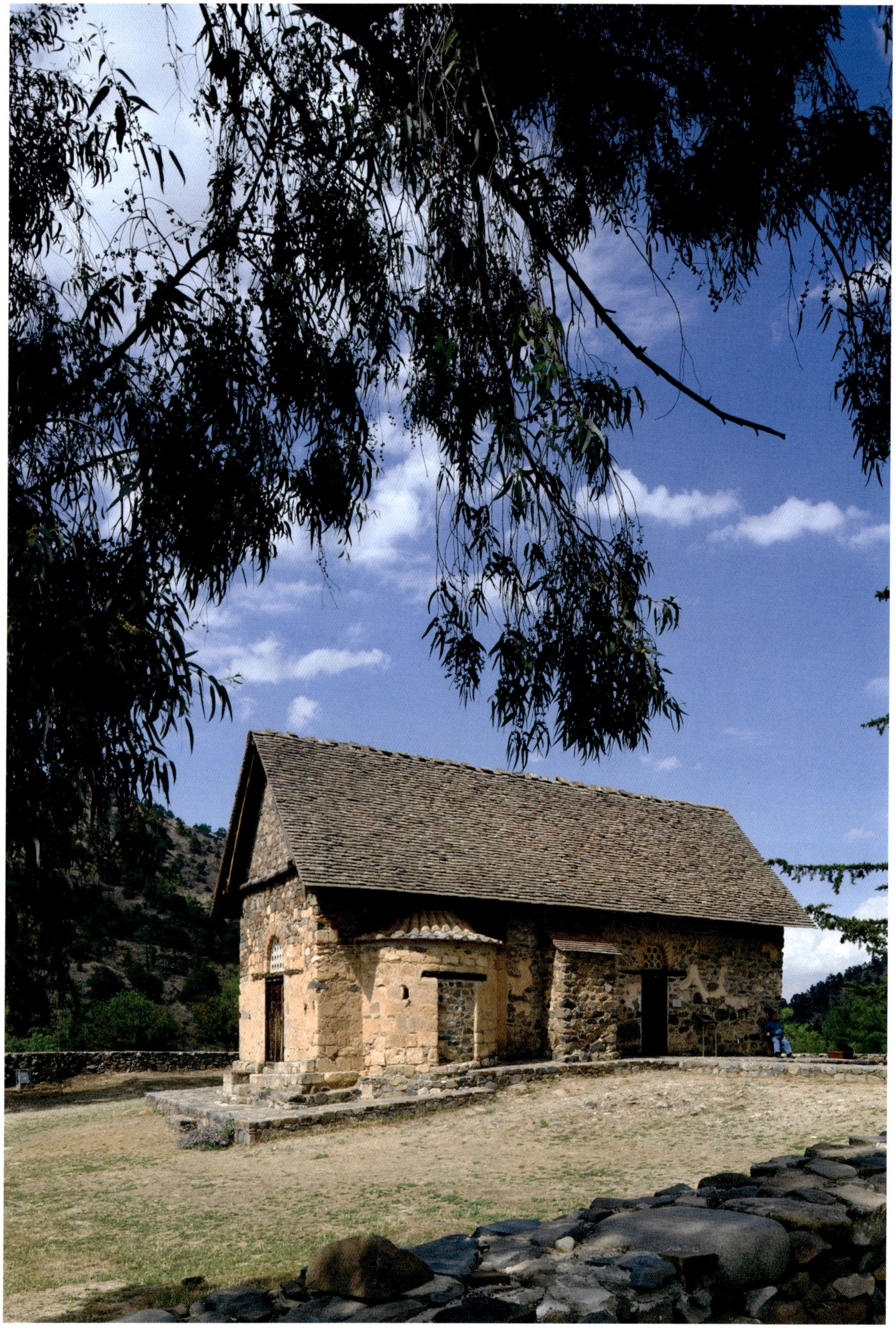

The church of Panagia Phorbiotissa from the southwest (photo courtesy of G. L. Carr)

Conclusion

Annemarie Weyl Carr

The monastic church of the Mother of God ton Phorbion (τῶν Φορβίων) has been approached in this book less for its initial mural cycle of 1105/6 than for its layer upon layer of ensuing life, registered in the surfaces and images that were added to it over the centuries. The authors, scholars of varied fields, have focused on the paintings from the two and a half centuries following the well-established date of 1105/6, when Asinou's first and most famous cycle of frescoes was completed. That cycle of paintings was produced at the behest of an otherwise unidentified magistrate by the name of Nikephoros Ischyrios. Nikephoros had his own portrait included among the mural images, and he had the fresco painters surround the space with poetic invocations for his salvation. We learn from the inscription accompanying his portrait that he had also sponsored the building of the church, but that inscription neither specifies the date nor explains the purpose of its construction. He may have built it for his own use as a private church or funerary chapel; on the other hand, he may have founded it as the katholikon of a monastery. Certainly the building had assumed this function within a decade of being frescoed, for the death of its founder, a certain lord Nicholas, is recorded in 1115 (see above, p. 17). Whether Nicholas was Nikephoros under a new, monastic name or another person altogether remains unresolved, and is the first of many questions this volume has had to leave open. The success of his foundation, however, is clear: the church of Asinou did serve as a katholikon for the next seven centuries. The monastery attracted new sponsors, their support registered visibly in the steady accretion of architectural modifications and mural paintings in the church. Each addition articulated the building's spaces anew, shaping them to new needs.

Most murals studied and documented in this book were painted on additions to the original structure. Oddly modest in light of its famous frescoes, the original building followed a simple plan, a long-established structural type, and rubble construction. Its accretions were more solidly built than the church itself. The first and most significant of these additions was the narthex, surely added to address the monastery's liturgical needs. Both its double-apse plan and its high-grade, reused material associate it with the churches of Cyprus based on Constantinopolitan models. Like the frescoes of 1105/6, the narthex is of higher quality than the original church, and it might be imagined as an improvement undertaken when the church assumed monastic status, a status it had earned by 1115. Its lightly pointed arches suggest a date no earlier than the mid-twelfth century, however, and the earliest evidence of painting that survives in the narthex belongs only to the last decades of the twelfth century. The awkwardly long span of some eighty years between the foundation of the monastery and the initial evidence of frescoes in the narthex leaves open questions about the date of the narthex's construction, its patronage, its purposes, and the period of its adornment. Athanasios Papageorgiou prefers to push the date of its construction as close as possible to that of its adornment (see Chapter 2).

The ensuing modifications to the church were not so much additions as repairs, prompted by one or more structural failures that cost the building its initial apse conch and destabilized the north side of the naos. These changes must have occurred in the thirteenth century, though their date(s), their cause(s), and even their number remain elusive. As Papageorgiou points out, had the apse collapsed in the twelfth century it would surely have been repainted when the late twelfth-century frescoes were introduced in the narthex, just as it was frescoed simultaneously with painting in the narthex in the late thirteenth century. It is impossible to know, however, how much time elapsed between the rebuilding of the conch and its late thirteenth-century adornment. Further reinforcements were built into the naos to redress the instability of the north wall. They are identical in technique to those in the apse, but may not have been installed at the same time, a possibility underscored by the frescoes on their lower portions. These are not far different in date from the frescoes in the apse, but they are not by the same hand. Once again, the interval between the installation of the reinforcements and their decoration remains unclear. The fact that they were only partially painted and remained largely unadorned for decades offers a salutary warning against identifying too closely the date of a construction with that of its painted adornment.

The repairs to Asinou's fabric tell us that the building was in use. Drawing on a vast knowledge of Cypriot culture and topography, Gilles Grivaud coaxes a coherent story of the monastery from images, inscriptions, scant documentary sources, glancing references in the margins of manuscripts, maps, tax records, and the physical, archaeological, and ethnographic testimony of the site (see Chapter 1). The monastery's efflorescence parallels the centuries between about 1100 and 1600, when pottery evidence in the valley attests its steady occupation.[1] This span embraces the centuries of Cyprus's Latin domination, when the monastery seems to have flourished. The structural collapses of the apse and the north wall tend to give the thirteenth century an aura of catastrophe that is easily aligned with the events of Crusader conquest and Latin implantation. To the contrary, the steady process of repair and the ever more ample redecoration register the institution's capacity to take such catastrophes in stride. Grivaud suggests what might have drawn the magistros Nikephoros to locate his little church in the Asinou Valley. He also proposes the sources of its vitality in the Lusignan and Venetian periods and demonstrates its survival deep into the Ottoman period. Additionally, he offers the clearest assessment of the likely date of the monastery's demise, near the year 1800. Perhaps Grivaud's most crucial gift lies in interlacing evidence of the monastery's personnel and patrons from the margins of Paris. gr. 1590 with evidence from Asinou's frescoes, thus shifting interest in the murals from painting to patronage. With their many portraits, the images at Asinou illustrate a shifting kaleidoscope of sponsorship and support. Representing different social classes, genders, ethnicities, and creeds, they demonstrate graphically how the little monastery of the

1. On the Asinou valley see Given, *Survey Project*; Sollars, "Settlement and Community," 101–51.

Mother of God ton Phorbion negotiated its survival by ceaselessly renegotiating its relationships with its neighbors and its sponsors. As a visual record of the monastery's patronage, the portraits diagram the shifting social matrix within which the monastery of the Phorbiotissa found the means for its survival.

The hopes and expectations that prompted these people to support the church of Asinou are expressed in the poetic inscriptions studied by Nancy Patterson Ševčenko in Chapter 3. Many of the church's poetic epigrams belong to the cycle of 1105/6 and reflect the sensibilities of the initial patron, the magistrate Nikephoros Ischyrios. But poetic invocations characterize each phase of painting and reveal interesting contrasts. There are shifts in invocation. Nikephoros Ischyrios appeals directly to the Mother of God with a confident "I–you" immediacy that is paralleled in no other invocation. The wealthy veterinarian Nikephoros of the mural icon of St. George in the narthex, by contrast, appeals to his chosen saint only indirectly, in the third person, invoking the intermediacy of the monastery in the hope that his generosity to the church will earn him the support of the great warrior whose portrait he has placed in its narthex. Where the veterinarian invokes the monastery from outside its community, the inscription of 1332/33 has lay and monastic patrons speaking together with one voice, appealing in unison regardless of calling. These contrasts in appeal are accompanied by contrasts in tone and expectation. Nikephoros Ischyrios speaks in a negotiatory tone that seems to anticipate Mary's direct and positive response to him; the veterinarian Nikephoros, in turn, speaks not in expectation but in hope; while the patrons of 1332/33 speak neither of expectation nor of hope but only of entreaty. The contrasts in appeal surely reflect the patrons' different social classes—neither the veterinarian Nikephoros nor the monk Theophilos, for all their likely genteel status, sets himself in a frame of courtly reference as Nikephoros Ischyrios did with his inscription naming Alexios I Komnenos, and none approaches sacred power with the magistros's confident sense of access. Nonetheless, all were men of substance, and the differences in their tone must also reflect shifts in the religious etiquette of the eras and the societies in which they lived.

That Asinou's frescoes span radical shifts in Cyprus's history and culture is clear from the frescoes' changing forms and iconography. Basic to the frescoes' historical analysis is their technical study by Ioanna Kakoulli (Chapter 7), who clarifies questions of their chronology. Along with her examination of painting techniques, plaster, pigments, metals, and binding media—the first such analysis of a frescoed Cypriot church to be published—Kakoulli confirms three crucial issues of chronology. The first concerns the initial adornment of the narthex, and it involves three factors. First, the image of the Mother of God Phorbiotissa over the door to the naos exhibits blue pigments in its background from both the early twelfth- and the fourteenth-century phases of painting. The image must belong—as David Winfield had suggested[2]—to the program of 1105/6, presumably as an exterior image over the western door, but it must have been repainted to some extent in 1332/33. As Andréas Nicolaïdès will show in a separate publication, this repainting also affected the word "Φορβιώτισσα." Second, Kakoulli's research shows that the plaster of the dado running from the east wall of the narthex into its southern apse—the earliest layer of plaster on the wall—is identical to that of the mural icon of St. George just above it in the apse. Thus the two layers belong to the same period of painting, and the work of this period not only covers the span of the immured door but also extends onto the eastern wall. Sophia Kalopissi-Verti and Andréas Nicolaïdès assign to this same period the other traces of painting preserved beneath the plaster of 1332/33 at the south side of the narthex, dating them together in the final quarter of the twelfth century, because they—like the dado—display patterns clearly paralleled in frescoes of this date. Nicolaïdès and Winfield concur in giving the same late twelfth-century date to the icon of St. George. Finally, Kakoulli distinguishes the figure of the archangel preserved under the layer of 1332/33

2. *Asinou: A Guide*, 23–24.

in the northern apse of the narthex from the late twelfth-century fragments and from the figure of St. George on the south, indicating that the archangel was not installed at the same time. It may, like the St. George, have constituted an independent votive.[3] These data suggest that the narthex was frescoed for the first time only in the late twelfth century. At the same time, they do not confirm the presence of a coherent program embracing the entire space at this date, and they cast no light on the relative role of lay and monastic patronage in initiating the work or selecting its subject matter.

The second area in which technical evidence confirms chronology is in the paintings surrounding the St. George in the south apse of the narthex. Here, Kakoulli clarifies the plaster sequence, with the votive panel of Anastasia Saramalina overlapping, and thereby following, the icon of St. George, and overlapped, in turn, by the image with the Latin lady. Kakoulli shows that the pigments and painting technique of Anastasia's panel are so nearly identical to those in the conch of the church's main apse that they must be by the same painter. The frescoes of SS. Peter and Paul in the naos, by contrast, cannot belong to this hand.

The relation of Anastasia's panel to the paintings in the apse and the naos are valuable for the chronology of the architecture: Athanasios Papageorgiou draws on the apse painting to date the collapse of the original conch, and—in questioning the contemporaneity of the repairs to conch and naos—refers to the disparity between the hands of the apse conch and the figures of Peter and Paul on the naos piers.

Finally, Kakoulli points to contrasts in both plastering techniques and the use of pigments between the paintings of 1332/33 in the narthex and the undated frescoes in the central bay of the naos. These contrasts need not require that the paintings in the narthex and naos were by distinct hands. But they do strongly suggest that the narthex was painted by one master or group, and the naos by a different and somewhat later one. This judgment is welcomed by Annemarie Weyl Carr in her study of the naos.

These conclusions do little to change the chronology given by David Winfield, but they do solidify it. A broadly acknowledged timeline has thus been clarified by the material presented in this volume. It is:

Final quarter of the twelfth century

Frescoes in the narthex:

(1) Mural icon of St. George in the south apse
(2) Dado running from the southeastern wall into the south apse of the narthex
(3) Paintings flanking the door from the narthex into the naos
(4) Ornament on the lintel of the same door
(5) Ornament below the fourteenth-century plaster with the portrait of George on the east face of the south apse

Between the late twelfth century and 1332/33

Fresco of the archangel Michael below the fourteenth-century image of the same figure in the north apse of the narthex

Final quarter of the thirteenth century

Frescoes in the narthex:

(1) Mural icon of St. Anastasia Pharmakolytria in the south apse
(2) Image of the Virgin of Mercy with Latin lady and two youths in the conch of the south apse

Frescoes in the bema by the hand of the mural icon of St. Anastasia:

(3) Mother of God Pantanassa and two archangels in the apse conch
(4) Sacrifice of Isaac and St. John of Damascus on the triumphal arch

3. The pigments used in the archangel are very close to those of the frescoes of 1332/33, as Ioanna Kakoulli confirmed in a letter to the author dated 12 September 2007, presumably placing it after, and not before, the paintings of the late twelfth century.

Frescoes in the naos:

(5) SS. Peter and Paul on the inner faces of the western responds of the central bay

1332/33

Remaining frescoes in the narthex, including some overpainting on the early twelfth-century Mother of God Phorbiotissa over the door to the naos

1340s

Frescoes in the central bay of the naos

Sixteenth century

Frescoes in the naos: figures of SS. Symeon Stylites, Onouphrios, and Nikephoros on the east face of the northwest respond in the central bay

1618–40

Fresco formerly on the reinforcing pilaster flanking the apse and now in the bema: Image of Christ in a Eucharistic chalice with fifteen signatures

Building an art history upon this chronology, the art historians Andréas Nicolaïdès, Sophia Kalopissi-Verti, and Annemarie Weyl Carr, in their chapters on the successive phases of Asinou's painted interiors, lay out shifting phases in the social history and culture of the site. The icon of St. George, the earliest of the images discussed here, is among the most opulent and skillful surviving examples of late twelfth-century Byzantine art, as David Winfield emphasizes. It is thoroughly metropolitan in material and taste. Yet its patron, the horse veterinarian Nikephoros, gives no intimation in his dedicatory words that he was himself aristocratic or associated with the court. Like other late twelfth-century patrons of means on Cyprus, he seems to have participated in a local Cypriot culture that was fully attuned to developments in the capital.

This is no longer the case with the later paintings in the narthex. Both the two votive murals of Anastasia Saramalina and the Latin lady in the south apse and the campaign of 1332/33 are rooted formally in the "maniera cypria," a manner of disputed origin but recognizably local to the Crusader Levant.[4] The style is variously inflected by local hands: the painter of Anastasia Saramalina applies it with a pungent, characterful sweetness that singles him out as one of Asinou's most distinctive artistic personalities, while the painters of 1332/33 practice a drier, harder, and probably considerably later variant. Nonetheless, it is an identifiably local manner, and it is accompanied by a number of local features. Thus the pigments and materials are local, the colors are somber in tone, and the richness achieved in the paintings of 1105/6 by the use of costly mineral colors—gold, silver, cinnabar, and ultramarine—is reclaimed by the textured relief of the raised-gesso haloes, which employ a locally specific technique. Especially interesting in this regard is the use of "auripetrum," a Western technique that underscores the mingling of sources distinctive to the Crusader states. By the same token, the saints in the narthex are predominantly local. The magistros Nikephoros in 1105/6 had had Cypriot hierarchs portrayed in the bema. But in the naos, where his own portrait must have been, he gathered saints of studied generality. This is what the patrons of the narthex did not do. Their protectors represent specific Cypriot cults. Along with their saints, their sins—as Sophia Kalopissi-Verti shows—are those of village communities. Yet these patrons include people of very high social standing. Especially interesting among them is the Latin lady. Her clothing designates her as noble; like Nikephoros Ischyrios, she was a member of the aristocracy. Yet in analyzing the style of the lady's panel, Kalopissi-Verti finds

4. Several scholars have wondered whether it should be called the "maniera tripolitana": see Immerzeel, "Holy Horsemen and Crusader Banners"; Carr, "Perspectives on Visual Culture," 108–10; Nelson and Collins, *Holy Image, Hallowed Ground*, 251–53, entry on the bilateral icon at Sinai of warrior saints and the Mother of God by R. W. Corrie.

kinships not to France but to the local "maniera cypria." The lady's nobility, if anything, binds her to her Cypriot setting as a member of the feudal nobility "overseas," that is, in Outremer. Even the aristocracy, in short, is local at this point. Rather than conversant with an imperial center, Cyprus is a part of the eastern Mediterranean community of autonomous Crusader states, with a local artistic culture.

The paintings in the naos are no longer local in the same way. Though they draw on a strong local vocabulary of forms, these are forms rooted in the old Byzantine art of the late twelfth century, when Cyprus belonged to an imperial culture, and they use these forms to make modern statements that draw upon current, Palaiologan inspiration. The style, too, reflects the light-shot colorism of Palaiologan painting, though not its delicacy. These features point to a Cyprus conversant once again with metropolitan Byzantine production, but as a state in its own right, not as a province of the empire. The yet later figures of SS. Symeon and Onouphrios and the Patriarch Nikephoros on the northwest respond of the naos show the eventual result of Cyprus's place at a nexus of Mediterranean cultures, displaying conversancy with both Byzantine and European high styles. Thus the frescoes show Cyprus with a shifting cultural character.

Asinou's frescoes are especially informative about the interplay of communities within this broad social picture. The narthex has drawn particular attention for its diversity. The integration of the votive painting with the Latin lady into the later, fourteenth-century cycle has been of recurrent interest to historians of Crusader societies. Cross-creedal benefactions are not infrequent in bequests from the Lusignan period on Cyprus.[5] Especially informative, because it reflects a monastic community like Asinou in the Troodos mountains, is the synaxarion Paris. gr. 1588, from the Greek Orthodox monastery of the Priests.[6] The book's margins record gifts from a number of Latin men and women, ranging from royalty to free peasants, offering a counterpart to Asinou's Latin votive. Asinou's inclusivity may have been yet greater if, as Gilles Grivaud tentatively proposes (above, p. 27), the Anna Lachana portrayed in the narthex was in some way related to the rich Nestorian merchant family of the Lacha.[7] A Syrian

5. Cross-creedal donations, attested as early as a royal decree of 1220—see Coureas and Schabel, *Cartulary of the Cathedral*, no. 84—continue and broaden in the fourteenth and fifteenth centuries. See the gifts of the Lusignan kings, the testament of the Genoese Peter of St. Donatus in 1307 and Walter of Brienne in 1354, all cited in Schabel, "Religion," 182; the inventory of accounts for 1422–24 compiled in Paris. gr. 1381 for a person of Latin faith but including donations to Greek monks and priests (Richard, *Chypre sous les Lusignans*, 22); and the artistic evidence, offered not just by the figure of the Latin lady at Asinou but also by the icon of ca. 1300 of St. Nicholas with a Latin knight and his family; the fourteenth-century Latin portraits in the Holy Cross, Pelendri; and, even more intriguingly, the Latin couple portrayed in the narthex at St. Nicholas of the Roof on either side of an inscription in local Greek recording the gift of a *χανούτι* or workshop to the monastery (Stylianou and Stylianou, "Επανεξέτασις τῆς ἐν τῷ νάρθηκι"). For a vivid example of a Latin lady's munificence to a Greek institution, see the church of the Stavros Phaneromenos built and fully outfitted with icons, vessels, and appropriate vestments by Mary of Ibelin after her relative, Queen Alix, was healed by the recovered cross of Tochni, as recounted by Leontios Machairas: *Recital*, 1: §67–77.

6. Darrouzès, "Un obituaire chypriote," and Constantinides and Browning, *Dated Greek Manuscripts*, 74–81. The Latin bequests include gifts of King Janus (Darrouzès, 31, 32, 22, 35; Constantinides and Browning, 78); a gift of Sir Balian of Soissons [?] (Darrouzès, 31); a gift of King Peter II de Lusignan (Darrouzès, 39; Constantinides and Browning, 78); a gift recorded in awkward Greek in what Darrouzès, 49, suggests is a Latin hand by a certain Bertin Bodin; and a benefaction of John de Montolif (Darrouzès, 51–52; Constantinides and Browning, 80).

7. A good view of cross-creedal largesse by a Syrian Orthodox family, in this case the Audeths, is offered by Richard, "Une famille de 'Vénetiens blancs'." The patronage of the Lacha is illustrated—perhaps exaggerated—by the case of Francis Lacha, who with his own money built a Nestorian church in Famagusta, often identified as the present SS. Peter and Paul (Schabel, "Religion," 165).

was also among the benefactors of the monastery τῶν Ἱερέων,[8] and surviving accounts of the Syrian Audeth family include donations to both Greek and Catholic as well as Syrian churches. While the relationship of Anna and the Latin lady to Asinou's fathers remains to be understood, there can be little question but that their portraits make visible a kind of cross-creedal benefaction that the texts suggest was current in practice.

Along with creedal diversity, the diversity of gender in Asinou's narthex has drawn the attention of Sophia Kalopissi-Verti and, before her, of Carolyn Connor and Sharon Gerstel. The number of women in Asinou's narthex—both living female donors and female saints—is striking. The association of women with funerary rites and mourning has been used to explain the appearance of women saints in the narthex, where funeral rites were conducted, and this use might have been a factor in the significant roster of women saints at Asinou.[9] Along with the saints, however, Asinou also bears portraits of prominent female donors. The funerary role of their portraits is questionable, especially in the case of the Latin lady—and possibly also Anna—who did not share the monastery's Orthodox rite.[10] The widowed status of the Latin lady raises the question whether Anastasia Saramalina and Anna Lachana were also widows with wealth of their own, and draws attention to the role of women in the inheritance and management of wealth in Lusignan Cyprus. Latin law is known to have responded to the fragility of life in the warrior states of the Levant by giving women a more significant role in the transmission of wealth and title than in the West, and this legal status may have played a role in the participation of the Latin lady at Asinou. On the other hand, because Greek family law in Cyprus remained in the domain of the Church, it was less subject to change.[11] Thus, the prominence of women in Asinou's narthex invites inquiry into the role of women, wealth, and monastic sponsorship in the mixed society of a Crusader state.

Whether the narthex at Asinou also drew attention to social diversity, as perhaps suggested by the conspicuous juxtaposition of the two rider saints—the rural Mamas and the aristocratic George—is hard to judge.[12] It does, however, offer

8. Darrouzès, "Un obituaire," 51–52 (folio 245v). This was the clerk Thomas, known in his religious life as Theodosios.

9. Connor, "Female Saints," 219; see also Gerstel, "Painted Sources for Female Piety," 103: "The placement of female saints in close proximity to the dead, whether in the church narthex or flanking arcosolia, suggests that Byzantine monumental decoration responded to the important role of female vigil and female lamentation in the eternal life of the deceased."

10. The major work on Latin burial in Cyprus is now Imhaus, *Lacrimae Cypriae*; see also Ivison, "Mortuary Practices in Byzantium"; Carr, "Cypriot Funerary Icons." Certain artifacts indicate that funerary customs did cross creedal lines: tomb slabs inscribed in Greek and engraved with portraits of the deceased in Greek gestures of piety, the bowl burials at Episkope (Ivison, 1:282), and the funerary icons. Latin burials at Greek churches—suggested by the tomb slab of Lady Simone de Gibilet (+1302) at Kiti, and the Latin portraits from the third quarter of the fourteenth century at the church of the Holy Cross, Pelendri—may have occurred at first only where there were Latin chapels. There do seem to have been Latin burials at the monastery of the Priests by the end of the fourteenth century, however (see above). On the opposite issue—Greek burial in Latin churches—see p. 29 and n. 93 above, citing the concern in 1452 of the Greek Cypriot nobleman Hugh Podocataro that "force la giesia cathedrale fara dificulta a lasarmi sopellir in grego": Rudt de Collenberg, "Les premiers Podocataro," 143.

11. On the social role of Latin women, see Schein, "Women in Medieval Colonial Society"; J. Richard, "Le statut de la femme." A study of the legal and economic status of Greek women under the Lusignans has not been made. One does, however, note the recurrent references in the margins of Paris. gr. 1588, to gifts made during the fourteenth and fifteenth centuries to the monastery of the Priests by women, both lay and monastic: Darrouzès, "Un obituaire chypriote."

12. Mamas was a protector of taxpayers (Stylianou and Stylianou, *Παναγία Φορβιώτισσα Ἀσίνου*, 29–31, 67–68). Thus one expects him to be a protector of the ordinary person. Yet, as Gilles Grivaud shows ("Pèlerinages grecs et latins," 74–76), the cult of St. Mamas was espoused

extensive insight into the relationship of two other communities of key importance to Asinou's life: the lay patrons and the monastic fathers. It is not clear whether Asinou was a katholikon from the beginning, or assumed that status after initially serving as a private church. As a private chapel, the building would have been accessible to the living members and retainers, male and female, of the family that founded and supported it, and its naos might well have housed the tombs of its deceased members. As the church of a male monastery, on the other hand, lay access would have been curtailed, especially for women, who were characteristically excluded from male monastic churches, as males were normally excluded from convents.[13] Yet increasingly, through the late eleventh and twelfth centuries, the monastery embraced the needs of its lay supporters. Aristocratic and landed families tended to turn to small, private churches for their spiritual needs,[14] and many of these needs were best met by staffing the churches with monks.[15] Family property could be secured by consecrating it to the use of a monastic house. Such houses served as hubs of family loyalty and identity, including family members among their overseers and housing the family tombs; the monastic offices assured regular prayers for the living patrons and commemorations for their dead; monasteries oversaw funerals and burials; and monks were widely cultivated as spiritual advisers. The Cypriot St. Neophytos found himself literally beleaguered by members of the lay gentry craving his counsel or the thrill of his presence.[16] These functions blurred the boundaries between lay and monastic access to the spaces of the church, as attested in the accounts of saints' lives and in foundation documents.[17] The clearest architectural sign of a church's monastic status was its narthex, added to accommodate monastic rituals; yet, more and more, the narthex became the selvage where lay and monastic met.

We know only a limited amount about the initial adornment of the narthex at Asinou, but we do know that its most impressive image was sponsored by a lay contributor to the monastery. The enigmatic addition of the name "Nikephoros Kallias,"[18] clearly a layman and perhaps a pilgrim to the site, could indicate that the image was accessible for veneration by other laypeople—as its dramatic embellishment with flanking sconces may imply. From the very beginning, then, the narthex offered recognition and even access to laypeople. When its adornment resumed in the late thirteenth century, moreover, it resumed in much the same way, with votive icons of lay donors. In this case the donors were women, and rather than identifying themselves in poetic inscriptions, as did the veterinarian Nikephoros, they had themselves portrayed.

Greek monasteries on Cyprus grew in number during the Lusignan era and surely served as

by Latin pilgrims and cultivated by the Lusignan court. Sophia Kalopissi-Verti points out (above, p. 163) the extravagantly Gothic ornament on his tomb at Morphou. Three large icons on the tomb show Mamas on his lion flanked by equestrian figures of George and Demetrios. The panels themselves are modern, but most probably reflect medieval ones. They imply parity among the riders. Whether this was an appropriation by the Lusignans, coopting Mamas as one of their own, or a reflection of popular perceptions remains a question posed for me already long ago by Elizabeth Nightlinger. I am indebted to Gilles Grivaud for sending his article to me.

13. On women's access to monastic churches, see Maguire, "*Abaton* and *Oikonomia*," 102–3, and Talbot, "Women's Space in Byzantine Monasteries." Both Taft, "Women at Church," and Gerstel, "Painted Sources," 111, presume minimal presence of women in male monastic institutions.

14. Mathews, "'Private' Liturgy in Byzantine Architecture."

15. See especially Morris, "Byzantine Aristocracy and the Monasteries"; eadem, "Monasteries and Their Patrons."

16. Galatariotou, *Making of a Saint*, 170–71.

17. See G. Constable, "Preface," in *BMFD*, 1:xix: "There are countless references to travelers, pilgrims, beggars, strangers, servants, laymen, and all sorts of hangers-on, and, in spite of efforts to exclude them, to women and boys in male houses and to men and girls in female houses."

18. See p. 82, above.

focal points of Orthodox solidarity.[19] For the local gentry, no less than for the Komnenian aristocrats two centuries earlier, the monastery offered an effective answer to their needs for intercession through regular, professional services of prayer, for burial, and for commemoration. In their case, however, the monastery served to unite less the family than the locale. It was above all in the narthex that these people's engagements with the institution must have taken place. How often the laypeople sought access to the naos of the monastic church is unclear; the women especially must have limited their presence to the narthex. In time, the village church would absorb the pious munificence of such people, as Gilles Grivaud notes. The monastery, however, seems still to have played a major role in serving the needs of lay worshippers in the fourteenth century. Asinou gives a valuable glimpse into the processes by which the Orthodox monastery served its faithful.

The program of 1332/33, with its portraits of three lay people and seven monks—six living and one deceased—is a vivid picture of the union of lay and monastic communities in support of the monastery and its church. The way the iconographic program echoes the customary imagery of the naos with its central Pantokrator, in essence likening the narthex to a church, shows how significant the narthex was as a space of sacred encounter. In important ways the decorative cycle at Asinou continues what the votive icons of Anastasia Saramalina and the Latin lady had begun: with its many portraits, it is a giant votive icon, with many, rather than one, donors/devotees. But in notable ways, too, it is different. The monks are numerically dominant now—indeed, the six living monks may represent the full community of the monastery; six would be a respectable number. Moreover, they dominate the message of the program. As Sophia Kalopissi-Verti shows, the lay portraits are clustered at the left hand of the Pantokrator, under the minatory images of the paradigmatic sins. The cycle is designed to elicit their awe. It turns the donors—the givers upon whose munificence the monastery depended—into supplicants, compelled to plead for heavenly grace. It is, in its way, a declaration of religious control over the increasingly visible lay community.

Notable in this regard is the fact that the narthex was adorned in 1332/33. The naos, the core of the building for its monastic members, had been only skimpily decorated in the late thirteenth century, and in 1332/33 was still somewhat shabby with its intrusive, unpainted masonry repairs. The narthex, however, not the naos, was the core of the building for the lay donors, whom the fathers needed both to please and to control. The narthex was given priority. The decision to focus on this area was apparently successful, for the largesse that ensued was adequate to allow the repainting of the naos, too, including the lavish reclamation of the portrait of Nikephoros Ischyrios, with his courtly nobility and legal authority emphatically enhanced.

In the slow jockeying for place and exposure, one watches the dominant themes of the church being successively reshaped and reformulated. Among the most elegant components of the program of 1105/6 is the imagery of the bema, a meditation on the Eucharist expressed through the body of Mary (Fig. 6.11): its advent, its presentation, and its incorporation of Emmanuel—God with us. Its incarnational immediacy echoes the immediacy of Nikephoros's first-person invocations that had ringed the space. The Eucharist continues to dominate the imagery of the later, thirteenth-century bema, but in very different and paternalistic terms that center on sacrifice. The Virgin, in turn, takes her place in the naos, but now in ways that stress less her immediacy than her mediacy. Her role on the transverse arches is essentially allegorical, speaking in the words of Old Testament prophecy about her role in the Incarnation, while her figures on the bema respond and the south wall are intermediary, less bringing God to humankind than bringing human pleas to God. The pleas she conveys are pleas in the face of judgment, and judgment, too, is a cardinal theme that runs from phase to phase of Asinou's adornment. It is integral to the single most persistent

19. Schabel, "Religion," 200.

theme of the building: protection in the face of death. As Sophia Kalopissi-Verti argues, Asinou's narthex, and very plausibly the church from the very beginning, was the site of funerals. Naos and narthex alike are governed by the awed concern of human devotees faced with their own mortality and the judgment that awaits them. Portraits, postures, inscriptions, and imagery are designed together to convey both the minatory force of divine engagement with humankind, and the human expectation of grace. Judgment is a fulcrum in each.

This theme plays itself out with telling differences. For the magistros Nikephoros it is an individual drama, played out in a context of incarnational intensity and divine passion and performed in first-person dialogues. For the figures in the narthex, on the other hand, that theme is played out together in the communal experience of a cosmic drama that subsumes individuals in a chorus of multiple voices that are most nearly blessed when they are most uniform. The interplay of imagery and space varies accordingly. The naos foregoes the iconic central image of the All-ruler, and seems to have found its focus in the incarnation and the figure of Mary. The multiplicity of the donors in the narthex, by contrast, seeks a forceful center in the Pantokrator, the traditional center point of the naos. Rather than the personally composed poetic pleas of the patron, the words that wreathe the space and tie it together are taken from the liturgy itself. As Sophia Kalopissi-Verti's text brings out so beautifully, these phrases reverberate around the narthex with the same fragmentary but compelling force as the phrases etched in the memories of devotees over a lifetime of attendance at the feasts and funerals that must have marked out the passage of time in Asinou's community.

How truly these themes and their images lived in the imaginations of the people who gathered in the space below is echoed poignantly in the obituaries inscribed in the margins of Paris. gr. 1590: on folio 97v, for instance, the notice recording the death of the hierodeacon and priest Michael on 27 November 1320 closes with the plea to the reader to pray for him to the Lord so that he might find mercy on the day of judgment;[20] on folio 204r, the death notice of Father Leon asks that God speed his spirit to Abraham, Isaac, and Joseph (*sic*).[21] As if materialized from such pleas, the three patriarchs now preside from the north apse of the narthex. In place since 1333, their laps full of safely garnered souls, they have attended the obsequies of others like Leon and guarded their remains. Three centuries later, in the 1620s, the archbishop Christodoulos and sixteen others assured that the little monastery church of Asinou could continue to furnish much the same protection. Today it is the building itself that deserves protection. It is a task we commend to our readers.

20. Constantinides and Browning, *Dated Greek Manuscripts*, 52: κ(αι) οἱ εντυχόντ(ες) αὐτοῦ, ευχεσθαι αυτὸν δϊὰ τὸν κ(ύριο)ν· ὅπ(ως) ἐύρι ἑλε(ος) ἐν ημέρ(α) κρΐσ(εως).
21. Ibid.: ὡ θ(εο)ς τάξι το πν(ευμ)α αυτου μετ(α) αββρααμ ισαακ κ(αι) ϊοσηφ:–.

APPENDIX

Inventory of Paleographic Forms in the Thirteenth- and Fourteenth-Century Murals

Annemarie Weyl Carr and
Sophia Kalopissi-Verti

The following pages inventory the letterforms and ligatures used in labeling the figures and writing the inscriptions in each of the discrete phases of painting from the late thirteenth and fourteenth centuries in Asinou. This is the first comprehensive inventory of letterforms in a Cypriot mural program to be published. The murals are examined in five clusters: the panel with Anastasia Saramalina in the narthex; the apse conch and triumphal arch in the bema; the figures of Saints Peter and Paul on the initial fresco layer of the western piers of the central bay; the paintings of 1332/33 in the narthex; and the paintings of the fourteenth century in the central bay. In each cluster, the letters and ligatures are aligned in alphabetical order; by reading across the charts the reader can readily compare the letterforms of any one cluster with those of the others. The inventory of letterforms serves a twofold purpose. Most immediately, it provides evidence drawn upon in this book. Variations in letterforms helped to clarify the kinships and contrasts among the frescoes painted in different parts of the church's interior, and these groupings served in turn to define authorship and chronology. Thus shared letterforms helped to confirm the attribution of the paintings in the apse conch and triumphal arch to the same late thirteenth-century hand as the Anastasia panel in the narthex. The recurrence in the inscriptions accompanying SS. Peter and Paul of the forms found in the apse and Anastasia panel made it possible in turn to assign the figures of the Apostle Princes to much the same date, though they were painted by a different hand or shop. By contrast, variations in the range especially of ligatures contributed to the conclusion that an interval of some span must have separated the frescoes of 1332/33 in the narthex from those of the central bay. The charts that follow present that evidence for scrutiny.

Beyond its utility in the arguments of this book, however, the inventory of letterforms has the broader purpose of laying the basis for a more systematic inclusion of epigraphic forms in the study of Byzantine mural painting. Letterforms have played a minimal role in art historical studies of mural painting hitherto, and it is not entirely clear who was responsible for producing them—the figure painters, or specialists in inscription. Nonetheless, letterforms shift together with shifts in painting style, as Maria Panayotidi has shown in studying painters' literacy, and she is surely right to conclude from this that in most cases the painter was the scribe, as well.[1] As such, letterforms should be a diagnostic in assessing the relationships among

1. Panayotidi, "Le peintre en tant que scribe," 72; eadem, "Οι γραμματικές γνώσεις των ζωγράφων" (with English summary).

different phases of work within a single church, as at Asinou, and between fresco campaigns in different churches. Identifying generic features of chronology and idiosyncratic features of particular campaigns will facilitate assessments of dates, hands, and workshops.

The seven churches with fourteenth-century frescoes akin to those of Asinou invite precisely such examination. Should their murals be understood as the product of a coherent workshop, as a loosely shared period manner, or as the legacy of one or two powerful personalities who left their imprint on many commissions the way the Asinou Master had done long before; should they be seen as the product of a compact decade or two dominated by a single style, or as the decades-long afterlife of one among several available manners? How painters functioned as a trade is not well known: whether they operated out of stable workshops that trained them and then assigned them their commissions, or worked as independent professionals who assembled in teams only on an ad hoc basis as commissions dictated, must be assessed anew for each era and region. As research continues to probe the social and cultural dimensions of the frescoed churches, epigraphic features should play a role in clarifying the grouping, attribution, chronology, and authorship of their paintings and the trade practices of their painters, both in Cyprus itself, and in the Byzantine oikoumene more broadly.

	NARTHEX LATE 13TH C. PAGES 115–30	NARTHEX 1332/33 PAGES 131–90	APSE CONCH AND TRIUMPHAL ARCH PAGES 213–23	SS. PETER AND PAUL, FIRST LAYER PAGES 211–13	NAOS 14TH C. PAGES 223–90
α	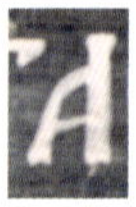 Donor Anastasia, line 1, char. 13 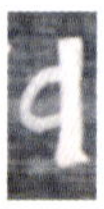 Donor Anastasia, line 1, char. 10	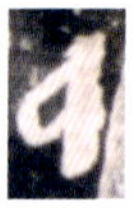 Donor Barnabas, line 2, char. 6 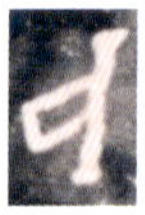 Donor Barnabas, line 3, char. 2 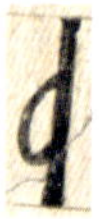 Scroll of St. John the Baptist, line 4, char. 2 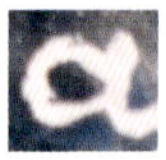 Donor Barnabas, line 4, char. 1 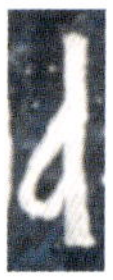 Donor Theophilos, line 2, char. 7	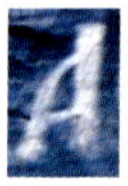 Apse conch, The Pantanassa, char. 4 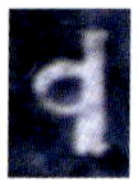 Triumphal arch, Sacrifice of Isaac, Angel's command: line 1, char. 3	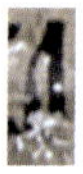 Scroll of St. Paul: line 3, char. 2	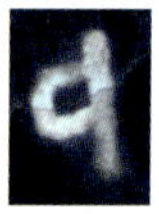 Donor inscription, line 2, char. 2 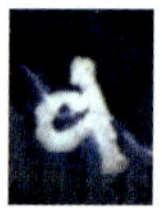 Donor inscription, line 3, char. 13 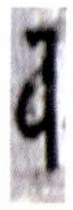 St. Paul, scroll: char. 1
αβ		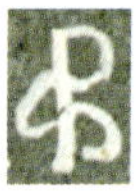 Donor Laurentios, line 1, char. 8	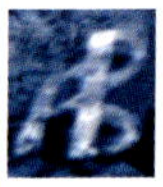 Apse conch, Archangel Gabriel: char. 4		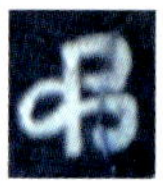 Enthroned Mother of God, The Archangel Gabriel: char. 4

	NARTHEX LATE 13TH C. PAGES 115–30	NARTHEX 1332/33 PAGES 131–90	APSE CONCH AND TRIUMPHAL ARCH PAGES 213–23	SS. PETER AND PAUL, FIRST LAYER PAGES 211–13	NAOS 14TH C. PAGES 223–90
αβ			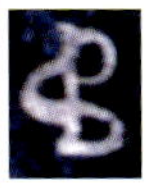 Triumphal arch, Sacrifice of Isaac, The Prophet Abraham: char. 5		
αγ		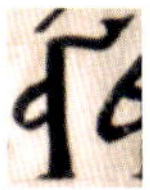 Scroll of Virgin Eleousa, line 2, char. 4 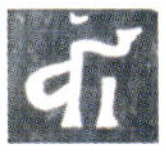 St. Eudokia			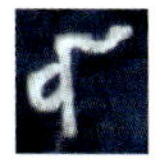 Donor inscription, line 2, char. 1
αι		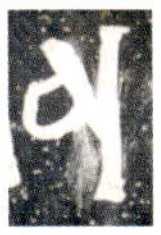 Donor Leontios, char. 8 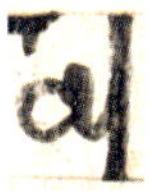 Scroll of St. John the Baptist, line 2, char. 3			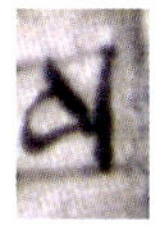 Ezekiel, scroll: line 4, char. 3
αις		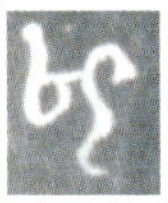 Last Judgment, Trumpeting angel, line 3, char. 6			
αμ	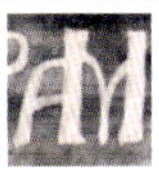 Donor Anastasia, line 2, char. 5	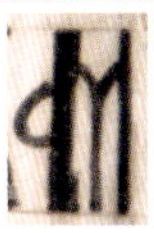 Scroll of Virgin Eleousa, line 6, char. 4	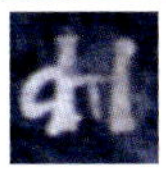 Triumphal arch, Sacrifice of Isaac, Angel's command: line 1, char. 4		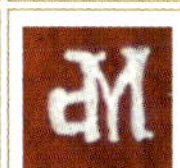 St. Abibos: column 2, char. 1
αν	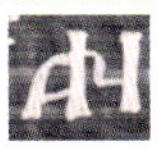 Donor Anastasia, line 1, char. 9	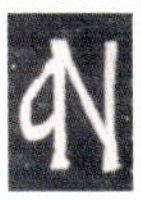 Donor Germanos, char. 11 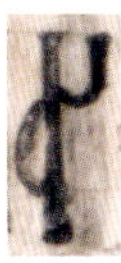 Scroll of Virgin Eleousa, line 8, char. 7	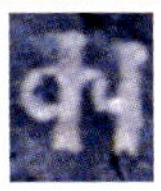 Triumphal arch, Sacrifice of Isaac, Angel's command: line 3, char. 5		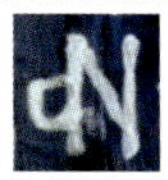 Donor inscription, line 5, char. 24
ανμ					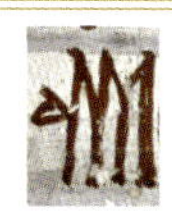 Virgin Paraklesis, scroll, line 6, char. 3
ανν		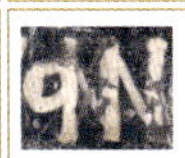 Donor Anna, line 2, char. 2			
απ					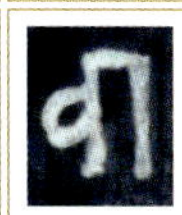 Donor inscription, line 5, char. 20

	NARTHEX LATE 13TH C. PAGES 115–30	NARTHEX 1332/33 PAGES 131–90	APSE CONCH AND TRIUMPHAL ARCH PAGES 213–23	SS. PETER AND PAUL, FIRST LAYER PAGES 211–13	NAOS 14TH C. PAGES 223–90
αρ	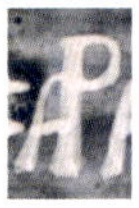 Donor Anastasia, line 2, char. 4	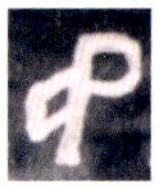 Donor Barnabas, line 2, char. 4 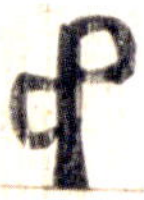 Scroll of St. John the Baptist, line 3, char. 4	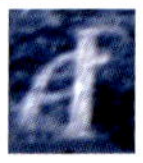 Apse conch, The Archangel Michael: char. 2 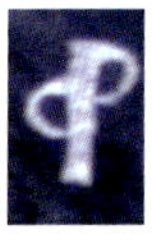 Triumphal arch, Sacrifice of Isaac, Angel's command: line 4, char. 2		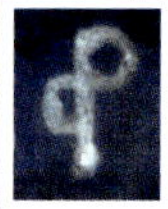 Donor inscription, line 4, char. 2 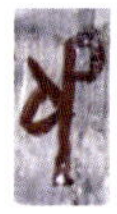 Virgin Paraklesis, scroll, line 5
ας	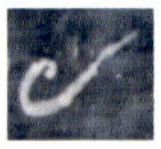 Donor Anastasia, line 1, char. 15	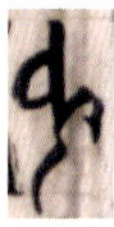 Scroll of Virgin Eleousa, line 3, char. 5 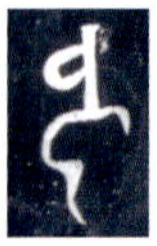 St. Cosmas			
ατ					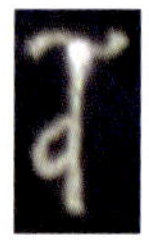 St. Theodore Stratelates, char. 2
αυ		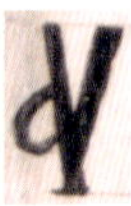 Scroll of Virgin Eleousa, line 6, char. 1			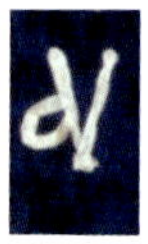 St. Paul: column 2, char. 2
β		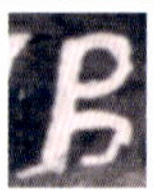 Donor Barnabas, line 2, char. 3 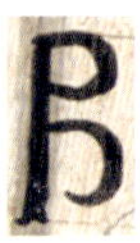 Scroll of St. John the Baptist, line 4, char. 1	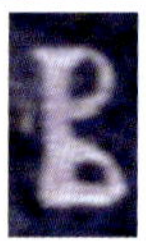 Triumphal arch, Sacrifice of Isaac, Angel's command: line 2, char. 9 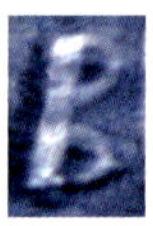 Apse Conch, The Archangel Gabriel: char. 4		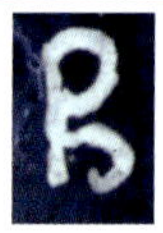 Donor inscription, line 2, char. 11
γ	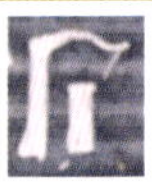 St. Anastasia the Poison Curer, left, vertical, char. 3	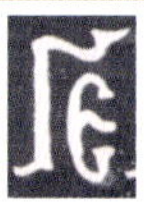 Donor Germanos, char. 7	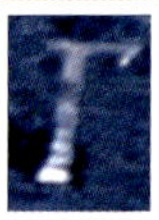 Apse Conch, The Archangel Gabriel: char. 3	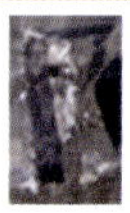 Scroll of St. Peter: line 2, char. 3	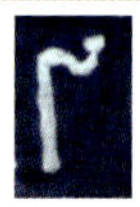 Donor inscription, line 3, char. 8
δ	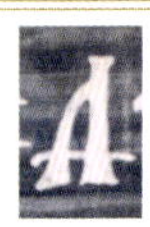 Donor Anastasia, line 1, char. 4	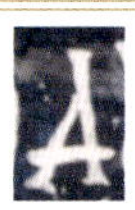 Donor Theophilos, line 1, char. 8	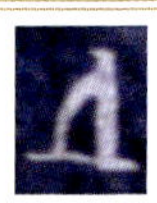 Triumphal arch, Sacrifice of Isaac, Angel's command: line 4, char. 1		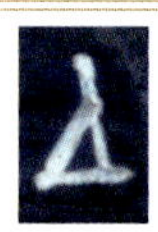 Donor inscription, line 5, char. 10

	NARTHEX LATE 13TH C. PAGES 115–30	NARTHEX 1332/33 PAGES 131–90	APSE CONCH AND TRIUMPHAL ARCH PAGES 213–23	SS. PETER AND PAUL, FIRST LAYER PAGES 211–13	NAOS 14TH C. PAGES 223–90
δ		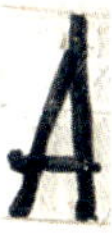 Codex of Christ Eleemon, left, line 3, char. 2	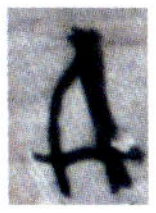 Triumphal arch, John of Damascus, scroll: line 4, char. 1		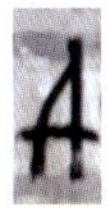 St. Paul, scroll, char. 2 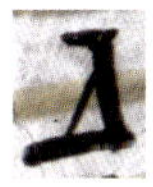 The Holy Mandylion: column 2, char. 3
δη					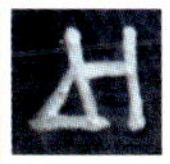 Donor inscription, line 7, char. 12
δου		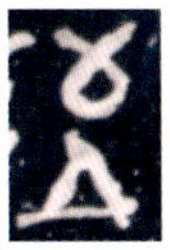 Donor Barnabas, line 1, char. 3			
ε		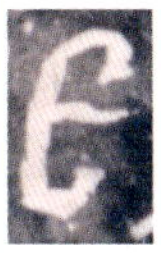 Donor Barnabas, line 3, char. 4 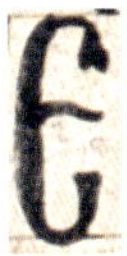 Scroll of St. John the Baptist, line 1, char. 2	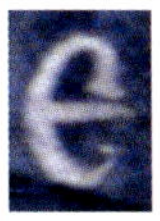 Triumphal arch, Sacrifice of Isaac, Angel's command: line 3, char. 9 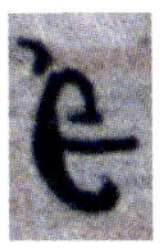 Triumphal arch, John of Damascus, scroll: line 2, char. 1	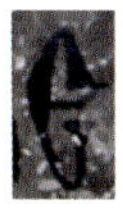 Scroll of St. Peter: line 2, char. 2	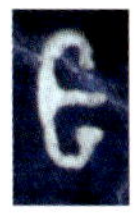 Donor inscription, line 1, char. 9 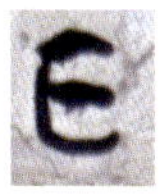 Virgin Paraklesis, scroll, line 4, char. 3
ει		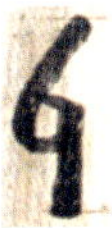 Scroll of St. John the Baptist, line 2, char. 1			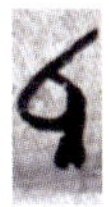 Virgin Paraklesis, scroll, line 2, char. 6
ερ					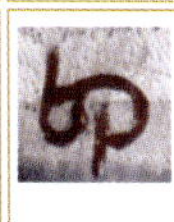 Virgin Paraklesis, scroll, line 4, char. 2
ες					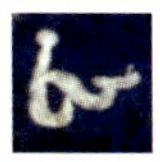 Women at the Tomb, the Maries: char. 4
ευ		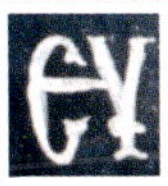 St. Eudokia			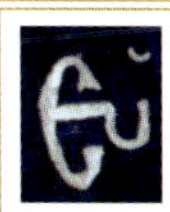 St. Eustathios: column 2, char. 1
ζ		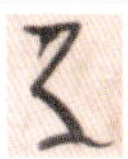 Cross on southern jamb of west entrance, line 5 right 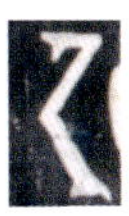 St. Sozomenos			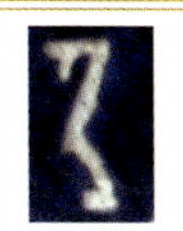 Gephyra, memorial inscription: line 1, final char.

	NARTHEX LATE 13TH C. PAGES 115–30	NARTHEX 1332/33 PAGES 131–90	APSE CONCH AND TRIUMPHAL ARCH PAGES 213–23	SS. PETER AND PAUL, FIRST LAYER PAGES 211–13	NAOS 14TH C. PAGES 223–90
η	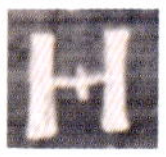 St. Anastasia the Poison Curer, left, vertical, char. 1	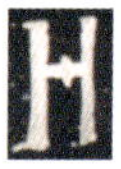 Donor Theophilos, line 2, char. 3 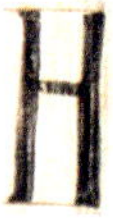 Scroll of St. John the Baptist, line 3, char. 5	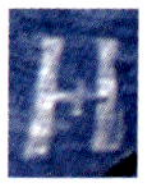 Apse conch: The Archangel Gabriel: char. 7 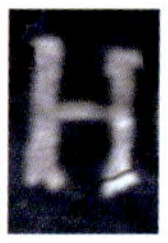 Triumphal arch, Sacrifice of Isaac, Angel's command: line 2, char. 11	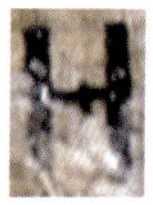 Scroll of St. Paul: line 3, char. 6	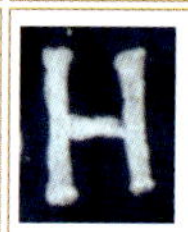 Donor inscription: line 1, char. 11
ηβ					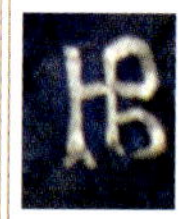 Burning Bush, title of scene: char. 1
ηγ		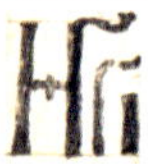 Scroll of St. John the Baptist, line 2, char. 4			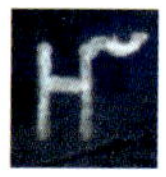 Donor inscription: line 5, char. 4
ηλ					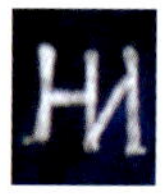 Closed Gate, The Prophet Ezekiel: final char.
ημ		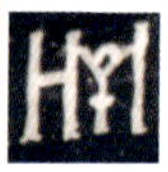 Donor Theophilos, line 1, char. 3 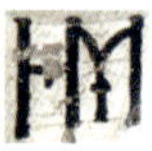 Codex of Christ Eleemon, right, line 1, char. 1			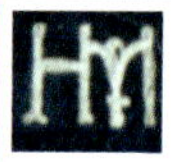 Christ Eleemon: line 2, char. 5
ην		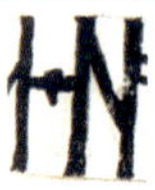 Codex of Christ Eleemon, left, line 2, char. 2	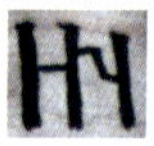 Triumphal arch, John of Damascus, scroll: line 4, char. 2		
ηπ		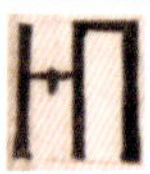 Scroll of Virgin Eleousa, line 4, char. 1	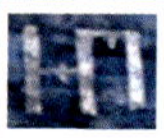 Apse conch, The Pantanassa: char. 1		
ης	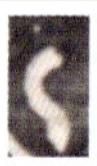 Donor Anastasia, line 1, char. 5				
θ		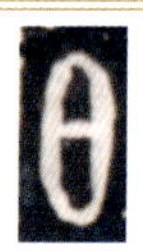 Donor Theophilos, line 1, char. 5	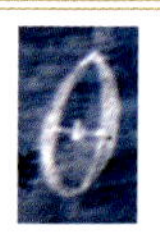 Apse conch, Mother of God, char. 2		
ι	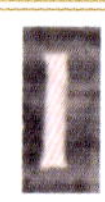 St. Anastasia the Poison Curer, left, horizontal, char. 7	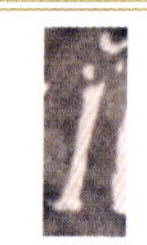 Donor Barnabas, line 3, char. 3	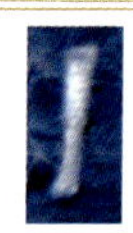 Apse conch, The Archangel Gabriel: char. 6	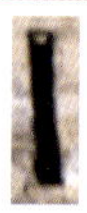 Scroll of St. Paul: line 3, char. 3	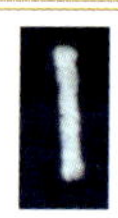 Donor inscription: line 1, char. 6

	NARTHEX LATE 13TH C. PAGES 115–30	NARTHEX 1332/33 PAGES 131–90	APSE CONCH AND TRIUMPHAL ARCH PAGES 213–23	SS. PETER AND PAUL, FIRST LAYER PAGES 211–13	NAOS 14TH C. PAGES 223–90
ι		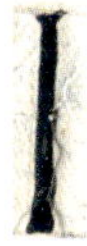 Codex of Christ Eleemon, left, line 3, char. 3	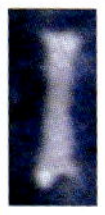 Triumphal arch, Sacrifice of Isaac, Angel's command: line 3, char. 9		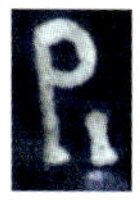 Donor inscription: line 3, char. 7 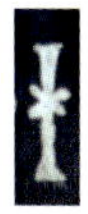 St. Eustathios: column 2, char. 5 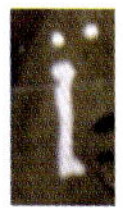 Burning Bush, The Prophet Moses: column 2, char. 3
ις					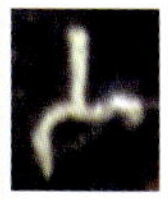 St. Theodore Stratelates, Stratilatis [sic]: char. 8
κ	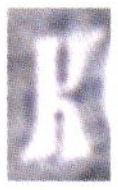 St. Anastasia the Poison Curer, right, line 5, char. 1	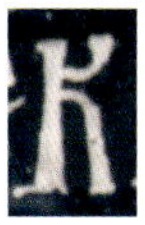 Donor Theophilos, line 1, char. 2	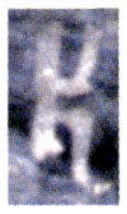 Triumphal arch, St. John of Damascus: line 2, char. 1	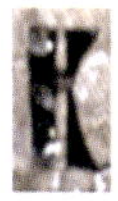 Scroll of St. Paul: line 3, char. 1	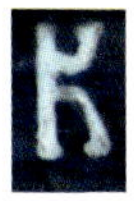 Donor inscription: line 4, char. 9 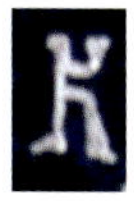 Closed gate, The Prophet Ezekiel: char. 7
και					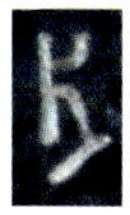 Donor inscription: line 5, char. 1
λ	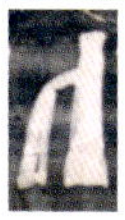 Donor Anastasia, line 2, char. 7	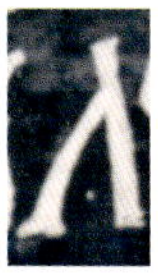 Donor Theophilos, line 1, char. 10 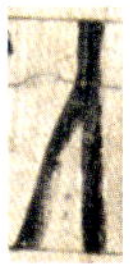 Scroll of St. John the Baptist, line 4, char. 4	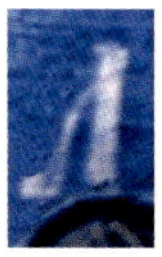 Apse conch: The Archangel Gabriel: char. 8	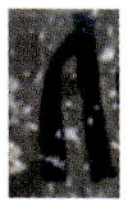 Scroll of St. Peter: line 2, char. 1	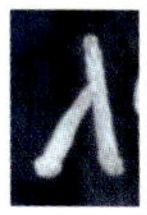 Donor inscription: line 1, char. 3
λη		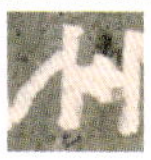 Donor Kallinikos, line 2, char. 2 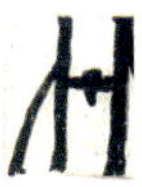 Codex of Christ Eleemon, left, line 2, char. 1	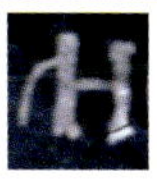 Triumphal arch, Sacrifice of Isaac, Angel's command: line 2, char. 11		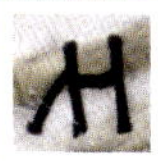 The Holy Mandylion: column 2, char. 5
λου		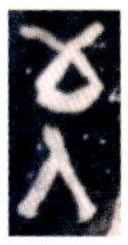 Donor Barnabas, line 1, char. 4			

	NARTHEX LATE 13TH C. PAGES 115–30	NARTHEX 1332/33 PAGES 131–90	APSE CONCH AND TRIUMPHAL ARCH PAGES 213–23	SS. PETER AND PAUL, FIRST LAYER PAGES 211–13	NAOS 14TH C. PAGES 223–90
μ	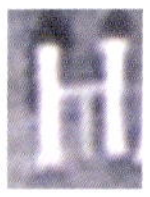 St. Anastasia the Poison Curer, right, line 4, char. 1	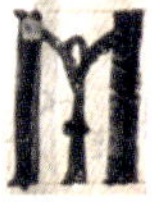 Scroll of St. John the Baptist, line 1, char. 1 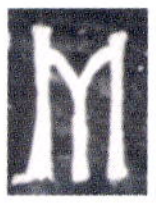 Donor Germanos, char. 10 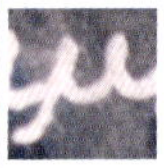 Donor Barnabas, line 4, char. 2	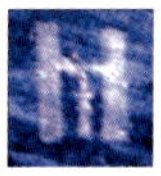 Apse conch: Mother of God, char. 1 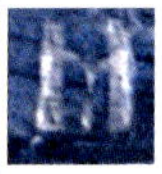 Apse conch: The Archangel Michael: char. 3 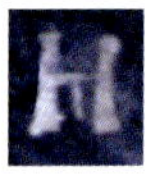 Triumphal arch, Sacrifice of Isaac, title of scene: char. 14	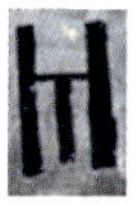 Scroll of St. Peter: line 1, char. 4	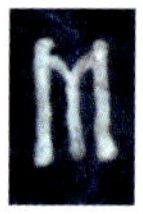 Donor inscription, line 4, char. 16 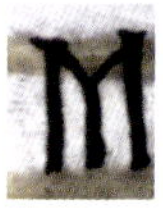 The Holy Mandylion: column 2, char. 1 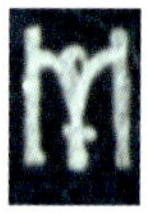 Christ Eleemon: line 2, char. 5 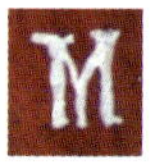 St. Abibos: column 2, char. 1 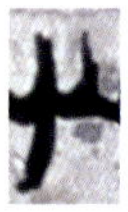 Virgin Paraklesis, scroll: line 6, char. 6
μη		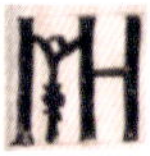 Scroll of Virgin Eleousa, line 3, char. 1	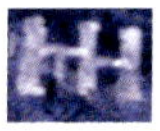 Triumphal arch, Sacrifice of Isaac, Angel's command: line 2, char. 5		
μην		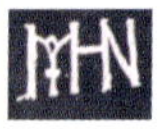 Donor Theophilos, line 3, char. 10			
ν	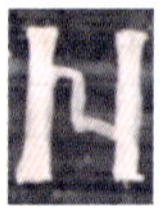 Donor Anastasia, line 2, char. 9	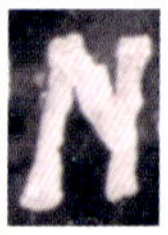 Donor Barnabas, line 2, char. 5 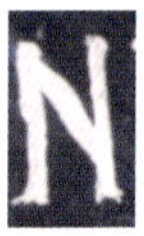 Donor Theophilos, line 2, char. 15 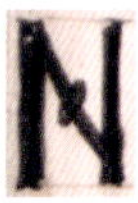 Scroll of Virgin Eleousa, line 5, char. 1	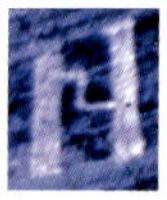 Apse conch, The Pantanassa: char. 5 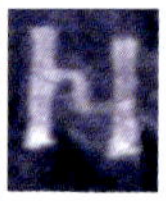 Triumphal arch, Sacrifice of Isaac, Angel's command: line 4, char. 5	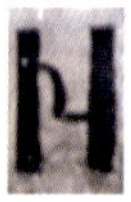 Scroll of St. Paul: line 2, char. 4	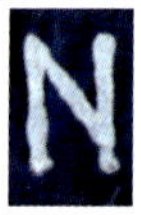 Donor inscription, line 4, char. 8 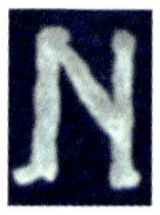 St. Nicholas: column 2, char. 1
νγ		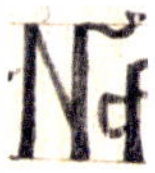 Scroll of St. John the Baptist, line 3, char. 3			
νηκ		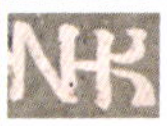 Donor Kallinikos, line 1, char. 3			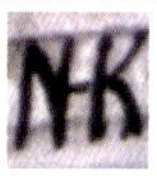 Closed Gate: Ezekiel, scroll: line 4, char. 2

	NARTHEX LATE 13TH C. PAGES 115–30	NARTHEX 1332/33 PAGES 131–90	APSE CONCH AND TRIUMPHAL ARCH PAGES 213–23	SS. PETER AND PAUL, FIRST LAYER PAGES 211–13	NAOS 14TH C. PAGES 223–90
νημ					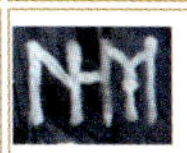 Donor inscription: line 6, penultimate char.
νμ					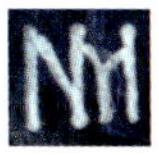 Donor inscription: line 5, char. 15
νην		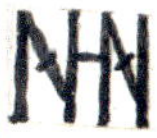 Codex of Christ Eleemon, left, line 3, char. 1			
νκ		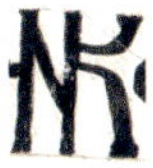 Codex of Christ Eleemon, left, line 2, char. 3			
ξ		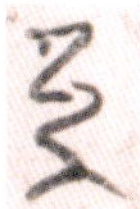 Cross on southern jamb of west entrance, line 5 left	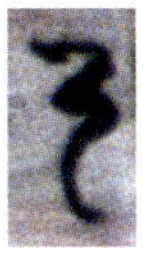 Triumphal arch, John of Damascus, scroll: line 2, char. 4		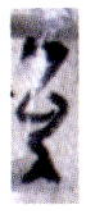 Virgin Paraklesis, scroll: line 1, char. 3
ο	 St. Anastasia the Poison Curer, right, line 5, char. 2	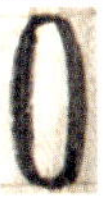 Scroll of St. John the Baptist, line 1, char. 5 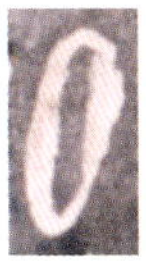 Donor Barnabas, line 3, char. 6	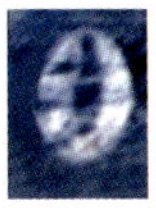 Apse conch, The Archangel Michael: char. 1 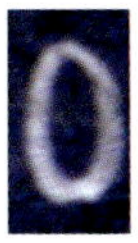 Triumphal arch, Sacrifice of Isaac, Angel's command: line 4, char. 4 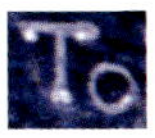 Triumphal arch, Sacrifice of Isaac, Angel's command: line 3, chars. 12 and 13	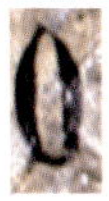 Scroll of St. Paul: line 2, char. 3	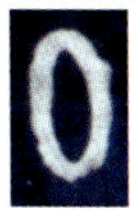 Donor inscription: line 1, char. 2 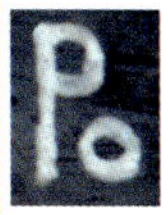 Donor inscription: line 6, char. 7
ος		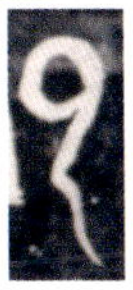 Donor Theophilos, line 1, char. 11			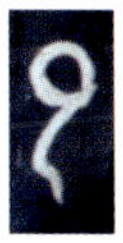 Donor inscription: line 4, penultimate char. 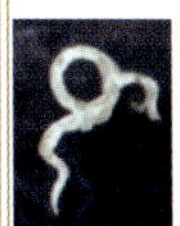 St. Eustathios: column 2, final char.

	NARTHEX LATE 13TH C. PAGES 115–30	NARTHEX 1332/33 PAGES 131–90	APSE CONCH AND TRIUMPHAL ARCH PAGES 213–23	SS. PETER AND PAUL, FIRST LAYER PAGES 211–13	NAOS 14TH C. PAGES 223–90
ου	 Donor Anastasia, line 1, char. 7	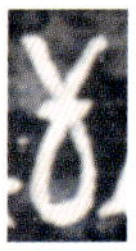 Donor Theophilos, line 1, char. 9 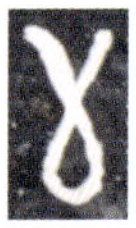 Donor Germanos, char. 12			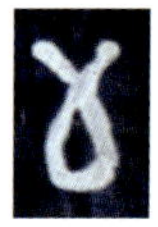 Donor inscription, line 5, final char.
ους		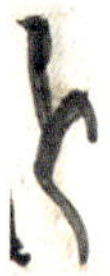 Codex of Christ Eleemon, right, line 4, char. 6			
π		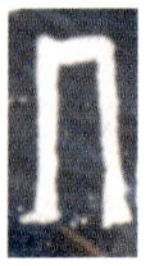 Donor Theophilos, line 2, char. 13	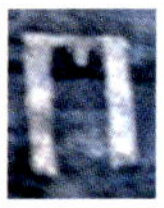 Apse conch, The Pantanassa: char. 2 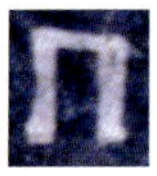 Triumphal arch, Sacrifice of Isaac, Angel's command: line 3, char. 9		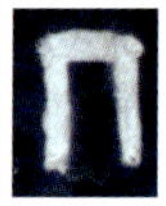 Donor inscription: line 1, char. 1
πρ		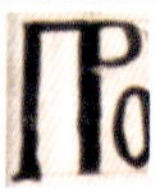 Scroll of Virgin Eleousa, line 2, char. 1			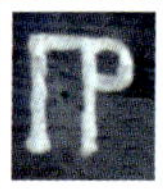 Donor inscription: line 6, char. 6
ρ		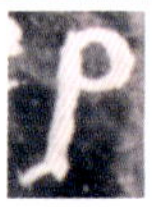 Donor Barnabas, line 3, char. 5 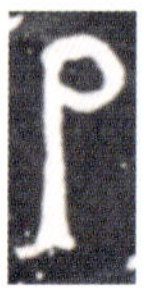 Donor Germanos, char. 9	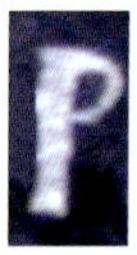 Triumphal arch, Sacrifice of Isaac, Angel's command: line 1, char. 2	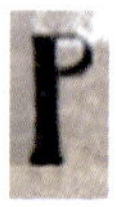 Scroll of St. Paul: line 2, char. 2	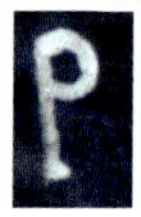 Donor inscription: line 3, char. 3
ργ					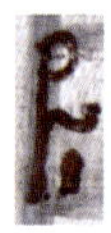 Virgin Paraklesis, scroll: line 6, char. 1
σ/ς	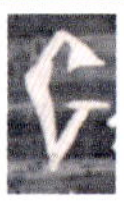 Donor Anastasia, line 1, char. 3	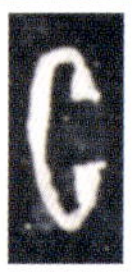 Donor Theophilos, line 2, char. 18	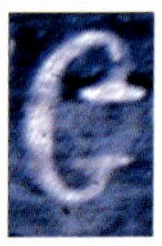 Apse conch, The Pantanassa: char. 7 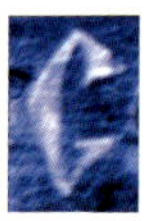 Apse conch, The Pantanassa: char. 8		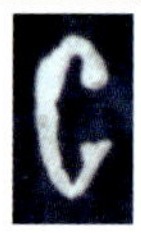 Donor inscription: line 1, char. 7 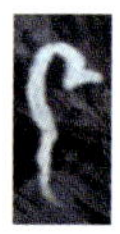 Donor inscription: line 7, final char.

	NARTHEX LATE 13TH C. PAGES 115–30	NARTHEX 1332/33 PAGES 131–90	APSE CONCH AND TRIUMPHAL ARCH PAGES 213–23	SS. PETER AND PAUL, FIRST LAYER PAGES 211–13	NAOS 14TH C. PAGES 223–90
σ/ς			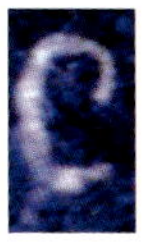 Triumphal arch, Sacrifice of Isaac, Angel's command: line 3, char. 6		
σι		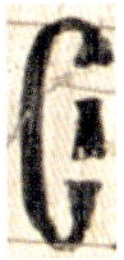 Scroll of St. John the Baptist, line 4, char. 3			
στ		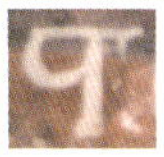 Dedicatory inscription on east lunette, line 2, char. 14			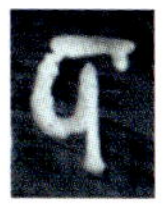 Donor inscription: line 6, char. 8
στρ		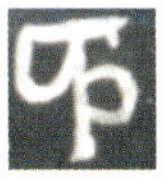 Last Judgment, She who refuses to nurse her children (ἡ ἀποστρέφουσα τὰ νήπια), line 1, char. 4			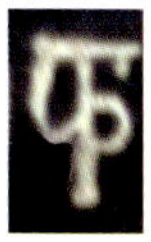 St. Theodore Stratelates, char. 1
συμ					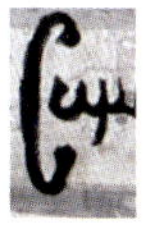 Virgin Paraklesis, scroll: line 6, char. 5
συν					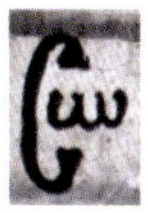 Virgin Paraklesis, scroll: line 2, char. 4
τ	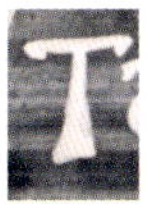 Donor Anastasia, line 1, char. 6	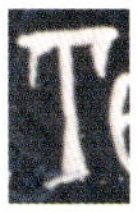 Donor Theophilos, line 2, char. 16 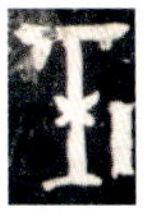 Donor Leontios, char. 11 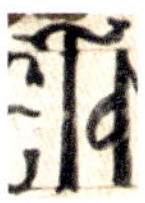 Scroll of St. John the Baptist, line 1, char. 3	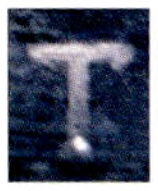 Apse conch, The Pantanassa: char. 3 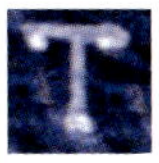 Triumphal arch, Sacrifice of Isaac, Angel's command: line 3, char. 12	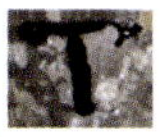 Scroll of St. Peter: line 3, penultimate char.	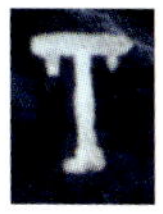 Donor inscription: line 1, char. 8
τε					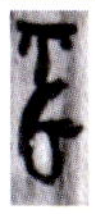 Virgin Paraklesis, scroll: line 2, char. 7
τει					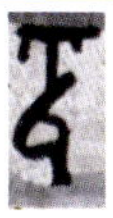 Virgin Paraklesis, scroll: line 2, char. 5

	NARTHEX LATE 13TH C. PAGES 115–30	NARTHEX 1332/33 PAGES 131–90	APSE CONCH AND TRIUMPHAL ARCH PAGES 213–23	SS. PETER AND PAUL, FIRST LAYER PAGES 211–13	NAOS 14TH C. PAGES 223–90
τη	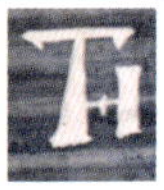 Donor Anastasia, line 1, char. 2	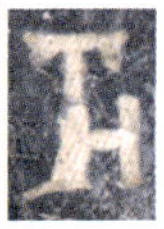 Donor Anna, line 1, char. 2	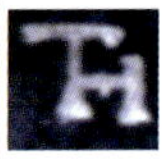 Triumphal arch, Sacrifice of Isaac, Angel's command: line 2, char. 13		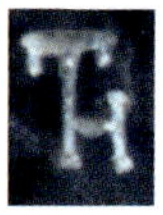 Donor inscription: line 5, char. 2
το		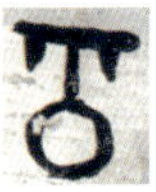 Codex of Christ Eleemon, left, line 1, char. 3 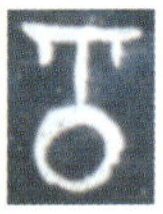 Last Judgment, The Outer Darkness (τὸ σκότος τὸ ἐξώτερον), char. 1			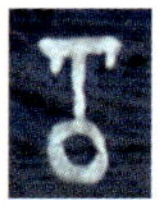 Donor inscription: line 6, char. 5
του		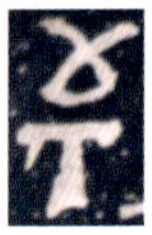 Donor Barnabas, line 1, char. 2 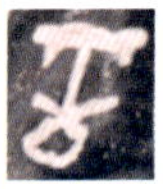 Donor Barnabas, line 2, char. 1			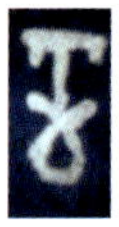 Gephyra, memorial inscription: line 2, char. 6
τρ	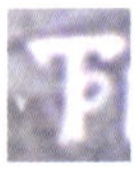 St. Anastasia the Poison Curer, right, line 7, char. 1	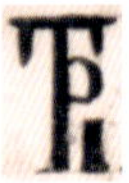 Scroll of Virgin Eleousa, line 2, char. 2			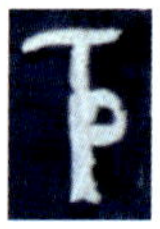 Donor inscription: line 4, char. 24 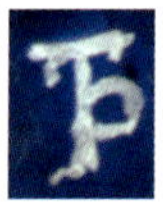 St. Tryphon: column 2, char. 1
τυν					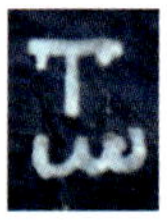 Donor inscription: line 6, char. 10
τω					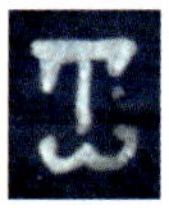 Donor inscription: line 5, char. 8
των		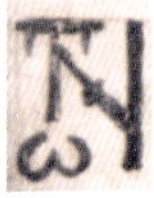 Scroll of Virgin Eleousa, line 8, char. 1 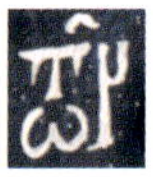 Donor Theophilos, line 3, char. 7			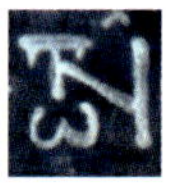 Donor inscription: line 5, char. 12
τωνβ					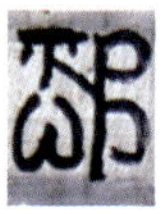 Virgin Paraklesis, scroll: line 4, char. 6

	NARTHEX LATE 13TH C. PAGES 115–30	NARTHEX 1332/33 PAGES 131–90	APSE CONCH AND TRIUMPHAL ARCH PAGES 213–23	SS. PETER AND PAUL, FIRST LAYER PAGES 211–13	NAOS 14TH C. PAGES 223–90
υ	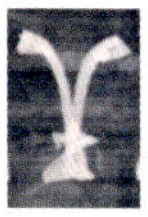 Donor Anastasia, line 2, char. 8	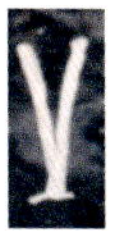 Donor Theophilos, line 1, char. 18	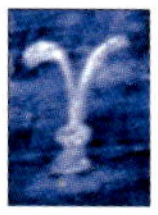 Apse conch: Mother of God: char. 3 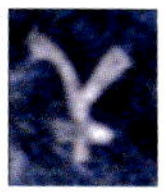 Triumphal arch, Sacrifice of Isaac, Angel's command: line 3, char. 8		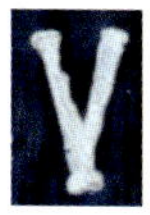 Donor inscription: line 3, final char.
υι					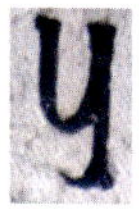 Northeast jamb, magic cross: left column, char. 3
φ	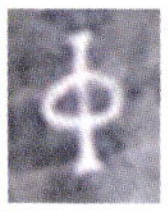 St. Anastasia the Poison Curer, right, line 2	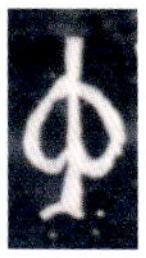 Donor Theophilos, line 1, char. 17		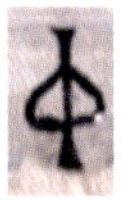 Scroll of St. Paul: line 2, char. 1	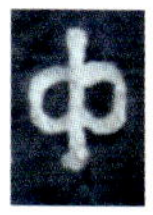 Donor inscription: line 7, char. 7  St. Tryphon: column 2, char. 3
χ		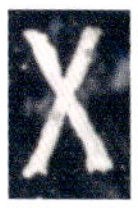 Donor Theophilos, line 2, char. 21	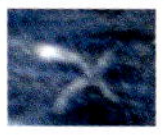 Apse conch, The Archangel Michael: chars. 1–2 above 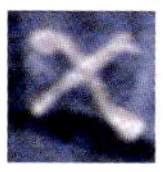 Triumphal arch, Sacrifice of Isaac, Angel's command: line 3, char. 1		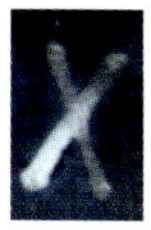 Donor inscription: line 3, char. 4
ψ		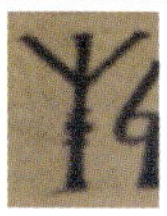 North couch, Paradise, inscription from Matthew's Gospel (25: 34–35)			
ω		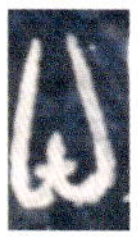 Donor Theophilos, line 2, char. 14 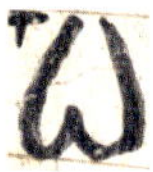 Scroll of St. John the Baptist, line 5, char. 2	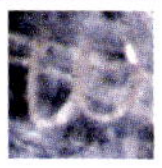 Triumphal arch, St. John of Damascus: line 1, char. 4 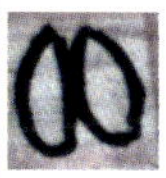 Triumphal arch, St. John of Damascus, scroll: line 3, char. 3		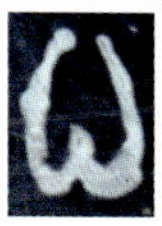 Donor inscription, line 7, char. 11 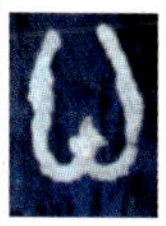 Donor inscription, line 2, char. 10 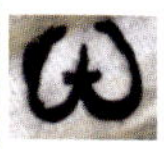 The Holy Mandylion: column 2, final char.

	NARTHEX LATE 13TH C. PAGES 115–30	NARTHEX 1332/33 PAGES 131–90	APSE CONCH AND TRIUMPHAL ARCH PAGES 213–23	SS. PETER AND PAUL, FIRST LAYER PAGES 211–13	NAOS 14TH C. PAGES 223–90
ω					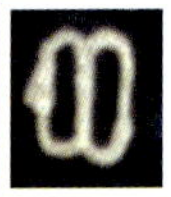 St. Theodore Tyro: char. 4 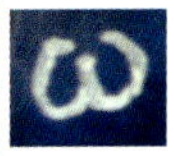 St. Tryphon: column 2, char. 4

	NARTHEX LATE 13TH C. PAGES 115–30	NARTHEX 1332/33 PAGES 131–90	APSE CONCH AND TRIUMPHAL ARCH PAGES 213–23	NAOS 14TH C. PAGES 223–90
ὁ ἅγιος		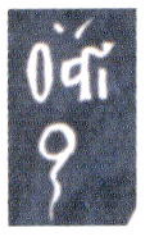 St. John of Damascus 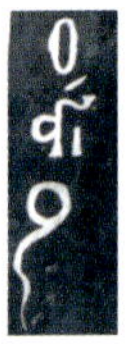 St. Sozomenos		
ὁ ἀρχάγγελος		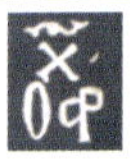 Archangel Michael		
δέησις	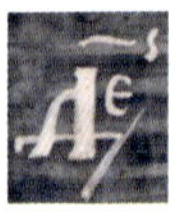 Donor Anastasia, line 1, char. 1	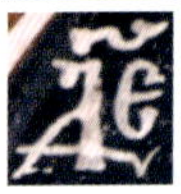 Donor Barnabas, line 1, char. 1 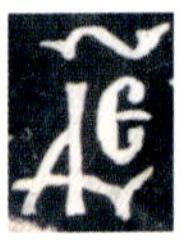 Donor Leontios, char. 1		
		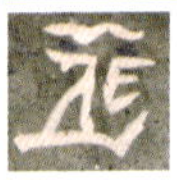 Donor Kallinikos, line 1, char. 1 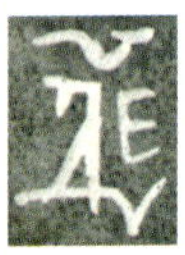 Donor Laurentios, line 1, char. 1 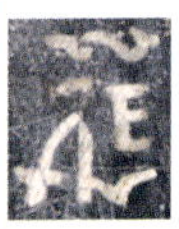 Donor Anna, line 1, char. 1		
δούλης	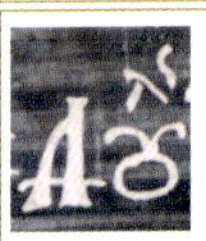 Donor Anastasia, line 1, char. 5			

	NARTHEX LATE 13TH C. PAGES 115–30	NARTHEX 1332/33 PAGES 131–90	APSE CONCH AND TRIUMPHAL ARCH PAGES 213–23	NAOS 14TH C. PAGES 223–90
Θεοῦ	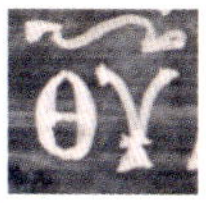 Donor Anastasia, line 1, char. 8	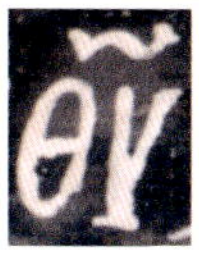 Donor Barnabas, line 2, char. 2		
Ἰησοῦς		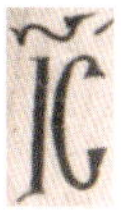 Cross on northern jamb of west entrance, line 1 left		
Ἰησοῦς Χριστός				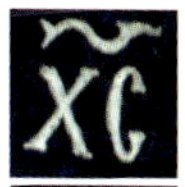 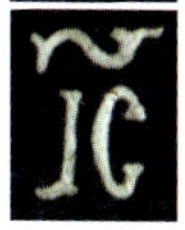 Christ Eleemon
Ἰωάννης		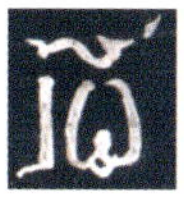 St. John of Damascus		
Μήτηρ Θεοῦ			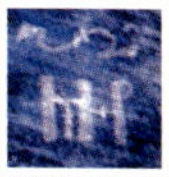 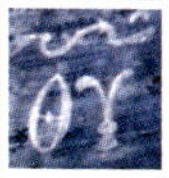 Apse conch	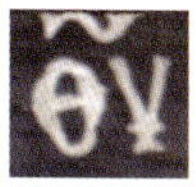 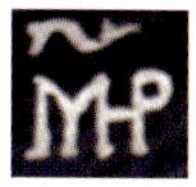 Enthroned Mother of God 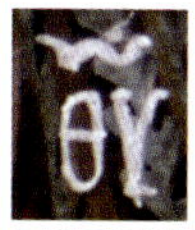 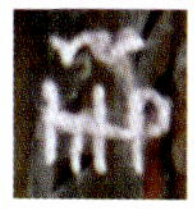 Burning Bush
ὁ Πρόδρομος				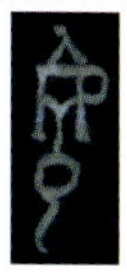 John the Baptist, bema pier
ὁ προφήτης			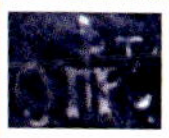 Triumphal arch, Sacrifice of Isaac, The Prophet Abraham: chars. 1–4	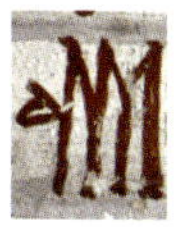 Prophet Solomon 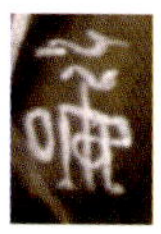 The Burning Bush, Prophet Moses  Closed Gate, Prophet Ezekiel

Abbreviations

AASS	*Acta sanctorum*. Paris, 1863–1940.
AB	*Analecta Bollandiana*
AJA	*American Journal of Archaeology*
ARDAC	*Annual Report of the Department of Antiquities, Cyprus*
ArtB	*Art Bulletin*
Ἀρχ.Δελτ.	*Ἀρχαιολογικὸν Δελτίον*
BCH	*Bulletin de correspondance hellénique*
BHG	*Bibliotheca hagiographica graeca*, 3rd ed., ed. F. Halkin, SubsHag 47. Brussels, 1957; repr. 1969.
BMFD	*Byzantine Monastic Foundation Documents: A Complete Translation of the Surviving Founders'* Typika *and Testaments*. Edited by J. Thomas and A. C. Hero. Dumbarton Oaks Studies 35. 5 vols. Washington, D.C., 2000.
BMGS	*Byzantine and Modern Greek Studies*
BNJ	*Byzantinisch-Neugriechische Jahrbücher*
BS	*Bibliotheca sanctorum*. 12 vols. Rome, 1961–70.
BSl	*Byzantinoslavica*
ByzF	*Byzantinische Forschungen*
BZ	*Byzantinische Zeitschrift*
CahArch	*Cahiers archéologiques*
CFHB	Corpus fontium historiae byzantinae
DACL	*Dictionnaire d'archéologie chrétienne et de liturgie*. 15 vols. Paris, 1907–53.
DOP	*Dumbarton Oaks Papers*
DOS	Dumbarton Oaks Studies
DOSeals	*Catalogue of Byzantine Seals at Dumbarton Oaks and in the Fogg Museum of Art*. Edited by N. Oikonomides and J. Nesbitt. Washington, DC, 1991–.
Δελτ.Χριστ.Ἀρχ.Ἑτ.	*Δελτίον τῆς Χριστιανικῆς Ἀρχαιολογικῆς Ἑταιρείας*
EChR	*Eastern Churches Review*
EO	*Echos d'Orient*
Ἐπ.Ἑτ.Βυζ.Σπ.	*Ἐπετηρὶς Ἑταιρείας Βυζαντινῶν Σπουδῶν*
Ἐπ.Κέν.Ἐπιστ.Ἐρ.	*Ἐπετηρὶς τοῦ Κέντρου Ἐπιστημονικῶν Ἐρευνῶν*
GOTR	*Greek Orthodox Theological Review*

ΘΗΕ	*Θρησκευτικὴ καὶ Ἠθικὴ Ἐγκυκλοπαίδεια*. 12 vols. Athens, 1962–68.
JbAC	*Jahrbuch für Antike und Christentum*
JHS	*Journal of Hellenic Studies*
JÖB	*Jahrbuch der Österreichischen Byzantinistik*
JÖBG	*Jahrbuch der Österreichischen Byzantinischen Gesellschaft*
JSAH	*Journal of the Society of Architectural Historians*
Κυπρ.Σπ.	*Κυπριακαὶ Σπουδαί*
LCI	*Lexikon der christlichen Ikonographie*. 8 vols. Rome–Freiburg, 1968–76.
OCP	*Orientalia Christiana Periodica*
ODB	*The Oxford Dictionary of Byzantium*. Edited by A. Kazhdan et al. New York–Oxford, 1991.
OrChr	*Orientalia christiana*
OrChrP	*Orientalia christiana periodica*
PG	Patrologiae cursus completus, Series graeca. Edited by J.-P. Migne. Paris, 1857–66.
PL	Patrologiae cursus completus, Series latina. Edited by J.-P. Migne. Paris, 1844–80.
RAC	*Reallexikon für Antike und Christentum*. Stuttgart, 1950–.
RÉArm	*Revue des études arméniennes*
REB	*Revue des études byzantines*
RBK	*Reallexikon zur byzantinischen Kunst*. 7 vols. Ed. K. Wessel. Stuttgart, 1963–.
RDAC	*Report of the Department of Antiquities, Cyprus*
REB	*Revue des études byzantines*
REG	*Revue des études grecques*
RIASA	*Rivista dell'Istituto nazionale d'archeologia e storia dell'arte*
SA	State Archives of Cyprus, Nicosia
SemKond	*Seminarium Kondakovianum*
StVen	*Studi Veneziani*
TM	*Travaux et mémoires*
VizVrem	*Vizantiiskii vremennik*
ZbLikUmet	*Zbornik za likovne umetnosti*
ZRVI	*Zbornik radova Vizantološkog instituta, Srpska akademija nauka*

Bibliography

Abraseys, N. *The Seismicity of Cyprus*. London, 1992.

Acheimastou-Potamianou, M., ed. *From Byzantium to El Greco: Greek Frescoes and Icons*. Exh. cat., Royal Academy of Arts, London, 27 March – 21 June 1987. Athens, 1987.

———, ed. *Holy Image, Holy Space: Icons and Frescoes from Greece*. Exh. cat., Walters Art Gallery, Baltimore, 21 August – 16 October 1988. Athens, 1988.

Ἁγίου Νεοφύτου τοῦ Ἐγκλείστου Συγγράμματα. Vol. 3, *Πανηγυρικὴ Α′*, ed. N. Papatriantaphyllou-Theodoride and T. X. Yiangos. Paphos, 1999.

Aidoni, S., et al. *Journeys on the Seas of Byzantium*. Athens, 1997.

Albani, J. "Οι τοιχογραφίες του ναού του Αγίου Ιωάννου στην Αξό Μυλοποτάμου." In *Ο Μυλοπόταμος από την αρχαιότητα ως σήμερα*, volume 5, *Βυζαντινοί χρόνοι*, ed. I. Gavrilaki and Y. Tziphopoulos, 159–96. Rethymno, 2006.

Aliprantis, T. C. *Moses auf dem Berge Sinai: Die Ikonographie der Berufung des Moses und des Empfangs der Gesetzestafeln*. Munich, 1986.

Alivizatos, A. S. "Ἡ κουρὰ τῶν κληρικῶν καὶ μοναχῶν κατὰ τὸ κανονικὸν δίκαιον τῆς Ὀρθοδόξου ἐκκλησίας." *Ἐπ.Ἑτ.Βυζ.Σπ.* 23 (1953): 233–39.

Amantos, K. "Σύμμεικτα." *Ἑλληνικά* 11 (1939): 330–31. Repr. Thessalonike, 1971.

Andaloro, M. "Note sui temi iconografici della Deesis e dell'Haghiosoritissa." *RIASA*, n.s. 17 (1970): 85–153.

Anderson, J. *The New York Cruciform Lectionary*. University Park, Pa., 1992.

Andreescu, I. "Torcello." *DOP* 26 (1972): 183–223; 30 (1976): 245–341.

Angelidi, C. "Ὁ βίος τοῦ Ὁσίου Βασιλείου τοῦ Νέου." Ph.D. diss., University of Ioannina, 1980.

———. "La version longue de la vision du moine Cosmas." *AB* 101 (1983): 73–99.

Angheben, M. "Les Jugements derniers byzantins des XIe–XIIe siècles et l'iconographie du jugement immédiat." *CahArch* 50 (2002): 105–34.

Arbel, B. "Ἡ Κύπρος ὑπὸ ἐνετικῆς κυριαρχίας." In *Ἱστορία τῆς Κύπρου*, 5 vols., ed. Th. Papadopoullos, 4:355–536. Nicosia, 1995.

Archontopoulos, Th. *Παναγία η Φιλόστοργος: μία εικόνα από τον ναό του Ευαγγελισμού στ' Ασφενδιού Κω*. In *Χάρις Χαίρε: Μελέτες στη μνήμη Χάρης Κάντζια*, ed. A. Giannikouri et al., 1:317–28. Athens, 2004.

Argyrou, C., and D. Myriantheus. *The Church of the Holy Cross of Ayiasmati*. Trans. D. Whitehouse. Nicosia, 2006.

Arranz, M. *L'Eucologio costantinopolitano agli inizi del secolo XI*. Hagiasmatarion e Archieratikon. Rome, 1996.

———. "Les grandes étapes de la liturgie byzantine: Paléstine–Byzance–Russie." In *Liturgie de l'église particulière, liturgie de l'église universelle*, 43–72. Rome, 1976.

Asdracha, A. "Ἡ Κύπρος ὑπὸ τοὺς Κομνηνούς." In *Ἱστορία τῆς Κύπρου*, volume 3, *Βυζαντινή Κύπρος*, ed. Th. Papadopoullos, 1:293–347, 2:349–412. Nicosia, 2005.

Aspra-Vardavaki, M. "Observations on a Thirteenth-Century Sinaitic Diptych Representing St. Prokopios, the Virgin Kykkotissa, and Saints along the Border / Παρατηρήσεις σε δίπτυχο του 13ου αιώνα στο Σινά με τον άγιο Προκόπιο, την Παναγία Κυκκώτισσα και αγίους στο πλαίσια." In *Βυζαντινές εικόνες: Τέχνη, τεχνική και τεχνολογία / Byzantine Icons: Art, Technique, and Technology*, ed. M. Vassilaki, 89–98. Iraklion, 2002.

Auzépy, M.-F. *La vie d'Etienne le Jeune par Etienne le Diacre: Introduction, édition et traduction*. Birmingham Byzantine and Ottoman Monographs 3. Aldershot, 1997.

Babić, G. *Les chapelles annexes des églises byzantines: Fonction liturgique et programmes iconographiques*. Paris, 1969.

———. "Les croix à cryptogrammes peintes dans les églises serbes des XIIIe et XIVe siècles." In *Byzance et les Slaves: Études de civilisation (Mélanges Ivan Dujcev)*, ed. S. Dufrenne, 1–13. Paris, 1979.

———. "La décoration en fresques des clôtures de choeur." *ZbLikUmet* 11 (1975): 3–49.

———. "L'Image symbolique de la 'porte fermée' à Saint-Clément d'Ohrid." In *Synthronon: Art et archéologie de la fin de l'Antiquité et du Moyen Age; Recueil d'études*, ed. A. Grabar and J. Hubert, 145–51. Bibliothèque des Cahiers archéologiques 2. Paris, 1968.

Bacci, M. "La Madonna della Misericordia individuale." *Acta ad archaeologiam et artium historiam pertinentia*, n.s. 7, 21 (2009): 171–95.

———. "Syrian, Palaiologan, and Gothic Murals in the 'Nestorian' Church of Famagusta." *Δελτ.Χριστ.Ἀρχ.Ἑτ.*, ser. 4, 27 (2006): 207–20.

———. "Tra Pisa e Cipro: La committenza artistica di Giovanni Conti (†1332)." *Annali della Scuola Normale Superiore di Pisa*, ser. 4, 5 (2000): 343–86.

Bache, F. "La fonction funéraire du narthex dans les églises byzantines du XIIe au XIVe siècle." *Histoire de l'Art* 7 (1989): 25–33.

Bagnoli, A., et al., eds. *Duccio: Alle origini della pittura senese*. Exh. cat., Santa Maria della Scala–Museo dell'Opera del Duomo, Siena, 4 October 2003 – 11 January 2004. Milan, 2003.

Bakalova, E. "A Cycle of the Holy Archangels in a Thirteenth-Century Rock-Cut Chapel near Ivanovo." In *Byzantine East, Latin West: Art-Historical Studies in Honor of Kurt Weitzmann*, ed. C. Moss and K. Kiefer, 215–28. Princeton, 1995.

———. "Hymnography and Iconography: Images of Hymnographers in Twelfth- and Thirteenth-Century Church Paintings in Bulgaria." In *Ritual and Art: Byzantine Essays for Christopher Walter*, ed. P. Armstrong, 246–73. London, 2006.

———. "La vie de sainte Parascève de Tirnovo dans l'art balkanique du Bas Moyen Age." *Byzantinobulgarica* 5 (1978): 175–209.

Bakirtzis, C. "Le culte de Saint Démétrius." In *Akten des XII. Internationalen Kongresses für Christliche Archäologie Bonn 22.–28. September 1991 = JbAC*, Ergänzungsband 20, 1:58–68. Münster, 1995.

———. "Warrior Saints or Portraits of Members of the Family of Alexios I Komnenos?" In *Mosaic: Festschrift for A. H. S. Megaw*, ed. J. Herrin, M. Mullett, and C. Otten-Froux, 85–88. London, 2001.

al-Baladhuri, abu'l-'Abbas Ahmad ibn Jabir. *Kitab Futuh al-Buldan*. Trans. P. K. Hitti. New York, 1916; repr. Beirut, 1966.

Ball, J. L. *Byzantine Dress: Representations of Secular Dress in Eighth- to Twelfth-Century Painting*. New York, 2005.

Bank, A. *Byzantine Art in the Collections of Soviet Museums*. 2nd ed. Leningrad, 1985.

Barber, C. "Mimesis and Memory in the Narthex Mosaics of the Nea Moni, Chios." *Art History* 24 (2001): 323–37.

Bars'kyj, V. *A Pilgrim's Account of Cyprus: Bars'kyj's Travels in Cyprus*. Ed. and trans. A. D. Grishin. Sources for the History of Cyprus 3. Altamont, New York, 1996.

Baschet, J. *Le sein du père: Abraham et la paternité dans l'Occident médiéval*. Paris, 2000.

Bauckham, R. "The Four Apocalypses of the Virgin Mary." In idem, *The Fate of the Dead: Studies on the Jewish and Christian Apocalypses*, 332–62. Leiden, 1998.

Baun, J. "The Apocalypse of Anastasia in its Middle Byzantine Context." Ph.D. diss., Princeton University, 1997.

———. "Middle Byzantine 'Tours of Hell': Outsider Theodicy?" In *Strangers to Themselves: The Byzantine Outsider; Papers from the Thirty-Second Spring Symposium of Byzantine Studies, University of Sussex, Brighton, March 1998*, ed. D. C. Smythe, 47–60. Aldershot, 2000.

———. *Tales from Another Byzantium: Celestial Journey and Local Community in the Medieval Greek Apocrypha*. Cambridge, 2007.

Beaudouin, M. *Étude du dialecte chypriote moderne et médiéval*. Paris, 1884.

Beck, H.-G. *Kirche und theologische Literatur im byzantinischen Reich*. Munich, 1977.

Beihammer, A. D. "Audiatur et altera pars: Η Βυζαντινοαραβική συγκυριαρχία στην Κύπρο υπό το πρίσμα των Αραβικών πηγών." *Κυπρ.Σπ.* 64–65 (2000–2001): 157–76.

———. "Zypern und die byzantinisch-arabische Seepolitik von 8. zu Beginn des 10. Jahrhunderts." In *Aspects of Arab Seafaring: An Attempt to Fill in the Gaps of Maritime History*, ed. Y.Y. Al-Hijj and V. Christides, 41–63. Athens, 2002.

Belting, H. *Das Illuminierte Buch in der spätbyzantinischen Gesellschaft*. Heidelberg, 1970.

Belting, H., C. Mango, and D. Mouriki. *The Mosaics and Frescoes of St. Mary Pammakaristos (Fethiye Camii) at Istanbul*. Ed. C. Mango. DOS 15. Washington, D.C., 1978.

Belting-Ihm, C. *"Sub Matris tutela": Untersuchungen zur Vorgeschichte der Schutzmantelmadonna*. Heidelberg, 1976.

Benaki Museum. *The Conservation of Icons in the Velimezis Collection*. Athens, 1998. CD-ROM.

Bentchev, I., and E. Haustein-Bartsch. *Gottesmutterikonen*. Recklinghausen, 2000.

Bernardini, L. "Les donateurs des églises de Cappadoce." *Byzantion* 62 (1992): 118–40.

Bitha, I. "Ενδυματολογικές μαρτυρίες στις τοιχογραφίες της μεσαιωνικής Ρόδου (14ος αι.–1523): Μία πρώτη προσέγγιση." In *Ρόδος 2.400 χρόνια: Η πόλη της Ρόδου από την ίδρυσή της μέχρι την κατάληψη από τους Τούρκους (1523); Πρακτικά*, 2:429–48. Athens, 2000.

Bogyay, T. von. "Deesis und Eschatologie." In *Polychordia: Festschrift Franz Dölger zum 75. Geburtstag*, ed. P. Wirth, 2:59–72. Amsterdam, 1967.

———. "Zur Geschichte der Hetoimasie." In *Akten des XI. Internationalen Byzantinistenkongresses München 1958*, 58–61. Munich, 1960.

Bolman, E. S., ed. *Monastic Visions: Wall Paintings in the Monastery of St. Antony at the Red Sea*. New Haven, 2002.

Borboudakis, M. *Panaghia Kera: Byzantine Wall-Painting at Kritsa*. Athens, n. d.

———. "Παρατηρήσεις στη ζωγραφική της εκκλησίας του Σκλαβεροχωρίου." In *Πεπραγμένα τοῦ ΣΤ′ Διεθνοῦς Κρητολογικοῦ Συνεδρίου*, 2:355–63. Chania, 1991.

Boucher, F. *Histoire du costume en Occident de l'Antiquité à nos jours*. 2nd ed. Paris, 1983.

Bougrat, M. "Trois Jugements derniers de Crète occidentale." *Cahiers Balkaniques* 6 (1984): 13–67.

Bouras, Ch. *Βυζαντινή και μεταβυζαντινή αρχιτεκτονική στην Ελλάδα*. Athens, 2001.

Bouras, Ch., and L. Boura. *Η Ελλαδική ναοδομία κατά τον 12° αιώνα*. Athens, 2002.

Bouras, Ch., A. Kalogeropoulou, and R. Andreade. *Εκκλησίες της Αττικής*. Athens, 1969.

Boyd, S. A. "The Church of the Panagia Amasgou, Monagri, Cyprus, and Its Wallpaintings." *DOP* 28 (1974): 277–328.

———. "Ex-Voto Therapy: A Note on a Copper Plaque with St. Hermolaus." In *ΑΕΤΟΣ: Studies in Honour of Cyril Mango*, ed. I. Ševčenko and I. Hutter, 15–27. Stuttgart–Leipzig, 1998.

Brenk, B. "Die Anfänge der byzantinischen Weltgerichtsdarstellung." *BZ* 57 (1964): 106–26.

———. *Tradition und Neuerung in der christlichen Kunst des ersten Jahrtausends*. Vienna, 1966.

Brightman, F. E. *Liturgies Eastern and Western*. Volume 1, *Eastern Liturgies*. Oxford, 1896.

Brock, S. P. *The Bible in the Syriac Liturgy*. 2nd ed. Piscataway, N.J., 2006.

———. "Ephrem's Letter to Publius." *Le Muséon* 89 (1976): 261–305.

———. "Passover, Annunciation, and Epiclesis: Some Remarks on the Term *aggen* in the Syriac Versions of Luke 1:35." *Novum Testamentum* 24 (1982): 222–33. Repr. in idem, *Fire From Heaven: Studies in Syriac Theology and Liturgy*, art. XII. Aldershot, 2006.

———, trans. *Saint Ephrem, Hymns on Paradise*. New York, 1990.

Brooks, E. W. "Byzantines and Arabs in the Time of the Early Abbasids." *English Historical Review* 15 (1900): 728–47.

Brosh, N. "Between East and West: Glass and Minor Arts in the Crusader Kingdom." In *Knights of the Holy Land: The Crusader Kingdom of Jerusalem*, ed. S. Rozenberg, 267–71. Jerusalem, 1999.

Browning, R. "Byzantium and Islam in Cyprus in the Early Middle Ages." *Ἐπ.Κέν.Ἐπιστ.Ἐρ.* 9 (1977–79): 101–16.

———. "Ἡ Κύπρος καὶ οἱ Ἄραβες." In *Ἱστορία τῆς Κύπρου*, ed. Th. Papadopoullos, 3:235–91. Nicosia, 2005.

———. "An Unpublished Corpus of Byzantine Poems." *Byzantion* 33 (1963): 289–316. Repr. in idem, *Studies on Byzantine History, Literature and Education*, art. 8. London, 1977.

Brubaker, L. *Vision and Meaning in Ninth-Century Byzantium: Image as Exegesis in the Homilies of Gregory of Nazianzus*. Cambridge, 1999.

Bryer, A. A. M., and G. S. Georghallides, eds. *The Sweet Land of Cyprus: Papers Given at the Twenty-Fifth Jubilee Spring Symposium of Byzantine Studies, Birmingham, March 1991*. Nicosia, 1993.

Buchthal, H. *Miniature Painting in the Latin Kingdom of Jerusalem*. Oxford, 1957.

Buckton, D., ed. *Byzantium: Treasures of Byzantine Art and Culture from British Collections*. Exh. cat., British Museum, 1994. London, 1994.

———. *The Treasury of San Marco*. Exh. cat., Metropolitan Museum of Art, New York, 1984. Milan, 1984.

Bustron, F. *Historia overo commentarii de Cipro*. Ed. R. de Mas Latrie. Paris, 1886. Repr. Leukosia, 1998.

Butler, H. C. *Early Churches in Syria, Fourth to Seventh Centuries*. Princeton, 1929.

Butyrskij, M. "Bogomater' Paraklesis u altarnoj pregrady: proischoždenie i lityrgičeskoe soderžanie obraza." In *Ikonostas: Proischoždenie—Razvitie—Simvolik*, ed. A. M. Lidov, 207–22. Moscow, 2000.

Buxton, H., V. Seymer, W. H. Buckler, and Mrs. W. H. (G.) Buckler. "The Church of Asinou, Cyprus, and Its Frescoes." *Archaeologia* 83 (1933): 327–50.

Το Βυζάντιο ως Οικουμένη: Ώρες Βυζαντίου; Έργα και Ημέρες στο Βυζάντιο. Exh. cat., Byzantine and Christian Museum, Athens, October 2001 – January 2002. Athens, 2001. [English translation with identical pagination, Athens, 2002.]

Byzance: L'art byzantin dans les collections publiques françaises. Exh. cat., musée du Louvre, Paris, 3 November 1992–1 February 1993. Paris, 1992.

Canivet, P. "Le Michaelion de Huarte (Ve s.) et le culte Syrien des anges." *Byzantion* 50 (1980): 85–117.

Carboni, S., and D. Whitehouse. *Glass of the Sultans*. Exh. cat., Corning Museum of Glass, Corning, New York, 24 May–3 September 2001; Metropolitan Museum of Art, New York, 2 October 2001 – 13 January 2002; Benaki Museum, Athens, 20 February–15 May 2002. New York, 2001.

Carli, E. *La pittura Senese del Trecento*. Milan, 1981.

Carr, A. W. "Art." In Nicolaou-Konnari and Schabel, *Cyprus: Culture and Society*, 285–328.

———. "Art in the Court of the Lusignan Kings." In *Η Κύπρος και οι Σταυροφορίες—Cyprus and the Crusades*, ed. N. Coureas and J. Riley-Smith, 239–74. Nicosia, 1995. Repr. in eadem, *Cyprus and the Devotional Arts*, art. VII.

———. *Byzantine Illumination 1150–1250: The Study of a Provincial Tradition*. Chicago, 1987.

———. "Byzantines and Italians on Cyprus: Images from Art." *DOP* 49 (1995): 339–57. Repr. in eadem, *Cyprus and the Devotional Arts*, art. XI.

———. "Correlative Spaces: Art, Identity, and Appropriation in Lusignan Cyprus." *Modern Greek Studies Yearbook, University of Minnesota* 14–15 (1998–99): 59–80. Repr. in eadem, *Cyprus and the Devotional Arts*, art. VI.

———. "Cypriot Funerary Icons: Questions of Convergence in a Complex Land." In *Medieval Paradigms: Essays in Honor of Jeremy DuQuesnay Adams*, ed. S. Hayes, 1:153–74. New York, 2005.

———. "Cyprus and the Decorative Style." *Ἐπ.Κέν.Ἐπιστ.Ἐρ.* 17 (1987–88): 123–67.

———. *Cyprus and the Devotional Arts of Byzantium in the Era of the Crusades*. Aldershot, 2005.

———. "The Holy Icons: A Lusignan Asset?" In *France and the Holy Land: Frankish Culture at the End of the Crusades*, ed. D. H. Weiss and L. Mahoney, 315–35. Baltimore, 2004.

———. "The 'Holy Sepulcher' of St. John Lampadistes, Cyprus." In *New Jerusalems: Hierotopy and Iconography*, ed. A. Lidov, 475–88. Moscow, 2009.

———. "Iconography and Identity: Syrian Elements in the Art of Crusader Cyprus." In *Religious Origins of Nations? The Christian Communities of the Middle East*, ed. R. B. ter Haar Romeny = *Church History and Religious Culture* 89, nos. 1–3 (2009): 127–51.

———. "Icon-tact: Byzantium and the Art of Cilician Armenia." In *Treasures in Heaven: Armenian Art, Religion and Society*, ed. T. F. Mathews and R. S. Wieck, 73–102. New York, 1998. Repr. in eadem, *Cyprus and the Devotional Arts*, art. VIII.

———. "The Mural Paintings of Abu Ghosh and the Patronage of Manuel Comnenus in the Holy Land." In Folda, *Crusader Art in the Twelfth Century*, 215–44.

———. "A Palaiologan Funerary Icon from Gothic Cyprus." In *Πρακτικὰ τοῦ τρίτου διεθνοῦς κυπρολογικοῦ συνεδρίου*, 2:599–619. Repr. in eadem, *Cyprus and the Devotional Arts*, art. IX.

———. "Perspectives on Visual Culture in Early Lusignan Cyprus: Balancing Art and Archaelogy." In *Archaeology and the Crusades*, ed. P. Edbury and S. Kalopissi-Verti, 83–110. Aldershot, 2006.

———. "The Presentation of an Icon on Sinai." *Δελτ.Χριστ. Ἀρχ.Ἑτ.*, ser. 4, 17 (1993–94): 239–48.

———. Review of *Icons of Cyprus, 7th to 20th Century*, by S. Sophocleous. *Speculum* 68 (1993): 1025–26.

———. "Thoughts on Seeing Christ Helkomenos: An Icon from Pelendri." In Koch, *Byzantinische Malerei*, 405–20. Repr. in eadem, *Cyprus and the Devotional Arts*, art. X.

Carr, A. W., and L. J. Morrocco. *A Byzantine Masterpiece Recovered: The Thirteenth-Century Murals of Lysi, Cyprus.* Austin, Texas, 1991.

Castelnuovo, E., ed. *La pittura in Italia: Il Duecento e il Trecento.* 2 vols. Milan, 1986.

Cavazzana Romanelli, F., and G. Grivaud. *Cyprus 1542: The Great Map of the Island by Leonida Attar.* Cyprus Cartography Lectures 7. Nicosia, 2006.

Cennini, C. A. *"Il libro dell' arte": The Craftsman's Handbook of Cennino d'Andrea Cennini*. Trans. and ed. D. V. Thompson, Jr. New Haven, 1933; repr. New York, 1960.

Chasiotes, I. K. *Ἰσπανικὰ ἔγγραφα τῆς κυπριακῆς ἱστορίας (ΙϚ'–ΙΖ' αἰ.):* Πηγαὶ καὶ μελέται τῆς κυπριακῆς ἱστορίας 3. Nicosia, 1972.

Chassoura, O. *Les peintures murales byzantines des églises de Longanikos–Laconie*. Athens, 2002.

Chatzidakis, M. "Ἐκ τῶν Ἐλπίου τοῦ Ρωμαίου." *Ἐπ.Ἑτ.Βυζ. Σπ.* 14 (1938): 393–414.

———. *Έλληνες Ζωγράφοι μετά την Άλωση (1450–1830).* Vol. 1. Athens, 1987.

———. "L'Évolution de l'icone aux 11e–13e siècles et la transformation du templon." In *XVe Congrès international d'études byzantines, Rapports et co-rapports,* volume 3, *Art et archéologie*, 159–91. Athens, 1976.

———. *Mystras: The Medieval City and the Castle; A Complete Guide to the Churches, Palaces, and the Castle.* Athens, 1985.

———. "Τοιχογραφίες στὴ Μονὴ τῆς Ἁγίας Αἰκατερίνης στὸ Σινᾶ." *Δελτ.Χριστ.Ἀρχ.Ἑτ.*, ser. 4, 6 (1970–72): 205–32.

Chatzidakis, M., and I. Bitha. *Ευρετήριο βυζαντινών τοιχογραφιών Ελλάδος: Κύθηρα*. Athens, 1997.

Chatzidakis, N. "Icon Painting in Crete during the Fifteenth and Sixteenth Centuries." In *From Byzantium to El Greco: Greek Frescoes and Icons*, ed. M. Acheimastou-Potamianou, 48–50. Exh. cat., Royal Academy of Arts, London. Athens, 1987.

———. *Εἰκόνες Κρητικῆς Σχολῆς 15ος–16ος αἰώνας.* Exh. cat., Benaki Museum. Athens, 1983.

Chatzidakis, T. "Particularités iconographiques du décor des chapelles occidentales de Saint-Luc en Phocide." *CahArch* 22 (1972): 89–113.

Chatzidakis-Bacharas, T. *Les peintures murales de Hosios Loukas: Les chapelles occidentales*. Athens, 1982.

Chatzioannou, K. P. "Αἱ παραστάσεις τῶν κολαζομένων εἰς τοὺς βυζαντινοὺς καὶ μεταβυζαντινοὺς ναοὺς τῆς Κύπρου." *Ἐπ.Ἑτ.Βυζ.Σπ.* 23 (1953): 290–303.

Chatzipsaltes, K. "Ἡ Κύπρος κατὰ τὸ δεύτερον ἥμισυ τοῦ ἐνάτου καὶ τὰς ἀρχὰς τοῦ δεκάτου αἰῶνος." In *Πεπραγμένα τοῦ IX διεθνοῦς βυζαντινολογικοῦ Συνεδρίου*, 2:327–41. Thessalonike, 1959.

———. "Ἡ Κύπρος, τὸ Βυζάντιον καὶ τὸ Ἰσλάμ: Ἡ ναυτικὴ σπουδαιότης τῆς Κύπρου κατὰ τὴν περίοδον τῶν ἀραβοβυζαντινῶν συγκρούσεων (648–965 μ.Χ.)." *Κυπρ.Σπ.* 20 (1956): 13–29.

Chatzoule, G. M. "Αμφίγραπτη εικόνα του Αγίου Νικολάου από την Πτελέα Καστοριάς." *Βυζαντινά* 18 (1995–96): 381–403.

Chiavari, G., D. Fabbri, S. Prati, R. Mazzeo, D. Bikiaris, Sister Daniilia, and Y. Chryssoulakis. "Analytical Pyrolysis: Application to the Chemical Characterisation of Byzantine Painting Layers." In *Proceedings of the 6th International Conference on Non-Destructive Testing and Microanalysis for the Diagnostics and Conservation of the Cultural and Environmental Heritage, Rome, 17–20 May 1999*, 2:1145–62. Rome, 1999.

Chiovaro, F., et al., eds. *Histoire des saints et de la sainteté Chrétienne.* 11 vols. Paris, 1986–88.

Cholet, D. de. "Fresque du Jugement dernier dans l'église de Saint-Héraclide au monastère de Saint-Jean Lampadistis à Chypre." *Cahiers Balkaniques* 6 (1984): 107–15.

Chotzakoglou, Ch. G. "Βυζαντινή αρχιτεκτονική και τέχνη στην Κύπρο." In *Ιστορία της Κύπρου,* volume 3, *Βυζαντινή Κύπρος*, ed. Th. Papadopoullos, 1:465–787 and vol. 2 (plates). Nicosia, 2005.

Christe, Y. *Jugements derniers.* Saint-Léger-Vauban, 1999.

Christides, V. *The Image of Cyprus in the Arabic Sources.* Nicosia, 2006.

Christodoulou, M., and K. Konstantinidis. *A Complete Gazetteer of Cyprus*. Nicosia, 1987.

Christoforaki, I. "Cyprus between Byzantium and the Levant: Eclecticism and Interchange in the Cycle of the Life of the Virgin in the Church of the Holy Cross at Pelendri." *Ἐπ.Κέν.Ἐπιστ.Ἐρ.* 21 (1996): 215–55.

———. "Displaying the Liturgy: The Apse Decoration of the Church of Archangel Michael at Lefkara, Cyprus." Paper read at the Twenty-first International Congress of Byzantine Studies, London, 23 August 2006.

———. "Female Dress in Cyprus during the Medieval Period." In *Female Costume in Cyprus from Antiquity to the Present Day*, ed. V. Karageorghis and L. L. Hadjigavriel, 13–19. Nicosia, 1999.

———. "Η Τέχνη στην Κύπρο την εποχή του Μαχαιρά και του Βουστρώνιου." In *Πρακτικά συμποσίου "Λεόντιος Μαχαιράς—Γεώργιος Βουστρώνιος, Δύο χρονικά της μεσαιωνικής Κύπρου,"* 87–96. Nicosia, 1996.

———. "An Unusual Representation of the Incredulity from Lusignan Cyprus." *CahArch* 48 (2000): 71–87.

———. "Χορηγικές μαρτυρίες στους ναούς της μεσαιωνικής Ρόδου (1204–1522)." In *Ρόδος 2.400 χρόνια: Η πόλη της Ρόδου από την ίδρυσή της μέχρι την κατάληψη από τους Τούρκους (1523), Πρακτικά*, 2:449–64. Athens, 2000.

Clédat, J. *Le monastère et la nécropole de Baouît.* Mémoires publiés par les membres de l'Institut français d'archéologie orientale du Caire 12. Cairo, 1904.

———. *Le monastère et la nécropole de Baouît*. Mémoires publiés par les membres de l'Institut français d'archéologie orientale du Caire 39. Cairo, 1916.

Collins, K. M. "Visual Piety and Institutional Identity at Sinai." In *Holy Image, Hallowed Ground: Icons from Sinai*, ed. R. S. Nelson and K. M. Collins, 95–119. Exh. cat., The J. Paul Getty Museum, Los Angeles, 14 November 2006 – 4 March 2007. Los Angeles, 2006.

Connor, C. L. *Art and Miracles in Medieval Byzantium: The Crypt of Hosios Loukas*. Princeton, 1991.

———. "Female Saints in Church Decoration of the Troodos Mountains in Cyprus." In *Medieval Cyprus: Studies in Art, Architecture, and History in Memory of Doula Mouriki*, ed. N. P. Ševčenko and C. Moss, 211–40. Princeton, 1999.

Constable, G. "Dumbarton Oaks and Byzantine Field Work." *DOP* 37 (1983): 171–76.

Constantine VII Porphyrogenitus. *De Cerimoniis*. Ed. and trans. A. Vogt as *Le livre des cérémonies*. 2 vols. Paris, 1935–39.

Constantinides, C. N. *Η διήγησις της θαυματουργής εικόνας της Θεοτόκου Ελεούσας του Κύκκου*. Nicosia, 2002.

Constantinides, C. N., and R. Browning. *Dated Greek Manuscripts from Cyprus to the Year 1570*. DOS 30; Texts and Studies of the History of Cyprus 18. Washington, D.C.–Nicosia, 1993.

Constantinides, E. C. *The Wall Paintings of the Panagia Olympiotissa at Elasson in Northern Thessaly*. 2 vols. Athens, 1992.

Constantoudaki-Kitromelides, M. *The Churches of the Virgin Podythou and of the Theotokos (or of the Archangel) in Galata*. Nicosia, 2007. In collaboration with D. Myrianthefs.

———. *Οι ναοί της Παναγίας Ποδύθου και της Θεοτόκου (ή του Αρχαγγέλου) στη Γαλάτα*. Nicosia, 2005.

———. "La pittura di icone a Creta Veneziana (secoli XV e XVI): Questioni di mecenatismo, iconografia e preferenze estetiche." In *Venezia e Creta: Atti del Convegno Internazionale di Studi, Iraklion–Chanià, 30 settembre – 5 ottobre 1997*, 459–507. Venice, 1998.

———. "Taste and the Market in Cretan Icons in the Fifteenth and Sixteenth Centuries." In *From Byzantium to El Greco: Greek Frescoes and Icons*, ed. M. Acheimastou-Potamianou, 51–53. Exh. cat., Royal Academy of Arts–London. Athens, 1987.

Cormack, R. *Writing in Gold: Byzantine Society and Its Icons*. London, 1985.

Cormack, R., and S. Mihalarias. "A Crusader Painting of St. George: 'Maniera greca' or 'Lingua franca'?" *The Burlington Magazine* 126 (1984): 132–41.

Corrie, R. "The Political Meaning of Coppo di Marcovaldo's Madonna and Child in Siena." *Gesta* 29 (1990): 61–75.

Cotsonis, J. "The Contribution of Byzantine Lead Seals to the Study of the Cult of the Saints (Sixth–Twelfth Century)." *Byzantion* 75 (2005): 383–497.

———. "The Virgin and Justinian on Seals of the *Ekklesiekdikoi* of Hagia Sophia." *DOP* 56 (2002): 41–55.

Coumbaraki-Pansélinou, N. *Saint-Pierre de Kalyvia-Kouvara et la chapelle de la Vierge de Mérenta: Deux monuments du XIIIe siècle en Attique*. Thessalonike, 1976.

Coureas, N. *The Latin Church in Cyprus, 1195–1312*. Aldershot, 1997.

———. "The Place to Be: Migrations to Lusignan and Venetian Cyprus." *Κυπρ.Σπ.* 66 (2002): 125–45.

Coureas, N., and C. Schabel, eds. *The Cartulary of the Cathedral of Holy Wisdom of Nicosia*. Texts and Studies of the History of Cyprus 25. Nicosia, 1997.

Couroupou, M., and P. Géhin, "Nouveaux documents chypriotes extraits des manuscrits." *REB* 59 (2001): 147–64.

Cramer, J. A. *Anecdota Graeca e Codd. Manuscriptis Bibliothecae Regiae Parisiensis.* Vol. 4. Oxford, 1841; repr. Hildesheim, 1967.

Cumont, F. "Les vents et les anges psychopompes." In *Pisciculi: Studien zur Religion und Kultur des Altertums, Franz Ioseph Dölger zum 60. Geburtstag*, 70–75. Münster, 1939.

Ćurčić, S. "Architectural Significance of Subsidiary Chapels in Middle Byzantine Churches." *JSAH* 36, no. 2 (1977): 94–110.

———. *Middle Byzantine Architecture on Cyprus, Provincial or Regional?* Nicosia, 2000.

———. "The Twin-Domed Narthex in Paleologan Architecture." *ZRVI* 13 (1971): 333–44.

Cutler, A. *The Aristocratic Psalters in Byzantium*. Paris, 1984.

———. "Under the Sign of the Deesis: On the Question of Representativeness in Medieval Art and Literature." *DOP* 41 (1987): 145–54.

Cutler, A., and J.-M. Spieser. *Byzance médiévale: 700–1240*. Paris, 1996.

Cvetković, B. "Prilog proučavanju vizantijskog dvorskog kostima—γρανάτζα, λαπάτζας." *ZRVI* 34 (1995): 143–56.

Dagron, G. "Hériter de soi-même." In *La transmission du patrimoine: Byzance et l'aire méditerranéenne,* ed. J. Beaucamp and G. Dagron, 81–99. Travaux et mémoires du Centre de recherche d'histoire et civilisation de Byzance: Monographies 11. Paris, 1998.

Damianos (Archbishop) of Sinai. "The Medieval Saints of the Orthodox Church in Byzantine Art." In *Material Culture and Well-Being in Byzantium (400–1453):*

Proceedings of the International Conference (Cambridge, 8–10 September 2001), ed. M. Grünbart et al., 41–50. Vienna, 2007.

Daniilia (Sister), and E. Minopoulou. "A Study of Smalt and Red Lead Discolouration in *Antiphonitis* Wall Paintings in Cyprus." *Applied Physics A: Materials Science and Processing* 96, no. 3 (2009): 701–11.

Daniilia (Sister), E. Minopoulou, D. Demosthenous, and G. Karagiannis. "A Comparative Study of Wall Paintings at the Cypriot Monastery of Christ Antiphonitis: One Artist or Two?" *Journal of Archaeological Science* 35, no. 6 (2008): 1695–1707.

Daniilia (Sister), S. Sotiropoulou, D. Bikiaris, C. Salpistis, G. Karagiannis, Y. Chryssoulakis, B. A. Price, and J. H. Carlson. "Panselinos' Byzantine Wall Paintings in the Protaton Church, Mount Athos, Greece: A Technical Examination." *Journal of Cultural Heritage* 1, no. 2 (2000): 91–110.

Darrouzès, J. "Autres manuscrits originaires de Chypre." *REB* 15 (1957): 131–68. Repr. in idem, *Littérature et histoire*, art. XII. London, 1972.

———. *Littérature et histoire des textes byzantins*. London, 1972.

———. "Le mouvement de fondations monastiques au XIe siècle." *TM* 6 (1976): 159–76.

———. "Notes pour servir à l'histoire de Chypre." *Κυπρ.Σπ.* 17 (1953): 81–102. Repr. in idem, *Littérature et histoire*, art. XIV.

———. "Notes pour servir à l'histoire de Chypre, deuxième article." *Κυπρ.Σπ.* 20 (1956): 31–63. Repr. in idem, *Littérature et histoire*, art. XV.

———. "Notes pour servir à l'histoire de Chypre, troisième article." *Κυπρ.Σπ.* 22 (1958): 221–50. Repr. in idem, *Littérature et histoire*, art. XIII.

———. "Un obituaire chypriote: Le *Parisinus Græcus* 1588." *Κυπρ.Σπ.* 15 (1951): 23–62. Repr. in idem, *Littérature et histoire*, art. XIII.

David-Danel, M. L. *Iconographie des saints médecins Côme et Damien*. Lille, 1958.

Davidov-Temerinski, A. "Ciklus strašnog suda." In *Zidno slikarstvo manastira Dečana: Gradja i studije*, ed. V. Djurić, 191–211. Belgrade, 1995.

Deer, W. A., R. A. Howie, and J. Zussman. *An Introduction to the Rock-Forming Minerals*. 2nd ed. London, 1992.

Deichmann, F. W. *Frühchristliche Bauten und Mosaiken von Ravenna*. Baden-Baden, 1958.

Delamare, F. "Les terres vertes et leur utilisation en peinture murale romaine." In *Datation-Caractérisation des peintures pariétales et murales*, ed. F. Delamare, T. Hackens, and B. Helly, 345–73. PACT 17. Ravello, 1987.

Delatte, A., ed. "Traité de Magie de Salomon." In *Anecdota Atheniensia*, ed. idem, 1:397–445. Liège–Paris, 1927.

Delehaye, H. "L'Invention des reliques de Saint Menas à Constantinople." *AB* 29 (1910): 117–50.

———, ed. *Les légendes grecques des saints militaires*. Paris, 1909.

———. "Saints de Chypre." *AB* 26 (1907): 161–301.

———, ed. *Synaxarium Ecclesiae Constantinopolitanae: Propylaeum ad Acta sanctorum Novembris*. Brussels, 1902.

Demetrokalles, G. *Βυζαντινή ναοδομία στη Νάξο*. Athens, 2000.

———. *Οἱ δίκογχοι χριστιανικοὶ ναοί*. Athens, 1976.

———. "Ὁ ναός τοῦ Ἁγίου Γεωργίου τοῦ Διασορίτου τῆς Τραγαίας Νάξου." *Τεχνικά Χρονικά* 217 (1962): 29–58. Repr. Athens, 1972.

Demus, O. *Byzantine Mosaic Decoration: Aspects of Monumental Art in Byzantium*. London, 1949.

———. *The Mosaics of Norman Sicily*. London, 1949.

———. *The Mosaics of San Marco in Venice*. 2 vols. in 4 parts. Chicago, 1984.

———. "Das Paradies von San Marco." In *Festschrift für Herbert von Einem zum 16. Februar 1965*, ed. G. von der Osten and G. Kauffmann, 51–59. Berlin, 1965.

Denninger, E. "What is 'Bianco di San Giovanni' of Cennino Cennini?" *Studies in Conservation* 19 (1974): 185–87.

Der Nersessian, S. *Armenian Manuscripts in the Freer Gallery of Art*. Washington, D.C., 1963.

———. "Deux exemples arméniens de la Vierge de Miséricorde." *RÉArm* 7 (1970): 187–202.

———. "The Illustrations of the Homilies of Gregory of Nazianzus: Par. gr. 510." *DOP* 16 (1962): 195–228.

———. *Miniature Painting in the Armenian Kingdom of Cilicia*. 2 vols. DOS 31. Washington, D.C., 1993.

———. "Program and Iconography of the Frescoes of the Parecclesion." In *The Kariye Djami*, volume 4, *Studies in the Art of the Kariye Djami and Its Intellectual Background*, ed. P. A. Underwood, 303–49. Bollingen Series 70. Princeton, 1975.

———. "Two Images of the Virgin in the Dumbarton Oaks Collection." *DOP* 14 (1960): 69–86.

Derbes, A. *Picturing the Passion in Late Medieval Italy: Narrative Painting, Franciscan Ideologies, and the Levant*. New York, 1996.

———. "Siena and the Levant in the Later Dugento." *Gesta* 28 (1989): 190–204.

Derrick, M. R. "Infrared Microspectroscopy in the Analysis of Cultural Artifacts." In *Practical Guide to Infrared Microspectroscopy*, ed. H. J. Humecki, 287–322. New York, 1995.

Detorakes, Th. "Η λαϊκὴ λατρεία τοῦ Ἁγίου Μάμα στὴν Κρήτη." *Ὕδωρ ἐκ Πέτρας* 5–6 (1982–83): 107–34.

Deubner, L. *Kosmas und Damian: Texte und Einleitung*. Leipzig–Berlin, 1907.

Deuchler, F. *Duccio*. Milan, 1984.

Dianoux de la Perrotine, H. J. de. "Saint Louis à Chypre." In *Πρακτικὰ τοῦ πρώτου διεθνοῦς κυπρολογικοῦ συνεδρίου*, 2:13–16.

Diez, E., and O. Demus. *Byzantine Mosaics in Greece: Hosios Lucas and Daphni*. Cambridge, Mass., 1931.

Dikigoropoulos, A. I. "The Political Status of Cyprus A.D. 648–965." In *RDAC* (1940–48): 94–114. Nicosia, 1958.

Dionysios of Fourna. *Ἑρμηνεία τῆς ζωγραφικῆς τέχνης*. Ed. A. Papadopoulos-Kerameus. St. Petersburg, 1909.
———. *Hermeneia*. Trans. P. Hetherington as *The Painter's Manual of Dionysius of Fourna*. London, 1974.
The Divine Liturgy of Our Father among the Saints Basil the Great. Brookline, Mass., 1988.
Djordjević, I. M. "Der heilige Demetrios in den serbischen adligen Stiftungen aus der Zeit der Nemaniden." In *L'art de Thessalonique et des pays balkaniques et les courants spirituels au XIVe siècle: Recueil des rapports du IVe colloque serbo-grec, Belgrade 1985*, 67–73. Belgrade, 1987.
Djordjević, I. M., and M. Marković. "On the Dialogue Relationship Between the Virgin and Christ in East Christian Art." *Zograf* 28 (2000–2001): 13–48.
Djurić, V. I. *Icônes de Yougoslavie*. Belgrade, 1961.
———. *Sopoćani*. Leipzig, 1967.
———. *Byzantinische Fresken in Jugoslawien*. Munich, 1976.
Dmitrievskij, A. *Opisanie liturgičeskich rukopisej*. 3 vols. Kiev, 1895–1917; repr. Hildesheim, 1965.
Dodd, E. C. *The Frescoes of Mar Musa al-Habashi: A Study in Medieval Painting in Syria*. Toronto, 2001.
———. *Medieval Painting in the Lebanon*. Wiesbaden, 2004.
Dölger, F. "Justinians Engel an der Kaisertür der H. Sophia." *Byzantion* 10 (1935): 1–4.
Drakopoulou, E. *Η Πόλη της Καστοριάς τη βυζαντινή και μεταβυζαντινή εποχή (12ος–16ος αι.). Ιστορία—τέχνη—επιγραφές*. Athens, 1997.
———. "Οι φόβοι της τιμωρίας στη βυζαντινή και μεταβυζαντινή ζωγραφική." In *Οι Συλλογικοί Φόβοι στην Ιστορία*, 93–110. Athens, 2000.
Drandakes, N. V. *Βυζαντινές τοιχογραφίες της Μέσα Μάνης*. Athens, 1995.
———. "Πόκος ή νεφέλη: Ἀσυνήθιστη λεπτομέρεια της παραστάσεως του Εὐαγγελισμού στη βυζαντινή εἰκονογραφία." *Ἐπιστημονική Ἐπετηρίς της Φιλοσοφικής Σχολής του Πανεπιστημίου Ἀθηνών* 26 (1977–78): 258–67.
Drandaki, A., ed. *Pilgrimage to Sinai: Treasures from the Holy Monastery of Saint Catherine*. Exh. cat., Benaki Museum, 20 July–26 September 2004. Athens, 2004.
Drewer, L. "Saints and their Families in Byzantine Art." *Δελτ.Χριστ.Ἀρχ.Ἑτ.*, ser. 4, 16 (1991–92): 259–70.
Drossoyianni, P. "Some Observations on the Asinou Frescoes." *Κληρονομία* 10 (1978): 53–77.
———. *Σχόλια στὶς τοιχογραφίες τῆς ἐκκλησίας τοῦ Ἁγίου Ἰωάννου τοῦ Προδρόμου στὴ Μεγάλη Καστάνια Μάνης*. Athens, 1982.
Duba, W. "The Afterlife in Medieval Frankish Cyprus." *Ἐπ.Κέν.Ἐπιστ.Ἐρ.* 26 (2000): 167–94.
Dunn, K. "The Reverend Flock: A Monastic Reading of the Cult of the Forty Martyrs of Sebasteia." Paper presented at the Medieval Studies Graduate Student Colloquium, Cornell University, spring 2002.
Edbury, P. W. *The Kingdom of Cyprus and the Crusades 1191–1374*. Cambridge, 1991.
Emmanouelides, N. E. *Το δίκαιο της ταφής στο Βυζάντιο*. Forschungen zur byzantinischen Rechtsgeschichte, Athener Reihe 3. Athens, 1989.
Emmanuel, M. "Hairstyles and Headdresses of Empresses, Princesses, and Ladies of the Aristocracy in Byzantium." *Δελτ.Χριστ.Ἀρχ.Ἑτ.*, ser. 4, 17 (1993–94): 113–20.
———. "Monumental Painting in Cyprus during the Last Phase of the Lusignan Dynasty, 1374–1489." In Ševčenko and Moss, *Medieval Cyprus*, 241–62.
———. "Ο ναός της Παναγίας στο Μουτουλλά της Κύπρου. Οι τοιχογραφίες της μεταβυζαντινής εποχής." *Κυπρ.Σπ.* 61 (1997): 107–37.
———. *Οἱ τοιχογραφίες τοῦ Ἁγ. Δημητρίου στὸ Μακρυχώρι καὶ τῆς Κοιμήσεως τῆς Θεοτόκου στὸν Ὀξύλιθο τῆς Εὔβοιας*. Athens, 1991.
———. "Οι τοιχογραφίες του Αγίου Νικολάου στην Αγόριανη της Λακωνίας." *Δελτ.Χριστ.Ἀρχ.Ἑτ.*, ser. 4, 14 (1987–88): 107–50.
Englezakis, B. *Studies on the History of the Church of Cyprus, 4th–20th Centuries*. Trans. N. Russell, ed. S. Ioannou and M. Ioannou. Aldershot, 1995.
Enlart, C. *Gothic Art and the Renaissance in Cyprus*. Ed. and trans. D. Hunt. London, 1987.
Epstein, A. "The Middle Byzantine Sanctuary Barrier: Templon or Iconostasis." *Journal of the British Archaeological Association* 134 (1981): 1–27.
———. "The Political Content of the Paintings at Saint Sophia at Ohrid." *JÖB* 29 (1980): 315–30.
———. *Tokalı Kilise: Tenth-Century Metropolitan Art in Byzantine Cappadocia*. DOS 22. Washington, D.C., 1986.
Esbroeck, M. van. "La diffusion orientale de la légende de saints Cosme et Damien." In *Hagiographie, cultures et sociétés*, 61–77. Paris, 1981.
———. "La légende 'romaine' des SS. Côme et Damien (BHG 373d) et sa métaphrase géorgiennne par Jean Xiphilin." *OrChrP* 47 (1981): 389–425; 48 (1982): 29–64.
Ettinghausen, R. *Arab Painting*. Geneva, 1962.
Eustratiades, S. *Ἁγιολόγιον τῆς Ὀρθοδόξου Ἐκκλησίας*. Athens, n.d.
———. *Θεοτοκάριον*. Vol. 1. Chennevières-sur-Marne, 1931.
Evangelatou-Notara, F. "ΑΔΕΛΦΑΤΟΝ ΨΥΧΙΚΟΝ: Evidence from Notes on Manuscripts." *Byzantion* 75 (2005): 164–70.
———. *Χορηγοί–Κτήτορες–Δωρητές σε σημειώματα κωδίκων: Παλαιολόγειοι χρόνοι*. Athens, 2000.
Evans, H. C., ed. *Byzantium, Faith and Power (1261–1557)*. Exh. cat., The Metropolitan Museum of Art, New York, 23 March–4 July 2004. New York, 2004.
Evans, H. C., and W. D. Wixom, eds. *The Glory of Byzantium: Art and Culture of the Middle Byzantine Era, A.D. 843–1261*. Exh. cat., The Metropolitan Museum, New York, 11 March–6 July 1997. New York, 1997.
Falla Castelfranchi, M. "Culto e immagini dei Santi Medici nell'Italia meridionale bizantina e normana." In *La cultura scientifica e tecnica nell'Italia meridionale bizantina: Atti della sesta giornata di studi bizantini; Arcavacata di*

Rende, 8–9 febbraio 2000, ed. F. Buzgarella and A. M. Ieraci Bio, 59–95. Soveria Mannelli, 2006.

Farmer, V. C., ed. *The Infrared Spectra of Minerals.* Mineralogical Society, Monograph 4. London, 1974.

Fedwick, P. J. "Death and Dying in Byzantine Liturgical Traditions." *EChR* 8 (1976): 152–61.

Feissel, D., and A. Philippidis-Braat. "Inventaires en vue d'un recueil des inscriptions historiques de Byzance: III. Inscriptions du Péloponnèse." *TM* 9 (1985): 267–395.

Festugière, A.-J., ed. and trans. *Sainte Thècle, saints Côme et Damien, saints Cyr et Jean (extraits), saint Georges.* Paris, 1971.

Finney, P. C. "Abraham and Isaac Iconography on Late Antique Amulets and Seals: The Western Evidence." *JbAC* 38 (1995): 140–66.

Fischer, C., and I. Kakoulli. "An Innovative Noninvasive and Nondestructive Multidisciplinary Approach for the Technical Study of the Byzantine Wall Paintings in the Enkleistra of St. Neophytos in Paphos, Cyprus." Project Grant Report. Washington, D.C., 2009. http://www.doaks.org/research/byzantine/doaks_eid_2424.html [accessed 4 March 2012].

———. "In Situ Reflectance and X-Ray Fluorescence Spectroscopy for the Study of the 12th Century Rock-Cut Paintings in the Enkleistra of St. Neophytos in Cyprus." In preparation.

———. "Multispectral and Hyperspectral Imaging Technologies in Conservation: Current Research and Potential Applications." *Reviews in Conservation* 7 (2006): 3–16.

Folda, J. *The Art of the Crusaders in the Holy Land, 1098–1187.* New York, 1995.

———. *Crusader Art in the Holy Land, From the Third Crusade to the Fall of Acre, 1187–1291.* New York, 2005.

———. "Crusader Art in the Kingdom of Cyprus, c. 1275–1291: Reflections on the State of the Questions." In *Η Κύπρος και οι Σταυροφορίες / Cyprus and the Crusades,* ed. N. Coureas and J. Riley-Smith, 209–37. Nicosia, 1995.

———, ed. *Crusader Art in the Twelfth Century.* BAR International Series 152. Oxford, 1982.

———. *Crusader Manuscript Illumination at Saint-Jean d'Acre, 1275–1291.* Princeton, 1976.

———. "The Figural Arts in Crusader Syria and Palestine, 1187–1291: Some New Realities." *DOP* 58 (2004): 315–31.

———. "The Saint Marina Icon: Maniera Cypria, Lingua Franca, or Crusader Art?" In *Four Icons in the Menil Collection,* ed. B. Davezac, 106–33. Houston, 1992.

Follieri, E. *I calendari in metro innografico di Cristoforo Mitileneo.* 2 vols. Brussels, 1980.

———. "Il calendario giambico di Cristoforo di Mitilene secondo i mss. Palat. gr. 383 e Paris. gr. 3041." *AB* 77 (1959): 245–304.

———. "Un carmine giambico in onore di Davide." *Studi bizantini e neoellenici* 9 (1957): 101–16.

———. *Initia Hymnorum Ecclesiae Graecae.* 5 vols. Vatican City, 1962.

Foskolou, V. "Αναζητώντας την εικόνα του Ελκομένου της Μονεμβασίας: Το χαμένο παλλάδιο της πόλης και η επίδρασή του στα υστεροβυζαντινά μνημεία του νότιου ελλαδικού χώρου." *Σύμμεικτα* 24 (2001): 229–55. [English summary, 256, as "Tracing the Monemvasia Icon of Christ Helkomenos: The City's Lost Palladium and Its Influence on the Late Byzantine Monuments of Southern Greece."]

Fotić, A. "The Official Explanations for the Confiscation and Sale of Monasteries (Churches) and their Estates at the Time of Selim II." *Turcica* 26 (1994): 33–54.

Foulias, A. *The Church of Our Lady Angeloktisti, Larnaka.* Nicosia, 2004.

Frantz, A. "Byzantine Illuminated Ornament: A Study in Chronology." *ArtB* 16 (1934): 43–76.

Frieden, V. "The Wall Paintings of the Church of Agios Ioannis Prodhromos, Askas, Cyprus: A Technical Study." Diploma diss., Courtauld Institute of Art, University of London, 1997.

Frigerio, F. "Una raffigurazione post-bizantina della Terra come Πότνια Θηρών, ad Asinou de Cipro." *Conoscenza Religiosa* 3 (1977): 218–23.

Frigerio-Zeniou, S. *L'art "italo-byzantin" à Chypre au XVIe siècle: Trois témoins de la peinture religieuse: Panagia Podithou, la Chapelle Latine et Panagia Iamatikê.* Bibliothèque de l'Institut hellénique d'études byzantines et post-byzantines de Venise 20. Venice, 1998.

———. "Οι δωρητές στην εκκλησία της Παναγίας Ποδίθου στη Γαλάτα και στο λατινικό παρεκκλήσι του Καλοπαναγιώτη." *Κυπρ.Σπ.* 51 (1997): 97–102.

———. "Κυπριώτισσες Κυράδες: Reflets de la mode féminine à Chypre au XVIe siècle." *Κυπρ.Σπ.* 67–68 (2003–4): 245–315.

———. "Μονὴ τῶν Φορβίων à Asinou de Chypre." In *ΒΟΥΚΟΛΕΙΑ: Mélanges offerts à Bertrand Bouvier,* ed. A. D. Lazaridis, V. Barras, and T. Birchler, 191–99. Geneva, 1995.

Frolow, A. "IC XC NI KA." *BSl* 17 (1956): 98–113.

Gabelić, S. "The Church of the Virgin near Kophinou, Cyprus." *Κυπρ.Σπ.* 48 (1984): 143–60.

———. "Contribution to the Iconography of Saint Mamas and Saints with Attributes." In *Πρακτικὰ τοῦ δευτέρου διεθνοῦς κυπρολογικοῦ συνεδρίου,* 2:577–81.

———. "Linearno slikarstvo sisojevca." In *Papers of the Third Yugoslav Byzantine Studies Conference, Kruševac 10–13 May 2000,* 417–40. Belgrade–Kruševac, 2002.

———. *Manastir Lesnovo: Istorija i slikarstvo.* Belgrade, 1998.

———. "Predstave Sv. Mamanta u zidnom slikarstvu na Kipru." *Zograf* 15 (1984): 69–75.

Gaetani, M. C., U. Santamaria, and C. Seccaroni. "The Use of Egyptian Blue and Lapis Lazuli in the Middle Ages: The Wall Paintings of the San Saba Church in Rome." *Studies in Conservation* 49, no. 1 (2004): 13–22.

Gagniers, J. des, and T. T. Tinh. *Soloi: Dix campagnes des fouilles (1964–1974).* Volume 1, *La basilique.* St. Foye, 1985.

Galadza, P. "The Evolution of Funerals for Monks in the Byzantine Realm: From the Tenth to the Sixteenth Century." *OCP* 70 (2004): 225–57.

Galatariotou, C. "Byzantine Ktetorika Typika: A Comparative Study." *REB* 45 (1987): 77–138.
———. *The Making of a Saint: The Life, Times and Sanctification of Neophytos the Recluse*. Cambridge, 1991.
Galavaris, G. *An Eleventh Century Hexaptych of the Saint Catherine's Monastery at Mount Sinai*. Venice–Athens, 2009.
Gallas, K., K. Wessel, and M. Borboudakis. *Byzantinisches Kreta*. Munich, 1983.
Gamillscheg, E. "Zypern oder nicht Zypern?" *JÖB* 47 (1997): 239–43.
Garides, M. K. *Études sur le Jugement dernier post-byzantin du XVe à la fin du XIXe siècle: Iconographie–Esthéthique*. Thessalonike, 1985.
———. "Icônes du XIIIe et du XIVe siècles dans l'aire du Patriarchat de Jérusalem." In *ΕΥΨΥΧΙΑ: Mélanges offerts à Hélène Ahrweiler*, 225–38. Byzantina sorbonensia 16. Paris, 1998.
———. "Les punitions collectives et individuelles des damnés dans le Jugement dernier (du XIIe au XIVe siècle)." *ZbLikUmet* 18 (1982): 1–17.
Gavrilović, Z. "Discs Held by Angels in the Anastasis at Dečani." In *Byzantine East, Latin West: Art-Historical Studies in Honor of Kurt Weitzmann*, ed. C. Moss and K. Kiefer, 225–30. Princeton, 1995. Repr. in eadem, *Studies in Byzantine and Serbian Medieval Art*, 184–89. London, 2001.
———. "St. Ephraim the Syrian's Thought and Imagery as an Inspiration to Byzantine Artists." In eadem, *Studies in Byzantine and Serbian Medieval Art*, 244–70. London, 2001.
Georgiou, S. "Περί του κτίτορος της Μονής της Παναγίας της Ασίνου Νικηφόρου Ισχυρίου." *Επετηρίδα Κέντρου Μελετών Ιεράς Μονής Κύκκου* 7 (2006): 191–98.
Georgitsoyanni, E. N. *Les Peintures murales du vieux Catholicon du monastère de la Transfiguration aux Météores (1483)*. Athens, 1993.
Gerola, G. *Monumenti Veneti nell'isola di Creta*. 4 vols. Venice, 1905–32.
Gerola, G., and K. Lassithiotakes. *Τοπογραφικὸς κατάλογος τῶν τοιχογραφημένων ἐκκλησιῶν τῆς Κρήτης*. Herakleion, 1961.
Gerov, G. "The Narthex as Desert: The Symbolism of the Entrance Space in Orthodox Church Buildings." In *Ritual and Art: Byzantine Essays for Christopher Walter*, ed. P. Armstrong, 144–59. London, 2006.
Gerstel, S. E. J. "An Alternate View of the Late Byzantine Sanctuary Screen." In eadem, *Thresholds of the Sacred*, 135–61.
———. "Art and Identity in the Medieval Morea." In *The Crusades from the Perspective of Byzantium and the Muslim World*, ed. A. Laiou and R. P. Mottahedeh, 263–85. Washington, D.C., 2001.
———. *Beholding the Sacred Mysteries: Programs of the Byzantine Sanctuary*. College Art Association Monographs on the Fine Arts 56. Seattle–London, 1999.
———. "The Byzantine Village Church: Observations on its Location and on Agricultural Aspects of its Program." In *Les villages dans l'empire byzantin (IVe–XVe siècle)*, ed. J. Lefort, C. Morrisson, and J.-P. Sodini, 165–78. Réalités Byzantines 11. Paris, 2005.
———. "Painted Sources for Female Piety in Medieval Byzantium." *DOP* 52 (1998): 89–111.
———. "Saint Eudokia and the Imperial Household of Leo VI." *ArtB* 79, no. 4 (1997): 699–707.
———. "The Sins of the Farmer: Illustrating Village Life (and Death) in Medieval Byzantium." In *Word, Image, Number: Communication in the Middle Ages*, ed. J. Contreni and S. Casciani, 205–17. Florence, 2002.
———, ed. *Thresholds of the Sacred: Architectural, Art Historical, Liturgical, and Theological Perspectives on Religious Screens, East and West*. Washington, D.C., 2006.
Gerstel, S. E. J. and S. Kalopissi-Verti. "Female Church Founders: The Agency of the Village Widow in Late Byzantium." *Wiener Jahrbuch für Kunstgeschichte* 2012 (forthcoming).
Gettens, R. J., and G. L. Stout. *Painting Materials: A Short Encyclopaedia*. London, 1942; repr. New York, 1966.
Gettens, R. J., R. L. Feller, and W. T. Chase. "Vermilion and Cinnabar." *Studies in Conservation* 17, no. 2 (1972): 45–69.
Giotto e i Giotteschi in Assisi. Rome, 1969.
Given, M. *Troodos Archaeological and Environmental Survey Project*. University of Glasgow, Department of Archaeology. http://www.gla.ac.uk/departments/archaeology/research/projects/taesp/. Accessed 30 March 2009.
Gkioles, N. *Βυζαντινή ναοδομία, 600–1204*. Athens, 1992.
———. "Οἱ λειτουργικὲς πηγὲς τῆς Ἀνάληψης στὸ ναὸ τοῦ Ἁγίου Ἡρακλειδίου τῆς Μονῆς τοῦ Ἁγίου Ἰωάννη τοῦ Λαμπαδιστῆ." In *Πρακτικὰ τοῦ δευτέρου διεθνοῦς κυπρολογικοῦ συνεδρίου*, 2:513–21.
———. *Η χριστιανική τέχνη στήν Κύπρο*. Nicosia, 2003.
Gligorijević-Maksimović, M. "Slikani kalendar u Treskavac i stixovi Christofora Mitilenskog." *Zograf* 8 (1977): 48–54.
Goar, J., ed. *Euchologion sive rituale graecorum*. Venice, 1730; repr. Graz, 1960.
Goldhill, S. "The Naive and Knowing Eye: Ecphrasis and the Culture of Viewing in the Hellenistic World." In *Art and Text in Ancient Greek Culture*, ed. S. Goldhill and R. Osborne, 197–223. Cambridge, 1994.
Goodwin, J. C. *Toponymy of Cyprus*. 2nd ed. Nicosia, 1977.
Gordon, D. "A Perugian Provenance for the Franciscan Double-sided Altar-piece by the Maestro di S. Francesco." *The Burlington Magazine* 126 (February 1982): 70–77.
Gounares, G. G. *Χριστός Βέροιας*. Thessalonike, 1991.
Grabar, A. *L'art de la fin de l'Antiquité et du Moyen Age*. 3 vols. Paris, 1968.
———. *Byzantine Painting*. Geneva, 1963.
———. "Deux notes sur l'histoire de l'iconostase d'après des monuments de Yougoslavie." In idem, *L'Art de la fin*

de l'Antiquité et du Moyen-Age, 1:403–10. Paris, 1968. Originally publ. in *ZRVI* 7 (1961): 13–22.

———. *L'église de Boïana: Architecture—peinture.* Sofia, 1924.

———. *Martyrium: Recherches sur le culte des reliques et l'art chrétien antique.* 2 vols. London, 1972.

———. *Les miniatures du Grégoire de Nazianze de l'Ambrosienne (Ambrosianus 49–50).* Paris, 1943.

———. "Un nouveau reliquaire de saint Démétrius." *DOP* 8 (1954): 307–13.

———. "Zur Geschichte von Sphaira, Globus und Reichsapfel." In *L'art de la fin de l'Antiquité et du Moyen Age*, 1:103–11. Paris, 1968.

Greenhill, F. A. *Incised Effigial Slabs: A Study of Engraved Stone Memorials in Latin Christendom, c. 1100 to c. 1700.* 2 vols. London, 1976.

Greilsammer, M, ed. *Le livre au Roi*. Paris, 1995.

Grigoriadou, H. "Peintures murales du 12e siècle en Grèce." Paris, Positions Thèses 3e cycle, 1968.

Grigoriadou-Cabagnols, H. "Le décor peint de l'église de Samari en Messénie." *CahArch* 20 (1970): 177–96.

Grivaud, G. "Un état des comptes du royaume de Chypre en 1412–1413." *BCH* 122, no. 1 (1998): 377–401.

———. "Formes et mythe de la *strateia* à Chypre." *Études balkaniques, Cahiers Pierre Belon* 5 (1998): 33–54.

———. "Grecs et Francs dans le royaume de Chypre (1191–1474): Les voies de l'acculturation." Dissertation for the *habilitation à diriger les recherches*, Université de Paris I, 2001.

———. "Le monastère de Kykkos et ses revenus en 1553." *StVen* n.s. 19 (1990): 225–54.

———. "Pèlerinages grecs et latins dans le royaume de Chypre (1192–1474): Concurrence ou complémentarité?" In *Identités pèlerines*, ed. C. Vincent, 67–76. Rouen, 2004.

———. *Villages désertés à Chypre (fin XIIe–fin XIXe siècle).* Μελέται και Υπομνήματα 3. Nicosia, 1998.

Grosdidier de Matons, J., ed. *Romanos le Mélode: Hymnes; Introduction, texte critique, traduction et notes.* 5 vols. Paris, 1964–81.

Grossmann, J. "Zur nicht erhaltenen Nordtür der Dornbuschkapelle des Klosters der Hl. Aikaterina im Sinai." *JÖB* 50 (2000): 243–65.

Grozdanov, C., and L. Hadermann-Misguich. *Kurbinovo.* Skopje, 1992.

Guilland, R. "Études sur l'histoire administrative de l'Empire byzantin: L'ordre (τάξις) des Maîtres (τῶν μαγίστρων)." *Ἐπ.Ἑτ.Βυζ.Σπ.* 39–40 (1972–73): 14–28.

Gunnis, R. *Historic Cyprus: A Guide to Its Towns and Villages, Monasteries and Castles.* London, 1936.

Hackett, J. *A History of the Orthodox Church of Cyprus.* London, 1901.

Hadermann-Misguich, L. *Kurbinovo: Les fresques de Saint-Georges et la peinture byzantine du XIIe siècle.* 2 vols. Bibliothèque de Byzantion 6. Brussels, 1975.

———. "Tissus de pouvoir et de prestige sous les Macédoniens et les Comnènes: A propos des coussins-de-pieds et de leur représentations." *Δελτ.Χριστ.Ἀρχ.Ἑτ.*, ser. 4, 17 (1993–94): 121–28.

Hadjichristodoulou, C., and D. Myrianthefs. *The Church of Our Lady of Asinou.* Nicosia, 2002.

———. *Ο ναός της Παναγίας της Φορβιώτισσας στην Ασίνου / L'église de la Vierge Phorbiotissa à Asinou.* 2nd ed. Nicosia, 2009.

Hadjichristodoulou, C., and K. Papaioakeim. "Φορητὲς Εἰκόνες στὴν Ἱερὰ Μητρόπολη Μόρφου (12ος–19ος Αἰώνας)." In *Ἱερὰ Μητρόπολις Μόρφου*, 127–58.

Hadjisavvas, S. "Chronique des fouilles et découvertes archéologiques à Chypre en 2001." *BCH* 126, no. 2 (2002): 691–727.

———. "Chronique des fouilles et découvertes archéologiques à Chypre en 2002." *BCH* 127, no. 2 (2003): 649–82.

Halkin, F., ed. *Légendes grecques de "martyres Romaines."* Subsidia hagiographica 55. Brussels, 1973.

Hamann-MacLean, R. "Der Berliner Codex Graecus Quarto 66 und seine nächsten Verwandten als Beispiele des Stilwandels in frühen 13. Jahrhundert." In *Studien zur Buchmalerei und Goldschmiedekunst des Mittelalters: Festschrift für Hermann Usener*, ed. F. Detweiler et al., 225–50. Marburg an der Lahn, 1967.

Hamann-MacLean, R., and H. Hallensleben. *Die Monumentalmalerei in Serbien und Makedonien vom 11. bis zum frühen 14. Jahrhundert: Bildband.* Osteuropastudien der Hochschulen des Landes Hessen, Reihe II, Marburger Abhandlungen zur Geschichte und Kultur Osteuropas, Band 3–5. Gießen, 1963.

Havice, C. "The Hamilton Psalter in Berlin, Kupferstichkabinett 78.A.9." Ph.D. diss., Pennsylvania State University, 1978.

———. "The Marginal Miniatures in the Hamilton Psalter, Kupferstichkabinett 78.A.9." *Jahrbuch der Berliner Museen* 26 (1984): 79–142.

Hawkins, E. J. W. "Summary of Work Carried out at Asinou 1965." *RDAC* (1969): 80–81.

Hein, E., A. Jakovljević, and B. Kleidt. *Cyprus, Byzantine Churches and Monasteries: Mosaics and Frescoes.* Trans. J. M. Deasy. Ratingen, 1998.

Heiser, L. *Die Engel im Glauben der Orthodoxie.* Trier, 1976.

Hélou, N. "L'icône bilatérale de la Vierge de Kaftoun au Liban: une oeuvre d'art syro-byzantin à l'époque des croisés." *Chronos* 7 (2003): 101–31.

Hemmerdinger-Iliadou, D. "Les données archéologiques dans la version grecque des sermons de St. Ephrem le Syrien." *CahArch* 13 (1962): 29–37.

———. "Éphrem le Syrien." In *Dictionnaire de Spiritualité*, 4:788–819. Paris, 1960.

Hendy, M. F. *Catalogue of the Byzantine Coins in the Dumbarton Oaks Collection and in the Whittemore Collection*, vol. 4, pt. 1. Washington, D.C., 1999.

———. *Coinage and Money in the Byzantine Empire, 1081–1261.* DOS 12. Washington, D. C., 1969.

Herman, E. "Die Regelung der Armut in den byzantinischen Klöstern." *OCP* 7, nos. 3–4 (1941): 406–60.

———. "Ricerche sulle istituzioni monastiche bizantine: Typika ktetorika, caristicari e monasteri 'liberi'." *OCP* 6, nos. 3–4 (1940): 293–375.
Hetherington, P. "The Byzantine Reliquary at the Cathedral Museum." In *Portable Altars in Malta*, ed. J. Azzopardi, 39–56. Malta, 2000.
———. "Byzantine Steatites in the Possession of the Knights of Rhodes." *The Burlington Magazine* 120 (1978): 811–20.
Hill, G. F. *A History of Cyprus*. 4 vols. Cambridge, 1940–52.
Himmelfarb, M. *Tours of Hell: An Apocalyptic Form in Jewish and Christian Literature.* Philadelphia, 1983.
Hirschbichler, M. "The Crusader Painting in the Frankish Gate at Nauplia, Greece: A Historical Construct in the Latin Principality of Morea." *Gesta* 44, no. 1 (2005): 13–30.
Hörandner, W. "Das byzantinische Epigramm und das heilige Kreuz: einige Beobachtungen zu Motiven und Typen." In *La Croce: Iconografia e interpretazione (sec. I–inizio XVI); Atti del convegno internazionale di studi (Napoli, 6–11 dicembre 1999),* ed. B. Ulianich, 3:107–25. Naples, 2007.
———. "A Cycle of Epigrams on the Lord's Feasts in Cod. Marc. Gr. 524." *DOP* 48 (1994): 117–33.
———. "Randbemerkungen zum Thema Epigramme und Kunstwerke." In *Πολύπλευρος Νοῦς: Miscellanea für Peter Schreiner zu seinem 60. Geburtstag*, ed. C. Scholz and G. Makris, 69–82. Byzantinisches Archiv 19. Munich–Leipzig, 2000.
———. "Ein Zyklus von Epigrammen zu Darstellungen von Herrenfesten und Wunderszenen." *DOP* 46 (1992): 107–15.
Hörandner, W., and A. Rhoby, eds. *Die kulturhistorische Bedeutung byzantinischer Epigramme: Akten des internationalen Workshop (Wien, 1.–2. Dezember 2006).* Vienna, 2008.
Houston, M. G. *Medieval Costume in England and France: The 13th, 14th and 15th Centuries.* London, 1939; repr. New York, 1996.
Howard, H. "Blue in the Lewes Group." In *Early Medieval Wall Painting and Painted Sculpture in England*, ed. S. Cather, D. Park, and P. Williamson, 195–203. BAR British Series 216. Oxford, 1990.
———. "Church of Archangel Michael, Monagri, Cyprus: Scientific Examination of the Wall Paintings." Unpublished report, Courtauld Institute of Art, University of London, 1992.
Hunger, H. "Ελιγήσεται ὁ οὐρανὸς ὡς βιβλίον." *Κληρονομία* 1 (1969): 79–82.
———. "Gregorios von Korinth, Epigramme auf die Feste des Dodekaorton." *AB* 100 (1982): 637–51.
Hunt, L.-A. "Christian Art in Greater Syria and Egypt: A Triptych of the Ascension with Military Saints Reattributed." *Al-Masāq: Islam and the Medieval Mediterranean* 12 (2000): 1–36.
———. "Christian-Muslim Relations in Painting in Egypt of the Twelfth to Mid-Thirteenth Centuries: Sources of Wallpainting at Deir es-Suriani and the Illustration of the New Testament MS Paris, Copte-Arabe 1/Cairo, Bibl. 94." *CahArch* 33 (1985): 111–56. Repr. in eadem, *Byzantium, Eastern Christendom and Islam: Art at the Crossroads of the Medieval Mediterranean*, 1:205–81 (art. VIII). London, 1998–2000.
———. "The Fine Incense of Virginity: A Late Twelfth-Century Wall Painting of the Annunciation at the Monastery of the Syrians, Egypt." *BMGS* 19 (1995): 182–232.
———. "A Woman's Prayer to St. Sergios in Latin Syria: Interpreting a Thirteenth-Century Icon at Mount Sinai." *BMGS* 15 (1991): 96–145. Repr. in eadem, *Byzantium, Eastern Christendom and Islam: Art at the Crossroads of the Medieval Mediterranean*, 2:78–126 (art. XIV). London, 1998–2000.
Hutter, I. *Corpus der byzantinischen Miniaturenhandschriften*. Vol. 5, *Oxford College Libraries*. 2 parts. Stuttgart, 1997.
———. "The Magdalen College 'Musterbuch': A Painter's Guide from Cyprus at Oxford." In Ševčenko and Moss, *Medieval Cyprus*, 117–46.
———. *El Menologio de Oxford (Ms. Gr. th. f. 1, Bodleian Library, Oxford).* Libro de Estudios. Madrid, 2007.
Ἱερὰ Μητρόπολις Μόρφου: 2000 χρόνια τέχνης καὶ ἁγιότητος. Exh. cat., Cultural Foundation of the Bank of Cyprus. Nicosia, 2000.
Imhaus, B. *Un document démographique et fiscal vénitien concernant le casal du Marethasse (1549).* Μελέται και Υπομνήματα 1. Nicosia, 1984.
———, ed. *Lacrimae Cypriae: Les larmes de Chypre ou Recueil des inscriptions lapidaires pour la plupart funéraires de la période franque et vénitienne de l'île de Chypre.* 2 vols. Nicosia, 2004.
Immerzeel, M. "Divine Cavalry: Mounted Saints in Middle Eastern Christian Art." In *East and West in the Crusader States: Context—Contacts—Confrontations III; Acta of the Congress held at Hernen Castle, September 2000*, ed. K. Ciggaar and H. Teule, 265–86. Leuven, 2003.
———. "Holy Horsemen and Crusader Banners: Equestrian Saints in Wall Paintings in Lebanon and Syria." *East Christian Art* 1 (2004): 29–60.
Immerzeel, M., and N. Hélou. "Icon Painting in the County of Tripoli of the Thirteenth Century." In *Interactions: Artistic Interchange between the Eastern and Western Worlds in the Medieval Period*, ed. C. P. Hourihane, 67–83. Princeton, 2007.
Innemée, K. C. *Ecclesiastical Dress in the Medieval Near East*. Leiden–New York–Köln, 1992.
Ivanov, S. A. "'Dushepoleznaya istoriya' o raskayavshemsya razboĭnike (BHG, 1450m)." *VizVrem* 60 (85) (2001): 247–53.
Ivison, E. A. "Mortuary Practices in Byzantium (c. 950–1453): An Archaeological Contribution." 2 vols. Ph.D. diss., University of Birmingham, 1993.

James, L. "'And Shall These Mute Stones Speak?' Text as Art." In *Art and Text in Byzantine Culture*, ed. L. James, 188–206. Cambridge, 2007.
James, M. R., ed. *Apocrypha Anecdota: A Collection of Thirteen Apocryphal Books and Fragments*. Texts and Studies: Contributions to Biblical and Patristic Literature, vol. 2, no. 3. Cambridge, 1893.
Janc, Z. *Ornamenti fresaka iz Srbje i Makedonije od XII do seredine XV veka*. Belgrade, 1961.
Janin, R. *La géographie ecclésiastique de l'Empire byzantin*, vol. 1, *Le siège de Constantinople et le patriarcat oecuménique*, part 3, *Les églises et les monastères*. 2nd ed. Paris, 1969.
———. "Le monachisme byzantin au Moyen Age: Commende et typica (X^{e}–XIVe siècle)." *REB* 22 (1964): 5–44.
———. "Les sanctuaires byzantins de St. Michel (Constantinople et banlieue)." *EO* 33 (1934): 28–52.
Jeffery, G. *A Description of the Historic Monuments of Cyprus*. Nicosia, 1918; repr. London, 1983.
Jennings, R. C. *Christians and Muslims in Ottoman Cyprus and the Mediterranean World, 1571–1640*. New York, 1993.
Jerphanion, G. de. "Les caractéristiques et les attributs des saints dans la peinture cappadocienne." *AB* 55 (1937): 1–28.
———. *Une nouvelle province de l'art byzantin: Les églises rupestres de Cappadoce*. 3 vols. in 5. Paris, 1925–42.
John Lydus. *De Mensibus*. Ed. I. Bekker. Corpus Scriptorum Historiae Byzantinae. Bonn, 1837.
John of Ibelin. *Le Livre des Assises*. Ed. P. W. Edbury. Leiden, 2003.
Johnson, M. "The Lost Royal Portraits of Gerace and Cefalù Cathedrals." *DOP* 53 (1999): 237–62.
Jolivet-Lévy, C. *La Cappadoce médiévale: Images et spiritualité*. Paris, 2001.
———. "Çarıklı Kilise, l'église de la précieuse croix à Göreme (Korama), Cappadoce: Une fondation des Mélissènoi?" In *ΕΥΨΥΧΙΑ: Mélanges offerts à Hélène Ahrweiler*, 301–12. Byzantina sorbonensia 16. Paris, 1998. Repr. in eadem, *Études cappadociennes*. London, 2002.
———. "Culte et iconographie de l'archange Michel dans l'Orient byzantin: Le témoignage de quelques monuments de Cappadoce." *Les Cahiers de Saint-Michel de Cuxà 28* (1997): 187–98.
———. *Les Églises byzantines de Cappadoce: Le programme iconographique de l'abside et de ses abords*. Paris, 1991.
———. *Études cappadociennes*. London, 2002.
———. "Hagiographie cappadocienne: À propos de quelques images nouvelles de saint Hiéron et de saint Eustathe." In *Ευφρόσυνον: Αφιέρωμα στο Μανόλη Χατζηδάκη*, 1:205–18. Athens, 1991.
———. "Images et espace cultuel à Byzance: l'exemple d'une église de Cappadoce (Karşı kilise, 1212)." In *Le Sacré et son inscription dans l'éspace à Byzance et en Occident: Études comparées*, ed. M. Kaplan, 163–81. Byzantina Sorbonensia 18. Paris, 2001. Repr. in eadem, *Études cappadociennes*.
———. "Note sur la représentation des archanges en costume impérial dans l'iconographie byzantine." *CahArch* 46 (1998): 121–28.
———. "Nouvelle découverte en Cappadoce: les églises de Yüksekli." *CahArch* 35 (1987): 113–41. Repr. in eadem, *Études cappadociennes*.
———. "Premières images du Jugement dernier en Cappadoce byzantine (Xe s.)." In Pace, *Jugement dernier*, 47–52.
———. "Les programmes iconographiques des églises de Cappadoce au Xe siècle: Nouvelles recherches." In *Constantine VII Porphyrogenitus and his Age: Second International Byzantine Conference (Delphi, 22–26 July 1987)*, 247–84. Athens, 1989.
Kakoulli, I. "Late Classical and Hellenistic Painting Techniques and Materials: A Review of the Technical Literature." *Reviews in Conservation* 3 (2002): 56–67.
———. "Philaretos' Akra Tapeinosis at Monagri: Its Technique, Condition, and Cleaning in the Context of Late Byzantine Wall Paintings in Cyprus." Diploma diss., Courtauld Institute of Art, University of London, 1994.
Kakoulli, I., and S. Cather. "Houghton-on-the-Hill: Technical Examination." Unpublished report, Courtauld Institute of Art, University of London, 2000.
Kakoulli, I., and D. Michaelides. "Technological Investigation of Monumental Graeco-Roman Tomb Paintings in Cyprus." In *Proceedings of the 32nd International Symposium on Archaeometry, Mexico City, 15–19 May 2000*. CD-ROM.
Kalamara, P. "Το ένδυμα στο Μυστρά κατά την όψιμη παλαιολόγεια περίοδο: στοιχεία από την ανασκαφή των τάφων της Αγίας Σοφίας." In *Parure d'une princesse byzantine: Tissus archéologiques de Sainte-Sophie de Mistra*, 113–18. Geneva, 2000. [French translation, 105–10.]
———. *Le système vestimentaire à Byzance du IVe jusqu'à la fin du XIe siècle*. Villeneuve d'Ascq, 1997.
———. "Le vêtement byzantin ou syrien en Chypre d'après les pierres tombales." In Imhaus, *Lacrimae Cypriae*, 2:107–37.
Kalavrezou-Maxeiner, I. *Byzantine Icons in Steatite*. 2 vols. Byzantina Vindobonensia 15. Vienna, 1985.
———. "Eudokia Makrembolitissa and the Romanos Ivory." *DOP* 31 (1977): 305–25.
Kalokyris, K. D. *Τὸ Ἄστρον τῆς Βηθλεέμ εἰς τὴν Βυζαντινὴν τέχνην*. Thessalonike, 1969.
Kalopissi-Verti, S. "Church Foundations by Entire Villages (13th–16th c.): A Short Note." *ZRVI* 44 (2007): 333–40.
———. "Church Inscriptions as Documents: Chrysobulls–Ecclesiastical Acts–Inventories–Donations–Wills." *Δελτ.Χριστ.Ἀρχ.Ἑτ.*, ser. 4, 24 (2003): 79–88.
———. "Collective Patterns of Patronage in the Late Byzantine Village: The Evidence of Church Inscriptions." In *Donation et Donateurs dans le monde byzantin: Actes du colloque international organisé à l'Université de Fribourg (Fribourg 13–15 mars 2008)*, ed. J.-M. Spieser and E. Yota, 125–40. Réalités Byzantines 14. Paris, 2012.

———. *Dedicatory Inscriptions and Donor Portraits in Thirteenth-Century Churches of Greece*. Vienna, 1992.
———. "Διακοσμημένοι φωτοστέφανοι σὲ εἰκόνες καὶ τοιχογραφίες τῆς Κύπρου καὶ τοῦ Ἑλλαδικοῦ χώρου." In *Πρακτικὰ τοῦ δευτέρου διεθνοῦς κυπριολογικοῦ συνεδρίου*, 2:555–60.
———. "Επιπτώσεις της Δ΄ Σταυροφορίας στη μνημειακή ζωγραφική της Πελοποννήσου και της Ανατολικής Στερεάς Ελλάδας ως τα τέλη του 13ου αιώνα" / "The Impact of the Fourth Crusade on Monumental Painting in the Peloponnese and Eastern Central Greece up to the End of the Thirteenth Century." In *Η βυζαντινή τέχνη μετά την τέταρτη σταυροφορία: Η τέταρτη σταυροφορία και οι επιπτώσεις της / Byzantine Art in the Aftermath of the Fourth Crusade: The Fourth Crusade and Its Consequences*, ed. P. L. Vocotopoulos, 63–104. International Congress, March 9–12, 2004. Athens, 2007.
———. *Die Kirche der Hagia Triada bei Kranidi in der Argolis (1244): Ikonographische und stilistische Analyse der Malereien*. Miscellanea Byzantina Monacensia 20. Munich, 1975.
———. "Painters in Late Byzantine Society: The Evidence of Church Inscriptions." *CahArch* 42 (1994): 139–58.
———. "The Proskynetaria of the Templon and Narthex: Form, Imagery, Spatial Connections, and Reception." In Gerstel, *Thresholds of the Sacred*, 107–34.
———. "Representations of the Virgin in Lusignan Cyprus." In Vassilaki, *Images of the Mother of God*, 305–19.
Karageorghis, V. *The A. G. Leventis Foundation and the Cultural Heritage of Cyprus*. Athens, 1990.
———. "Chronique des fouilles et découvertes à Chypre en 1959." *BCH* 84 (1960): 242–99.
Karakatsanis, A. A., ed. *Treasures of Mount Athos*. Exh. cat., Museum of Byzantine Culture, Thessalonike, 1997. 2nd ed. Thessalonike, 1997.
Karapidakis, L. "Le Jugement dernier de l'église de Saint-Jean-de-Séli." *Cahiers Balkaniques* 6 (1984): 67–106.
Kartsonis, A. *Anastasis: The Making of an Image*. Princeton, 1986.
Kasiere, O. G., and A. X. Koumparidou. "Λαογραφικά από τα Σπήλια: Ασίνου." *Λαογραφική Κύπρος* 17 (1987): 28.
Katsaros, V. "Η παράσταση της Βάπτιστης στην Παλαιά Μητρόπολη Βεροίας." *Δελτ.Χριστ.Ἀρχ.Ἑτ.*, ser. 4, 27 (2006): 169–80. [English summary, 180.]
Katselake, A. "Ο Χριστός Ελκόμενος επί Σταυρού. Εικονογραφία και τυπολογία της παράστασης στη βυζαντινή τέχνη (4ος αι.–15ος αι.)." *Δελτ.Χριστ.Ἀρχ.Ἑτ.*, ser. 4, 19 (1996–97): 167–200. English summary, 200.
Kazamia-Tsernou, M. *Ιστορώντας τη "Δέηση" στις βυζαντινές εκκλησίες της Ελλάδος*. Thessalonike, 2005.
Kazanaki-Lappa, M. "Η βυζαντινή παράδοση και η σχέση με τη δυτική τέχνη." *Cretan Studies* 6 (1998): 51–70.
Kazhdan, A. "The List of Saints of the 1st–10th Centuries in a Chronological Order." 3 vols. Unpublished 1993 typescript held at Dumbarton Oaks, Washington, D.C.
Kazhdan, A., and H. Maguire. "Byzantine Hagiographical Texts as Sources on Art." *DOP* 45 (1991): 1–22.
Kazhdan, A., and S. Ronchey. *L'aristocrazia bizantina dal principio dell'XI alla fine del XII secolo*. Palermo, 1997.
Kedar, B. "Gerald of Nazareth, A Neglected Twelfth-Century Writer in the Latin East: A Contribution to the Intellectual and Monastic History of the Crusader States." *DOP* 37 (1983): 55–77.
Kelly, H. A. *The Devil at Baptism: Ritual, Theology and Drama*. Ithaca and London, 1985.
Kepetzi, V. "Autour d'une inscription métrique et de la représentation des apôtres Pierre et Paul dans une église en Élide." In *Ritual and Art: Byzantine Essays for Christopher Walter*, ed. P. Armstrong, 160–81. London 2006.
———. "Empereur, piété et rémission des péchés dans deux *ekphraseis* byzantines: Image et rhétorique." *Δελτ.Χριστ.Ἀρχ.Ἑτ.*, ser. 4, 20 (1998): 231–44.
———. "À propos d' une représentation du Jugement dernier d'une église de Laconie." In *Λαμπηδών: Αφιέρωμα στη μνήμη της Ντούλας Μουρίκη*, ed. M. Aspra-Vardavaki, 1:395–420. Athens, 2003.
———. "Quelques remarques sur le motif de l'enroulement du ciel dans l'iconographie byzantine du Jugement dernier." *Δελτ.Χριστ.Ἀρχ.Ἑτ.*, ser. 4, 17 (1993–1994): 99–112.
Kessler, H., ed. *The Holy Face and the Paradox of Representation*. Villa Spelman Colloquia 6. Bologna, 1998.
Kitchener, H. H. *Trigonometrical Survey of the Island of Cyprus*. London, 1885.
Kitzinger, E. "The Descent of the Dove: Observations on the Mosaic of the Annunciation in the Cappella Palatina in Palermo." In *Byzanz und der Westen*, ed. I. Hutter, 99–115. Vienna, 1984.
———. "The Mandylion at Monreale." In *Arte profana e arte sacra a Bisanzio*, ed. A. Iacobini and E. Zanini, 575–602. Rome, 1995.
———. *I mosaici del periodo normanno in Sicilia*, fasc. 1, *La Cappella Palatina di Palermo, I mosaici del presbyterio*. Palermo, 1992.
———. *I mosaici del periodo normanno in Sicilia*, fasc. 4, *Il Duomo di Monreale, I mosaici del transetto*. Palermo, 1995.
———. *The Mosaics of St. Mary's of the Admiral in Palermo*. DOS 27. Washington, D.C., 1990.
Klein, C., and C. S. Hurlbut, Jr. (after J. D. Dana). *Manual of Mineralogy*. 21st ed. New York, 1993.
Kleinschmidt, B. *Die heilige Anna: Ihre Verehrung in Geschichte, Kunst und Volkstum*. Forschungen zur Volkskunde 1–3. Düsseldorf, 1930.
Klerides, N. *25 μοναστήρια στὴν Κύπρο*. 2 vols. Nicosia, 1968.
———. "Ὁ Ἅγιος Σωζόμενος: Προλεγόμενα καὶ κείμενον τῆς ἀκολουθίας." *Κυπρ.Σπ.* 2 (1938): 105–20.
———. "Προλεγόμενα καὶ κείμενον τῆς ἀκολουθίας τοῦ ἁγίου ἐνδόξου μεγαλομάρτυρος Μάμαντος τοῦ Θαυματουργοῦ." *Κυπρ.Σπ.* 15 (1951): 89–145.
———. *Χωριά καὶ πολιτείες τῆς Κύπρου*. Nicosia, 1961.

Koch, G., ed. *Byzantinische Malerei: Bildprogramme–Ikonographie–Stil; Symposion in Marburg 25.–29.6.1997.* Wiesbaden, 2000.

Kokkinoftas, K., and I. Theocharides. "Μοναστηριακά δεδομένα σύμφωνα με το κατάστιχο VI της Αρχιεπισκοπής Κύπρου (1825)." *Επετηρίδα Κέντρου Μελετῶν Ιεράς Μονής Κύκκου* 4 (1999): 241–309.

Kokosalakis, N. "The Political Significance of Popular Religion in Greece." *Archives des sciences sociales des religions* 64 (1987): 37–52.

Kollias, E. *The City of Rhodes and the Palace of the Grand Master.* Athens, 1988.

Komodikes, K. "Θεομηνίες και Θεοσημίες στην Κύπρο κατά την ύστερη μεσαιωνική περίοδο." *Επετηρίδα κέντρου μελετών Ιεράς Μονής Κύκκου* 7 (2006): 125–56.

Komroff, M., ed. *The Apocrypha or Non-Canonical Books of the Bible: The King James Version.* New York, 1936.

Konidaris, I. M. *Νομική θεώρηση των μοναστηριακών τυπικών.* Athens, 1984.

Kono, K. "The Personifications of the Jordan and the Sea: Their Function in the Baptism in Byzantine Art." In *Αφιέρωμα στη μνήμη του Σωτήρη Κίσσα*, ed. X. Mauropoulou-Tsiume and E. Kyriakoudes, 161–212. Thessalonike, 2001.

Kotoula, D. "'Maniera Cypria' and Thirteenth-Century Icon Production on the Island of Cyprus: A Critical Approach." *BMGS* 28 (2004): 89–100.

Koukiares, S. *Ὁ κύκλος τοῦ βίου τῆς ἁγίας Παρασκευῆς τῆς Ρωμαίας καὶ τῆς ἐξ Ἰκονίου στὴ χριστιανικὴ τέχνη.* Athens, 1994.

———. "Τὰ ζεύγη τῶν Ἁγίων Ἀναργύρων σὲ ὁμάδα: Μερικὲς παρατηρήσεις." *Βυζαντινά* 28 (2008): 307–30.

Koukoules, Ph. *Βυζαντινῶν βίος καὶ πολιτισμός.* 4 vols. Athens, 1948–51.

Koumoussi, A. *Les peintures murales de la Transfiguration de Pyrgi et de Sainte-Thècle en Eubée: Rapports avec l'art occidental.* Athens, 1987.

Kourres, Ch. "Ἅγιος Μάμας ὁ μεγάλος Ἅγιος τῆς Μόρφου." In *Ἱερὰ Μητρόπολις Μόρφου*, 229–39.

Krautheimer, R. *Early Christian and Byzantine Architecture.* Harmondsworth, 1986.

Kretzenbacher, L. *Griechische Reiterheilige als Gefangenenretter.* Vienna, 1983.

Kühnel, B. *Crusader Art of the Twelfth Century: A Geographical, an Historical or an Art-Historical Notion?* Berlin, 1994.

Kühnel, G. *Wall Painting in the Latin Kingdom of Jerusalem.* Berlin, 1988.

Κύπρια Μηναῖα. Currently 10 vols. Nicosia, 1994–.

Kurtz, E. *Die Gedichte des Christophoros Mitylenaios.* Leipzig, 1903.

Kyprianos (Archimandrite). *Ἱστορία χρονολογικὴ τῆς νήσου Κύπρου.* Venice, 1788; repr. Nicosia, 1971.

Kyriakakis, J. "Byzantine Burial Customs: Care of the Deceased from Death to the Prothesis." *GOTR* 19 (1974): 37–72; 29 (1984): 115–95.

Kyriazes, N. G. *Τὰ μοναστήρια ἐν Κύπρῳ.* Nicosia, 1950.

Kyritses, D. "The Late Byzantine Aristocracy, 13th–Early 14th Centuries." Ph.D. dissertation, Harvard University, 1997.

Kyrris, K. P. "Δύο Κυπριακὰ ἁγιολογικὰ μελετήματα." *Επετηρίδα Κέντρου Μελετών Ιεράς Μονής Κύκκου* 5 (2001): 87–119.

———. "The Nature of the Arab-Byzantine Relations in Cyprus from the Middle of the 7th to the Middle of the 10th Century." *Graeco-Arabica* 1 (1982): 144–75.

———. "Ελένη, αγία, και Κύπρος." In *Μεγάλη κυπριακή εγκυκλοπαιδεία*, 14 vols., 5:39–41. Nicosia, 1986.

———. "Ἡ Κύπρος, τὸ Βυζάντιον καὶ οἱ Ἄραβες ἀπὸ τὸν 7ο μέχρι τὶς ἀρχὲς τοῦ 8ου αἰῶνα." *Ἐπ.Ἑτ.Βυζ.Σπ.* 49 (1994–98): 185–236.

———. "The 'Three Hundred Alaman Saints' of Cyprus: Problems of Origin and Identity: A Summary." In Bryer and Georghallides, *Sweet Land of Cyprus*, 203–35.

Lafontaine-Dosogne, J. *Iconographie de l'enfance de la Vierge dans l'Empire byzantin et en Occident.* 2 vols. Brussels, 1964–65.

———. "Un thème iconographique peu connu: Marina assommant Belzébuth." *Byzantion* 32 (1962): 251–59.

Lagarde, P. de, ed. *Ioannis Euchaitorum metropolitae quae in Codice Vaticano Graeco 676 supersunt.* Göttingen, 1882; repr. Amsterdam, 1979.

Lampros, S. P. "Ὁ Μαρκιανὸς κῶδιξ 524." *Νέος Ἑλληνομνήμων* 8 (1911): 3–59, 123–92.

———. "Τὰ ὑπ᾽ ἀριθμὸν ΡΙΖ' καὶ ΡΓ' κατάλοιπα." *Νέος Ἑλληνομνήμων* 16 (1922): 30–59.

Lamy-Lasalle, C. "Les archanges en costume impérial dans la peinture murale italienne." In *Synthronon: Art et archéologie de la fin de l'Antiquité et du Moyen Age*, 189–98. Paris, 1968.

Landström, B. *Das Schiff.* Munich, 1961.

Laourdas, B. "Βυζαντινὰ καὶ μεταβυζαντινὰ ἐγκώμια εἰς τὸν Ἅγιον Δημήτριον." *Makedonika* 4 (1955–60): 47–162.

Lasithiotakis, K. "Κυριαρχοῦντες τύποι χριστιανικῶν ναῶν ἀπὸ τὸν 12ον αἰώνα καὶ ἐντεῦθεν στὴ Δυτικὴ Κρήτη." *Κρητικὰ Χρονικά* 15–16 (1961–62): 175–201.

Last, J. S. "Kourion: The Ancient Water Supply." *Proceedings of the American Philosophical Society* 119 (1975): 39–72.

Latyšev, B. *Menologii Anonymi Byzantini saeculi X quae supersunt.* 2 vols. St. Petersburg, 1911–12; repr. Leipzig, 1970.

Lauxtermann, M. D. "The Byzantine Epigram in the Ninth and Tenth Centuries." 2 vols. Ph.D. diss., Universiteit van Amsterdam, 1994.

———. *Byzantine Poetry from Pisides to Geometres: Texts and Contexts.* Vol. 1. Wiener Byzantinische Studien 24. Vienna, 2003.

Lazarev, V. *Old Russian Murals and Mosaics.* London, 1966.

———. "Regard sur l'art de la Russie prémongole, II: Le système de la décoration murale de Sainte-Sophie de Kiev." *Cahiers de civilisation médiévale* 14 (1971): 221–38.

———. *Storia della pittura bizantina.* Turin, 1967.

Lehmann, K. "The Dome of Heaven." *ArtB* 27 (1945): 1–27.

Lemerle, P. *Les plus anciens recueils des miracles de Saint Démétrius*. 2 vols. Paris, 1979–81.

Leontios Machairas. *See under* Machairas.

Lepage, C. "L'ornementation végétale fantastique et le pseudo-réalisme dans la peinture byzantine." *CahArch* 19 (1969): 191–211.

Leroy, J. *Les Manuscrits syriaques à peintures conservés dans les bibliothèques d'Europe et d'Orient*. 2 vols. Paris, 1964.

———. *Les peintures des couvents du Ouadi Natroun*. Peinture murale chez les Coptes 2. Cairo, 1982.

Liares, H. *Μεσαιωνικὰ μνημεῖα Εὐβοίας*. Athens, 1971.

Lidov, A. M., ed. *Ikonostas: Proiskhozhdenie, Razvitie, Simvolika*. Moscow, 2000.

Lidov, A., and G. Sidorenko, eds. *The Miraculous Image: The Icons of Our Lady in the Tretyakov Gallery*. Moscow, 1999.

The Life and Martyrdom of Saint Anastasia and Those Who Were Martyred with Her. Translated by Holy Transfiguration Monastery. Seattle, 1987.

Lipsmeyer, E. "The Donor and His Church Model in Medieval Art from Early Christian Times to the Late Romanesque Period." Ph.D. diss., Rutgers University, 1981.

Loon, G. J. M. van. *The Gate of Heaven: Wall Paintings with Old Testament Scenes in the Altar Room and the Ḫūrus of Coptic Churches*. Leiden, 1999.

Lowden, J. *Illuminated Prophet Books*. London, 1988.

Lusignan, Estienne de. *Description de toute l'isle de Chypre*. Paris, 1580. Repr. Nicosia, 2004.

Lymberopoulou, A. *The Church of the Archangel Michael at Kavalariana: Art and Society on Fourteenth-Century Venetian-Dominated Crete*. London, 2006.

Maas, P. "Der byzantinische Zwölfsilber." *BZ* 12 (1903): 278–323.

Machairas, Leontios. *Χρονικό της Κύπρου: Παράλληλη διπλωματική έκδοση των χειρογράφων*. Ed. and trans. M. Pieris and A. Nicolaou-Konnari. Nicosia, 2003.

———. *Recital Concerning the Sweet Land of Cyprus Entitled "Chronicle."* Trans. and ed. R. M. Dawkins. 2 vols. Oxford, 1932.

Maderakes, S. "Αναζητήσεις των κρητικών αγιογράφων στην παράσταση του γυμνού στο θέμα των Ποινών σε τρεις εκκλησίες των Χανίων." *Chania* (1984): 80–91.

———. "Ἡ κόλαση καὶ οἱ ποινὲς τῶν κολασμένων σὰν θέματα τῆς Δευτέρας Παρουσίας στὶς ἐκκλησίες τῆς Κρήτης." *Ὕδωρ ἐκ Πέτρας* 2 (1978): 185–236; 3–4 (1979): 21–80; 5–6 (1980–81): 51–130.

Maguire, H. "*Abaton* and *Oikonomia*: St. Neophytos and the Iconography of the Presentation of the Virgin." In Ševčenko and Moss, *Medieval Cyprus*, 95–105. Princeton, 1999.

———. *Art and Eloquence in Byzantium*. Princeton, 1981.

———. "The Depiction of Sorrow in Middle Byzantine Art." *DOP* 31 (1977): 123–74.

———. "The Iconography of Symeon with the Christ Child in Byzantine Art." *DOP* 34–35 (1980–81): 161–69.

———. *The Icons of their Bodies: Saints and their Images in Byzantium*. Princeton, 1996.

———. *Image and Imagination: The Byzantine Epigram as Evidence for Viewer Response*. Toronto, 1996.

———. "A Murderer among the Angels: The Frontispiece Miniatures of Paris. Gr. 510 and the Iconography of the Archangels in Byzantine Art." In *The Sacred Image East and West*, ed. R. Ousterhout and L. Brubaker, 63–71. Urbana, Ill., 1995.

Makin, Jirjis ibn al-ʿAmid. *Historia saracenica, qua res gestae Muslimorum, inde a Muhammede primo imperij & religionis muslimicae auctore, usque ad initium imperij Atabacaei, per XLIX imperatorem successionem fidelissime explicantur*. Trans. T. Erpenius. Leiden, 1625.

Malamut, É. *Les îles de l'Empire byzantin: VIII*[e]*–XII*[e] *siècles*. 2 vols. Byzantina Sorbonensia 8. Paris, 1988.

Maliaras, N. *Βυζαντινά Μουσικά Όργανα*. Athens, 2007.

Mango, C. *The Art of the Byzantine Empire, 312–1453: Sources and Documents*. Englewood Cliffs, N.J., 1972; repr. Toronto, 1986.

———. *The Brazen House: A Study of the Vestibule of the Imperial Palace of Constantinople*. Arkaeologisk-kunsthistoriske Meddelelser udgivet af Det Kongelige Danke Videnskabernes Selskab, Bind 4, 4. Copenhagen, 1959.

———. "Chypre, carrefour du monde byzantin." In *XV*[e] *Congrès international des études byzantines: Rapports et co-rapports*, 5:3–13. Athens, 1976. Repr. in idem, *Byzantium and Its Image*, art. 17. London, 1984.

———. "The Date of the Narthex Mosaics of the Church of the Dormition at Nicaea." *DOP* 13 (1959): 245–52.

———. "The Monastery of St. Chrysostomos at Koutsovendis (Cyprus) and Its Wall Paintings: Part I: Description, with the collaboration of E. J. W. Hawkins and Susan Boyd." *DOP* 44 (1990): 63–94.

———. "On the Cult of Saints Cosmas and Damian at Constantinople." In *Θυμίαμα στη μνήμη Λασκαρίνας Μπούρα*, 1:189–92. Athens, 1994.

———. "On the History of the Templon and the Martyrion of St. Artemios at Constantinople," *Zograf* 10 (1979): 40–44.

———. "St. Michael and Attis." *Δελτ.Χριστ.Ἀρχ.Ἑτ.*, ser. 4, 12 (1984): 39–62.

———. "Summary of Work Carried out by the Dumbarton Oaks Byzantine Center in Cyprus 1959–1969." *RDAC* (1969): 98–104.

Mango, C., and E. J. W. Hawkins. "The Hermitage of St. Neophytos and Its Wall Paintings." *DOP* 20 (1966): 119–206.

———. "Report on Field Work in Istanbul and Cyprus 1962–1963." *DOP* 18 (1964): 319–40.

Mantas, A. G. *Die Ikonographie der Gleichnisse Jesu in der ostkirchlichen Kunst (5.–15. Jh.)*. Leiden, 2010.

———. "Überlegungen zur Deesis in der Hauptapsis mittelbyzantinischer Kirchen Griechenlands." In Koch, *Byzantinische Malerei*, 165–82.

Marankou, A., ed. *Η ζωή στην Κύπρο στα χρόνια της Φραγκοκρατίας και της Βενετοκρατίας: Χορηγία Ιδρύματος*

Αναστασίου Λεβέντη. Exh. cat., Famagusta Gate, Nicosia, 14–30 September 1985. Nicosia, 1985.
Marava-Chatzinikolaou, A. *Ο Ἅγιος Μάμας*. 2nd ed. Athens, 1995.
———. "Εὐλογία τοῦ Ἁγίου Μάμα." *Δελτ.Χριστ.Ἀρχ.Ἑτ.*, ser. 4, 2 (1960–61): 131–37.
———. "Η ψηφιδωτὴ εἰκόνα τῆς Πάτμου." *Δελτ.Χριστ.Ἀρχ. Ἑτ.*, ser. 4, 1 (1959): 127–34.
Marinis, V. "Tombs and Burials in the Monastery *tou Libos* in Constantinople." *DOP* 63 (2009): 147–66.
Martin-Hisard, B. "Le culte de l'archange Michel dans l'empire byzantin (VIIIe–XIe siècles). " In *Culto e insediamenti micaelici nell'Italia meridionale fra tarda antichità e medioevo: Atti del convegno internazionale Monte Sant'Angelo 18–21 novembre 1992,* ed. C. Carletti and G. Otranto, 351–73. Bari, 1994.
Mary (Mother), and K. Ware. *The Festal Menaion.* London 1977.
Mas-Latrie, L. de. *Histoire de l'île de Chypre sous le règne des princes de la maison de Lusignan*. 3 vols. Paris, 1852–61.
Mathews, T. F. "The Epigrams of Leo Sacellarios and an Exegetical Approach to the Miniatures of Vat. Reg. Gr. 1." *OCP* 43 (1977): 91–133. Repr. in idem, *Art and Architecture in Byzantium and Armenia: Liturgical and Exegetical Approaches*, art. VIII. Aldershot, 1995.
———. "'Private' Liturgy in Byzantine Architecture: Toward a Reappraisal." *CahArch* 30 (1982): 125–38.
Mavrodinof, M. *L'église à nef unique et l'église à coupôle en pays Bulgare*. Sofia, 1931.
McCabe, A. *A Byzantine Encyclopaedia of Horse Medicine: The Sources, Compilation and Transmission of the Hippiatrica*. Oxford 2007.
McKay, G. K. "The Eastern Christian Exegetical Tradition of Daniel's Vision of the Ancient of Days." *Journal of Early Christian Studies* 7 (1999): 139–61.
Meester, P. de. *Liturgia Bizantina: Studi di rito bizantino*. Book 2, part 6, *Rituale–Benedizionale Bizantino.* Rome, 1930.
Megaw, A. H. S. "Byzantine Architecture and Decoration in Cyprus, Metropolitan or Provincial?" *DOP* 28 (1974): 57–88.
———. "Supplementary Excavations on a Castle Site at Paphos, Cyprus, 1970–1971." *DOP* 26 (1972): 322–43.
———. "Three Vaulted Basilicas in Cyprus." *JHS* 66 (1946): 48–56.
Megaw, A. H. S., and E. J. W. Hawkins. "The Church of the Holy Apostles at Perachorio, Cyprus, and Its Frescoes." *DOP* 16 (1962): 277–348.
———. *The Church of the Panagia Kanakariá at Lythrankomi in Cyprus: Its Mosaics and Frescoes.* DOS 14. Washington, D.C, 1977.
Megaw, A. H. S., and A. Stylianou. *Cyprus: Byzantine Mosaics and Frescoes*. Greenwich, Conn., 1963.
Meinardus, O. F. A. "Der Erzengel Michael als psychopompos." *OrChr* 62 (1978): 166–68.
———. "Relics in the Churches and Monasteries of Cyprus." *Ostkirchliche Studien* 19 (1970): 19–43.
Menaion = *Μηναῖα τοῦ ὅλου ἐνιαυτοῦ*. 6 vols. Rome, 1888–1902.
Menardos, S. "Η Ἁγία Ἑλένη εἰς τὴν Κύπρον." *Λαογραφία* 2 (1910): 316–17.
Menologio Basilio II. Città del Vaticano, 1907.
Mentzos, A. *Το προσκύνημα του Αγίου Δημητρίου Θεσσαλονίκης στα βυζαντινά χρόνια*. Athens, 1994.
Meyendorff, J. "L'Iconographie de la Sagesse divine dans la tradition byzantine." *CahArch* 10 (1959): 259–77.
Michael the Syrian. *Chronique de Michel le Syrien, Patriarche Jacobite d'Antioche (1166–1199)*. 4 vols. Ed. and trans. J. B. Chabot. Paris, 1899–1910; repr. Brussels, 1963.
Mijatev, K. *Die Mittelalterliche Baukunst in Bulgarien*. Sofia, 1974.
Mijović, P. "La personnification de la Mer dans le Jugement dernier à Gračanica." In *Χαριστήριον εἰς Ἀναστάσιον Κ. Ὀρλάνδον*, 4:208–19. Athens, 1967–68.
Milanović, V. "The Tree of Jesse in the Byzantine Mural Painting of the Thirteenth and Fourteenth Centuries." *Zograf* 20 (1989): 48–59.
Miljković-Pepek, P. "La fresque de la Vierge avec le Christ du pilier situé au nord de l'iconostase de Sainte-Sophie à Ohrid." In *Akten des XI. internationalen byzantinischen Kongresses, 1958*, 388–91. Munich, 1960.
Miller, E., ed. *Manuelis Philae Carmina*. 2 vols. Paris, 1855.
Millet, G. "L'art des Balkans et d'Italie au XIIIe siècle." In *V Congresso internazionale di studi bizantini*, 2:275–88. Rome, 1940.
———. *La Dalmatique du Vatican*. Paris, 1945.
———. *La peinture du Moyen Âge en Yougoslavie (Serbie, Macédoine et Monténégro).* 4 vols. Paris, 1956–69.
———. *Monuments byzantins de Mistra*. Paris, 1910.
———. *Monuments de l'Athos.* Volume 1, *Les peintures*. Paris, 1927.
———. *Recherches sur l'iconographie de l'Évangile aux XIVe, XVe, et XVIe siècles.* Bibliothèque des écoles françaises d'Athènes et de Rome 109. Paris, 1916.
Millet, G., J. Pargoire, and L. Petit. *Recueil des inscriptions chrétiennes du Mont Athos.* Paris, 1904.
Mills, J. S. "The Gas Chromatographic Examination of Paint Media: Part I, Fatty Acid Composition and Identification of Dried Oil Films." *Studies in Conservation* 11 (1966): 92–107.
Mills, J. S., and R. White. "Organic Mass Spectrometry of Art Materials: Work in Progress." *National Gallery Technical Bulletin* 6 (1982): 3–16.
Milošević, D. *Das jüngste Gericht.* Recklinghausen, 1963.
Mitchel, V. A. *The Mariology of Saint John Damascene*. Kirkwood, Mo., 1930.
Mitsakis, K. "Byzantine and Modern Greek Parahymnography." *Studies in Eastern Chant* 5 (1990): 28–36.
Mitsides, A. N. *Η παρουσία τῆς Ἐκκλησίας τῆς Κύπρου εἰς τὸν ἀγῶνα ὑπὲρ τῶν εἰκόνων.* Nicosia, 1989.
Moorsel, P. van. *Les peintures du monastère de Saint-Antoine près de la Mer Rouge*. 2 vols. Peinture murale chez les Coptes 3. Cairo, 1995.

Mora, P., L. Mora, and P. Philippot. *Conservation of Wall Paintings*. London, 1984.
Morello, G., ed. *Splendori di Bisanzio: Testimonianze e riflessi d'arte e cultura bizantina nelle chiese d'Italia*. Exh. cat., Ravenna, 1990. Milan, 1990.
Morris, R. "The Byzantine Aristocracy and the Monasteries." In *The Byzantine Aristocracy, IX–XIII Centuries*, ed. M. Angold, 112–37. BAR International Series 221. Oxford, 1984.
———. "Monasteries and Their Patrons in the Tenth and Eleventh Centuries." *ByzF* 10 (1985): 185–231.
Moschos, J. *The Spiritual Meadow (Pratum Spirituale)*. Intro., trans., and notes by J. Wortley. Kalamazoo, Mich., 1992.
Mouriki, D. "Αἱ βιβλικαὶ προεικονίσεις τῆς Παναγίας εἰς τὸν τροῦλλον τῆς Περιβλέπτου τοῦ Μυστρᾶ." *Ἀρχ.Δελτ.* 25 (1970): 1:217–51.
———. "Οἱ βυζαντινὲς τοιχογραφίες τῶν παρεκκλησίων τῆς Σπηλιᾶς τῆς Πεντέλης." *Δελτ.Χριστ.Ἀρχ.Ἑτ.*, ser. 4, 7 (1973–74): 79–119.
———. "The Cult of Cypriot Saints in Medieval Cyprus as Attested by Church Decorations and Icon Painting." In Bryer and Georghallides, *Sweet Land of Cyprus*, 237–77.
———. "A Deesis Icon in the Art Museum." *Record of the Art Museum (Princeton)* 28 (1968): 13–28.
———. "Four Thirteenth-Century Sinai Icons by the Painter Peter." In *Studenica et l'art byzantin autour de l'année 1200*, ed. V. Korać, 331–41. Colloques scientifiques de l'Académie Serbe des sciences et des arts 41, classe des Sciences historiques 11. Belgrade, 1988.
———. "Icons from the 12th to the 15th Century." In *Sinai: Treasures of the Monastery of Saint Catherine*, ed. K. A. Manafes, 102–24. Athens, 1990.
———. *The Mosaics of Nea Moni on Chios*. 2 vols. Athens, 1985.
———. "Portraits de donateurs et invocations sur les icônes du XIIIe siècle au Sinaï." *Études Balkaniques, Cahiers Pierre Belon* 2 (1995): 105–37.
———. "Revival Themes with Elements of Daily Life in Two Palaeologan Frescoes Depicting the Baptism." In *Okeanos: Essays Presented to Ihor Ševčenko on His Sixtieth Birthday by His Colleagues and Students = Harvard Ukrainian Studies* 7 (1983), ed. C. Mango and O. Pritsak, 458–88.
———. "Thirteenth-Century Icon Painting in Cyprus." *The Griffon*, n.s., 1–2 (1985–86): 9–112.
———. "Οἱ τοιχογραφίες τοῦ Παρεκκλησίου τῆς Μονῆς Ἰωάννου τοῦ Θεολόγου στὴν Πάτμο." *Δελτ.Χριστ.Ἀρχ.Ἑτ.*, ser. 4, 14 (1987/88): 205–63.
———. *Οἱ τοιχογραφίες τοῦ Σωτήρα κοντὰ στὸ Ἀλεποχώρι Μεγαρίδος*. Δημοσιεύματα τοῦ Ἀρχαιολογικοῦ Δελτίου 25. Athens, 1978.
———. "An Unusual Representation of the Last Judgment in a Thirteenth Century Fresco at St. George near Kouvaras in Attica." *Δελτ.Χριστ.Ἀρχ.Ἑτ.*, ser. 4, 8 (1975–76): 145–71.
———. "The Wall Paintings of the Church of the Panagia at Moutoullas, Cyprus." In *Byzanz und der Westen*, ed. I. Hutter, 171–214. Vienna, 1984.
———. "Ὁ ζωγραφικός διάκοσμος τοῦ τρούλλου τοῦ Ἁγίου Ἱεροθέου κοντά στά Μέγαρα." *Ἀρχαιολογικά Ἀνάλεκτα ἐξ Ἀθηνῶν* 11 (1978): 115–42.
Moutsopoulos, N. K. *Καστοριά: Παναγία ἡ Μαυριώτισσα*. Athens, 1967.
———. *Ἡ Παληαχώρα τῆς Αἰγίνης: Ἱστορικὴ καὶ μορφολογικὴ ἐξέτασις τῶν μνημείων*. Athens, 1962.
Moutsopoulos, N. K., and G. Demetrokalles. *Γεράκι. Οἱ ἐκκλησίες τοῦ οἰκισμοῦ*. Thessalonike, 1981.
Mutafov, E. "Epigrafikata na svetija krŭsti krŭstŭt kato epigrafski znak." *Trudove na katedrite po istorija i bogoslovie* 6 (2004): 230–47.
Mylopotamitake, K. "Η βυζαντινή γυναικεία φορεσιά στη βενετοκρατούμενη Κρήτη." *Κρητική Εστία* 1 (1987): 110–18.
———. "Παρατηρήσεις στὶς τοιχογραφημένες παραστάσεις τῶν κτητόρων-ἀφιερωτῶν τῆς Κρήτης." In *Εἰλαπίνη: Τόμος τιμητικὸς γιὰ τὸν καθηγητὴ Νικόλαο Πλάτωνα*, 1:139–50, 2: pls. 1–11. Herakleion, 1987.
Myriantheas, K. *Μελέται Κώστα Μυριανθέα*. Nicosia, 1991.
Nadolny, J. "The Technical and Stylistic Context of the Relief Backgrounds of the Thornham Parva Retable and the Cluny Frontal." In *The Thornham Parva Retable: Technique, Conservation and Context of an English Medieval Painting*, ed. A. Massing, 174–88. Turnhout, 2003.
———. "The Techniques and Use of Gilded Relief Decoration by Northern European Painters, c. 1200–1500." Ph.D. diss., Courtauld Institute of Art, University of London, 2001.
Nasrallah, J. *Saint Jean de Damas: Son époque, sa vie, son oeuvre*. Harissa, Lebanon, 1950.
Naumann, R., and H. Belting. *Die Euphemia-Kirche am Hippodrom zu Istanbul und ihre Fresken*. Berlin, 1966.
Nelson, R. S. "Text and Image in a Byzantine Gospel Book in Istanbul (Ecumenical Patriarchate, cod. 3)." Ph.D. diss., New York University, 1978.
Nelson, R. S., and K. M. Collins, eds. *Holy Image, Hallowed Ground: Icons From Sinai*. Exh. cat., J. Paul Getty Museum, Los Angeles, 14 November 2006–4 March 2007. Los Angeles, 2006.
Nicholl, G. "A Contribution to the Archaeological Interpretation of *Typika*: The Case of the Narthex." In *Work and Worship at the Theotokos Evergetis 1050–1200*, ed. M. Mullett and A. Kirby, 285–308. Belfast, 1997.
Nicolaïdès, A. "L'église de la Panagia Arakiotissa à Lagoudéra, Chypre: Étude iconographique des fresques de 1192." *DOP* 50 (1996): 1–138.
———. "L'église de la Panagia Arakiotissa à Lagoudéra et la peinture Byzantine du XIIe à l'aube du XIIIe siècle à Chypre." 3 vols. Ph.D. diss., Université de Provence, 1993.
———. "Le Jugement dernier de l' église de la Panagia de Moutoullas à Chypre." *Δελτ.Χριστ.Ἀρχ.Ἑτ.*, ser. 4, 18 (1995): 71–77.

———. *Η κομνήνεια και υστεροκομνήνεια μνημειακή τέχνη στην Κύπρο*. Nicosia, 2003.
———. "Les *ktitores* dans la peinture au XIIe siècle à Chypre: une remise au point." In *Artistes, artisans et production artistique au moyen age: Rapports provisoires*, ed. X. Barral i Altet, 1:679–86. Rennes, 1983.
Nicolaïdès, A., and C. Vanderheyde. "La topographie cultuelle chrétienne de la région de Potamia–Agios Sozoménos." *Cahier du Centre d'Études Chypriotes* 34 (2004): 251–66.
Nikolaou-Konnari, A. "Η Κύπρος στις απαρχές της Τουρκοκρατίας· τα ιστορικά σημειώματα στα φφ. 239v–240r του κώδικα Ven. Marc. Gr. VII.16.1080." *Ἐπ.Κέν.Ἐπιστ.Ἐρ.* 31 (2005): 193–238.
Nicolaou-Konnari, A., and C. Schabel, eds. *Cyprus: Society and Culture, 1191–1374*. Leiden, 2005.
Nikonanos, N. K. *Βυζαντινοὶ ναοὶ τῆς Θεσσαλίας ἀπὸ τὸν 10ον αἰώνα ὡς τὴν κατάκτηση τῆς περιοχῆς ἀπὸ τοὺς Τούρκους τὸ 1393*. Athens, 1979.
Nordiguian, L., and J.-C. Voisin. *Châteaux et églises du moyen âge au Liban*. Beirut, 1999.
Obolensky, D. "The Cult of St. Demetrius of Thessaloniki in the History of Byzantine-Slav Relations." *Balkan Studies* 15 (1974): 3–20. Repr. in idem, *The Byzantine Inheritance of Eastern Europe*, art. IV. London, 1982.
O'Connor, R. "The Mediaeval History of the Double-Axe Motif." *AJA* 24 (1920): 151–70.
Oikonomakes, N. "Η Κύπρος και οι Άραβες." *Μελέται και Υπομνήματα* 1 (1984): 1–142.
Olster, D. M. "Byzantine Hermeneutics after Iconoclasm: Word and Image in the Leo Bible." *Byzantion* 64 (1994): 419–58.
———. "The Construction of a Byzantine Saint: George of Choziba." *GOTR* 38 (1993): 309–22.
Omont, H. *Evangiles avec peintures byzantines du XIe siècle*. 2 vols. Paris, 1908.
———. *Missions archéologiques en Orient aux XVIIe et XVIIIe siècles*. 2 vols. Paris, 1902.
Onasch, K. "Paraskeva-Studien." *Ostkirchliche Studien* 6 (1957): 121–41.
Onasch, K., and A. Schnieper. *Icons: The Fascination and the Reality*. Trans. D. G. Conklin. New York, 1997.
Oppenheim, P. *Das Mönchskleid im christlichen Altertum*. Römische Quartalschrift 28, Supplementheft. Freiburg im Breisgau, 1931.
Opstall, E. Van. "Verses on Paper, Verses Inscribed? A Case Study, with Epigrams of John Geometres." In *Die kulturhistorische Bedeutung byzantinischer Epigramme: Akten des internationalen Workshop (Wien, 1.–2. Dezember 2006)*, ed. W. Hörandner and A. Rhoby, 55–60. Vienna, 2008.
Orlandos, A. K. *Ἡ ἀρχιτεκτονικὴ καὶ αἱ βυζαντιναὶ τοιχογραφίαι τῆς Μονῆς τοῦ Θεολόγου Πάτμου*. Athens, 1970.
Otten-Froux, C. "Un notaire vénitien à Famagouste au XIVe siècle: Les actes de Simeone, prètre de San Giacomo dell'Orio (1362–1371)." *Θησαυρίσματα* 33 (2003): 15–159.
Ousterhout, R. G. *The Architecture of the Kariye Camii in Istanbul*. DOS 25. Washington, D.C., 1987.
———. "Observations on the 'Recessed Brick' Technique during the Palaeologan Period." *Ἀρχαιολογικὸν Δελτίον* 39 (1984), Μελέται: 163–70.
———. "Some Notes on the Construction of Christos Ho Pantepoptes (Eski Imaret Camii) in Istanbul." *Δελτ. Χριστ.Ἀρχ.Ἑτ.*, ser. 4, 16 (1991–92): 47–56.
Ovcharova, O. "Images of the Holy Hymnographers in the Iconographic Programme of the Church of St. Panteleimon in Nerezi, Macedonia (1164)." *Al-Masāq: Islam and the Medieval Mediterranean* 16 (2004): 131–46.
Pace, V., ed. *Le Jugement dernier entre Orient et Occident*. Paris, 2007.
Pallas, D. I. *Die Passion und Bestattung Christi in Byzanz: Der Ritus–Das Bild*. Miscellanea Byzantina Monacensia 2. Munich, 1965.
Panagi, N. *Ο Ιερός ναός Παναγίας Φανερωμένης στη Λευκωσία της Κύπρου*. Nicosia, 2002.
Panayotidi, M. "Οι γραμματικές γνώσεις των ζωγράφων: Ένα παράδειγμα σχετικού προβληματικού από την Μάνη." *Δελτ.Χριστ.Ἀρχ.Ἑτ.*, ser. 4, 24 (2003): 185–93. [English summary, 193–94.]
———. "Le peintre en tant que scribe des inscriptions d'un monument et la question du niveau de sa connaissance grammaticale et orthographique." In *L'artista a Bisanzio e nel mondo cristiano-orientale*, ed. M. Bacci, 71–116. Pisa, 2007.
———. "La peinture monumentale en Grèce de la fin de l'Iconoclasme jusqu'à l'avènement des Comnènes (843–1081)." *CahArch* 34 (1986): 75–108.
———. "The Question of the Role of the Donor and of the Painter: A Rudimentary Approach." *Δελτ.Χριστ.Ἀρχ.Ἑτ.*, ser. 4, 17 (1993–94): 143–56.
———. "The Wall-Paintings in the Church of the Virgin Kosmosoteira at Ferai (Vira) and Stylistic Trends in 12th-Century Painting." *ByzF* 14 (1989): 457–84.
———. "Η ζωγραφική του 12ου αιώνα στην Κύπρο και το πρόβλημα των τοπικών εργαστηρίων." In *Πρακτικά του τρίτου διεθνούς κυπρολογικού συνεδρίου*, 2:411–39.
Panić, D., and G. Babić. *Bogorodica Ljeviška*. 2nd ed. Belgrade, 1988.
Papacostas, T. "Byzantine Cyprus: The Testimony of Its Churches, 650–1200." 3 vols. Ph.D. diss., Oxford University, 1999.
———. "The History and Architecture of the Monastery of Saint John Chrysostom at Koutsovendis, Cyprus." *DOP* 61 (2007): 25–156.
Papadaki-Oekland, S. "Το Αγιο Μανδήλιο ως το νέο σύμβολο σε ένα αρχαίο εικονογραφικό σχήμα." *Δελτ.Χριστ.Ἀρχ.Ἑτ.*, ser. 4, 14 (1987–88): 283–296.
———. "Οἱ τοιχογραφίες τῆς Ἁγίας Ἄννας στὸ Ἀμάρι: Παρατηρήσεις σὲ μία παραλλαγὴ τῆς Δεήσεως." *Δελτ. Χριστ.Ἀρχ.Ἑτ.*, ser. 4, 7 (1973–74): 31–57.
Papademetriou, E. *Κυπριακές Εθνογραφικές Συλλογές σε Βρεττανικά Μουσεία*. Nicosia, 2000.
———. *Ηλαϊκή τέχνη της Κύπρου*. Nicosia, 1996.

Papadopoullos, Th. "Ἡ Ἐκκλησία Κύπρου κατὰ τὴν περίοδο τῆς Φραγκοκρατίας." In *Ἱστορία τῆς Κύπρου*, ed. idem, 4.1:543–665. Nicosia, 1995.
Papadopoulos, K. *Die Wandmalereien des XI. Jahrhunderts in der Kirche Παναγία τῶν Χαλκέων in Thessaloniki.* Byzantina Vindobonensia 2. Graz, 1966.
Papadopoulos-Kerameus, A., ed. *Manuel d'iconographie chrétienne.* St. Petersburg, 1909.
Papaevangelou, P. S. *Ἡ διαμόρφωση τῆς ἐξωτερικῆς ἐμφανίσεως τοῦ ἀνατολικοῦ καὶ ἰδίᾳ τοῦ ἑλληνικοῦ κλήρου.* Thessalonike, 1965.
Papageorgiou, A. "Αμιροὺς Παναγίας μοναστήρι." In *Μεγάλη Κυπριακή Εγκυκλοπαιδεία*, 2:30–31. Nicosia, 1985.
———. "L'art byzantin de Chypre et l'art des Croisés: Influences réciproques." *RDAC* (1982): 217–26.
———. "Ασίνου." In *Μεγάλη Κυπριακή Εγκυκλοπαιδεία*, 2:14. Nicosia, 1985.
———. *"Βασιλικὸ παρεκκλήσι" Πυργά: Ὁδηγός.* Nicosia, n. d.
———. "Βυζαντινή επιγραφική στην Κύπρο." In *Κύπρος, το πολιτιστικό της πρόσωπο δια μέσου των αιώνιων*, 97–119. Nicosia, 2003.
———. *Christian Art in the Turkish-Occupied Part of Cyprus.* Nicosia, 2010.
———. "Constantinopolitan Influence on the Architecture of Cyprus." *JÖB* 32, no. 4 (1982): 469–78.
———. "Η ἐκκλησία τοῦ Ἀρχαγγέλου, Κάτω Λευκάρα." *RDAC* (1990): 189–230.
———. "Ἡ Ἐπισκοπή τῶν Σόλων." *Επετηρίδα Κέντρου μελετών Ιεράς Μονής Κύκκου* 5 (2001): 9–41.
———. "Ἔρευνα ἐν τῷ ναῷ τοῦ Ἁγίου Σπυρίδωνος ἐν Τρεμετουσιᾷ: Πρώτη προκαταρκτικὴ ἔκθεσις." *Κυπρ.Σπ.* 30 (1966): 17–33.
———. *Icons of Cyprus.* Geneva, 1969.
———. *Icons of Cyprus.* Nicosia, 1992.
———. "Ἰδιάζουσαι βυζαντιναὶ τοιχογραφίαι τοῦ 13ου αἰώνος ἐν Κύπρῳ." In *Πρακτικὰ τοῦ πρώτου διεθνοῦς κυπρολογικοῦ συνεδρίου*, 2:201–12.
———. *Ιερά Μητρόπολις Πάφου: Ιστορία και Τέχνη.* Nicosia, 1996.
———. "Ὁ καθεδρικὸς ναὸς τοῦ Ἰωάννου τοῦ Θεολόγου. Προβλήματα τῆς Μονῆς τοῦ Ἁγίου Ἰωάννου τοῦ Πίπι καὶ τῆς εἰκονογράφησης τοῦ ναοῦ." *Κυπρ.Σπ.* 61 (1997): 47–96.
———. "Κηρύκου και Ἰουλίττης Ἁγίων Ἐκκλησία Λετύμπου." In *Μεγάλη Κυπριακή Ἐγκυκλοπαιδεία*, 7:777–78. Nicosia, 1987.
———. "Ἡ Κύπρος κατὰ τοὺς βυζαντινοὺς χρόνους." In *Κύπρος, Ἱστορία, προβλήματα καὶ ἀγῶνες τοῦ λαοῦ της*, ed. G. Tenekides and G. Kranidiotes, 33–80. Athens, 1981.
———. "Λαξευτά ἀσκητήρια καί μοναστήρια τῆς Κύπρου." *Ἐπετηρίδα Κέντρου Μελετῶν Ἱερᾶς Μονῆς Κύκκου* 4 (1999): 33–70.
———. *Masterpieces of the Byzantine Art of Cyprus.* Nicosia, 1965.
———. "Μία σύγχρονη πηγὴ γιὰ τὶς δύο πρῶτες Ἀραβικὲς ἐπιδρομὲς ἐναντίον τῆς Κύπρου." *Στασῖνος* 9 (1986–88). 167–75.
———. "Η μονὴ Ἀψινθιωτίσσης." *RDAC* (1963): 73–83.
———. *Η μονή του Αγίου Ιωάννου του Λαμπαδιστού στον Καλοπαναγιώτη.* Nicosia, 2007.
———. "The Narthex of the Churches of the Middle Byzantine Period in Cyprus." In *Rayonnement Grec: Hommages à Charles Delvoye*, ed. L. Hadermann-Misguich and G. Raepsaet, 437–48. Brussels, 1982.
———. "The Paintings in the Dome of the Church of the Panagia Chryseleousa, Strovolos." In Ševčenko and Moss, *Medieval Cyprus*, 147–60. Princeton, 1999.
———. *Ἡ παλαιοχριστιανικὴ καὶ βυζαντινὴ ἀρχαιολογία καὶ τέχνη ἐν Κύπρῳ κατὰ τὸ 1963.* Nicosia, 1964.
———. *Ἡ παλαιοχριστιανικὴ καὶ βυζαντινὴ ἀρχαιολογία καὶ τέχνη ἐν Κύπρῳ κατὰ τὸ 1964.* Nicosia, 1965.
———. *Ἡ παλαιοχριστιανικὴ καὶ βυζαντινὴ ἀρχαιολογία καὶ τέχνη ἐν Κύπρῳ κατὰ τὸ 1965–1966.* Nicosia, 1967.
———. *Ἡ παλαιοχριστιανικὴ καὶ βυζαντινὴ ἀρχαιολογία καὶ τέχνη ἐν Κύπρῳ κατὰ τὸ 1967–1968.* Nicosia, 1970.
———. "Ἡ Παλαιοχριστιανικὴ τέχνη στὴν Κύπρο κατὰ τὴν πρώτη χριστιανικὴ χιλιετία." In *Ἐκκλησία Κύπρου, 2000 χρόνια χριστιανισμοῦ*, ed. Th. X. Giankou, 283–362. Nicosia, 2002.
———. "Les premières incursions Arabes à Chypre et leurs conséquences." In *Αφιέρωμα εις τον Κωνσταντίνον Σπυριδάκιν*, ed. K. Chrysanthis, 152–58. Nicosia, 1964.
———. "Ο σταυρός των Λευκάρων." In *Θυμίαμα στη μνήμη της Λασκαρίνας Μπούρα*, 1:245–50, 2: pls. 132–35. Athens, 1994.
———. *Οἱ ξυλόστεγοι ναοί τῆς Κύπρου.* Nicosia, 1975.
Papagiannis, G. *Theodoros Prodromos: Jambische und hexametrische Tetrasticha auf die Haupterzählungen des Alten und des Neuen Testaments.* 2 vols. Meletemata 7/1 and 7/2. Wiesbaden, 1997.
Papamastorakes, T. *Ὁ διάκοσμος τοῦ τρούλου τῶν ναῶν τῆς Παλαιολόγειας περιόδου στὴ Βαλκανικὴ Χερσόνησο καὶ τὴν Κύπρο.* Athens, 2001.
———. "Ένα εικαστικό εγκώμιο του Μιχαήλ Η' Παλαιολόγου: οι εξωτερικές τοιχογραφίες στο καθολικό της Μονής της Μαυριώτισσας στην Καστοριά." *Δελτ.Χριστ.Ἀρχ.Ἑτ.*, ser. 4, 15 (1989–90): 221–38. [English summary, 239–40.]
———. "Η ένταξη των προεικονίσεων της Θεοτόκου και της Ύψωσης του Σταυρού σε ένα ιδιότυπο εικονογραφικό κύκλο στον Άγιο Γεώργιο Βιάννου Κρήτης." *Δελτ.Χριστ. Ἀρχ.Ἑτ.*, ser. 4, 14 (1987–88): 315–27.
———. "Επιτύμβιες παραστάσεις κατά τη μέση και ύστερη βυζαντινή περίοδο." *Δελτ.Χριστ.Ἀρχ.Ἑτ.*, ser. 4, 19 (1996–97): 285–303. [English summary, 304.]
———. "Ιστορίες και ιστορήσεις βυζαντινών παλληκαριών." *Δελτ.Χριστ.Ἀρχ.Ἑτ.*, ser. 4, 20 (1998): 213–30.
Papanikola-Bakirtzi, D. *Medieval Cypriot Pottery in the Pierides Foundation Museum.* Larnaca, 1989.
Papanikola-Bakirtzi, D., and M. Iacovou, eds. *Βυζαντινή μεσαιωνική Κύπρος.* Nicosia, 1997.

Papas, T. *Studien zur Geschichte der Messgewänder im byzantinischen Ritus*. Miscellanea Byzantina Monacensia 3. Munich, 1965.
Papaskevopoulou, M. *Researches into the Traditions of the Popular Religious Feasts of Cyprus*. Nicosia, 1982.
Papatheophanous-Tsoure, E. "Οι βυζαντινές τοιχογραφίες δύο μνημείων της Κω: Παναγία των Καστριανών και Ζωοδόχος Πηγή στο Μονάγρι." In *Ιστορία—τέχνη—ἀρχαιολογία της Κω. Α' διεθνές επιστημονικό συνέδριο (Κως, 2–4 Μαίου 1997)*, ed. G. Kokkorou-Alevra, A. A. Laimou, and E. Simantoni-Bournia, 357–64. Athens, 2001.
Παρακλητικὴ ἤτοι Ὀκτώηχος ἡ Μεγάλη. Rome, 1885.
Parani, M. *Reconstructing the Reality of Images: Byzantine Material Culture and Religious Iconography (11th–15th Centuries)*. Leiden–Boston, 2003.
Patlagean, E. "L'histoire de la femme déguisée en moine et l'évolution de la sainteté féminine à Byzance." *Studi Medievali*, 3rd ser., 17 (1976): 597–623. Repr. in eadem, *Structure sociale, famille, chrétienté à Byzance: IVe–XIe siècle*, art. 11. London, 1981.
Patterson [Ševčenko], N. "Byzantine Frescoes at Pherrai." M.A. thesis, Columbia University, 1964.
Peers, G. *Subtle Bodies: Representing Angels in Byzantium*. Berkeley, 2001.
Peeters, P. "St. Romain le Neomartyr (+11 Mai 780) d'après un document géorgien." *AB* 30 (1911): 393–427.
Pelekanides, S. M. *Καλλιέργης, ὅλης Θετταλίας ἄριστος ζωγράφος*. Library of the Athenian Archaeological Society 75. Athens, 1973.
———. *Καστορία*. Volume 1, *Βυζαντιναὶ τοιχογραφίαι: Πίνακες*. Thessalonike, 1953.
Pelekanides, S., and M. Chatzidakes. *Καστοριά*. Athens, 1984.
———. *Kastoria*. Athens, 1985.
Pelekanides, S. M., P. K. Christou, C. Mavropoulou-Tsioume, S. N. Kadas, and A. Katsarou. *The Treasures of Mount Athos*. Series 1, *Illuminated Manuscripts*. Volume 1, *The Protaton and the Monasteries of Dionysiou, Koutloumousiou, Xeropotamou, and Gregoriou*. Athens, 1974.
———. *The Treasures of Mount Athos*. Series 1, *Illuminated Manuscripts*. Volume 2, *The Monasteries of Iveron, St. Panteleimon, Esphigmenou, and Chilandari*. Athens, 1975.
———. *Οἱ θησαυροὶ τοῦ Ἁγίου Ὄρους*. Series 1, *Εἰκονογραφημένα χειρόγραφα*. Volume 3, *Μ. Μεγίστης Λαύρας, Μ. Παντοκράτορος, Μ. Δοχειαρίου, Μ. Καρακάλλου, Μ. Φιλοθέου, Μ. Ἁγίου Παύλου*. Athens, 1979.
Pennas, Ch. *Η βυζαντινή Αίγινα*. Athens, 2004.
Pentcheva, B. *Icons and Power: The Mother of God in Byzantium*. University Park, Pa., 2006.
Πεντηκοστάριον Χαρμόσυνον. Ἔκδοσις τῆς Ἀποστολικῆς Διακονίας τῆς Ἐκκλησίας τῆς Ἑλλάδος. Athens, 1959.
Perdiki, O. "Les Peintures Murales (Xe–XIIIe siècle) de l'église de Saint-Antoine de Kellia à Chypre." Master 2 dissertation, Ecole Pratique des Hautes Etudes, Paris, 2009.
Perdrizet, P. "L'archange Ouriel." *SemKond* 2 (1928): 258–63.
Peristianes, H. K. *Μονογραφία τῆς ἀρχαίας πόλεως καὶ ἐκκλησίας τῆς Ἀσίνης (νῦν Ἀσίνους)*. Nicosia, 1922.
Pernot, H. "Descente de la Vierge aux enfers, d'après les manuscrits grecs de Paris." *REG* 13 (1900): 233–57.
Petković, V. R. *La peinture serbe du moyen âge*. 2 vols. Belgrade, 1934.
Philippou, L. "Ἡ ναυμαχία τῆς Κεραμαίας." *Κυπρ.Σπ.* 6 (1943): 1–5.
Philotheou, G. "Ἡ μνημειακὴ ζωγραφικὴ στὴν περιοχὴ τῆς μητροπολιτικῆς περιφέρειας Μόρφου." In *Ἱερὰ Μητρόπολις Μόρφου*, 109–26.
Piatnitsky, Y., et al. *Sinai, Byzantium, Russia: Orthodox Art from the Sixth to the Twentieth Century*. Exh. cat., The State Hermitage Museum, St. Petersburg, 2000. London–St. Petersburg, 2000.
Pinasa, D. *Costumes: Modes et manières d'être*. Paris, 1992.
Piponnier, F. "Le vêtement occidental à Chypre d'après les pierres tombales." In Imhaus, *Lacrimae Cypriae*, 2:89–106.
Pivovarova, N. *Freski crkvi Spasa na Neredice v Novgorode: ikonografičeskaja programma rospis*. St. Petersburg, 2002.
Plesters, J. "Cross-sections and Chemical Analysis of Paint Samples." *Studies in Conservation* 2 (1956): 110–57.
———. "Ultramarine Blue, Natural and Artificial." In *Artists' Pigments, A Handbook of Their History and Characteristics*, ed. A. Roy, 2:37–65. Washington, D.C., 1993.
Ploumides, G. S. "Ἔγγραφα ἀφορῶντα εἰς τὴν μονὴν Ἁγίου Νικολάου τῆς Στέγης (1558)." *Ἐπ.Κέν.Ἐπιστ.Ἐρ.* 4 (1970–71): 233–38.
Η Πολιτεία του Μυστρά. (Ώρες Βυζαντίου; Έργα και Ημέρες στο Βυζάντιο). Exh. cat., Mistra, August 2001 – January 2002. Athens, 2001.
Popović, D. *Pod okriljem svetosti: Kult svetih vladara i relikvija u srednjovekovnoj Srbiji*. Belgrade, 2006.
Πρακτικὰ τοῦ πρώτου διεθνοῦς κυπρολογικοῦ συνεδρίου. 3 vols. Nicosia, 1972–73.
Πρακτικὰ τοῦ δευτέρου διεθνοῦς κυπριολογικοῦ συνεδρίου. 3 vols. Nicosia, 1985–87.
Πρακτικά του τρίτου διεθνούς κυπρολογικού συνεδρίου. 3 vols. Nicosia, 2000–2001.
Probatakes, Th. *Ὁ Διάβολος εἰς τὴν βυζαντινὴν τέχνην*. Thessalonike, 1980.
Prokopiou, E. "Άγιος Παύλος, Κυπαρισσόβουνου." In *Ἱερά Μητρόπολις Κυρηνείας: Οδοιπορικό στα χριστιανικά μνημεία της Μητροπολιτικής περιφέρειας Κυρηνείας*, 230–33. Nicosia, 2006.
———. *Ο συνεπτυγμένος σταυροειδής εγγεγραμμένος ναός στην Κύπρο (9ος–12ος αιώνας)*. Μελέτες Βυζαντινής και Μεταβυζαντινής Αρχαιολογίας και Τέχνης 2. Nicosia, 2007.
Prolović, J. *Die Kirche des Heiligen Andreas an der Treska*. Vienna, 1997.
Radojičić, S. *Mileševa*. 2nd ed. Belgrade, 1971.

Raft, A. "About Theophilus' Blue Colour, 'Lazur'." *Studies in Conservation* 13 (1968): 1–6.

Ralles, G. A., and M. Potles. *Σύνταγμα τῶν θείων καὶ ἱερῶν κανόνων*. 6 vols. Athens, 1852–59.

Ramsay, W. M., and G. L. Bell. *The Thousand and One Churches*. London, 1909.

Rasolkoska-Nikolavska, Z. "Le Christ Antiphonitis d'après les monuments à Chypre." In *Πρακτικὰ τοῦ δευτέρου διεθνοῦς κυπριολογικοῦ συνεδρίου*, 2:523–27.

Restle, M. *Byzantine Wall Painting in Asia Minor.* Trans. I. R. Gibbons. 3 vols. Greenwich, Conn., 1968.

Rhoby, A. *Byzantinische Epigramme auf Fresken und Mosaiken*. Byzantinische Epigramme in inschriftlicher Überlieferung 1. Vienna, 2009.

Richard, J. *Chypre sous les Lusignans: Documents Chypriotes des Archives du Vatican (XIVe et XVe siècles)*. Paris, 1962.

———. "Une famille de 'Vénetiens blancs' dans le royaume de Chypre au milieu du XVe siècle: les Audeth et la seigneurie du Marethasse." *Rivista di studi bizantini e slavi* 1 = *Miscellanea Agostino Pertusi*, 1:90–91. Bologna, 1981. Repr. in idem, *Croisés, missionaires et voyageurs*, art. 10. London, 1983.

———, ed. *Le livre des remembrances de la Secrète du royaume de Chypre (1468–1469)*. Sources et études de l'histoire de Chypre 10. Nicosia, 1983.

———. "Un monastère grec de Palestine et son domaine chypriote: le monachisme orthodoxe et l'établissement de la domination franque." In *Πρακτικὰ τοῦ δευτέρου διεθνοῦς κυπριολογικοῦ συνεδρίου*, 2:61–75. Repr. in idem, *Croisades et Etats latins d'Orient: Points de vue et documents*, art. XIV. Aldershot, 1992.

———. "Le peuplement latin et syrien en Chypre au XIIIe siècle." *ByzF* 7 (1979): 157–73. Repr. in idem, *Croisés, missionaires et voyageurs*. London, 1983.

———. "Le statut de la femme dans l'Orient latin." *Recueils de la Société Jean Bodin* 12 (1962): 377–88. Repr. in idem, *Orient et Occident au moyen âge: Contacts et relations (XIIe–XVe s.)* art. XII. London, 1976.

Rizopoulou-Hegoumenidou, E. *Η αστική ενδυμασία της Κύπρου κατά τον $18^{ο}$ και τον $19^{ο}$ αιώνα*. Nicosia, 1996.

Rohland, J. P. *Der Erzengel Michael, Arzt und Feldherr: Zwei Aspekte des vor- und frühbyzantinischen Michaelskultes*. Leiden, 1977.

Ross, M. C., and G. Downey. "A Reliquary of St. Marina." *BSl* 23 (1962): 41–44.

Roueché, C. "The Prehistory of the Cyprus Department of Antiquities." In *Mosaic: Festschrift for A. H. S. Megaw*, ed. J. Herrin, M. Mullett, and C. Otten-Froux, 155–66. British School at Athens Studies 8. Athens, 2001.

Rudt de Collenberg, W. H. "Les premiers Podocataro: Recherches basées sur le testament de Hugues (1452)." *Θησαυρίσματα* 23 (1993): 130–82.

Rupprecht, E. *Cosmae et Damiani sanctorum medicorum vita et miracula*. Berlin, 1935.

Russell, J. D. "Infrared Methods." In *A Handbook of Determinative Methods in Clay Mineralogy*, ed. M. J. Wilson, 133–73. Glasgow–New York, 1987.

Rydén, L. "The Date of the Life of Andreas Salos." *DOP* 32 (1978): 127–55.

———, ed. and trans. *The Life of St. Andrew the Fool*. Studia Byzantina Upsaliensia 4. 2 vols. Uppsala, 1995.

———. "The Life of St. Basil the Younger and the Date of the Life of St. Andreas Salos." In *Okeanos: Essays Presented to Ihor Ševčenko*, ed. C. Mango and O. Pritsak, 568–86. Cambridge, Mass., 1983.

———. "A Note on Some References to the Church of St. Anastasia in Constantinople in the 10th Century." *Byzantion* 44 (1974): 198–201.

Sacopoulo, M. *Asinou en 1106 et sa contribution à l'iconographie*. Bibliothèque de Byzantion 2. Brussels, 1966.

Safran, L. "The Art of Veneration: Saints and Villages in the Salento and the Mani." In *Les villages dans l'Empire byzantin (IVe–XVe siècle)*, ed. J. Lefort, C. Morrisson, and J.-P. Sodini, 179–92. Paris, 2005.

Sajdak, J. "Spicilegium Geometreum." *Eos* 32 (1929): 191–98, 33 (1931): 521–34.

Sakellarios, A. A. *Τὰ Κυπριακά: Ἤτοι γεωγραφία, ἱστορία καὶ γλῶσσα τῆς νήσου Κύπρου ἀπὸ τῶν ἀρχαιοτάτων χρόνων μέχρι σήμερον*. 2 vols. Athens, 1891; repr. Nicosia, 1991.

Salaville, S. "Marie dans la liturgie byzantine ou gréco-slave." In *Maria: Études sur la Sainte Vierge*, ed. H. Du Manoir de Juaye, 1:247–326. Paris, 1952.

Salko, N., ed. *Early Russian Painting 11th to Early 13th Centuries: Mosaics, Frescoes, Icons / Zhivopis' drevnei Rusi XI–nachala XIII Veka: Mozaiki, freski, ikony*. Leningrad, 1982.

Savage, M. "The Interrelationship of Text, Imagery and Architectural Space in Byzantium." In *Die kulturhistorische Bedeutung byzantinischer Epigramme: Akten des internationalen Workshop (Wien, 1.–2. Dezember 2006)*, ed. W. Hörandner and A. Rhoby, 101–12. Vienna, 2008.

Schabel, C. "Religion." In Nicolaou-Konnari and Schabel, *Cyprus: Society and Culture*, 157–218.

———, ed. and trans. *The Synodicum Nicosiense and Other Documents of the Latin Church of Cyprus, 1196–1373*. Texts and Studies in the History of Cyprus 39. Nicosia, 2001.

Schein, S. "Between Mount Moriah and the Holy Sepulchre: The Changing Traditions of the Temple Mount in the Central Middle Ages." *Traditio* 40 (1984): 175–95.

———. "Women in Medieval Colonial Society: The Latin Kingdom of Jerusalem in the Twelfth Century." In *Engendering the Crusades*, ed. S. B. Edgington and S. Lambert, 140–53. New York, 2002.

Schiller, G. *Iconography of Christian Art*. 2 vols. Greenwich, Conn., 1971–72.

Schilling, M., and H. Khanjian. "Gas Chromatographic Analysis of Amino Acids as Ethyl Chloroformate Derivatives: III. Identification of Proteinaceous Binding Media by Interpretation of Amino Acid Composition Data." In *ICOM Committee for Conservation Preprints, 11th Triennial Meeting, Edinburgh, Scotland, 1–6 September 1996*, ed. J. Bridgland, 220–27. London, 1996.

Schirò, G., ed. *Analecta Hymnica Graeca, Canones Septembris*. Rome, 1966.
Schmidt, V. "La 'Madonna dei francescani' di Duccio: Forma, contenuti, funzione." *Prospettiva* 97 (2000): 30–44.
Schmidt-Colinet, A. "'Velum und Kolpos': Ein paganer Bildtopos und seine interpretatio christiana." *Mitteilungen zur Spätantiken Archäologie und Byzantinischen Kunstgeschichte* 1 (1998): 29–46.
Schreiner, P. *Die byzantinischen Kleinchroniken*. 3 vols. CFHB 12. Vienna, 1975–79.
Schwartz, E. "The Whirling Disc." *Zograf* 8 (1977): 24–29.
Seferis, G. *Collected Poems 1924–1955*. Trans., ed., and intro. by E. Keeley and P. Sheppard. Princeton, 1967.
Semoglou, A. "Portraits chypriotes de donateurs et le triomphe de l'élégance: Questions posées par l'étude des vêtements du XIVe au XVIe siècle." In *Αφιέρωμα στη μνήμη του Σωτήρη Κίσσα*, 485–509. Thessalonike, 2001.
———. *Le voyage outre-tombe de la Vierge dans l'art byzantin de la Descente aux Enfers à la Montée au Ciel*. Thessalonike, 2003.
Ševčenko, I. "Captions to a David Cycle in the Tenth-Century Oxford *Auct. D. 4. 1*." In *Πολύπλευρος Νοῦς: Miscellanea für Peter Schreiner zu seinem 60. Geburtstag*, ed. C. Scholz and G. Makris, 324–41. Byzantinisches Archiv 19. Munich–Leipzig, 2000.
———. "The Lost Panels of the North Door to the Chapel of the Burning Bush at Sinai." In *Aetos: Studies in Honour of Cyril Mango*, ed. I. Ševčenko and I. Hutter, 284–98. Stuttgart–Leipzig, 1998.
Ševčenko, N. P. "Close Encounters: Contact between Holy Figures and the Faithful as Represented in Byzantine Works of Art." In *Byzance et les images*, ed. A. Guillou and J. Durand, 255–84. Paris, 1994.
———. "The Five Hymnographers at Nerezi," *Palaeoslavica* 10, no. 2 (2002) = *Χρυσαῖ Πύλαι—Zlataia vrata: Essays Presented to Ihor Ševčenko on His Eightieth Birthday by His Colleagues and Students*, ed. P. Schreiner and O. Strakhov, 55–68. Cambridge, Mass., 2002.
———. "Icons in the Liturgy." *DOP* 45 (1991): 45–57.
———. *Illustrated Manuscripts of the Metaphrastian Menologion*. Chicago, 1990.
———. *The Life of Saint Nicholas in Byzantine Art*. Turin, 1983.
———. "The Painted Metrical Inscriptions at Asinou (Cyprus): A Preliminary Report." In *L'épistolographie et la poésie épigrammatique: Actes de la 16e Table ronde du XXe Congrès international des études byzantines*, 229–31. Dossiers byzantins 3. Paris 2003.
———. "The *Vita* Icon and the Painter as Iconographer." *DOP* 53 (1999): 149–65.
Ševčenko, N. P., and C. Moss, eds. *Medieval Cyprus: Studies in Art, Architecture, and History in Memory of Doula Mouriki*. Princeton, 1999.
Shchepkina, M. V. *Miniatiury Khludovskoĭ Psaltyri*. Moscow, 1977.
Shorr, D. C. "The Iconographic Development of the Presentation in the Temple." *ArtB* 28 (1946): 17–32.
Šimek, P., A. Heydová, and A. Jegorov. "High Resolution Capillary Gas Chromatography and Gas Chromatography–Mass Spectrometry of Protein and Non-protein Amino Acids, Amino Alcohols, and Hydroxycarboxylic Acids as Their *Tert*-butyldimethylsilyl Derivatives." *Journal of High Resolution Chromatography* 17 (1994): 145–52.
Sinkević, I. "Changes in the Composition of the Presentation of Christ in the Temple in Palaeologan Times." *Kulturno Nasledstvo/Patrimoine Culturel* 28–29 (2002–3): 33–38.
———. *The Church of St. Panteleimon at Nerezi: Architecture, Programme, Patronage*. Wiesbaden, 2000.
Siomkos, N. *L'église Saint-Etienne à Kastoria: Étude des différentes phases du décor peint (X^e–XIVe siècles)*. Byzantine Texts and Studies 38. Thessalonike, 2005.
Skalova, Z. "Mourning with Indigo: A Restored Medieval Passion Triptych in the Coptic Museum, Cairo." In *East and West in the Crusader States: Context—Contacts—Confrontations II*, ed. K. Ciggaar and H. Teule, 177–210. Leuven, 1999.
Skawran, K. M. *The Development of Middle Byzantine Fresco Painting in Greece*. Pretoria, 1982.
Skrobucha, H. *Kosmas und Damian*. Recklinghausen, 1965.
Smirnova, E. "Culte et image de St. Démètre dans la principauté de Vladimir à la fin du XIIe–début du XIIIe siècle." In *Βυζαντινή Μακεδονία 324–1430 μ.Χ: Διεθνές Συμπόσιο, Θεσσαλονίκη 29–31 Οκτωβρίου 1992*, 267–77. Thessalonike, 1995.
———. *Ikony Severo-Vostochnoĭ Rusi*. Moscow, 2004.
———. "Remarques sur l'iconographie de Saint Démétrios." In *Αφιέρωμα στη μνήμη Σωτήρη Κίσσα*, 537–47. Thessalonike, 2001.
Smyrlis, K. *La fortune des grands monastères byzantins (fin du Xe–milieu du XIVe siècle)*. Paris, 2006.
Sollars, L. H. "Settlement and Community: Their Location, Limits and Movement through the Landscape of Historical Cyprus." Ph.D. diss., University of Glasgow, 2005.
Sophocleous, S. *Cyprus the Holy Island: Icons through the Centuries, 10th–20th Century*. Exh. cat., The Hellenic Centre, London, 1 November – 17 December, 2000. Nicosia, 2000.
———. *Icônes de Chypre: Diocèse de Limassol 12e–16e siècle*. Nicosia, 2006.
———. *Icons of Cyprus, 7th–20th Century*. Nicosia, 1994.
Soteriou, G. A. *Τὰ βυζαντινὰ μνημεῖα τῆς Κύπρου*. Volume 1, *Λεύκωμα*. Athens, 1935.
———. "Ἡ εἰκὼν τῆς Παμμακαρίστου." *Πρακτικὰ τῆς Ἀκαδημίας Ἀθηνῶν* 8 (1933): 359–68.
Soteriou, G. A., and M. G. Soteriou. *Εἰκόνες τῆς Μονῆς Σινᾶ*. 2 vols. Athens, 1956–58.
Soteriou, M. G. "Ενταφιασμὸς—θρῆνος." *Δελτ.Χριστ.Ἀρχ. Ἑτ.*, ser. 4, 7 (1974): 139–48. [English summary, 147–48.]

———. "Αἱ τοιχογραφίαι τοῦ βυζαντινοῦ ναΰδρίου τῶν Ταξιαρχῶν Δεσφίνης." *Δελτ.Χριστ.Ἀρχ.Ἑτ.*, ser. 4, 3 (1962–63): 175–202.

Sotiropoulou, S., Sister Daniilia, C. Miliani, F. Rosi, L. Cartechini, and D. Papanikola-Bakirtzis. "Micro-analytical Investigation of Degradation Issues in Byzantine Wall Paintings," *Applied Physics A: Materials Science & Processing* 92, no. 1 (2008): 143–50.

Spanou, Ch. "Η τέχνη στη μητροπολιτική περιφέρεια Κιτίου από τον 6ο έως το 15ο αι. Μνημειακή ζωγραφική και φορητές εικόνες." In *Η κατά Κίτιον αγιογραφική τέχνη*, ed. eadem, 21–56. Larnaca, 2002.

Spatharakis, I. *Byzantine Wall Paintings of Crete: Rethymnon Province*. Volume 1. London, 1999.

———. *Dated Byzantine Wall Paintings of Crete*. Leiden, 2001.

———. *The Illustrations of the Cynegetica in Venice: Codex Marcianus Graecus Z 139*. Leiden, 2004.

———. "The Influence of the Lithos in the Development of the Iconography of the Threnos." In *Byzantine East, Latin West: Art-Historical Studies in Honor of Kurt Weitzmann*, ed. D. Mouriki, S. Ćurčić, G. Galavaris, H. L. Kessler, and G. Vikan, 435–46. Princeton, 1995.

———. *The Portrait in Byzantine Illuminated Manuscripts*. Byzantina Neerlandica 6. Leiden, 1976.

Spatharakis, I., A.A. T. van den Brink, and A. Verweij. "A Cycle of St. Mamas in a Cretan Church." *JÖB* 53 (2003): 229–38.

Speck, P. *Theodoros Studites Jamben auf verschiedene Gegenstände*. Supplementa Byzantina 1. Berlin, 1968.

Spyridakis, K., G. Papacharalampous, and N. Klerides. "Οἱ ἅγιοι Καρπασίας Φίλων, Συνέσιος, Θύρσος, Φωτεινή, Σωζόμενος." *Κυπρ.Σπ.* 11 (1947). [Entire issue.]

Staurobouniotes, Ch. "Οἱ ἅγιοι τῆς μητροπολιτικῆς περιφερείας Μόρφου." In *Ἱερὰ Μητρόπολις Μόρφου*, 207–28.

Sternbach, L. "Methodii patriarchae et Ignatii patriarchae carmina inedita." *Eos* 4 (1898): 150–63.

Stewart, C. *Demons and the Devil: Moral Imagination in Modern Greek Culture*. Princeton, 1991.

Stichel, R. *Studien zum Verhältnis von Text und Bild spät- und nachbyzantinischer Vergänglichkeitsdarstellungen*. Vienna, 1971.

Stornajolo, C. *Miniature delle Omilie di Giacomo Monaco (cod. Vatic. gr. 1162) e dell'Evangeliario greco urbinate (cod. Vatic. urbin. gr. 2)*. Rome, 1910.

Stratos, A. *Τὸ Βυζάντιο στὸν Ζ' αἰώνα*. Athens, 1977.

Strzygowski, J. *Die Miniaturen des Serbischen Psalters der königlichen Hof- und Staatsbibliothek in München*. 2 vols. Vienna, 1906.

Stubblebine, J. H. *Guido da Siena*. Princeton, 1964.

Stylianou, A., and J. A. Stylianou. "Donors and Dedicatory Inscriptions, Supplicants and Supplications in the Painted Churches of Cyprus." *JÖBG* 9 (1960): 97–128.

———. "Ἐπανεξέτασις τῆς ἐν τῷ νάρθηκι τοῦ ναοῦ τοῦ ἁγίου Νικολάου τῆς Στέγης κτητορικῆς ἐπιγραφῆς." *Κυπρ.Σπ.* 15 (1951): 83–88.

———. "The Militarization of the Betrayal and Its Examples in the Painted Churches of Cyprus." In *Ευφρόσυνον: Αφιέρωμα στον Μανόλη Χατζηδάκη*, 2:570–81. Athens, 1991.

———. "Ὁ ναὸς τοῦ Ἁγίου Νικολάου τῆς Στέγης παρὰ τὴν Κακοπετριάν." *Κυπρ.Σπ.* 10 (1946): 95–196.

———. *The Painted Churches of Cyprus: Treasures of Byzantine Art*. London, 1985. Rev. ed. Nicosia, 1997.

———. "Παναγία Φορβιώτισσα Ἀσίνου." *Κυπρ.Σπ.* 15 (1951): 147–52.

———. *Παναγία Φορβιώτισσα Ἀσίνου / Panagia Phorbiotissa Asinou*. Nicosia, 1973.

———. "Prophet Zechariah 'the Sickle'." *RDAC* (1984): 348–50, pl. 78.2.

Taft, R. F. "Women at Church in Byzantium: Where, When—and Why?" *DOP* 52 (1998): 27–87.

Talbot, A.-M. "The Byzantine Family and the Monastery." *DOP* 44 (1990): 119–29.

———. "Epigrams in Context: Metrical Inscriptions on Art and Architecture of the Palaiologan Era." *DOP* 53 (1999): 75–90.

———. "Epigrams of Manuel Philes on the Theotokos tes Peges and Its Art." *DOP* 48 (1994): 135–65.

———. "Healing Shrines in Late Byzantine Constantinople." In eadem, *Women and Religious Life in Byzantium*, art. XIV. Aldershot, 2001.

———. "Metaphrasis in the Early Palaiologan Period: The Miracula of Kosmas and Damian by Maximos the Deacon." In *The Heroes of the Orthodox Church: The New Saints, 8th–16th c.*, ed. E. Kountoura-Galake, 227–37. Athens, 2004.

———. "Women's Space in Byzantine Monasteries." *DOP* 52 (1998): 113–28.

Talbot Rice, D. *The Church of Haghia Sophia at Trebizond*. Edinburgh, 1968.

———. *The Icons of Cyprus*. Courtauld Institute Publications on Near Eastern Art 2. London, 1937.

Talbot Rice, T. "The Costume of Cyprus in the Middle Ages." In D. Talbot Rice, *The Icons of Cyprus*, 100–139. London, 1937.

Taousianes, Ch. N. *Εκκλησίες και μοναστήρια της Κύπρου. Λεύκωμα Θ': Εκκλησίες και μοναστήρια της Επαρχίας Λεμεσού*. Nicosia, 2010.

Tapkova-Zaimova, V. "Le culte de St. Démétrius à Byzance et aux Balkans (Problèmes d' histoire et de culture)." In *Das Christentum in Bulgarien und auf der übrigen Balkanhalbinsel in der Spätantike und im frühen Mittelalter*, volume 2, *Internationales Symposium Haskovo (Bulgarien), 10.–13. Juni 1986*, ed. V. Gjuselev and R. Pillinger, 139–46. Vienna, 1987.

Tatić-Djurić, M. "Archanges gardiens de porte à Dečani." In *Dečani i Vizantijska umetnost sredinom XIV veka*, ed. V. Djurić, 359–66. Belgrade, 1989.

———. *Das Bild der Engel*. Recklinghausen, 1962.

———. "Eleousa: A la recherche du type iconographique." *JÖB* 25 (1976): 259–67.

———. "Steatitska ikonica iz Kuršumlije." *ZbLikUmet* 2 (1966): 65–85.
Taylor, M. D. "A Historiated Tree of Jesse." *DOP* 34/35 (1980/81): 125–76.
Tchalenko, G. *Villages antiques de la Syrie du Nord: Le massif de Bélus à l'époque romaine*. Paris, 1953.
Teteriatnikov, N. "Burial Places in Cappadocian Churches." *GOTR* 29 (1984): 141–74.
———. "The Frescoes of the Chapel of St. Basil in Cappadocia: Their Date and Context Reconsidered." *CahArch* 40 (1992): 99–114.
———. *The Liturgical Planning of Byzantine Churches in Cappadocia*. Rome, 1976.
———. "Private Salvation Programs and Their Effect on Byzantine Church Decoration." *Arte Medievale* 7, no. 2 (1993): 47–63.
Theocharides, I. P. *Οθωμανικά έγγραφα*. 5 vols. Nicosia, 1993.
Theodore of Mopsuestia. *On the Lord's Prayer and on the Sacraments of Baptism and the Eucharist*. Ed. and trans. A. Mingana. Woodbrooke Studies 6. Cambridge, 1933.
Theophanes the Confessor. *Chronographia*. 2 vols. Ed. C. De Boor. Leipzig, 1883–85.
Theophilus, *On Divers Arts*. Trans. J. G. Hawthorne and C. S. Smith. Chicago, 1963; repr. New York, 1979.
Thierry, M., and N. Thierry. "Ayvalı Kilise ou Pigeonnier de Güllü Dere, église inédite de Cappadoce." *CahArch* 15 (1965): 97–154.
———. *Nouvelles églises rupestres de Cappadoce: Région du Hasan Daği*. Paris, 1963.
Thierry, N. "L'Apocalypse de Jean et l'iconographie byzantine." In *L'Apocalypse de Jean: Traditions exégétiques et iconographiques IIIe–XIIIe siècles; Actes du colloque de la Fondation Hardt, Genève, 29 février–mars 1976*, ed. R. Petraglio, 319–30. Geneva, 1979.
———. "A propos des peintures d'Ayvali köy (Cappadoce): Les programmes absidaux à trois registres avec Déïsis, en Cappadoce et en Géorgie." *Zograf* 5 (1974): 5–22.
———. "Aux limites du sacré et du magique: Un programme d'entrée d'une église en Cappadoce." In *La science des cieux: Sages, mages, astrologues*, 233–47. Res Orientales 12. Bures-sur-Yvette, 1999.
———. "Découvertes: La nécropole de Göreme (Cappadoce)." *Comptes rendus de l'Académie des inscriptions et belles-lettres* (1984): 656–91.
———. "Deux notes à propos du Mandylion." *Zograf* 11 (1980): 16–19.
———. "L'église au Jugement dernier de Göreme (Göreme No 2b)." In *Λαμπηδών: Αφιέρωμα στη μνήμη Ντούλας Μουρίκη*, ed. M. Aspra-Vardavaki, 815–28. Athens, 2002.
———. *Haut Moyen Age en Cappadoce: Les églises de la région de Çavuşin*. 2 vols. Paris, 1983.
———. "Le portrait funéraire byzantin: Nouvelles données." In *Ευφρόσυνον: Αφιέρωμα στον Μανόλη Χατζηδάκη*, 2:582–92. Athens, 1991.
———. "Vision d'Eustache, Vision de Procope: Nouvelles données sur l'iconographie funéraire byzantine." In *Άρμός: Τιμητικός τόμος στον Καθηγητή Ν. Κ. Μουτσόπουλο για τα 25 χρόνια πνευματικής του προσφοράς στο πανεπιστήμιο*, 3:1845–60. Thessalonike, 1991.
Thomas, J. P. *Private Religious Foundations in the Byzantine Empire*. DOS 24. Washington, D.C., 1987.
Thompson, D. V. *The Materials and Techniques of Medieval Painting*. New York, 1956. [Repr. of *The Materials of Medieval Painting*, 1936.]
Tischendorf, C., ed. *Apocalypses apocryphae Mosis, Esdrae, Pauli, Johannis item Mariae Dormitio*. Leipzig, 1866.
Todić, B. *Staro Nagoričino*. Belgrade, 1993.
Tomeković, S. "Contribution à l'étude du programme du narthex des églises monastiques (XIe–première moitié du XIIIe s.)." *Byzantion* 58 (1988): 140–54.
———. "Le Jugement dernier inédit de l'église d'Agètria (Magne)." In *16. Internationaler Byzantinistenkongress, Akten II, 5 = JÖB* 32, no. 5 (1982): 469–79.
Torraca, G. *Porous Building Materials*. Rome, 1988.
Trésors de Byzance: Manuscrits grecs de la Bibliothèque Nationale de France. Exh. cat., 20 August – 2 September 2001. Paris, 2001.
Triantaphyllopoulos, D. D. "Il culto e l'immagine di san Nicola a Cipro." In *San Nicola: Splendori d'arte d'Oriente e d'Occidente*, ed. M. Bacci, 117–26. Exh. cat., Castello Svevo, Bari, 7 December 2006 – 6 May 2007. Milan, 2006.
———. "Ἡ τέχνη στὴν Κύπρο ἀπὸ τὴν ἅλωση τῆς Κωνσταντινουπόλεως (1453) ἕως τὴν ἔναρξη τῆς Τουρκοκρατίας (1571): Βυζαντινή / Μεσαιωνική ἤ Μεταβυζαντινή." In *Πρακτικά του τρίτου διεθνούς κυπρολογικού συνεδρίου*, 2:621–50.
Τριώδιον Κατανυκτικόν. Ἔκδοσις τῆς Ἀποστολικῆς Διακονίας τῆς Ἐκκλησίας τῆς Ἑλλάδος. Athens, 1960.
Troianos, S. "Οι ποινές στο βυζαντινό δίκαιο." In *Έγκλημα και Τιμωρία στο Βυζάντιο*, ed. idem, 13–65. Athens, 1997.
Tsigaridas, E. N. "La peinture à Kastoria et en Macédoine grecque occidentale vers l'année 1200." In *Studenica et l'art Byzantin autour de l'année 1200*, ed. V. Korać, 309–20. Colloques scientifiques de l'Académie Serbe des sciences et des arts 41, classe des Sciences historiques 11. Belgrade, 1988.
———. "Τοιχογραφία του Αγίου Δημητρίου Θεσσαλονίκης." In *Δώρον: Τιμητικός τόμος στον καθηγητή Νίκο Νικονάνο*, 209–12. Thessalonike, 2006.
———. *Οι τοιχογραφίες της Μονής Λατόμου Θεσσαλονίκης και η βυζαντινή ζωγραφική του 12ου αιώνα*. Thessalonike, 1986.
Tsiknopoullos, I. P. "Ἅγιοι τῆς Κύπρου." *Κυπρ.Σπ.* 30 (1966): 131–61.
———. *Ἡ Ἱερὰ Μονὴ τοῦ Χρυσοστόμου τοῦ Κουτσοβέντη καὶ τὰ αὐτῆς κτίσματα*. Nicosia, 1959.
———. "Νεοφύτου πρεσβυτέρου, μοναχοῦ καὶ ἐγκλείστου, ἐγκώμιον εἰς Μαρῖναν." *Apostolos Barnabas* 16 (1955): 326–29.
Tsitouridou, A. *The Church of the Panagia Chalkeon*. Thessalonike, 1985.
———. *Ο ζωγραφικός διάκοσμος τοῦ Ἁγίου Νικολάου Ὀρφανοῦ στὴ Θεσσαλονίκη*. Thessalonike, 1986.

Tsuji, S. "The Headpiece Miniatures and Genealogy Pictures in Paris. Gr. 74." *DOP* 29 (1975): 166–203.

———. "The Study of the Byzantine Gospel Illustrations in Florence, Laur. Plut. VI 23 and Paris, Bibl. Nat. cod. gr. 74." Ph.D. diss., Princeton University, 1967.

Underwood, P. A. *The Kariye Djami*. 4 vols. Bollingen Series 70. New York, 1966–75.

———. "Some Problems in Programs and Iconography of Ministry Cycles." In idem, *The Kariye Djami*, 4:243–302. Princeton, 1975.

———. "Third Preliminary Report on the Restoration of the Frescoes in the Kariye Camii at Istanbul by the Byzantine Institute, 1956." *DOP* 12 (1958): 235–65.

Usener, H. *Acta S. Marinae et S. Christophori: Festschrift zur fünften Säcularfeier der Carl-Ruprecht-Universität zu Heidelberg*. Bonn, 1886.

Vaivre, J.-B. de, and P. Plagnieux, ed. *L'Art gothique en Chypre*. Paris, 2006.

Van der Marel, H. W., and H. Beutelspacher. *Atlas of Infrared Spectroscopy of Clay Minerals and Their Admixtures*. New York, 1976.

Van Rompay, L. "'Une faucille volante': La représentation du prophète Zacharie dans le codex de Rabbula et la tradition syriaque." In *La Spiritualité de l'univers byzantin dans le verbe et l'image: Hommages offerts à Edmond Voordeckers à l'occasion de son éméritat*, ed. K. Demoen and J. Vereecken, 343–54. Turnhout, 1997.

Varales, I. D. "Παρατηρήσεις για τη θέση του Ευαγγελισμού στη μνημειακή ζωγραφική κατά τη μεσοβυζαντινή περίοδο." *Δελτ.Χριστ.Ἀρχ.Ἑτ.*, ser. 4, 19 (1996–97): 201–20.

Vassilaki, M. "A Cretan Icon of Saint George." *The Burlington Magazine* 131 (1989): 208–14.

———. "Εἰκονογραφικοὶ κύκλοι ἀπὸ τὴ ζωὴ τοῦ Μεγάλου Κωνσταντίνου σὲ ἐκκλησίες τῆς Κρήτης." *Κρητικὴ Ἑστία*, ser. 4, 1 (1987): 60–84.

———, ed. *Images of the Mother of God: Perceptions of the Theotokos in Byzantium*. Aldershot, 2005.

———. "Καθημερινή ζωή και πραγματικότητα στη βενετοκρατούμενη Κρήτη: Η μαρτυρία των τοιχογραφημένων εκκλησιών." In *Ενθύμησις Νικολάου Μ. Παναγιωτάκη*, 57–80. Herakleion, 2000.

———, ed. *Mother of God: Representations of the Virgin in Byzantine Art*. Exh. cat., Benaki Museum, Athens, 20 Oct. 2000 – 20 Jan. 2001. Milan, 2000.

———. "Οἱ πλούσιοι πᾶνε στὴν Κόλαση;" In *Διεθνὲς Συμπόσιο Πλούσιοι καὶ Φτωχοὶ στὴν κοινωνία τῆς ἑλληνολατινικῆς Ἀνατολῆς*, ed. Ch. Maltezou, 473–82. Venice, 1998.

Vassis, I. *Initia carminum Byzantinorum*. Supplementa Byzantina 8. Berlin–New York, 2005.

Vees, N. A. "Σύνταγμα ἐπιγραφικῶν μνημείων Μετεώρων καὶ τῆς πέριξ Χώρας μετὰ σχετικῶν ἀρχαιολογημάτων." *Βυζαντίς* 1 (1909): 537–626.

Velmans, T. "L'arbre de Jessé en Orient chrétien." °, ser. 4, 26 (2005): 125–40.

———. "L'image de la Déisis dans les églises de Géorgie et dans celles d'autres régions du monde byzantin." *CahArch* 29 (1980–81): 47–102; 31 (1983): 129–73. Repr. in eadem, *L'art médiéval de l'Orient chrétien: Recueil d'études*, 2nd ed. Sofia, 2002.

———. *La peinture murale byzantine à la fin du Moyen Âge*. Bibliothèque des Cahiers archéologiques 11. Paris, 1978.

———. "Le portrait dans l'art des Paléologues." In *Art et société à Byzance sous les Paléologues*, 91–148. Bibliothèque de l'Institut hellénique d'études byzantines et post-byzantines de Venise 4. Venice, 1971.

———. "Quelques programmes iconographiques de coupoles chypriotes du XIIe au XVe siècle." *CahArch* 32 (1984): 137–62.

———. "Rayonnement de l'icône au XIIe et au début du XIIIe siècle." In *XVe Congrès international d'études byzantines, Rapports et co-rapports*, volume 3, *Art et archéologie*, 195–227. Athens, 1976.

———. *Le Tétraévangile byzantin de la Laurentienne, Laur. VI 23*. Bibliothèque des Cahiers archéologiques 6. Paris, 1971.

Ven, Paul van den. *La Légende de S. Spyridon, évêque de Trimithonte*. Louvain, 1953.

Venditti, A. *Architettura bizantina nell'Italia meridionale*. 2 vols. Naples, 1967.

Veselovskij, A. N., ed. "Razyskanija v oblasti russkogo duchovnogo sticha." *Sbornik Otdelenija russkogo jazyka i slovesnosti Imperatorskoj Akademii nauk* 46 (1889–90): supp. 3-89; 53 (1891–92): supp. 3-174.

Vilinskij, S. G. "Žitie sv. Vasilja novago v russkoj literature, II: Teksty žitia." *Zapiski imp. Novorossiskago universitete* 7. Odessa, 1911.

Viollet-le-Duc, E.-E. *Encyclopédie médiévale*. 2 vols. Ed. G. Bernage. Bayeux, 1978.

Vloberg, M. "Les types iconographiques de la mère de Dieu dans l'art byzantin." In *Maria: Études sur la Sainte Vierge*, ed. H. du Manoir de Juaye, 2:403–43. Paris, 1952.

Vocotopoulos, P. L. *Βυζαντινές Εικόνες: Ελληνική τέχνη*. Athens, 1995.

———. "The Concealed Course Technique: Further Examples and a Few Remarks." *JÖB* 28 (1979): 247–60.

———. *Ἡ ἐκκλησιαστικὴ ἀρχιτεκτονικὴ εἰς τὴν δυτικὴν Στερεὰν Ἑλλάδα καὶ τὴν Ἤπειρον, ἀπὸ τοῦ τέλους τοῦ 7ου μέχρι τοῦ τέλους τοῦ 10ου αἰῶνος*. Thessalonike, 1975.

———. "L'évangile illustré de Mytilène." In *Studenica et l'art byzantin autour de l'année 1200*, ed. V. Korać, 377–84. Colloques scientifiques de l'Académie Serbe des sciences et des arts 41, classe des Sciences historiques 11. Belgrade, 1988.

———. "Three Thirteenth-Century Icons at Moutoullas." In Ševčenko and Moss, *Medieval Cyprus*, 161–71, color pls. 9–12.

Vojvodić, D. "Kult i ikonografija svete Anastasije Farmakolitrije u zemljama vizantijskog kulturnog kruga." *Zograf* 21 (1990): 31–40.

Walter, C. *Art and Ritual of the Byzantine Church*. London, 1982.

———. "Bulletin on the Deësis and the Paraclesis." *REB* 38 (1980): 261–69.

———. "Further Notes on the Deësis." *REB* 28 (1970): 161–87. Repr. in idem, *Studies in Byzantine Iconography*, art. 2. London, 1977.
———. "IC XC NI KA: The Apotropaic Function of the Victorious Cross." *REB* 55 (1997): 193–220.
———. "A New Look at the Byzantine Sanctuary Barrier." *REB* 51 (1993): 203–28.
———. "The Origins of the Cult of St. George." *REB* 53 (1995): 295–326.
———. "The Portrait of St. Paraskeve." *BSl* 56 (1995): 753–58. Repr. in idem, *Pictures as Language: How the Byzantines Exploited Them*, art. 22. London, 2000.
———. "Two Notes on the Deësis." *REB* 26 (1968): 311–36. Repr. in idem, *Studies in Byzantine Iconography*, art. 1. London, 1977.
———. "St. Demetrius: The Myroblytos of Thessalonika." *EChR* 5 (1973): 157–78. Repr. in idem, *Studies in Byzantine Iconography*, art. 5.
———. *Studies in Byzantine Iconography*. London, 1977.
———. *The Warrior Saints in Byzantine Art and Tradition*. Aldershot, 2003.
Warland, R. "Deesis–Emmanuel–Maria: Bildkonzepte kappadokischer Höhlenkirchen des 13. Jahrhunderts." In Koch, *Byzantinische Malerei*, 365–86.
Wassiliou, A.-K. "Ο Άγιος Γεώργιος ο Διασορίτης auf Siegeln." *BZ* 90 (1997): 416–24.
Weissbrod, U. *"Hier liegt der Knecht Gottes . . .": Gräber in byzantinischen Kirchen und ihr Dekor (11. bis 15. Jahrhundert)*. Wiesbaden, 2003.
Weitzmann, K. *Die byzantinische Buchmalerei des IX. und X. Jahrhunderts*. Berlin, 1935; repr. Vienna, 1996.
———. "Four Icons on Mount Sinai: New Aspects in Crusader Art." *JÖB* 21 (1972): 279–93. Repr. in idem, *Studies in the Arts at Sinai*, art. 13.
———. "A Group of Early Twelfth-Century Sinai Icons Attributed to Cyprus." In *Studies in Memory of David Talbot Rice*, ed. G. Robertson and G. Henderson, 47–63. Edinburgh, 1975.
———. "Icon Painting in the Crusader Kingdom." *DOP* 20 (1966): 51–83. Repr. in idem, *Studies in the Arts at Sinai*, art. 12.
———. "Illustrations to the Lives of the Five Martyrs of Sebaste." *DOP* 33 (1979): 95–112.
———. "*Loca Sancta* and the Representational Arts of Palestine." *DOP* 28 (1974): 31–56. Repr. in idem, *Studies in the Arts at Sinai*, art. 2.
———. "A Metamorphosis Icon or Miniature on Mt. Sinai." *Starinar*, n.s., 20 (1969): 415–21.
———. *The Monastery of Saint Catherine at Mount Sinai: The Icons*. Volume 1, *From the Sixth to the Tenth Century*. Princeton, 1976.
———. "The Origin of the Threnos." In *De Artibus Opuscula XL: Essays in Honor of Erwin Panofsky*, ed. M. Meiss, 476–90. New York, 1961.
———. *The St. Peter Icon of Dumbarton Oaks*. Washington, D.C., 1983.
———. *Studies in Classical and Byzantine Manuscript Illumination*. Chicago, 1971.
———. *Studies in the Arts at Sinai*. Princeton, 1982.
———. "Thirteenth-Century Crusader Icons on Mount Sinai." *ArtB* 45, no. 3 (1963): 179–203. Repr. in idem, *Studies in the Arts at Sinai*, art. 11.
Weitzmann, K., and H. L. Kessler. *The Frescoes of the Dura Synagogue and Christian Art*. Washington, D.C., 1990.
Weitzmann, K., et al. *The Icon*. New York, 1982.
Westerink, L. G., ed. *Michael Psellus, Poemata*. Stuttgart, 1992.
Westphalen, S. "Byzantinisierende Wandmalereien in Syrien." In Koch, *Byzantinische Malerei*, 387–403.
———. "Das Kloster Mar Yakub und seine Wandmalereien." In *Christliche Wandmalereien in Syrien: Qara und das Kloster Mar Yakub*, ed. A. Schmidt and S. Westphalen, 69–153. Wiesbaden, 2005.
Wharton, A. J. *Art of Empire: Painting and Architecture of the Byzantine Periphery; A Comparative Study of Four Provinces*. University Park, Pa., 1988.
Whitaker, E. C. *Documents of the Baptismal Liturgy*. London, 1970.
Wilk, B. "Die Darstellung der Kreuztragung Christi und verwandter Szenen bis um 1300." Ph.D. diss., Eberhard-Karls-Universität, Tübingen, 1969.
Wilkinson, J. *Jerusalem Pilgrimage, 1099–1187*. London, 1988.
Winfield, D. *Asinou: A Guide*. Nicosia, 1969.
———. "The Church of the Panagia tou Arakos, Lagoudera: First Preliminary Report, 1968." *DOP* 23–24 (1969–70): 377–80. [Appendix by C. Mango.]
———. "Hagios Chrysostomos, Trikomo, Asinou: Byzantine Painters at Work." In *Πρακτικὰ τοῦ πρώτου διεθνοῦς κυπρολογικοῦ συνεδρίου*, 2:285–91. Nicosia, 1972.
———. *La Maniera Greca*. Nicosia, forthcoming.
———. "Middle and Later Byzantine Wall Painting Methods: A Comparative Study." *DOP* 22 (1968): 61–139.
Winfield, D. C., and E. J. W. Hawkins. "The Church of Our Lady at Asinou, Cyprus: A Report on the Seasons of 1965 and 1966." *DOP* 21 (1967): 260–66.
Winfield, D., and J. Winfield. *The Church of the Panaghia tou Arakos at Lagoudhera, Cyprus: The Paintings and their Painterly Significance*. DOS 37. Washington, D.C., 2003.
Winfield, J., and D. Winfield. *Proportion and Structure of the Human Figure in Byzantine Wall-Painting and Mosaic*. BAR International Series 154. Oxford, 1982.
Wittman, A. *Kosmas und Damian: Kultausbreitung und Volksdevotion*. Berlin, 1967.
Woerden, S. van. "The Iconography of the Sacrifice of Abraham." *Vigiliae Christianae* 15 (1961): 214–55.
Wollensen, J. T. *Patrons and Painters on Cyprus: The Frescoes in the Royal Chapel at Pyrga*. Toronto, 2010.
Woodfin, W. "An Officer and a Gentleman: Transformations in the Iconography of a Warrior Saint." *DOP* 60 (2006): 111–43.
Wunderlich, E. *Die Bedeutung der roten Farbe im Kultus der Griechen und Römer*. Gießen, 1925.

Xanthaki, Th. "Ο ναός της Αγίας Άννας στο Ανισαράκι Κανδάνου: Ο κύκλος της αγίας, οι αφιερωτές, η χρονολόγηση." *Δελτ.Χριστ.Άρχ.Έτ.* 31 (2010): 71–86.
Xyngopoulos, A. *Ὁ ἅγιος Δημήτριος ἐν τῇ βυζαντινῇ εἰκονογραφίᾳ*. Thessalonike, 1950.
———. "Τὸ ἀνάγλυφον τῶν Ἁγίων Ἀναργύρων εἰς τὸν Ἅγιον Μᾶρκον τῆς Βενετίας." *Ἀρχ.Δελτ.* 20 (1965): 1:84–95.
———. "Ἀρχάγγελος Μιχαὴλ ὁ Φύλαξ." *BNJ* 10 (1933): 184.
———. *Τὰ μνημεῖα τῶν Σερβίων*. Athens, 1957.
———. *Οἱ τοιχογραφίες τοῦ Ἁγίου Νικολάου Ὀρφανοῦ Θεσσαλονίκης*. Athens, 1964.
Yamshchikov, S., ed. *Pskov: Art Treasures and Architectural Monuments, 12th–17th Centuries*. St. Petersburg, 1978.
Yenipınar, H., and S. Şahin. *Paintings of the Dark Church*. Istanbul, 1998.
Yerasimou, K. "Η αγιογραφική τέχνη στη Μητρόπολη Κιτίου από τα μέσα του 15ου έως τα τέλη του 17ου αιώνα." In *Η κατά Κίτιον αγιογραφική τέχνη*, ed. Ch. Spanou et al., 57–94. Larnaca, 2002.
Yerasimou, K., K. Papaioakeim, and Ch. Spanou. *Η κατά Κίτιον αγιογραφική τέχνη*, ed. Ch. Spanou. Larnaca, 2002.
Young, S. H. "Byzantine Painting in Cyprus during the Early Lusignan Period." Ph.D. diss., Pennsylvania State University, 1983.
———. "The Iconography and Date of the Wall Paintings at Ayia Solomoni, Paphos, Cyprus." *Byzantion* 48 (1978): 91–111.
Zarras, N. *The Church of the Holy Cross at Pelendri*. Lefkosia, 2010.
Zervou Tognazzi, I. "Δέησις: Interpretazione del termine e sua presenza nell'iconografia bizantina." In *Costantinopoli e l'arte delle province orientali*, ed. F. de' Maffei, C. Barsanti, and A. Guiglia Guidobaldi, 391–416. Rome, 1990.
Zeses, Th. "Ἡ Ἁγία Παρασκευὴ ἡ Ἐπιβατηνὴ καὶ ἄγνωστος κανὼν τοῦ Μελετίου Συρίγου εἰς αὐτήν." *Kleronomia* 11 (1979): 317–39.
Zesiou, K. G. "Ἐπιγραφαὶ χριστιανικῶν χρόνων τῆς Ἑλλάδος." *Βυζαντίς* 1 (1909): 114–45, 422–60.
Živković, B. *Bogorodica Ljeviška*. Belgrade, 1991.
———. *Gračanica: Les dessins des fresques*. Belgrade, 1989.

About the Authors

Annemarie Weyl Carr is professor emerita of art history at Southern Methodist University. She has written four books and a number of articles on Byzantine icons, the role of women as artists in the Middle Ages, and the art of Byzantine and medieval Cyprus. She was editor of the journal *Gesta* from 1993 to 1996, was president of the International Center of Medieval Art (2002–2005), and has been a longstanding trustee of the Cyprus American Archaeological Research Institute in Nicosia, Cyprus.

Gilles Grivaud, professor of medieval Mediterranean history at the University of Rouen (Groupe de Recherche d'Histoire), specializes in research on medieval Greek territories, such as Cyprus, that came under Frankish and Venetian domination, from the twelfth to the fifteenth centuries. Among his recent publications are *Excerpta Cypria Nova: Voyageurs occidentaux à Chypre au XVe siècle* (1990); *Villages désertés à Chypre (fin XIIe–fin XIXe siècle)* (1998); and *Cyprus 1542: The Great Map of the Island by Leonida Attar* (2006).

Ioanna Kakoulli, associate professor in the Department of Materials Science and Engineering at UCLA and chair of the UCLA/Getty Conservation Program at the Cotsen Institute of Archaeology, is also the codirector of the Molecular and Nano Archaeology Laboratory and founder of the archaeomaterials group at UCLA. Her research intersects traditional and advanced scientific techniques and focuses on reverse engineering processing, studying the relation between microstructure and properties to understand ancient technology and trade in antiquity as well as environmental and diagenetic alterations and their effects in the preservation of artifacts. She has authored numerous scientific articles and chapters in books and has written *Greek Painting Techniques and Materials from the Fourth to the First Century BC* (London, 2009). She is a member of delegations on Science & Technology, a consultant in federal art-crime investigations, a foreign expert for UNESCO missions, and a member of the Board of Trustees of the Cyprus American Archaeological Institute (CAARI).

Sophia Kalopissi-Verti, professor of Byzantine Art and Archaeology at the University of Athens, is author of *Dedicatory Inscriptions and Donor Portraits in Thirteenth-Century Churches of Greece*. She is also coeditor of *Archaeology and the Crusades*. She has written some sixty articles on Byzantine painting, church inscriptions, and issues of patronage and painters. She has also served as codirector of excavations of an early Christian settlement on the island of Kos (Dodecanese, Greece) and of early Byzantine sites at Sinai.

Andréas Nicolaïdès is maître de conférence of Byzantine Art History and Archaeology at the Aix-Marseille Université and is a researcher at the Laboratoire d'Archéologie Médiévale et Moderne en Méditerranée, UMR 7298–CNRS. A native of Cyprus, he wrote his doctoral dissertation on the church of the Panagia Arakiotissa, Lagoudera, and its wall paintings, comparing them with Byzantine wall paintings in Cyprus from the end of the eleventh to the beginning of the thirteenth century. His current research focuses mainly on Byzantine art and iconography in Cyprus of the Comnenian period; Byzantine and post-Byzantine churches in the valley of Potamia-St. Sozomenos, Cyprus; and Byzantine icons and ceramic production (lamps) in Beirut.

Athanasios Papageorgiou was Curator of Ancient Monuments from 1962 to 1989, director of the Department of Antiquities of Cyprus from 1989 to 1991, and was founding director of the comprehensive photo archive of Byzantine and medieval antiquities on Cyprus at the Holy Archiepiscopate of Cyprus. He has written nine books on the Byzantine and medieval painting of Cyprus, curated exhibitions of Cypriot icons in Nicosia and Athens, and helped to edit both the fourteen-volume *Μεγάλη κυπριακή εγκυκλοπαιδεία* and the publication of the second and third volumes of the International Congress of Cypriot Studies.

Nancy P. Ševčenko is an independent scholar living in South Woodstock, Vermont. She is the author of *The Life of Saint Nicholas in Byzantine Art* and a book about illustrated manuscripts of Byzantine saints' lives, as well as numerous articles on Byzantine art and liturgy. With Christopher Moss, she edited *Medieval Cyprus: Studies in Art, Architecture, and History in Memory of Doula Mouriki*. She is an honarary vice-president of the Association Internationale des Études Byzantines and is vice-president of the International Center of Medieval Art.

David Winfield, an independent scholar who has divided his career between conservation work and Byzantine studies, has published work on both subjects. Among his many conservation projects was the church of the Panagia Phorbiotissa at Asinou in Cyprus. His monograph *The Church of the Panaghia tou Arakos at Lagoudhera, Cyprus: The Paintings and Their Painterly Significance*, coauthored by June Winfield, was published by Dumbarton Oaks in 2003. For his conservation work, he was named a member of the Order of the British Empire (M.B.E.).

INDEX

C

D

H

I

J

K